HANDBOOK OF CRANIOMAXILLOFACIAL SURGERY

HANDBOOK OF CRANIOMAXILLOFACIAL SURGERY

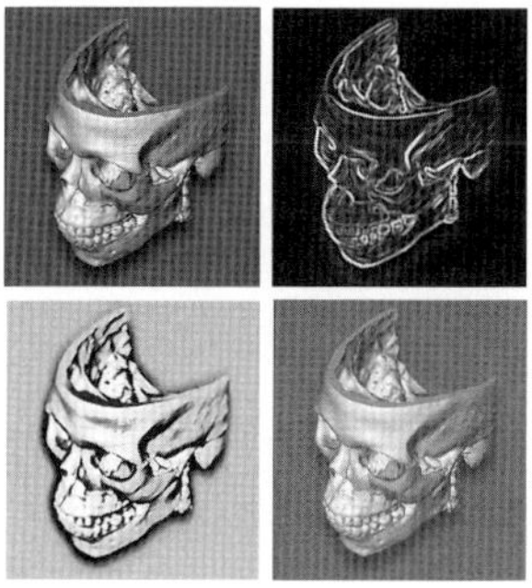

Edited by

James E. Zins, MD, FACS

Professor and Chairman

Cleveland Clinic Lerner College of Medicine

Department of Plastic Surgery, Cleveland Clinic

Cleveland, Ohio, USA

Chad R. Gordon, DO

Craniofacial Plastic Surgeon

Clinical Director, Facial Transplantation Program

The Johns Hopkins Hospital

Assistant Professor, Department of Plastic and Reconstructive Surgery

The Johns Hopkins University School of Medicine

Baltimore, Maryland, USA

World Scientific

NEW JERSEY • LONDON • SINGAPORE • BEIJING • SHANGHAI • HONG KONG • TAIPEI • CHENNAI

Published by

World Scientific Publishing Co. Pte. Ltd.
5 Toh Tuck Link, Singapore 596224
USA office: 27 Warren Street, Suite 401-402, Hackensack, NJ 07601
UK office: 57 Shelton Street, Covent Garden, London WC2H 9HE

Library of Congress Control Number: **2014941004**

British Library Cataloguing-in-Publication Data
A catalogue record for this book is available from the British Library.

HANDBOOK OF CRANIOMAXILLOFACIAL SURGERY

ISBN 978-981-4295-09-3

Typeset by Stallion Press
Email: enquiries@stallionpress.com

Printed in Singapore by FuIsland Offset Printing (S) Pte Ltd

FOREWORD

Can you be at the right place at the right time? Of course. I was the second of Dr. Linton Whitaker's craniofacial fellows in 1978. In these years craniofacial fellows were Hospital of Pennsylvania general surgery residents spending their general surgery research years with him. The year was spent part time in the research laboratory and part time scrubbing on the craniofacial cases at the University of Pennsylvania and Children's Hospital of Philadelphia. The field was so new and the pathology so profound that each day in the operating room was filled with adventure and often new discovery.

In addition to Dr. Whitaker, the first generation of craniofacial surgeons in the United States included Fernando Ortiz-Monasterio, Ken Salyer, Ian Munroe, Tony Wolfe, Ian Jackson, Henry Kawamoto and others. Their training consisted of making the trip to Paris to watch Paul Tessier operate. These craniofacial surgeons then set up their own units in Mexico, Canada and the United States.

Craniofacial surgery has evolved tremendously since those times. Fellowships have become postgraduate training experiences and a formalized match established. The field has exploded from one dealing predominantly with rare pediatric craniofacial anomalies to a discipline that has had a significant effect on facial trauma, tumor reconstruction and aesthetic surgery. Along the way literally thousands of pediatric and adult patients have been treated and their lives changed for the positive. Today nearly all major trauma programs have a fellowship-trained craniofacial surgeon on staff.

What follows is a primer of craniomaxillofacial surgery addressing a wide variety of pediatric and adult facial problems. This text is designed as a quick reference, summary and introduction to an ever-expanding field of plastic surgery. I hope that you enjoy this text and especially the field as much as I have.

James E. Zins, MD

To my father, Gene Zins, who was my role model throughout my life, to my mother, Adele Zins, the great Ambassador, to my wife, Cindy Kavouksorian Zins, my soul mate for the past 30 years, and to my residents and fellows, many of whom are or will become better plastic surgeons than I ever was.

James E. Zins, MD

I would like to dedicate this book to the Cleveland Clinic Faculty for teaching me the art of plastic surgery, and to Dr. Yaremchuk and Dr. Zins — both incredible surgeons and role models — for providing generous mentorship and opportunities for me to grow as a craniomaxillofacial surgeon — and to my wife Abbey and sons Austin and Sage for their unwaivering support and unconditional love in light of many late nights and busy weekends.

Chad R. Gordon, D.O.

CONTENTS

PRINCIPLES OF CRANIOFACIAL SURGERY 1

Anthony Wolfe, MD

1.1 Introduction

The field of craniofacial surgery owes its beginnings to Dr. Paul Tessier more than any other individual. After performing the first successful Le Fort III-type osteotomy in 1958, he went on to develop procedures for correcting virtually every major orbitocranial malformation: Crouzon's disease, Apert's syndrome, orbital hypertelorism and other orbital dystopias, Treacher Collins-Franceschetti syndrome, hemifacial microsomia, arrhinias, and orbitofacial clefts, with "spin-offs" having a profound effect on the primary treatment of trauma, excision of facial tumors and primary reconstruction, and aesthetic surgery. He could provide methods to correct these conditions because of his understanding of the underlying skeletal abnormality and his surgical ability to work with autogenous bone. His powers of observation and cataloguing of his patients led to his empiric classification of facial clefts, published in 1976, which is used throughout the world.[1]

Dr. Tessier, considered to be the father of craniofacial surgery, wrote relatively little in his career, perhaps because of his demanding surgical schedule. He worked in Paris, 6 days a week, often until midnight, and traveled extensively in the United States as an invited surgeon. What follows are some notes that he made in 2001.

1.2 Notes by Tessier

After 40 years, let us cast a glance back on our craniofacial adventure. From 1940 to 1960, reconstruction of the facial structures was done mostly for the lower jaw, nose, and zygoma. However, (1) skin flaps were often used to mask skeletal defects, (2) the orbital cavity was almost completely ignored except for fractures, (3) the cranial cavity was the exclusive game preserve of the neurosurgeons, and (4) the orbitofrontal bar (which I consider one of my significant contributions) was a barrier not crossed by ophthalmologists or plastic surgeons, and only rarely by neurosurgeons.

Such limitations made radical treatments impossible for all major disorders: Crouzon's disease, Apert's syndrome, the orbitofacial clefts, plagiocephaly, frontonasal dysplasia, all kinds of hypertelorism, basicranial tumors, and countless orbitocranial trauma cases.

1.2.1 *The clinical impulse to craniofacial surgery (1958–1963)*

Craniofacial surgery did not develop from an unarticulated desire for a new specialty, not at all. In fact, over a 5-year period, the impetus came from observing eight patients. By chance, all were mentally normal, although each one represented an extreme and monstrous form of a given type of malformation.

In none of these patients could form and function have been corrected by procedures in use at that time. Consequently, new procedures were developed after a careful evaluation of the skeletal disorder. But, in 1960, there was no CT scanner, no 3-D imaging for the skeletal structures, and no MRI for the brain and eyes. Animal experiments could not help, since the primate head has little in common with the human head.

1.2.2 *Five basic principles and two technical procedures*

Looking back, one can see that a few basic principles were joined in a short time. They emerged less from maxillofacial surgery than from orthopedic surgery of the limbs.

Five principles stand at the core of craniofacial surgery:

- One overriding concept is the priority given to bony structures over the soft-tissue coverage, since a form and several functions depend largely upon the underlying skeletal framework.
- The initial surgical step always consists of a sharp, aggressive elevation of the periosteum, which is necessary for both the protection of the overlying soft tissues and for facial bone healing.
- All the techniques used are based upon the displacement of large facial or cranial segments, which are easy to stabilize and more economical of available bone than onlay grafts. So far, this includes all synthetic bone substitutes.
- Stability requires that all bony defects resulting from clefts, trauma, or surgical displacements be filled with autogenous bone: iliac, tibial, costal, or now cranial.
- Surgical tactics pay no importance whatsoever to the time spent repairing a damaged or abnormal face. Whenever possible, depending upon the age of the patient or the strategy envisaged for a particular case, the operation is designed to be a one-stage correction of all components of that face.

Two technical procedures are specific to craniofacial surgery:

- First, a circumferential orbital dissection is carried out, deep beneath the periorbitum, which permits the displacement of the ocular globe while preserving the extraocular muscle function and motion.
- Second, the intracranial approach is used for all dissections, resections, displacements, and repairs to be made at the orbitofrontal level or between the orbits from the nose to the sphenoid bone. An extradural dissection for cranial surgery does not mean neurosurgery. When the intracranial route is combined with deep orbital dissections, there are no

longer any limitations for the possible correction of the Crouzon, the asymmetries of plagiocephaly, the hypertelorism of median dysraphias, the reduction of sphenoidal encephalocoeles and the repair of innumerable trauma cases. This becomes routine with experience.

1.2.3 *Seven basic techniques*

Seven basic techniques are applied to four different malpositions of facial components and to three situations where bone is lacking.

- *To move forward* the retruded midface of the Crouzon and Apert with exorbitism and class III dental malocclusion; this is the Le Fort III–type midfacial advancement (1958).
- *To move medially* the orbital complexes by an intracranial route for the resection of an excess of interorbital tissue in all hyperteloric syndromes (1962).
- *To move forward* the frontofacial complex and to split it sagittally, from the glabella to the palate, either for narrowing, bending, or stretching that framework (1970) or for spreading it apart as an approach to the body of the sphenoid (1984).
- *To move vertically* an orbit already made dystopic by clefts, either the No. 4 (orbitofacial) or the No. 10 (orbitofrontal) (1965); or, in children, to construct primarily with bone grafts the bony deficiencies of the No. 3 or No. 4 orbitofacial clefts in order to prevent an orbital prolapse (1958).
- *To resect* the extensive orbitocranial tumors and (when they are benign), to reconstruct the framework with autogenous bone grafts in the meningiomas, in fibrous dysplasia, and in spheno-ethmoidal encephalocoeles.
- *To adapt* the osteotomies, segmental displacements, and reconstructions to the unpredictable and differing situations encountered in craniofacial trauma.
- *To find new sources* for large amounts of bone graft material by splitting the parietal bones either extracranially (split *in situ*) or after a craniotomy (1972). This can provide as much bone as an entire iliac wing.

1.2.4 *Perspectives for the future*

Automotive trauma cases may continue to arrive at a regular rate, but more patients' faces will be restored completely because of the more widespread application of craniofacial principles and techniques.

Autogenous bone grafts, easy to harvest and cheap, will remain the gold standard for a long, long time. In the future, they might be replaced in part by bone substitutes, bone growth factors, or bone grown in tissue culture.

The Cephaloteque Project has been envisaged as an international library for the collection of 3-D images to be used in the teaching of all rare craniofacial disorders. From its present 300 cases, it realistically could grow in 10 years to 5,000 cases.

Children will benefit widely from the use of bone distraction methods, which over the past years have been extrapolated from the limbs to the mandible by Joseph McCarthy and later to other parts of the face by Fernando Ortiz-Monasterio. As for the few groups afflicted with total agenesis, we will have to wait for another decade, or perhaps even another century.

1.3 Conclusion

These words of Dr. Tessier still ring true. Craniofacial surgery deals with the essential — skeletal — nature of many malformations. It was through his study and understanding of this abnormal bony anatomy that Dr. Tessier was able to devise his various surgical procedures, deemed radical at the time, in which the abnormal skeletal anomaly was corrected.

- If it is in the wrong place, move it to the right place, and stabilize it there, either by bone stock formed by distraction osteogenesis or by autogenous bone grafts.
- Autogenous bone grafts — yes, autogenous bone grafts — are still the key to craniofacial reconstruction. A craniofacial surgeon should not try to avoid them by trying a potpourri of nonautogenous substances, but

rather should learn how to harvest bone grafts easily, quickly, and safely. One embraces them. One should *not always* be putting metal mesh or porous polyethylene into orbital defects simply because it is expedient or because one does not have the equipment or expertise to harvest an appropriate bone graft.
- If it is not there, build it, and then move it.

Craniofacial surgery, at its core, is also orbital surgery. Besides an ability to reconstruct and displace the bony orbit, the craniofacial surgeon must be a master of techniques for the periorbital structures (the medial and lateral canthus and the eyelids) and be adept at reconstruction of the structure between the orbits — the nose; the structure above the nose — the skull; and the structure below the orbits — the maxilla.

Reference

1. **Tessier P**. Anatomical classification facial, craniofacial and laterofacial clefts. *J Maxillofac Surg* 1976;4:69–92.

CRANIOFACIAL ANATOMY AND EMBRYOLOGY 2

Arun K. Gosain, MD; Ali Totonchi, MD and Stephanie Polites

2.1 Embryology

Understanding the embryologic processes of the human head and neck provides a foundation upon which craniofacial anatomy and related congenital anomalies could be studied. The keystone of head and neck development is the branchial arch system, analogous to the branchial apparatus that gives rise to gills for gas exchange in fish and amphibians. The human branchial arches are not used for gas exchange but instead contain cellular precursors of nearly all the structures of the head and neck. The arch system begins to develop during the 4th week, following creation of three germ layers — ectoderm, mesoderm, and endoderm — by gastrulation during the 3rd week.[1] The ectoderm layer differentiates into both surface ectoderm and neural ectoderm, which is the earliest cell lineage of the human central nervous system. The term *neural crest* is used to describe the interface of neural and surface ectoderm, and a population of pluripotent neural crest cells is created by interactions between the two adjacent types of ectoderm. Neural crest cells migrate along predetermined pathways while dividing and differentiating into one of many possible cell types. Products of neural-crest cell differentiation include muscle, connective tissue, nervous tissue, endocrine tissue, and melanocytes. Endoderm differentiates into select visceral structures, including gut epithelium. Upon interaction with pharyngeal endoderm, predestined neural crest cells cease migration and create "bulges" of tissue together with nearby mesoderm tissue. Such collections of mesenchymal tissue constitute the earliest branchial arches.

2.1.1 *Branchial arch system*

The human embryo develops a series of six paired arches where the first arch is most cranial and largest. The sixth arch is most caudal and smallest, although the fifth arch is commonly absent and considered vestigial in humans. Though derivatives of each arch are anatomically distinct, all arches are initially composed of cartilage, aortic arch artery, muscle, and nerve elements (Figure 2.1). The cartilaginous rod of each arch gives rise to bone, cartilage, and ligament derivatives of that arch. It is important to note that only bones formed by endochondral ossification are arch-cartilage derivatives.[1] Bones that undergo membranous ossification are derivatives of arch mesoderm. The mandible, for example, is derived from the first arch and has both cartilaginous (condyles) and mesodermal (body and ramus) origins. Additionally, only the first and second arches have ligamentous derivatives. The six aortic arch arteries serve to connect the embryonic heart, located ventral to the endoderm-lined pharynx, and the dorsal primitive aorta. The aortic arch arteries are initially named by their associated arch number but later contribute to arteries of the mature human circulation. The nervous tissue component of each arch gives rise to both motor and sensory fibers of a cranial nerve that is then associated with that arch. All human muscle development relies on adequate innervation to initiate formation of myoblasts from mesoderm. Therefore, the mesoderm-derived muscle component of each arch develops into muscles that retain motor innervation by the cranial nerve associated with that arch.

The branchial arch system consists of multiple tissue layers that essentially recapitulate the trilaminar disk formed by gastrulation. The

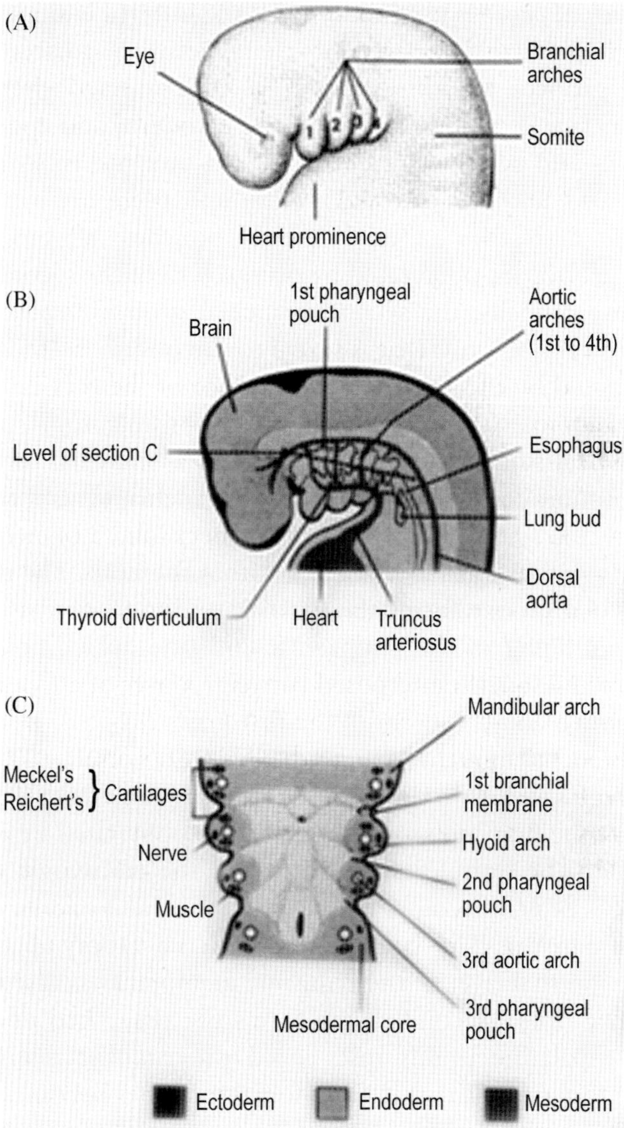

Figure 2.1. Each branchial arch has a cartilage, nerve, muscle, and aortic arch component.[1] Reprinted with permission from Wolters Kluwer (Ref. 1; p. 180).

term *branchial pouch* is used to describe the internal endoderm lining of the invaginated interface, or cleft, between adjacent arches. Branchial grooves are corresponding ectoderm-lined clefts on the external surface of the arch system. The ectoderm and endoderm of the grooves and pouches, respectively, also give rise to structures of the head and neck (Figure 2.2). Although there are anatomically identifiable derivatives of all branchial pouches, all but the first branchial groove are obliterated by overgrowth of the second groove. As it grows caudally, the second branchial groove creates an ectoderm-lined cervical sinus that is sealed to the outside by the 6th week and eliminated by the 7th week. Persistence of the cervical sinus is a congenital anomaly that results in a branchial fistula, sinus, or cyst.[1] A patent cervical sinus at birth is classified as a branchial fistula if the sinus communicates with the pharynx, a branchial sinus if communicating with the surface of the skin of the neck, and a branchial cyst if the patent cervical sinus is contained within the neck. The remaining first branchial groove forms the external auditory meatus as well as the external lining of the tympanic membrane, which consists of a thin layer of mesoderm interposed between a layer of endoderm from the first pouch and ectoderm of the first groove.

The branchial pouches can be divided into dorsal and ventral, as each area can give rise to different derivatives (Table 2.1). The ventral portions of the first and second pouches are obliterated by growth of the tongue. The dorsal first pouch forms the embryonic tubotympanic recess, which becomes the auditory tube and middle ear cavity of the human ear. The lateral surface of the tubotympanic recess forms the internal layer of the tympanic membrane, as discussed previously. The dorsal second pouch forms the tissue bed upon which the future palatine tonsils rest, called the *palatine tonsillar fossa*. Dorsal endoderm of the third and fourth pouches becomes the inferior and superior parathyroid glands, respectively. This counterintuitive process indicates that significant caudal migration of the inferior parathyroid glands occurs. As thymus tissue, derived from ventral endoderm of the third pouch, travels to the superior mediastinum, it effectively pulls the parathyroid tissue of the third pouch caudal to the parathyroid tissue of the fourth pouch.[2] Lastly, endoderm of the

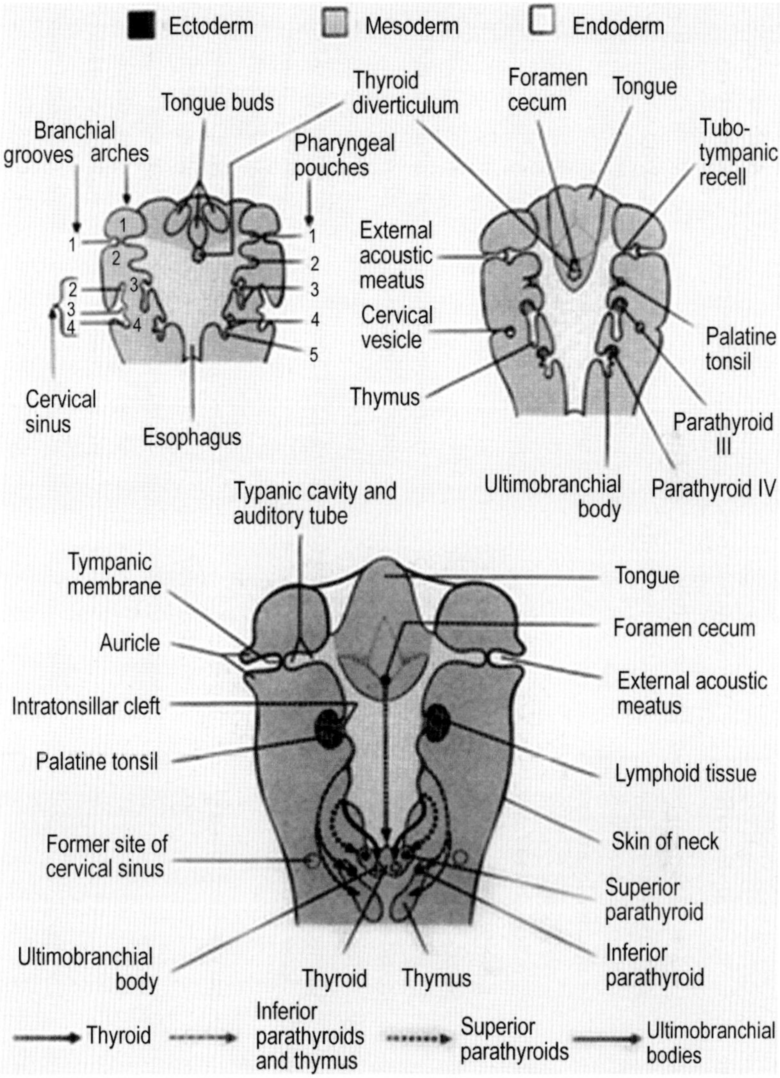

Figure 2.2. The internal endodermal surface and external ectoderm surface of the branchial apparatus gives rise to structures and organs of the head and neck.[1] Reprinted with permission from Wolters Kluwer (Ref. 1; 182).

Table 2.1. Summary of the Branchial Apparatus.

Arch	Nerve	Skeletal derivatives	Pouch derivatives	Muscle derivatives	Arch artery derivatives
First (mandibular)	Trigeminal	Greater wing of sphenoid, incus, malleus, maxilla, zygoma, mandible; anterior ligament of malleus, sphenomandibular ligament	Auditory tube, middle ear cavity	Muscles of mastication, anterior belly of digastrics, mylohyoid, tensor tympani, tensor veli palatine	Portion of external carotid and maxillary arteries
Second (hyoid)	Facial	Stapes, styloid process (temporal), lesser cornu and upper hyoid; stylohyoid ligament	Palatine tonsillar fossa	Muscles of facial expression, posterior belly of digastric, stylohyoid, stapedius	Tympanic branch of internal carotid artery
Third	Glosso-pharyngeal	Greater cornu and lower part of hyoid	Inferior parathyroids, thymus	Stylopharyngeus	Common carotid and proximal internal carotid arteries
Fourth	Superior laryngeal of vagus	Laryngeal cartilages	Superior parathyroids, lateral thyroid	Pharyngeal constrictors, cricothyroid, levator veli palatine, palatoglossus	Left arch of aorta, brachiocephalic and right subclavian arteries, distal pulmonary arteries
Fifth/Sixth	Recurrent laryngeal of vagus	Laryngeal cartilages	Ultimobranchial body	Laryngeal muscles except cricothyroid, striated muscle of esophagus	Proximal pulmonary arteries, ductus arteriosus

fifth branchial pouch forms the *ultimobranchial body*, from which parafollicular C cells originate. These cells become interspersed in the follicular epithelium of the thyroid gland and secrete calcitonin, a hormone with a minor role in calcium homeostasis.

2.1.2 *Development of human facial features*

Though the entire branchial arch system contributes to structures of the head and neck, the first branchial arch and mesenchyme ventral to the forebrain are responsible for development of the features characteristic of the human face (Figure 2.3).[3] During the 4th week, the primitive mouth, or stomodeum, is the first recognizable feature to appear. Initially it is formed by a central collection of mesenchyme ventral to the forebrain, known as the frontonasal prominence, and the paired cartilaginous maxillary and mandibular prominences of the first arch. The cephalic border of the stomodeum is formed by the frontonasal prominence, the lateral borders by the paired maxillary prominences, and the caudal border by the paired mandibular prominences. While the incus and greater wing of the sphenoid form from endochondral ossification of maxillary cartilage, the actual maxilla, zygoma, and squamous temporal bone form by membranous ossification within the maxillary prominence. Likewise, cartilage within the mandibular prominence forms only the malleolus of the mandible and serves as a template for membranous ossification of the body and ramus. The caudal face is the first region to take recognizable human form, as the paired mandibular prominences migrate and fuse medially early in the 4th week, forming the primitive chin, lower lip, lower jaw, and lower cheek. Migration and fusion of the primary facial prominences occurs largely from weeks 4 to 8, and an embryo has a distinctly human face by week 10.

By the end of the 4th week, nasal development begins with appearance of bilateral nasal placodes at the lateral, inferior surface of the frontonasal prominence (Figure 2.3). In human embryology, the term *placode* refers to thickening of surface ectoderm. As the nasal placodes enlarge, they develop distinct medial and lateral regions, which are termed *medial* and *lateral nasal prominences*. The central

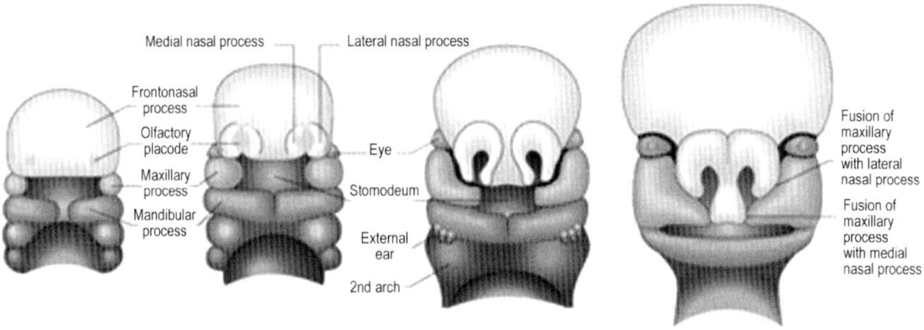

Figure 2.3. Human facial features develop from the paired maxillary and mandibular processes and the unpaired frontonasal process.[3] Reprinted with permission from Elsevier (Gray's Anatomy: The Anatomical Basis of Clinical Practice. 39th ed. Chapter 34, 2005:609). Copyright © 2005 Elsevier.

depressed regions of each placode, or nasal pits, are the earliest manifestations of nares. The bilateral nasal pits lie between their respective medial and lateral nasal prominences and are initially in contact with the stomodeum. This continuity is obliterated due to central migration of the paired maxillary prominences and bilateral medial and lateral nasal prominences.[1] This important migratory process creates a single nose, upper lip, and primary palate. Specifically, medial fusion of the medial nasal prominences creates the nasal septum, nasal tip, and philtrum of the lip. The lateral nasal prominences develop into the nasal alae. Fusion of the paired maxillary prominences forms the upper lip (excluding the philtrum), upper jaw, and upper cheek. The primary palate is created by fusion of the maxillary prominences with the medial nasal prominences. Failure of this fusion can result in a primary cleft palate.[4] The lateral nasal prominences are separated from the maxillary prominences by bilateral furrows in the mesenchyme, termed the *nasolacrimal grooves.* The grooves epithelialize and become sealed from the facial surface, forming paired nasolacrimal ducts. These ducts become patent after birth, to drain lacrimal gland secretions from the medial conjunctival sacs to the nares. The maxillary prominences also fuse with the mandibular prominences, creating the lateral commissure of the mouth.

The actual nasal cavities are created when the nasal pits deepen to form nasal sacs that are separated from the oral cavity by the oronasal membrane. This membrane ruptures, allowing communication between the oral and nasal cavities just posterior to the primary palate via primitive choanae. Upon formation of the secondary palate by fusion of the lateral palatine processes and nasal septum, the choanae are shifted posteriorly. In their final position, the choanae allow communication between the oral cavity and the pharynx. The lateral walls of each nasal cavity give rise to three elevations that become the superior, middle, and inferior conchae.

The nasal cavities are also responsible for creation of the paranasal air sinuses, which are created when diverticula of the lateral walls grow into the sphenoid, ethmoid, frontal, and maxillary bones. The maxillary sinuses are the first to develop, appearing in the 3rd fetal month, followed by the ethmoid sinuses in the 5th month. The sphenoid sinus appears at 5 months postnatally and the frontal sinuses between 5 and 6 years of life. The olfactory epithelium responsible for the sense of smell is derived from ectoderm in the roof of each nasal cavity. This epithelium is composed of several cell types that include olfactory cells, which are actually bipolar neurons of the olfactory nerve responsible for odor detection.[5]

In addition to forming the forehead, the frontonasal prominence is involved in early development of the eyes. As mentioned previously, placodes are formed by thickening of surface ectoderm. This process occurs within the lateral facets of the frontonasal prominence, forming bilateral lens placodes. Surface ectoderm is also notably responsible for the eyelids, which appear during the 8th week and overgrow the developed eyes. The lens placodes are induced to fold inwards by outgrowths of the forebrain, the optic stalks, thereby forming lens vesicles once the placodes lose contact with the surface (Figure 2.4). The optic vesicles are hollow bulbs enclosing the developing eyes at the distal ends of the optic stalks. The lens vesicles continue to differentiate into the lenses, the optic stalks into the optic nerves, and the optic vesicles into the optic cups. Though the optic nerve is also the second cranial nerve, its embryologic development indicates that it is actually a part of the central nervous system. Neural crest cells soon populate the region to become the sclera and choroid just superficial to the cup and the ciliary bodies at the medial and lateral

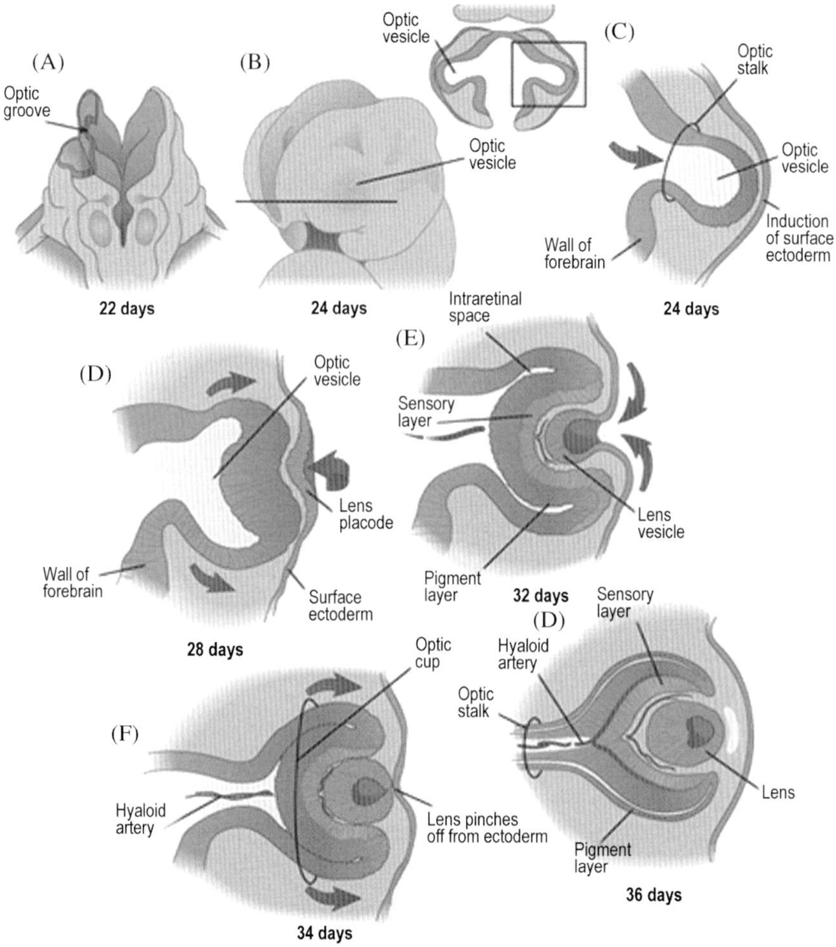

Figure 2.4. The eye begins as an evagination of the forebrain, which induces overlying ectoderm to become the lens.[6] Reprinted with permission from Elsevier (Ref. 6; p. 293). Copyright © 2004 Elsevier.

margins of each cup. The cornea is also derived from neural crest cells superficial to the lens. Though the eyes are initially placed eccentrically on the face, they undergo accelerated medial migration between the 5th and 9th week.

Development of the human tongue is initiated during the 4th week, when the median tongue bud appears from the floor of the pharynx. Subsequent development can be divided into that of the anterior two-thirds (oral) and posterior one-third (pharyngeal) tongue. The terminal sulcus is a V-shaped furrow visible in the adult tongue that superficially divides anterior from posterior tongue. The oral tongue is formed when two lateral lingual swellings overgrow the median tongue bud. Both the median tongue bud and lateral lingual swellings, also known as *distal tongue buds*, are derived from first-arch mesenchyme. The posterior tongue is initially formed by mesenchyme of the second arch, or the copula. The copula is soon overgrown by the hypobranchial eminence of the third and fourth arches. Innervation of the tongue is rooted in its embryologic origins, as the oral tongue receives sensory innervation from the mandibular branch of the trigeminal nerve and the pharyngeal tongue from the glossopharyngeal and superior laryngeal nerves. Only the muscular components of the tongue are not derived from the branchial arches, originating instead from occipital somites. All tongue muscles except the palatoglossus, which is innervated by the vagus nerve, receive motor innervation from the hypoglossal nerve. The dorsum of the tongue has a midline depression called the *foramen cecum* (Figure 2.5).

Also during the 4th week, endoderm of the foramen cecum proliferates to create the thyroid diverticulum. As this diverticulum descends within the neck, anterior to the hyoid bone, laryngeal cartilages, and trachea, it remains connected to the tongue via the thyroglossal duct. The diverticulum completes its descent when it reaches the second and third tracheal rings, usually by the 7th week. It solidifies and takes its adult form of bilateral lobes connected by a central isthmus. Asymptomatic anomalies of thyroid development include undescended thyroid tissue at the foramen cecum, known as a *lingual thyroid*, and persistence of thyroid tissue in the distal thyroglossal duct, forming a third lobe of the thyroid gland.[6]

The human palate is composed of a primary and secondary palate, each with distinct embryologic origins and processes.[4] The incisive foramen just posterior to the maxillary incisors indicates the intersection of primary and secondary palates in the adult palate. The primary palate is derived from the frontonasal prominence via the median palatine process, which forms upon the merging of the medial nasal

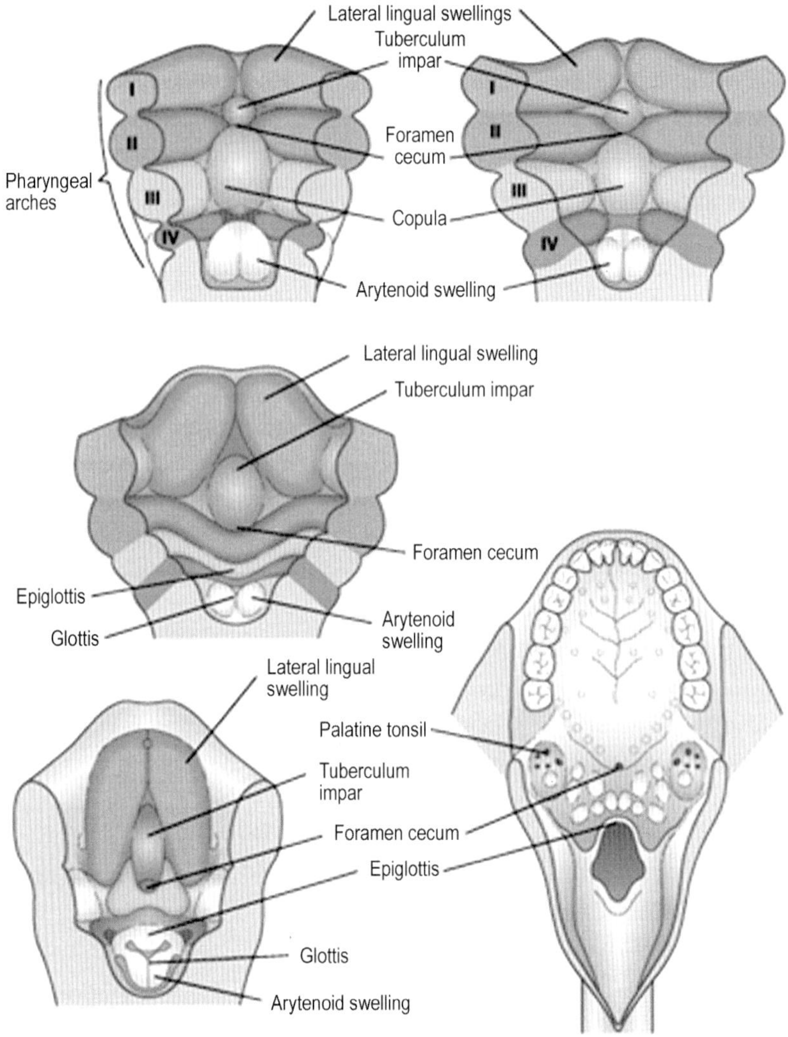

Figure 2.5. The anterior tongue is formed by derivatives of the first arch and the posterior tongue by derivatives of the third arch.[6] Reprinted with permission from Elsevier (Ref. 6; p. 344). Copyright © 2004 Elsevier.

prominences. The secondary palate is formed from the lateral palatine processes, which are bilateral outgrowths of the maxillary prominences. The lateral palatine processes are initially oriented vertically and evolve to the horizontal position during the 8th week, allowing medial migration. The developing tongue is interposed between the lateral palatine processes in their vertical stage, and micrognathia by pushing the tongue cephalad can delay or prevent the horizontal shift. Eventual midline fusion of the processes and creation of a single mesenchymal secondary palate depends on apoptosis of the epithelial cells lining the medial shelves during migration. The line of fusion, called the *palatine raphe,* can be seen in the adult palate (Figure 2.6). The palate is complete only upon fusion of mesenchyme of the medial and lateral palatine processes as well as fusion of the lateral palatine processes with the nasal septum. If any of the aforementioned steps are disrupted, preventing complete coalescence of appropriate mesenchymal processes, a cleft palate results. The embryology of the palate is clinically relevant, as the location and degree of clefting is directly related to the stage of development that was disrupted. The hard palate is named as such due to ossification of the primary and anterior secondary palates. The posterior portion of the secondary palate does not ossify and becomes the soft palate.

The external ear is composed of the auricle and the external acoustic meatus. Like most other elements of facial anatomy, the

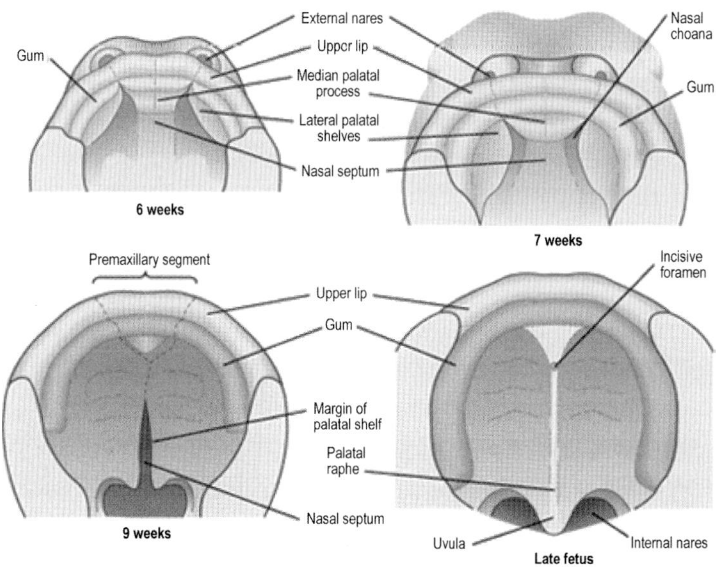

Figure 2.6. Development of the primary and secondary palate.[6] Reprinted with permission from Elsevier (Ref. 6; p. 326). Copyright © 2004 Elsevier.

external ear is derived from the branchial arch system. The first branchial groove lies between the first and second arches, and the auricle is created on its dorsal aspect by means of six mesenchymal swellings, or auricular hillocks. The caudal region of the first arch contributes three anterior hillocks, and three posterior hillocks arise from the cephalic portion of the second arch. The hillocks undergo progressive expansion and fusion to create a recognizable auricle by the end of the 8th week (Figure 2.7). Cutaneous sensation of the auricle recapitulates its embryology, as portions derived from first-arch hillocks are innervated by the trigeminal nerve (auriculotemporal branch) and portions from second-arch hillocks by the facial nerve and cervical plexus (great auricular nerve). The external auditory meatus is created during the 2nd month, when ectoderm of the dorsal region of the first branchial cleft grows inward. Initially, the meatus is occluded by a proliferation of ectoderm known as the *meatal plug*. This plug canalizes late in the 7th month of development. As the auricles and external auditory meatuses develop, they shift cranially and dorsally from the neck region to the lateral face. This is clinically significant because any aberration or arrest of branchial arch development results in caudally displaced auricles at birth.

Development of the cranium, or skull, can be divided into that of the neurocranium and viscerocranium. The neurocranium is the skeletal encasement of the brain and the viscerocranium is the facial skeleton. The neurocranium can further be divided into the skull base and the cranial vault. The skull base is termed the *chondrocranium*, as it is derived from cartilages that undergo endochondral ossification (Figure 2.8). Neural crest cells give rise to cartilages of

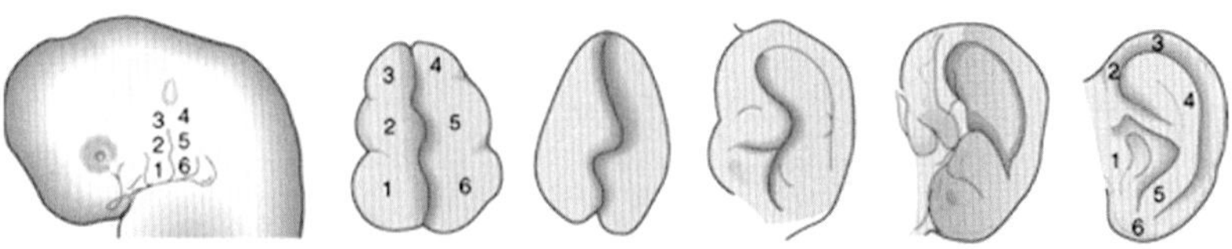

Figure 2.7. The auricle is formed by progressive growth and interaction of six mesenchymal swellings contributed by the first and second branchial arches.[6] Reprinted with permission from Elsevier (Ref. 6; p. 311). Copyright © 2004 Elsevier.

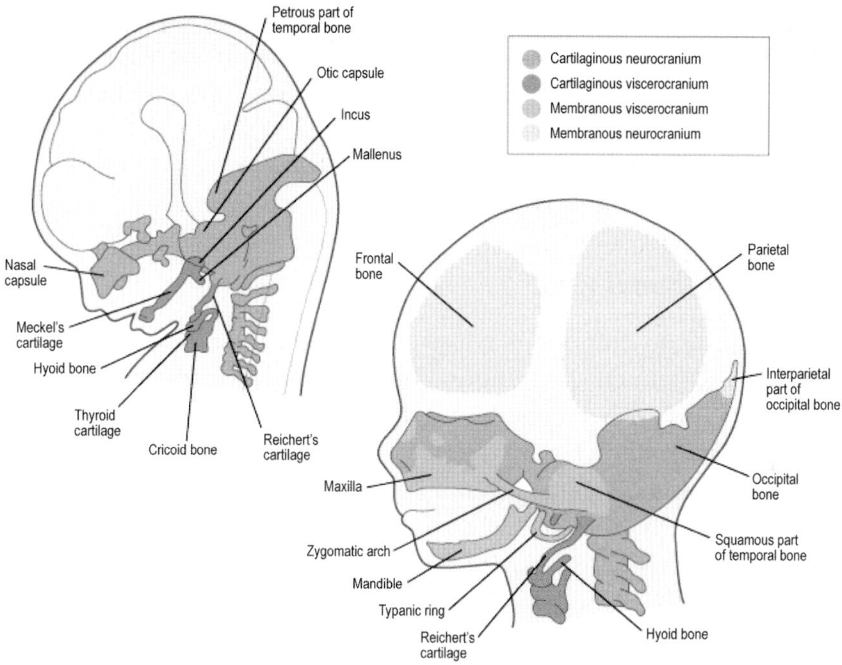

Figure 2.8. Bones of the cranial vault are derived from membranous neurocranium, whereas those of the skull base are from cartilaginous neurocranium. Facial bones are derived from membranous or cartilaginous viscerocranium.[6] Reprinted with permission from Elsevier (Ref. 6; p. 192). Copyright © 2004 Elsevier.

the chondrocranium that lie rostral to the sella turcica. Cartilages posterior to this landmark originate from paraxial mesoderm via occipital somites. Bones of the cranial vault, also known as flat bones, undergo membranous ossification, meaning that neural crest cell and paraxial mesoderm mesenchyme ossify directly without a cartilaginous stage. Development of the cranial vault is not complete at birth, as the flat bones are separated by connective tissue sutures. The term *fontanelle* is used to describe the connective tissue intersection of three or more bones. These flexible components of the cranial vault are necessary to allow shifting and overlap of the bones during childbirth and to accommodate the brain as it grows rapidly throughout childhood. The viscerocranium is also formed by both endochondral and membranous ossification of branchial arch contributions. Bones of the facial skeleton that undergo endochondral ossification are derived from neural crest cells that become arch cartilages, while bones undergoing membranous ossification form directly from arch mesenchyme.

2.2 Bones

2.2.1 *The cranial vault*

The entire neurocranium is constructed from six bones. The frontal bone, paired parietal and temporal bones, and the occipital bone form a cranial vault with a concave interior facade to encase the convex surface of the brain (Figure 2.9).[7] Since the frontal bone is the most anterior bone of the cranial vault, it is also important in facial anatomy, forming the forehead and roof of the orbit. The frontal bone is fused posteriorly to the paired parietal bones at the coronal suture. The parietal bones form the superior and lateral surfaces of the cranial vault, meeting in the midline at the sagittal suture and meeting the unpaired occipital bone posteriorly at the transverse lambdoid suture. The posterior fontanelle is formed by the intersection of the sagittal and lambdoid sutures. Upon ossification of the membranous fontanelle, the intersection is termed the *lambda*. Likewise, the anterior fontanelle is the membranous intersection of the coronal and sagittal sutures, becoming the *bregma* upon ossification. The vertex, or highest point, of the skull is usually found approximately halfway along the sagittal suture as it runs from anterior to posterior. The superior and inferior temporal lines arch across the exterior surface of the parietal bones. The former gives rise to the temporal fascia and the latter to the temporalis muscle. At their inferior edge, the parietal bones articulate with the superior aspect of the paired temporal bones, creating bilateral squamosal sutures.

An important bony landmark of the lateral cranium is the pterion, which marks the intersection of the frontal, parietal, temporal, and sphenoid bones. The temporal bone is divided into several regions, the squamous portion, temporal portion, mastoid process, and petrous portion, each representing a separate center of ossification.

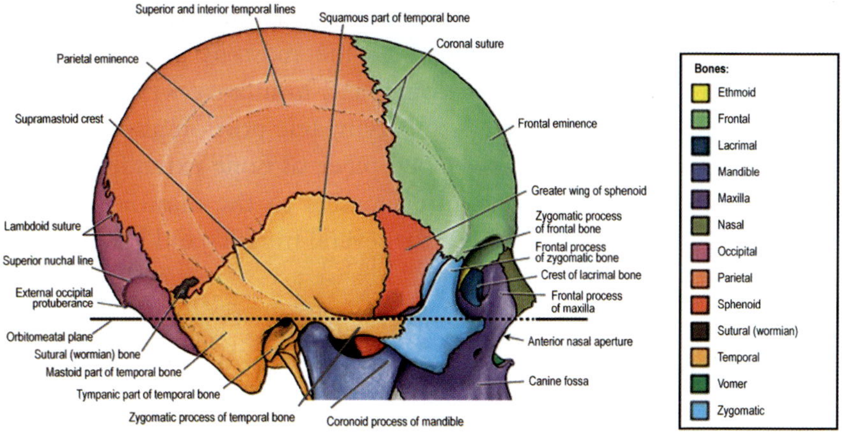

Figure 2.9. The cranial vault is a dome-shaped bony enclosure for the brain. It consists of the frontal, parietal, temporal, occipital, and sphenoid (greater wing) bones, which articulate at anatomically identifiable suture lines.[7] Reprinted with permission from Wolters Kluwer (Agur AMR, Dalley AF II, eds. Grant's Atlas of Anatomy. 12th ed. Philadelphia, PA: Lippincott Williams & Wilkins; 2009:613). Copyright © 2009 Lippincott Williams & Wilkins.

The squamous portion, or squama temporalis, represents the temporal bone's contribution to the cranial vault and gives rise to the zygomatic process. The squama also contains the mandibular fossa and the petrotympanic fissure. The former is a depression housing the mandibular condyles at the temporomandibular joint (TMJ) and the latter an opening containing the chorda tympani from the middle ear to the mandibular fossa, where it exits the skull. The tympanic portion of the temporal bone lies just inferior to the squama and anterior to the mastoid process. It blends medially with the petrous temporal bone and is attached laterally to the cartilaginous part of the external acoustic meatus. Only the outer one-third of the meatus is formed by cartilage; the inner two-thirds are formed by the tympanic portion of the temporal bone.

Just posterior to the opening of the external acoustic meatus is the mastoid process, which does not appear until after birth. This conical process extends inferiorly from the posterior temporal bone and completes development only at puberty, when it is filled with mastoid air cells. The motor branch of the facial nerve exits the skull through the stylomastoid foramen, just medial to the mastoid process, and is vulnerable to injury during childbirth and in infancy when the mastoid process has not developed. The tympanic portion also gives rise to the styloid process, a horn-shaped piece of bone extending inferiorly from the temporal bone anteromedial to the mastoid process. This process provides attachment for several muscles and ligaments of the head and neck.[5]

2.2.2 *External skull base*

The base of the cranium is formed by the inferior neurocranium, including the occipital, temporal, and sphenoid bones, and the viscerocranium excluding the mandible (Figure 2.10). The most anterior aspect of the external base of the cranium is formed by the maxilla. It communicates laterally with the zygomatic bone and posteriorly with the horizontal plates of the palatine bones. Superior to the posterior free edge of the hard palate is the posterior nasal apertures, or choanae, separated by the vertically oriented vomer bone. The vomer articulates inferiorly with the hard palate and posteriorly with the unpaired sphenoid bone. The sphenoid bone comprises a body and three sets of paired processes — the greater wings, lesser wings, and pterygoid processes. Each pterygoid process extends inferior and perpendicular to the cranial base, separating distally into a medial and lateral pterygoid plate. The latter allows attachment of the medial and lateral pterygoid muscles, two muscles of mastication. The greater wings articulate posteriorly with the petrous portion of the temporal bone, and there is a groove in the inferior aspect of the synchondrosis for the cartilaginous segment of the auditory (eustachian) tube. The posterior portion of the cranial base is formed by the occipital bone.

Visible on the external aspect of the occipital part of the cranial base is the foramen magnum, a large opening through which the spinal cord and its meninges pass, along with the vertebral arteries, spinal arteries, and accessory nerve. The skull articulates with the vertebral column at paired occipital condyles that lie on either side of the

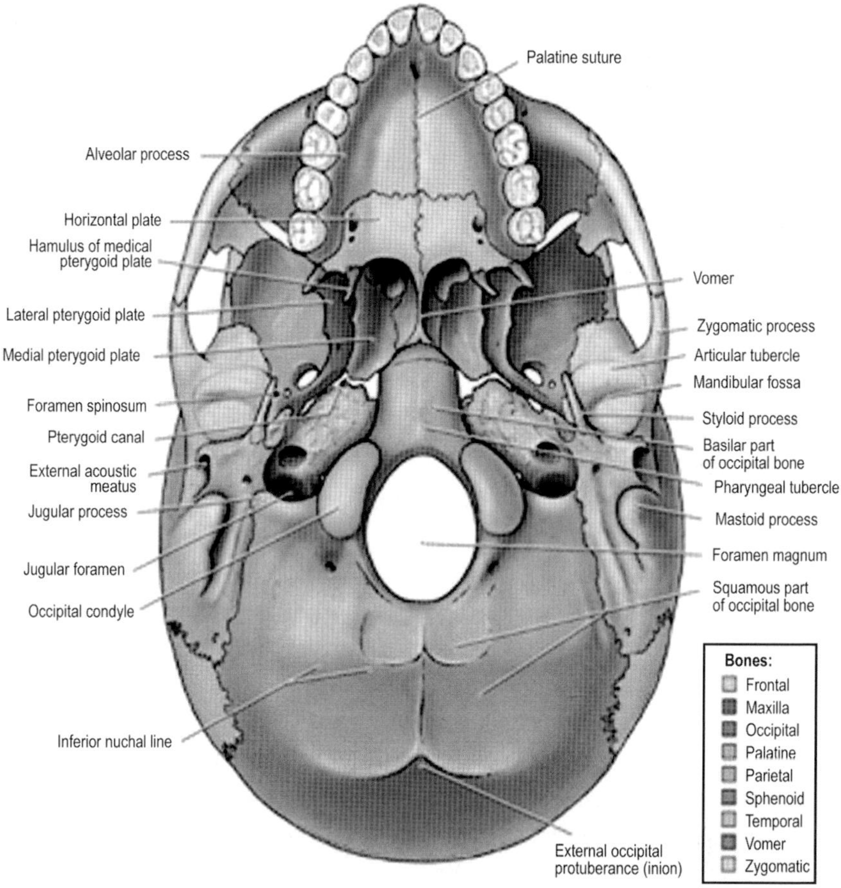

Figure 2.10. The external base of the skull includes bones of the facial skeleton except for the mandible, and transmits many intracranial neural and vascular structures to the face and neck.[7] Reprinted with permission from Wolters Kluwer (Agur AMR, Dalley AF II, eds. Grant's Atlas of Anatomy. 12th edn. Philadelphia, PA: Lippincott Williams & Wilkins; 2009:617). Copyright © 2009 Lippincott Williams & Wilkins.

foramen magnum. The jugular foramen is formed by a gap in the articulation between the occipital and petrous temporal bones. It contains the origin of the internal jugular vein from the sigmoid sinus and three cranial nerves: the glossopharyngeal, vagus, and accessory nerves.

There are several bony landmarks visible on the occipital portion of the external cranial base. The external occipital protuberance is a midline elevation that may be externally palpated on the human head. The superior and inferior nuchal lines are transverse elevations that provide attachment to muscles of the neck and the occipital body of the occipitofrontalis.

2.2.3 *Internal skull base*

The internal, or superior, face of the skull base can be divided into three spaces — the anterior, middle, and posterior cranial fossae (Figure 2.11). The anterior fossa comprises the frontal bone, the superior ethmoid bone, and the lesser wings of the sphenoid bone. The floor of the frontal bone contains depressions formed by ridges in the overlying frontal bone of the brain in addition to a hiatus, termed the *ethmoidal notch*, for the crista galli and cribriform plate of the ethmoid bone. The crista galli is a midline, upward projection from the ethmoid bone surrounded on either side by the porous cribriform plate. Axons composing the olfactory nerve pass through the cribriform plate, terminating in the olfactory bulb that lies atop this part of the ethmoid bone. The anterior midline of the frontal bone contains a protuberance, or frontal crest, that is formed by the underlying superior sagittal sinus. The foramen cecum is a small opening at the base of the crest that is usually closed in the adult but patent during fetal development. It is clinically significant because it may permit passage of a nasal emissary vein to the superior sagittal sinus, providing a route for cutaneous facial infection to reach the cranial cavity. The anterior cranial fossa is separated from the middle fossa by the sharp posterior edges of the lesser wings of the sphenoid (sphenoidal crests) and the sphenoidal limbus that lies between two anterior clinoid processes. Also of note is that the crista galli and frontal crest provide attachment for the falx cerebri and the anterior clinoid processes for the tentorium cerebelli.

The middle cranial fossa is formed by portions of the sphenoid and temporal bones. Centrally, the fossa contains the sella turcica atop the body of the sphenoid bone. The greater wings of the sphenoid,

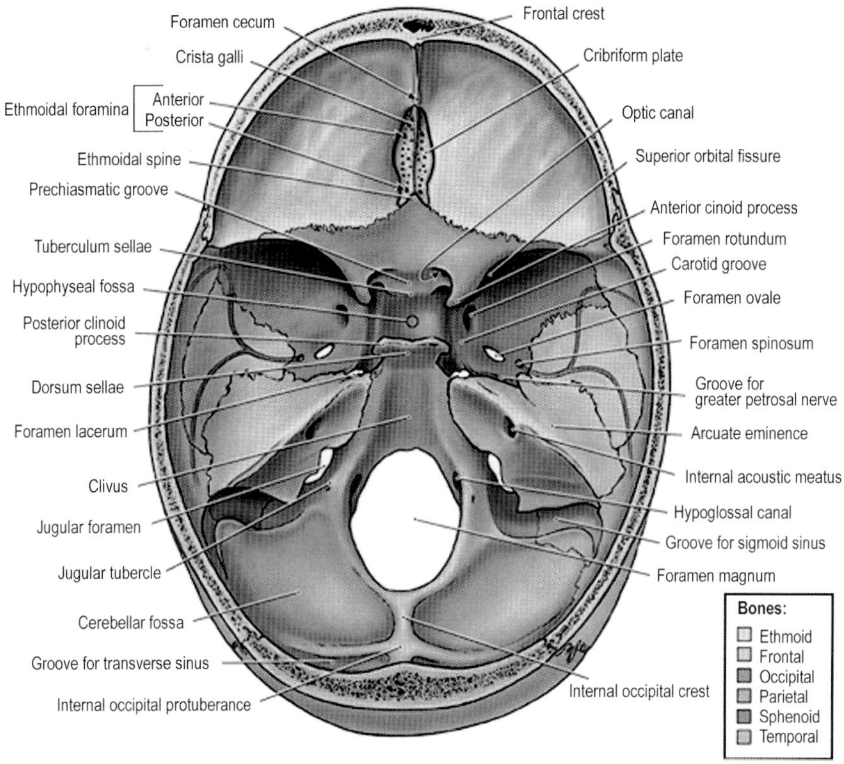

Figure 2.11. The skull base and its contents are divided into anterior, middle, and posterior cranial fossae.[7] Reprinted with permission from Wolters Kluwer (Agur AMR, Dalley AF II, eds. Grant's Atlas of Anatomy. 12th ed. Philadelphia, PA: Lippincott Williams & Wilkins; 2009:619). Copyright © 2009 Lippincott Williams & Wilkins.

the petrous temporal, and the squama temporalis bones are found on either side of the sella turcica, forming the lateral areas of the middle fossa. The fossa is bounded anteriorly by the lesser wings of the sphenoid and anterior clinoid processes as well as the chiasmatic groove, a transverse depression in the anterior body of the sphenoid for the optic chiasm. The groove leads into bilateral optic foramina on either side that transmits the optic nerves and ophthalmic arteries to each orbit. The posterior boundaries of the middle cranial fossa are the petrous crests laterally and the dorsum sellae medially. The former are elevations in the petrous temporal bones and the latter a single vertically orientated plate of bone that terminates bilaterally in the posterior clinoid processes. The sella turcica is a saddle-shaped structure formed by the superior surface of the body of the sphenoid. The "seat" of the saddle is a depression in the body of the sphenoid that is occupied by the hypophyseal fossa, or space for the pituitary gland. The sphenoid sinus, which drains to the posterior nasal cavity, is found in the body of the sphenoid just deep to the sella. Further clinical significance of the middle cranial fossa is attributed to multiple openings in the greater wing of the sphenoid that allow passage of nerves and vessels from the intracranial cavity (Table 2.2).

The posterior cranial fossa is formed by the occipital bone medially and the petrous temporal bone laterally. Its depth and size can be attributed to its containing the cerebellum, pons, and medulla

Table 2.2. Foramina and Fissures of the Skull Base.

Name	Location	Contents
Superior orbital fissure	Between greater and lesser wings of the sphenoid bone	Ophthalmic veins; ophthalmic nerve, oculomotor nerve, trochlear nerve, abducens nerve
Foramen rotundum	Anterior greater wing of sphenoid bone	Maxillary nerve
Foramen ovale	Posterolateral to foramen rotundum	Mandibular nerve
Foramen spinosum	Posterior angle of greater wing of the sphenoid	Middle meningeal vessels, meningeal branch of the mandibular nerve
Foramen lacerum (obliterated by cartilage)	Between greater wing of the sphenoid and petrous temporal bones	Internal carotid artery passes over superior aspect of foramen; deep petrosal nerve from carotid sympathetic plexus joins greater petrosal nerve within cartilage to form nerve of pterygoid canal[a]

[a]The pterygoid canal passes anteriorly through the medial pterygoid plate to the pterygopalatine ganglion.

oblongata. Its anterior boundaries are the petrous crests and dorsum sellae, from which there is a steep posterior incline leading to the most conspicuous structure of the fossa — the foramen magnum. As mentioned previously, this foramen contains the spinal cord as it originates from the brainstem and its meningeal covering, anterior and posterior spinal arteries, vertebral arteries, and the accessory nerve (XI). Posterior to the foramen magnum, the occipital bone is divided into bilateral cerebellar fossae by the internal occipital crest. The crest culminates in the internal occipital protuberance, which marks the location of the confluence of the sinuses. Several important dural venous sinuses come together at the confluence, which is drained by transverse, then sigmoid, sinuses. The posterior cranial fossa contains depressions for these two sinuses, the latter of which exits the cranium through the jugular foramen as the internal jugular vein. This foramen also transmits cranial nerves and meningeal branches of divisions of the external carotid artery (ECA). The internal acoustic meatus is located on the posterior margin of the petrous crest and transmits the vestibulocochlear and facial nerves to the inner ear. The hypoglossal nerve (XII) exits the skull through the hypoglossal canal, found on the anterolateral margin of the foramen magnum.

2.2.4 *Facial skeleton*

The facial skeleton, or splanchnocranium, is composed of the frontal bone, the orbit and zygomatic bone, the nose, the maxilla, and the mandible (Figure 2.12). The appearance of a human face depends on the meticulous arrangement of these bony components.

2.2.5 *Frontal bone/forehead*

At birth, the frontal bone consists of two pieces connected by the midline metopic suture, which is typically obliterated by the 8th year of life. The frontal sinuses also form by the 8th year; however, they do not complete development until puberty. The frontal bone can be

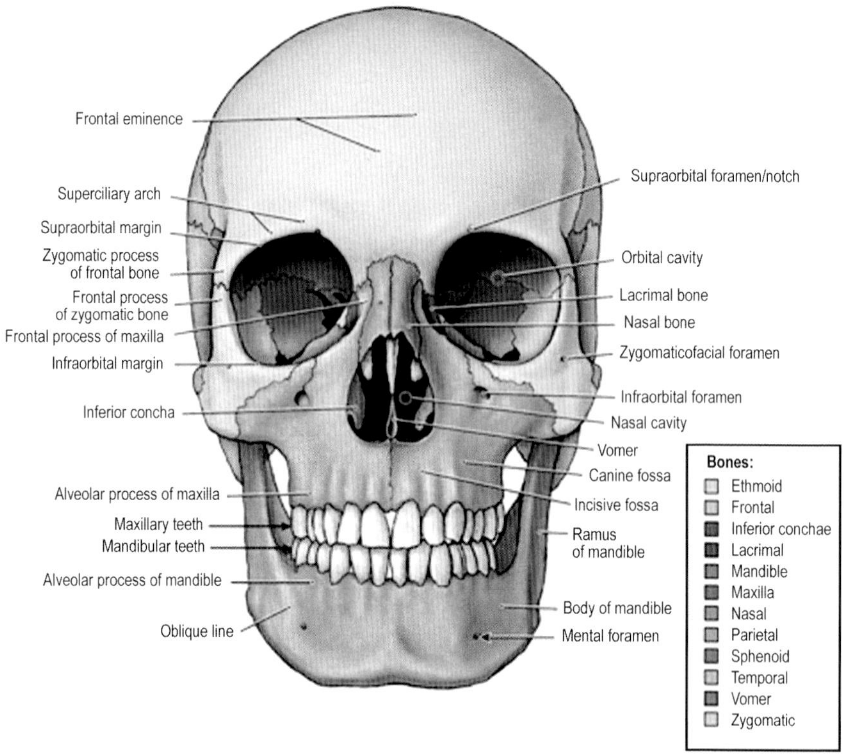

Figure 2.12. The facial skeleton (splanchnocranium).[7] Reprinted with permission from Wolters Kluwer (Agur AMR, Dalley AF II, eds. Grant's Atlas of Anatomy. 12th edn. Philadelphia, PA: Lippincott Williams & Wilkins; 2009:611). Copyright © 2009 Lippincott Williams & Wilkins.

divided into a squamous portion, or squama frontalis, and orbital portion, or pars orbitalis. The former creates the forehead and the latter forms the roof of the orbit and the anterior portion of the skull base. The supraorbital margin is the interface between squamous and orbital portions of the frontal bone. There is often a supraorbital notch along the margin that transmits the supraorbital nerve. Laterally, the supraorbital margins become the zygomatic processes of the frontal bone, which articulate with the zygomatic bones of the face. Superior to each supraorbital margin is a curved elevation called the *superciliary arch*, palpated deep to the eyebrows. They are most prominent medially, where they come together to form the glabella, a central elevation just superior to the nasal process of the frontal bone. The frontal sinuses are found deep to the arches and glabella, which tend to be more prominent in males. These sinuses drain into the nasal cavity via the frontonasal duct. The nasal process of the frontal bone articulates with the nasal bones centrally to form the bridge of the nose, or nasion. The nasal spine is a thin, vertical plate of the frontal bone that continues inferior to the frontonasal suture, contributing to the nasal septum.

2.2.6 *Orbit*

The orbits are bony sockets of the facial skeleton that accommodate the eyes, extraocular muscles, and neurovasculature needed for sight. Each orbit is pyramidal; the base is the anterior opening and the apex is the optic canal. The roof of the orbit, or everything superior to the optic canal, is formed by the pars orbitalis of the frontal bone and a small portion of the lesser wing of the sphenoid (Figure 2.13). The pars orbitalis has an anterolateral depression that accommodates the lacrimal gland and an anteromedial cartilaginous protrusion forming the trochlear spine. The inferior wall, or floor, of the orbit is formed by the maxilla and the maxillary process of the zygomatic bone. This surface also forms the roof of the maxillary sinus. The maxillary nerve (V_2) traverses the floor of the orbit in the infraorbital groove before exiting onto the face as the infraorbital nerve through the infraorbital foramen in the maxilla. The inferior orbital fissure separates the floor of the orbit from the lateral wall, which is formed by the frontal process of the zygomatic bone and the greater wing of the sphenoid. The medial wall of the orbit, from anterior to posterior, is composed of the frontal process of the maxilla, the lacrimal bone, the ethmoid bone, and a small portion of the sphenoid bone. The orbital portion of the lacrimal bone contains a depression for the lacrimal sac and nasolacrimal duct (lacrimal fossa). The lacrimal crest is an elevation just lateral to the fossa.

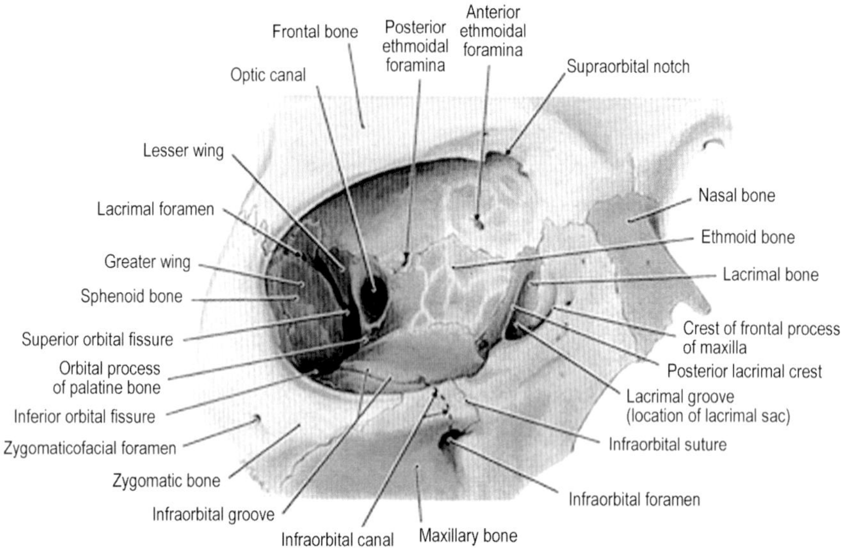

Figure 2.13. Detailed anatomy of the orbit.[7] Reprinted with permission from Wolters Kluwer (Agur AMR, Dalley AF II, eds. Grant's Atlas of Anatomy. 12th ed. Philadelphia, PA: Lippincott Williams & Wilkins; 2009:650). Copyright © 2009 Lippincott Williams & Wilkins.

2.2.7 *Nasal/midface region*

The nose is an intricate assembly of bone and cartilage that functions in both breathing and the sense of smell. The nose begins superiorly with the nasal process of the frontal bone. Paired nasal bones articulate with the nasal process of the frontal bone superiorly, each other medially, and the frontal processes of the maxillae laterally. The nasal bones are the ceiling of the superior nasal cavity and have free inferior edges that bound the anterior nasal aperture superiorly. The aperture, which represents the opening in the facial skeleton for the nasal cavities, is bounded laterally and inferiorly by the maxillae. Protruding from the lateral walls of the nasal cavities are three curved shelves of bone, or nasal conchae (Figure 2.14). The superior and middle conchae are part of the ethmoid bone while the inferior concha is a separate bone. The nasal cavities are divided by the nasal septum, which is formed by the perpendicular plate of the ethmoid bone superiorly, the

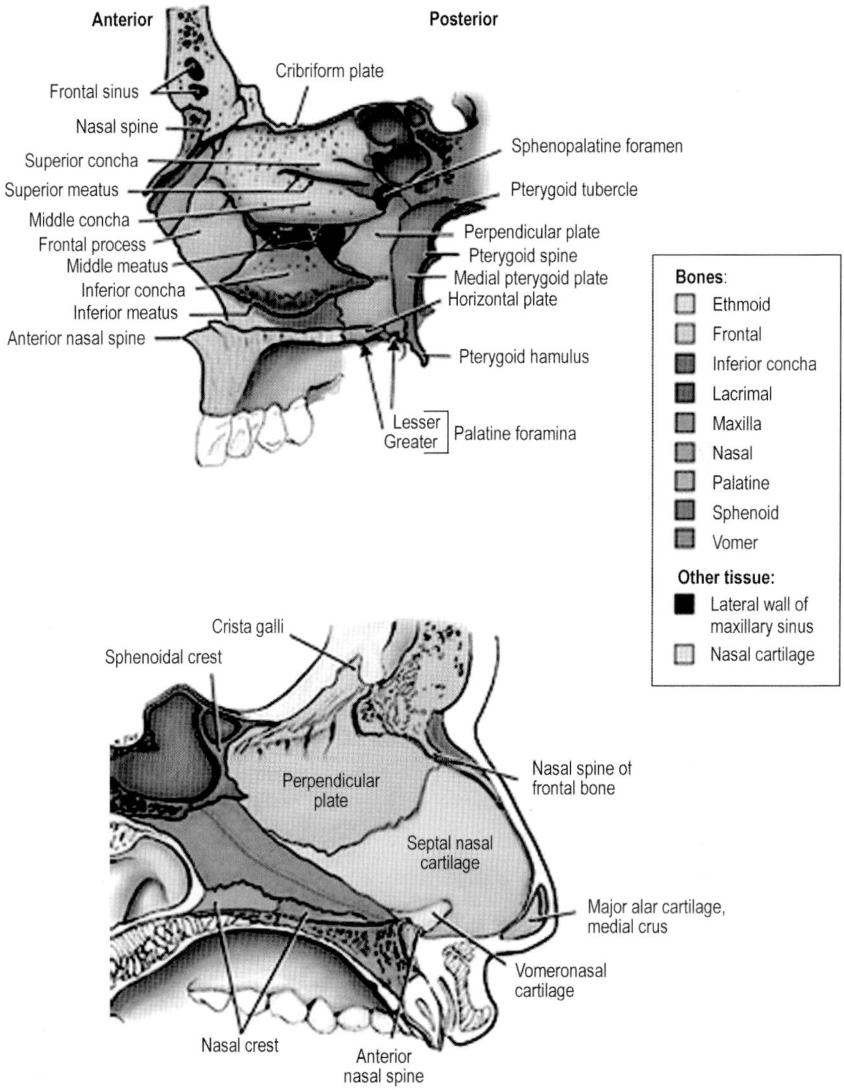

Figure 2.14. The lateral nasal wall (top) contains the conchae while the medial nasal wall (bottom) is formed by the nasal septum.[7] Reprinted with permission from Wolters Kluwer (Agur AMR, Dalley AF II, eds. Grant's Atlas of Anatomy. 12th ed. Philadelphia, PA: Lippincott Williams & Wilkins; 2009:691). Copyright © 2009 Lippincott Williams & Wilkins.

vomer posteriorly, and the septal cartilage anteriorly (Figure 2.14). The hard palate is the floor of the nasal cavity and separates it from the oral cavity. The nasal cavities are open to the face anteriorly and to the nasopharynx posteriorly through the external and internal choanae, respectively. The appearance of the human nose is completed by additional cartilaginous components, including the greater and lesser alar cartilages, which form the nasal alae.

The facial prominences commonly recognized as the cheek bones or malar bones are formed by the zygomatic bones. As mentioned previously, these bones articulate with the zygomatic processes of the frontal bones, the greater wings of the sphenoid, the maxilla, and the zygomatic processes of the parietal bones. The zygomatic bone contains a zygomaticofacial and zygomaticotemporal foramen laterally, which deliver the corresponding branches of the maxillary nerve to the face.

2.2.8 *Maxillae*

The paired maxillae are central to the facial skeleton, contributing to the orbit, the nasal cavities, and the jaw. Initially two bony processes that fuse centrally at the intermaxillary suture, each maxilla comprises a body and four bony processes — alveolar, palatine, zygomatic, and frontal. As discussed earlier, the zygomatic and frontal processes articulate with the zygomatic and frontal bones, respectively, and contribute to the walls of the orbit. The alveolar process is a tooth-bearing region found on the inferior aspect of the maxilla. Teeth are anchored to bony recesses, or sockets, in the alveolar processes by periodontal ligaments. The palatine processes are bilateral horizontal extensions of each maxilla, coming together centrally to form the anterior hard palate. The smaller, posterior portion of the hard palate is formed by paired palatine bones and contains greater and lesser palatine foramina on each side. The greater palatine nerve and vessels travel from the pterygopalatine fossa through the greater palatine canal in the posterior palatine bone and emerge from the greater palatine foramen to supply the hard palate. The greater palatine artery courses forward to anastomose with the sphenopalatine artery in the incisive foramen of the anterior hard palate. The lesser palatine foramen transmits the lesser palatine nerve. The body of the maxilla contains the maxillary sinus, which also forms recesses in the zygomatic, alveolar, and infraorbital regions of the bone. The cartilaginous medial wall of the sinus has an ostium that opens into the nasal cavity through an opening deep to the middle concha, the hiatus semilunaris. The maxillary sinus is prone to infection because the ostium is located high on the medial wall, making drainage difficult.[5]

2.2.9 Mandible

The mandible begins as two bilateral processes that fuse centrally at the mandibular symphysis. Both sides, however, are considered a single bone (Figure 2.15). The mandible consists of a horizontal body with a vertical ramus on either side, the exterior aspect of which provides inferior attachment to the masseter muscles. The superior aspect of the body contains an alveolar process, as the mandible is also a tooth-bearing bone. The inferior portion of the body is elevated anteriorly to form the mental protuberance, or chin. Mandibular canals run through the rami from the mandibular foramina on the superomedial aspect of the ramus to the mental foramina on either

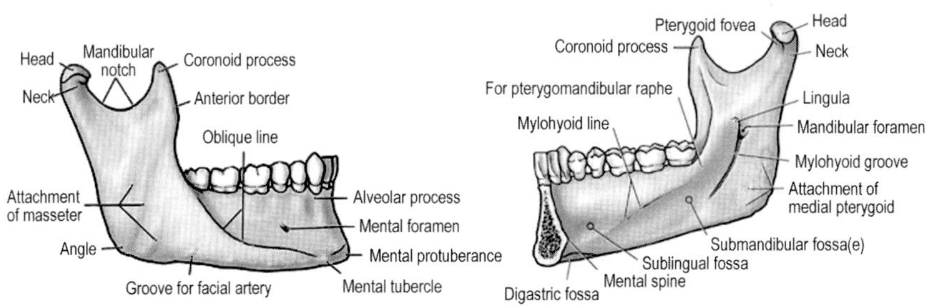

Figure 2.15. (Left) The external surface of the mandible contains a mental protuberance and mental foramina. (Right) The deep surface contains the mandibular foramina and several additional bony landmarks.[1] Reprinted with permission from Wolters Kluwer (Agur AMR, Dalley AF II, eds. Grant's Atlas of Anatomy. 12th ed. Philadelphia, PA: Lippincott Williams & Wilkins; 2009:664–665). Copyright © 2009 Lippincott Williams & Wilkins.

side of the mental protuberance. The lingula of the mandible is an irregular prominence just adjacent to and partially occluding the mandibular foramen. The mandible is involved in the TMJ with the temporal bone, allowing the mandible appropriate masticatory movement. The superior aspect of each mandibular ramus is composed of a coronoid process anteriorly and condylar head posteriorly with a depressed central region, the mandibular (sigmoid) notch. The coronoid process provides inferior attachment to the temporalis muscle and the condylar process is the mandible's contribution to the TMJ, articulating with the mandibular fossa of the temporal bone within a thick capsule (Figure 2.16). Besides the joint capsule, proper function of the TMJ relies on two ligaments that limit excessive joint

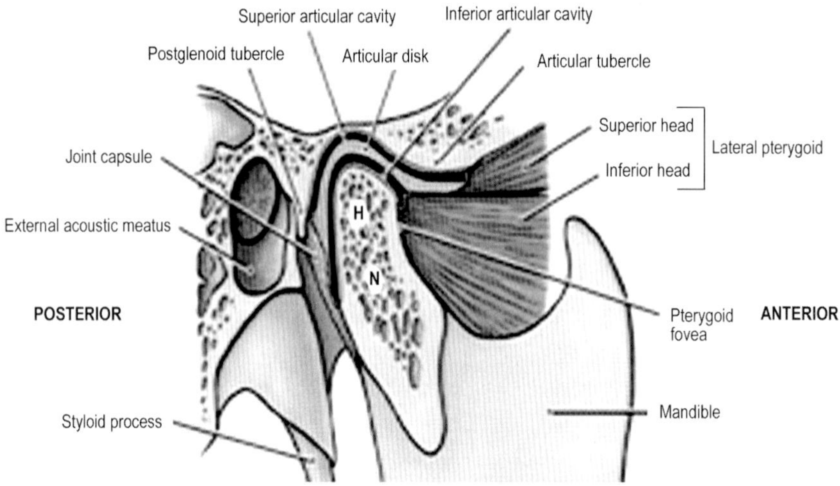

Figure 2.16. The TMJ is one of two synovial joints with a fibrocartilage articular disk dividing the joint into two parts. The lower portion, between the condylar head and disk, is purely rotational and is therefore responsible for opening and closing. The upper portion, between the disk and mandibular fossa, is involved in side-to-side and anterior–posterior movement of the mandible. With the temporalis and masseter muscles, the medial and lateral pterygoid muscles function to move the mandible via the TMJ. The medial pterygoid muscle attaches to the medial ramus and angle while the lateral pterygoid attaches to the coronoid process and the joint capsule of the TMJ.[7] Reprinted with permission from Wolters Kluwer (Agur AMR, Dalley AF II, eds. Grant's Atlas of Anatomy. 12th edn. Philadelphia, PA: Lippincott Williams & Wilkins; 2009:675). Copyright © 2009 Lippincott Williams & Wilkins.

movement — the sphenomandibular ligament, which is attached superiorly to the undersurface of the sphenoid bone and inferiorly to the lingula of the mandible, and the stylomandibular ligament, which runs from the styloid process to the angle of the mandible.

2.3 Craniofacial Vasculature

The face and scalp receive a rich vascular supply from the carotid system that is compounded by significant anastomoses of vessels. The venous drainage typically follows the arterial system, which is largely derived from the ECA.

2.3.1 *Arterial supply*

The common carotid arteries arise from the brachiocephalic trunk on the right and the aortic arch on the left, ascending bilaterally through the neck within the carotid sheath. The common carotid arteries divide into the internal carotid artery (ICA) and ECAs at approximately the level of the fourth cervical vertebra. The ICA continues directly upward after the bifurcation and enters the cranium through the carotid canal of the temporal bone without branches in the neck or face. The ICA is a major component of the cerebral circulation; however, it notably forms the ophthalmic artery just proximal to the circle of Willis. The ophthalmic artery enters the orbit through the optic canal and immediately gives rise to the central artery of the retina, which travels inferior to the optic nerve within its dural sheath to supply the internal portion of the retina. The ophthalmic artery also sends out muscular branches to supply the extraocular muscles; ciliary branches to supply the choroid, iris, and ciliary body; and several other branches supplying structures of the orbit and nearby face.[7] Distribution of the ophthalmic artery is outlined in Table 2.3 and illustrated in Figure 2.17.[8]

Unlike the ICA, the ECA contributes significantly to the facial vasculature, and all its branches are in the head and neck. The ECA initially travels upward at the anterior border of the sternocleidomastoid muscle, typically giving off the superior thyroid, ascending

Table 2.3. Distribution of the Ophthalmic Artery.

Branch of ophthalmic artery	Course and function
Supraorbital	Travels forward in orbit and emerges from supraorbital notch to supply skin of forehead and scalp, frontal sinus, and superior eyelid
Supratrochlear	Terminal branch of ophthalmic artery exits orbit medially and ascends to supply skin of forehead and scalp
Lacrimal	Passes forward in orbit with lateral rectus muscle to supply the lacrimal gland and eyelids
Dorsal nasal	Emerges from medial orbit and supplies dorsal surface of the nose
Anterior ethmoidal	Exits orbit medially through anterior ethmoidal foramen to supply anterior and middle ethmoid air cells, frontal sinus, and nose
Posterior ethmoidal	Exits orbit medially through posterior ethmoidal foramen to supply posterior ethmoid air cells

pharyngeal, lingual, facial, and occipital branches in the neck region (Figure 2.18). It continues superiorly and gives off the posterior auricular branch while coursing posterior to the mandibular ramus. In the substance of the parotid gland, the ECA divides into two terminal branches, the maxillary and superficial temporal arteries. The superior thyroid artery emerges at the level of the hyoid bone and runs anteroinferiorly to supply the thyroid gland and the larynx via its superior laryngeal branch. The ascending pharyngeal artery arises from the medial ECA and ascends deep to the ICA to supply many structures of the head and neck including the pharynx, middle ear, meninges of posterior fossa, and distal cranial nerves. The lingual artery emerges from the anterior ECA and passes deep to the muscles of the anterior neck before turning upward to supply the tongue.[5]

The facial artery usually originates just superior to the lingual artery and is the principal source of arterial blood for the face.[5] Initially shielded by the angle of the mandible, the facial artery turns inferior to pass beneath the body of the mandible before turning

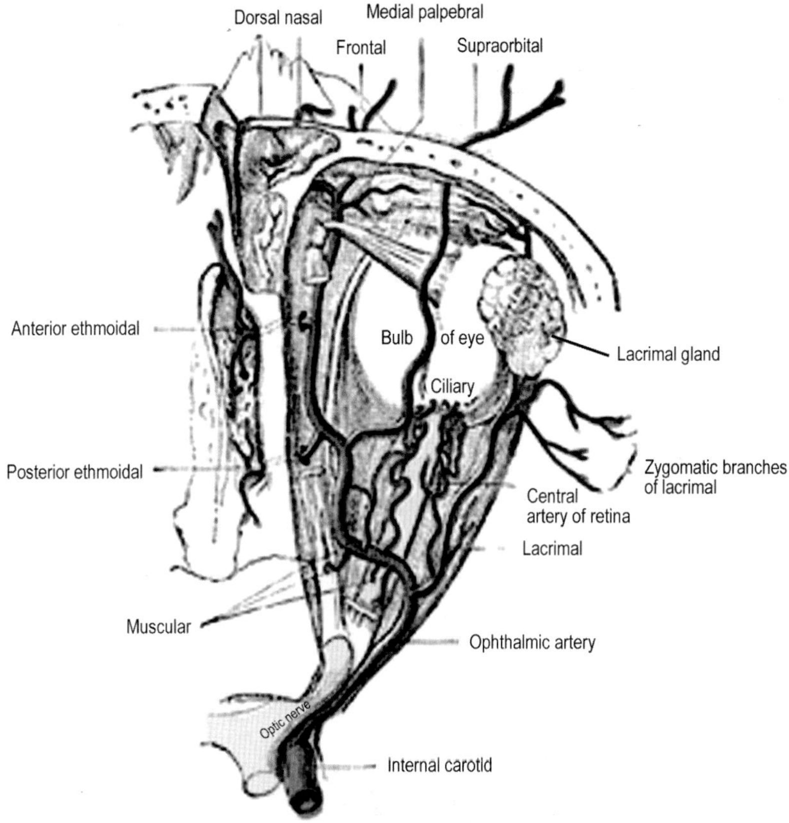

Figure 2.17. Distribution of the ophthalmic artery in the orbit.[8] Reprinted with permission from Bartleby.com, Inc. (Ref. 8). Copyright © 2000 Bartleby.com, Inc.

upward on the surface of the body. From here it passes anteromedially, coursing diagonally across the cheek to the angle of the mouth and then along the lateral nose to the medial eye, where it anastomoses with the dorsal nasal branch of the ophthalmic artery. The inferior and superior labial arteries are proximal branches of the facial artery, supplying the lower and upper lips, respectively. The lateral nasal branch supplies the nasal dorsum and ala. The facial artery is called the *angular artery* upon reaching the root of the nose, which supplies the inferior eyelid and superior cheek. The occipital branch of the ECA ascends to the posterior scalp deep to the sternocleidomastoid

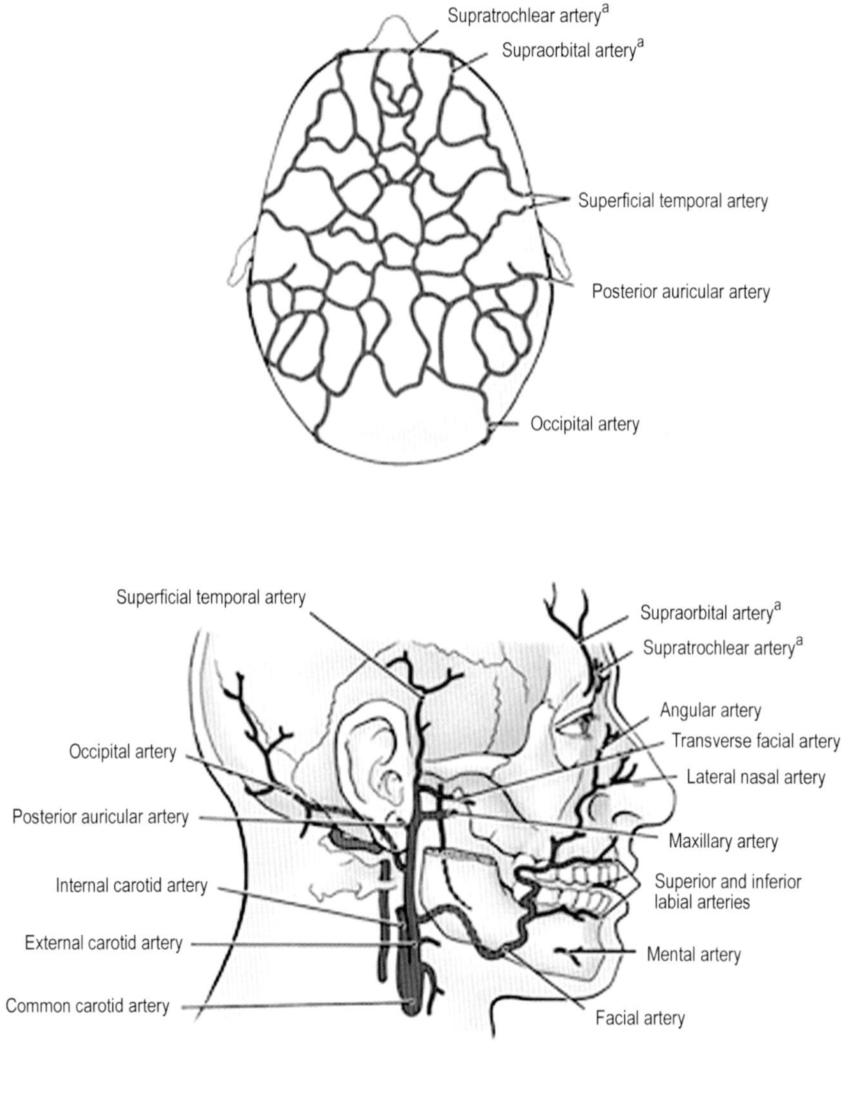

[a]Source = internal carotid artery (ophthalmic artery); all other labeled arteries are from external carotid

Figure 2.18. The ECA provides the blood supply to the face and scalp. It branches extensively in the cervical region before bifurcating into two terminal branches in the substance of the parotid gland.[7] Reprinted with permission from Wolters Kluwer (Agur AMR, Dalley AF II, eds. Grant's Atlas of Anatomy. 12th ed. Philadelphia, PA: Lippincott Williams & Wilkins; 2009:632). Copyright © 2009 Lippincott Williams & Wilkins.

muscle. The posterior auricular artery is usually the last branch of the ECA before the terminal branches. It is a posterior branch that ascends between the external acoustic meatus and the mastoid process to supply the posterior auricle and adjacent scalp.

The smaller terminal branch, the superficial temporal artery, courses anterior to the ear and over the zygomatic process of the temporal bone. On reaching the lateral surface of the parietal bone, the superficial temporal artery bifurcates into the frontal and parietal branches, which anastomose with other superficial arteries of the scalp to create an extensive collateral circulation. The larger maxillary artery runs horizontally from the bifurcation and can be divided into three parts by its relation to the lateral pterygoid muscle. Branches of the artery are shown and described in Figure 2.19 and Table 2.4, ordered from proximal to distal. The first, or mandibular, part is proximal to the lateral pterygoid and is found between the condyloid process and the stylomandibular ligament. The artery becomes the second, or pterygoid, part upon reaching the lateral pterygoid muscle. It may pass superficial or deep to the muscle but remains deep to the mandibular ramus. The third, pterygopalatine part begins when the artery passes medially through the pterygomaxillary fissure, formed by the posterior edge of the maxilla and the anterior edge of the lateral pterygoid plate, to enter the pterygopalatine fossa formed by the sphenoid and palatine bones.

2.3.2 *Venous drainage*

Venous drainage generally parallels the craniofacial arterial supply; however, vessel anastomoses and anatomic variability are more extensive in the venous system. The superficial drainage system is composed mainly of the facial, retromandibular, and external jugular veins (Figure 2.20). These veins anastomose with deep venous structures that include the cavernous sinus, pterygoid plexus of veins, and the internal jugular vein, forming effective collateral drainage. The superficial venous system begins superiorly with the supraorbital and supratrochlear veins, which begin on the forehead, anastomosing with each other and with the superficial temporal vein. These veins are also

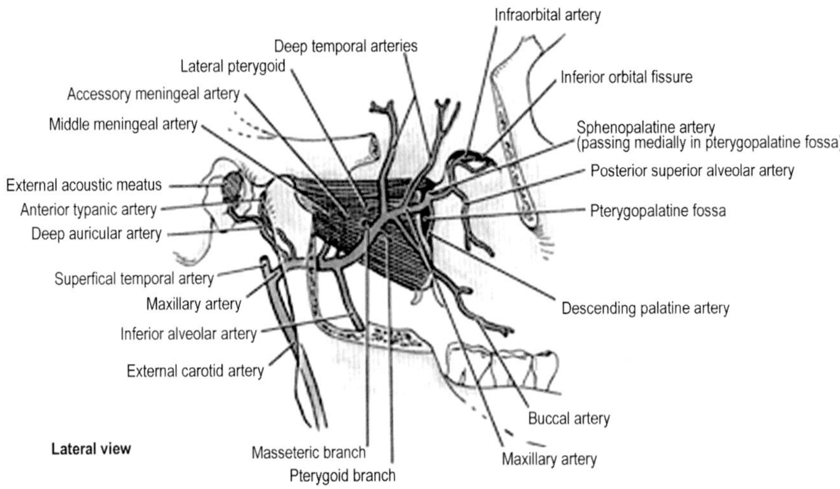

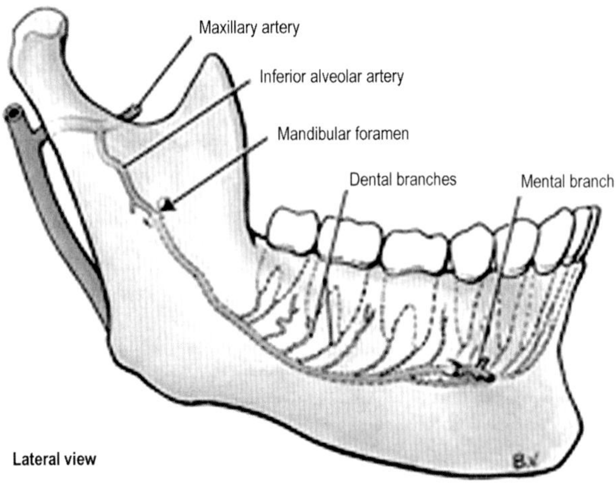

Figure 2.19. The maxillary artery branches extensively in the infratemporal fossa before entering the pterygopalatine fossa and then the orbit as the infraorbital artery. The inferior alveolar artery enters the mandibular canal.[7] Reprinted with permission from Wolters Kluwer (Agur AMR, Dalley AF II, eds. Grant's Atlas of Anatomy. 12th ed. Philadelphia, PA: Lippincott Williams & Wilkins; 2009:670). Copyright © 2009 Lippincott Williams & Wilkins.

Table 2.4. Distribution of the Maxillary Artery.

Branch	Distribution
Mandibular Part	
Deep auricular	External acoustic meatus to supply its lining and the external tympanic membrane
Anterior tympanic	Passes through petrotympanic fissure to supply tympanic cavity and internal tympanic membrane
Middle meningeal[a]	Through foramen spinosum to supply the skull, dura mater, and ganglia of the trigeminal and facial nerves
Accessory meningeal	Through foramen ovale; however, supplies mostly extracranial structures
Inferior alveolar	Enters mandibular canal through mandibular foramen, sends branches to mandibular teeth, mylohyoid muscle, chin (becomes mental nerve)
Pterygoid Part	
Masseteric	Through mandibular notch to supply masseter muscle
Deep temporal	Anterior and posterior branches ascend to supply temporalis muscle, ascend between muscle and cranium
Pterygoid	Variable number of branches; supplies medial and lateral pterygoid muscles
Buccal	Passes forward to buccinator muscle, buccal fat pad, and buccal oral mucosa
Pterygopalatine Part	
Posterior superior alveolar	Descends on posterior maxilla to enter alveolar canals and supply maxillary molars and premolars and maxillary sinus
Infraorbital	Traverses infraorbital canal and foramen to supply skin of infraorbital region; sends anterior superior alveolar branch to remaining maxillary teeth and orbital branches to inferior rectus and oblique muscles and the lacrimal sac; anastomoses medially with angular and dorsal nasal arteries
Artery of pterygoid canal	Enters pterygoid canal and is distributed to auditory tube, pharynx, and tympanic cavity

(Continued)

Table 2.4. *(Continued)*

Branch	Distribution
Descending palatine	Divides into greater and lesser palatine branches that enter respective palatine canals and foramina to supply hard and soft palate; greater palatine branch passes through incisive foramen to join sphenopalatine artery
Sphenopalatine	Enters posterosuperior nasal cavity through sphenopalatine foramen; supplies much of the nasal cavities and facial sinuses

[a]The intracranial portion of the middle meningeal artery is vulnerable to rupture upon injury to the side of the head, resulting in an epidural hematoma, because it lies just deep to the weakest part of the cranium — the pterion.

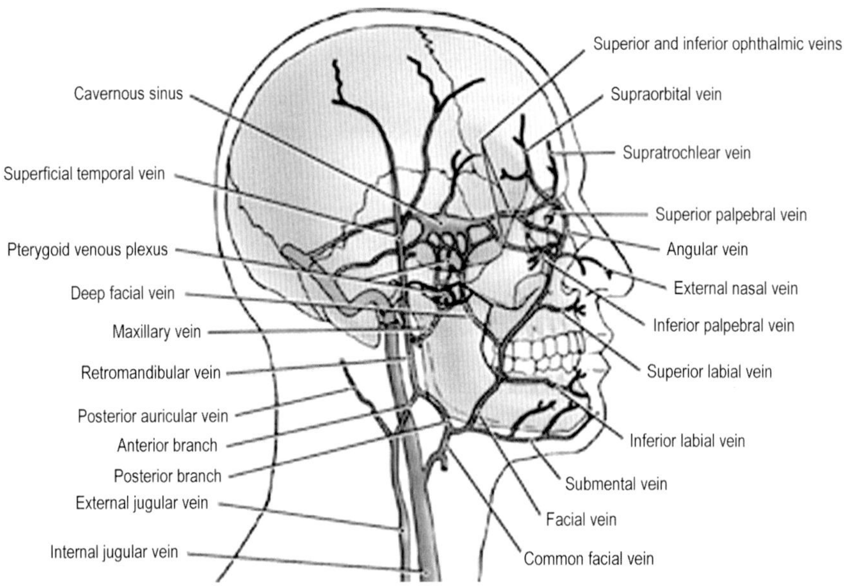

Figure 2.20. The facial and retromandibular veins drain the superficial face. However, they are redundantly connected to deep venous structures such as the pterygoid venous plexus, cavernous sinus, and internal jugular vein.[7] Reprinted with permission from Wolters Kluwer (Agur AMR, Dalley AF II, eds. Grant's Atlas of Anatomy. 12th ed. Philadelphia, PA: Lippincott Williams & Wilkins; 2009:633). Copyright © 2009 Lippincott Williams & Wilkins.

connected with the cavernous sinus through the superior and inferior ophthalmic veins. The supratrochlear and supraorbital veins join medially at the root of the nose to form the angular vein. This vein courses inferiorly along the side of the nose, becoming the facial vein at the inferior orbital margin. The facial vein continues on the side of the nose, receiving palpebral and external nasal branches, and then runs across the cheek to the inferior border of the mandible. It receives superior and inferior labial, deep facial, and submental branches before uniting with a communicating branch of the retromandibular vein to form the common facial vein. The deep facial vein drains the pterygoid plexus of veins within the infratemporal fossa and passes anteriorly on the maxilla to the facial vein. The retromandibular vein is formed posterior to the mandibular ramus by union of the superficial temporal vein, draining the lateral scalp, and the maxillary vein, also formed by the pterygoid venous plexus. It continues caudally and gives a communicating branch to the facial vein before joining with the posterior auricular vein to form the external jugular vein. The common facial vein drains into the cervical portion of the internal jugular vein and the external jugular vein drains into the subclavian vein just before it joins the internal jugular vein, forming the brachiocephalic vein.

2.4 Cranial Nerves

The cranial nerves comprise 12 sets of paired nerves that originate intracranially and pass to the head, neck, and even thoracic and abdominal viscera, supplying motor, sensory, and autonomic innervation to their target structures. Most of the cranial nerves have at least one corresponding nucleus in the brainstem gray matter, and many have anatomically identifiable peripheral ganglia. Although the nerves are numbered I through XII, they are also given names that reflect their function. The third (oculomotor), fourth (trochlear), sixth (abducens), eleventh (accessory), and twelfth (hypoglossal) nerves contain purely motor fibers; the first (olfactory), second (optic), and eighth (vestibulocochlear) nerves are solely sensory; and the fifth (trigeminal), seventh (facial), ninth (glossopharyngeal), and tenth (vagus) nerves are mixed nerves containing both motor and sensory fibers.[5] Several cranial nerves provide parasympathetic innervation, originating in the brainstem, and carry sympathetic fibers, which originate only in the thoracic and upper lumbar spinal cord.

The ***olfactory nerves*** (cranial nerve I) are essentially collections of olfactory receptor neurons from each nasal cavity and are responsible for the sense of smell, or olfaction. Their cell bodies are embedded within the olfactory mucosa, which is found on the roof, medial superior concha, and septum of the nasal cavity. Dendrites project tiny cilia that contain the actual olfactory G-protein–coupled receptors onto the mucosal surface. Axons of these neurons pass into the anterior cranial fossa through the cribriform plate to the olfactory bulb where they synapse on mitral cells. Axons of each olfactory bulb form an olfactory tract that travels along the undersurface of the frontal lobe before dividing into medial and lateral olfactory striae. The medial olfactory striae project olfactory information to the contralateral hemisphere whereas the lateral striae project to the ipsilateral temporal lobe. The integrity of the olfactory system can be assessed by placing a strong odor under one nostril while blocking the other and asking the patient to identify the odor. A diminished sense of smell can occur due to aging, fracture of the cribriform plate, or space-occupying lesion of the frontal lobe or anterior cranial fossa.[2]

The ***optic nerves*** (cranial nerve II) develop as outgrowths of the forebrain and are essentially collections of axons from retinal ganglion cells with a complete meningeal covering. The retina is a multilayered structure, and the cell bodies of these cells compose the most superficial layer. Axons are initially unmyelinated and travel within the orbit toward the posteromedial optic disk, where they become myelinated, aggregate to form the optic nerve, and leave the orbit through the optic canal. The two optic nerves converge at the optic chiasm, where axons from the medial half of each retina decussate and then diverge again as two optic tracts.[3] Since the medial half of each retina receives information from the lateral visual field and vice versa, each optic tract contains information from the ipsilateral medial visual field and the lateral half of the contralateral visual field. The optic tracts travel posteriorly, and most axons synapse in the lateral geniculate nucleus of the thalamus, a relay center for incoming sensory information. Second-order neurons then carry visual information to the visual cortex of the occipital lobe. Lesions to the above visual apparatus can be evaluated by testing one's visual fields. Damage to one of the optic nerves results in defects of the entire visual field of one eye. Damage to an optic tract will result in defects of one-half of both visual fields.[5]

The ***oculomotor nerve*** (cranial nerve III) provides motor innervation to four of six extraocular muscles and the levator palpebrae superioris.[5] Parasympathetic fibers originate in the Edinger–Westphal nucleus just cephalad to the somatic oculomotor nucleus in the midbrain and also travel in the oculomotor nerve to the sphincter pupillae muscle and ciliary body. The rectus muscles are named for the direction in which they move the eyeball, whereas the inferior oblique muscle paradoxically elevates the eyeball in addition to rotating laterally and abducting. The sphincter papillae muscle functions to constrict the pupil for near vision (accommodation) and to reduce visual input in bright light. Contraction of the ciliary body to adjust the shape of the lens is also required for near vision. The oculomotor nerves pass forward from the anterior surface of the midbrain and shed their meningeal coverings just in front of and lateral to the hypophyseal fossa. Before exiting the cranium through the superior orbital fissure, the oculomotor nerve traverses the lateral wall of the cavernous sinus. The nerve divides into superior and inferior rami as it enters the orbit below the trochlear nerve and above the abducens nerve (Figure 2.21). The former travels medially within the orbit to supply the superior rectus and levator palpebrae superioris muscles. The latter sends branches to the inferior rectus, medial rectus, and inferior oblique muscles. It also contains parasympathetic fibers that synapse in the ciliary ganglion before traveling on short ciliary nerves to sphincter papillae and ciliary body muscles. One can examine the function of a patient's oculomotor nerves by asking him or her to hold the head still while following your finger transcribing an "H" with their eyes alone. The oculomotor nerves also carry the efferent limb of the papillary reflex, causing the pupils to constrict upon the sensation of light by the optic nerves.[5]

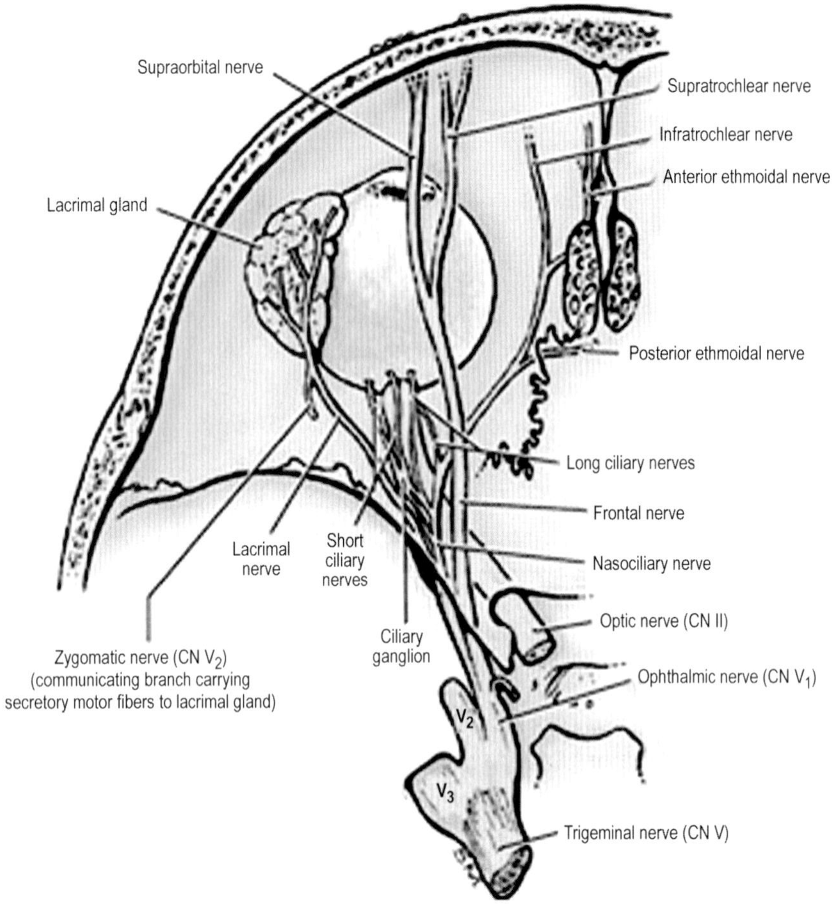

Figure 2.21. The frontal, nasociliary, and lacrimal nerves give rise to many branches as they pass from the superior orbital fissure to the anterior ocular opening.[7] CN = cranial nerve. Reprinted with permission from Wolters Kluwer (Agur AMR, Dalley AF II, eds. Grant's Atlas of Anatomy. 12th ed. Philadelphia, PA: Lippincott Williams & Wilkins; 2009:825). Copyright © 2009 Lippincott Williams & Wilkins.

The ***trochlear nerves*** (cranial nerve IV) provide somatic motor innervation to the superior oblique extraocular muscles. The associated nuclei are found in the midbrain just caudal to those of the oculomotor nerves, and the subsequent cranial nerves are unique in appearing from the posterior aspect of the midbrain before turning and passing forward toward the orbit.[3] It emerges from the meninges near the anterior edge of the tentorium and passes through the lateral wall of the cavernous sinus before entering the orbit through the superior orbital fissure. The trochlear nerve travels superior to the oculomotor nerve but inferior to the lacrimal and frontal branches of the ophthalmic nerve to supply its target muscle, located medially in the superior orbit. The trochlear nerve is particularly vulnerable to injury upon head trauma because of its long intracranial course, resulting in double vision (diplopia) when the person is performing activities such as reading or going downstairs that require intorsion and depression of the eye.[5]

The ***trigeminal nerve*** (cranial nerve V) is a large, paired cranial nerve that provides general sensation to the head as well as motor innervation to derivatives of the first branchial arch (branchial motor) including the muscles of mastication. The intracranial portion of the nerve is divided into a sensory and a motor root that emerge close to each other but distinctly separate from the lateral surface of the pons. The sensory root is composed of axons traveling centrally from the trigeminal ganglion, which sits, enclosed by dura (Meckel's cave), in an impression on the petrous ridge of the temporal bone.[8] It is here that the three peripheral divisions of the trigeminal nerve — the ophthalmic, maxillary, and mandibular nerves — converge after entering the cranium separately. The motor root passes adjacent to the trigeminal ganglion to join the peripheral mandibular nerve. Each division of the trigeminal nerve supplies cutaneous innervation to the area of the face for which it is named. Branches of each division are also responsible for distribution of postganglionic autonomic fibers.

The ophthalmic division passes forward to enter the orbit through the superior orbital fissure in which it trifurcates into frontal, nasociliary, and lacrimal divisions.[7] Distribution of these nerves is described in Table 2.5. Their paths and derivatives are illustrated in Figure 2.21. The long ciliary nerves, which also carry postganglionic sympathetic fibers, penetrate the posterior sclera to enter the oculus.[3] The lacrimal branch carries the terminal portions of parasympathetic secretomotor fibers to the lacrimal gland.

Table 2.5. Distribution of Branches of the Ophthalmic Nerve.

Branch	Distribution
Frontal	
Supratrochlear	Exits orbit medially and ascends to supply skin of medial forehead and skin and conjunctiva of medial upper eyelid
Supraorbital	Exits orbit through supraorbital notch and ascends to supply skin of lateral forehead, scalp, and pericranium
Nasociliary	
Long ciliary	Iris, cornea, dilator papillae muscle (sympathetic fibers)
Posterior ethmoidal	Sphenoid sinus, posterior ethmoid air cells
Anterior ethmoidal	Nasal cavities
Infratrochlear	Passes under trochlea to exit the orbit and supply conjunctiva, lacrimal sac and caruncle, skin of eyelid and root of nose
Lacrimal	Passes along lateral rectus muscle to lacrimal gland, skin and conjunctiva of superior eyelid

The *maxillary nerve* (cranial nerve V_2), responsible for sensation in the midface, enters the pterygopalatine fossa through the foramen rotundum.[7] It sends sensory sphenopalatine branches to the pterygopalatine ganglion, which also receives parasympathetic fibers from the greater petrosal nerve, a division of the facial nerve, and sympathetic fibers from the deep petrosal nerve, a division of the carotid plexus. Branches of the ganglion that carry sensory and secretomotor fibers are the nasopalatine, greater palatine, lesser palatine, and pharyngeal nerves. The nasopalatine nerve enters the nasal cavity and descends to the incisive foramen, where it communicates with the greater palatine nerve. The maxillary nerve enters the orbit through the inferior orbital fissure, sending out the zygomatic nerve and then the posterior superior alveolar nerve. The zygomatic nerve divides into the zygomaticotemporal and zygomaticofacial nerves, which exit the orbit through foramina in the zygomatic bone. The maxillary nerve then enters the infraorbital canal as the infraorbital nerve, where it sends out the middle superior alveolar nerve proximally and then the anterior superior alveolar nerve distally, just before exiting through the infraorbital foramen. Once on the face, the infraorbital nerve divides into cutaneous sensory branches to the maxillary region. Branches of the maxillary nerve are illustrated in Figure 2.22 and Table 2.6.

The *mandibular nerve* (cranial nerve V_3) supplies sensation to the mandibular region of the face and motor fibers to first-arch derivatives and masticatory muscles. This large nerve enters the infratemporal fossa through the foramen ovale and immediately sends off a sensory branch to the dura mater of the middle cranial fossa. Motor branches are given off to each of the four muscles of mastication (temporalis, masseter, lateral pterygoid, and medial pterygoid) and to tensor tympani and tensor veli palatini. The sensory branches of the mandibular nerve are the auriculotemporal, inferior alveolar, lingual, and buccal nerves (Figure 2.23 and Table 2.7). The auriculotemporal nerve runs posterior from its bifurcation, deep to the mandibular ramus and parotid gland, and emerges anterior to the external ear to

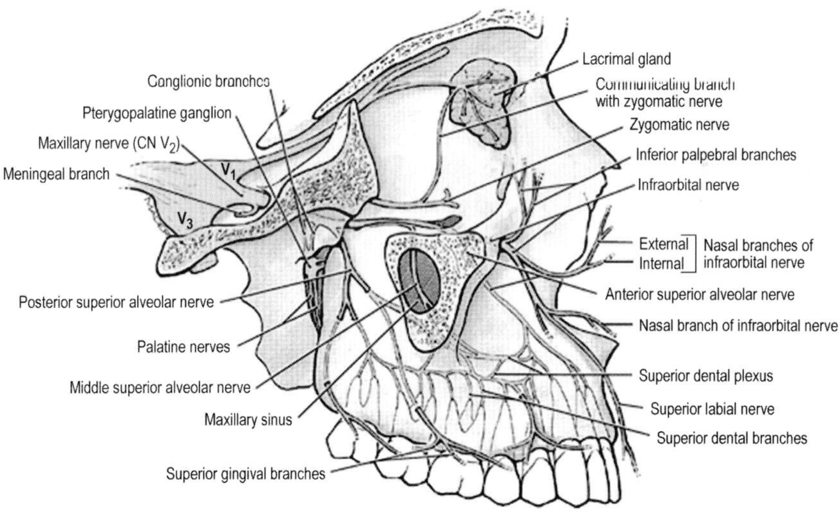

Figure 2.22. Distribution of the maxillary nerve (lateral view).[7] CN = cranial nerve. Reprinted with permission from Wolters Kluwer (Agur AMR, Dalley AF II, eds. Grant's Atlas of Anatomy. 12th edn. Philadelphia, PA: Lippincott Williams & Wilkins; 2009). Copyright © 2009 Lippincott Williams & Wilkins.

Table 2.6. Distribution of Branches of the Maxillary Nerve.[3]

Branch	**Distribution**
Nasopalatine	Nasal mucosa, hard palate, maxillary incisors and canines
Greater palatine	Branches to nasal mucosa, hard palate, maxillary gingiva
Lesser palatine	Branches to nasal mucosa, soft palate, uvula, palatine tonsils
Pharyngeal	Mucosa of nasopharynx
Zygomaticotemporal	Skin of lateral forehead, carries parasympathetic fibers to lacrimal nerve
Zygomaticofacial	Skin of cheek prominence
Posterior superior alveolar	Maxillary sinus mucosa, maxillary molars, maxillary gingival
Middle superior alveolar	Maxillary sinus mucosa, maxillary premolars
Anterior superior alveolar	Branches to inferior nasal mucosa, maxillary incisors and canines
Infraorbital	Maxillary sinus; skin of cheek, inferior eyelid (inferior palpebral branches), lateral nose (external nasal branches), nasal septum (internal nasal branches), and superior lip (superior labial branches)

ascend on the superficial temporal surface of the head. It passes through the otic ganglion and carries postganglionic parasympathetic fibers, originally from the glossopharyngeal nerve to the parotid gland.[1] The auriculotemporal nerve is closely associated with the TMJ and may be affected by injury to the joint. The inferior alveolar nerve enters the mandibular canal and emerges from the mental foramen as the mental nerve. The lingual nerve receives taste and preganglionic sympathetic fibers when it is joined by the chorda tympani of the facial nerve. The lingual nerve travels to the inferior oral cavity and sends parasympathetic fibers to synapse in the mandibular ganglion before delivering postganglionic fibers to the mandibular and sublingual salivary glands.[6]

The ***abducens nerve*** (cranial nerve VI) provides somatic motor innervation to the lateral rectus muscle, responsible for abduction of

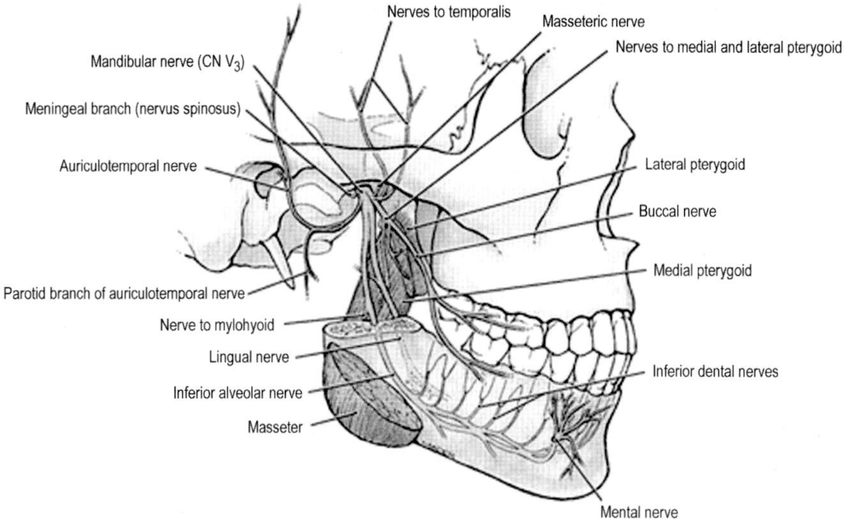

Figure 2.23. The mandibular nerve supplies sensation to the lower face and motor fibers to muscles of mastication.[7] Reprinted with permission from Wolters Kluwer (Agur AMR, Dalley AF II, eds. Grant's Atlas of Anatomy. 12th ed. Philadelphia, PA: Lippincott Williams & Wilkins; 2009:828). Copyright © 2009 Lippincott Williams & Wilkins.

Table 2.7. Distribution of Branches of Mandibular Nerve.

Branch	**Distribution**
Auriculotemporal	Skin anterior to auricle and of superficial temporal region, external acoustic meatus, tympanic membrane
Inferior alveolar	Mandibular teeth
Mental	Skin of chin, skin and oral mucosa of inferior lip
Lingual	Anterior two-thirds of tongue
Buccal	Buccal oral mucosa and skin, buccal gingival

the eye. Its nucleus is in the pons, and the nerve emerges on the anterior face of the brainstem from the pontomedullary junction. It ascends anterior to the brainstem and then turns forward to run along the base of the skull, passing over the petrous ridge and through the middle of the cavernous sinus, adjacent to the ICA. It is vulnerable to injury during its intracranial course, as aneurysms of the ICA within the cavernous sinus or fractures of the petrous ridge may cause damage to the nearby nerve.[5] It passes through the floor of the superior orbital fissure into the orbit and terminates along the medial side of the lateral rectus (Figure 2.24).

The ***facial nerve*** (cranial nerve VII) is a complex cranial nerve associated with the second branchial arch that contains multiple motor and sensory modalities. The facial nerve emerges laterally from the pontomedullary junction as two roots — the motor root containing fibers from the pontine motor nucleus of the facial nerve to the muscles of facial expression and the intermediate nerve containing parasympathetic and sensory fibers.[5] Preganglionic parasympathetic fibers from the superior salivatory nucleus travel with the facial nerve to facial ganglia that supply the lacrimal, submandibular, and sublingual glands. Branches of the trigeminal nerve then distribute postganglionic fibers to their glandular targets. Central axonal processes of taste neurons synapse in the nucleus of the solitary tract while those of general sensory neurons synapse in the spinal nucleus of the trigeminal nerve. The facial nerve enters the facial canal, which can be divided into three parts, within the petrous temporal bone through

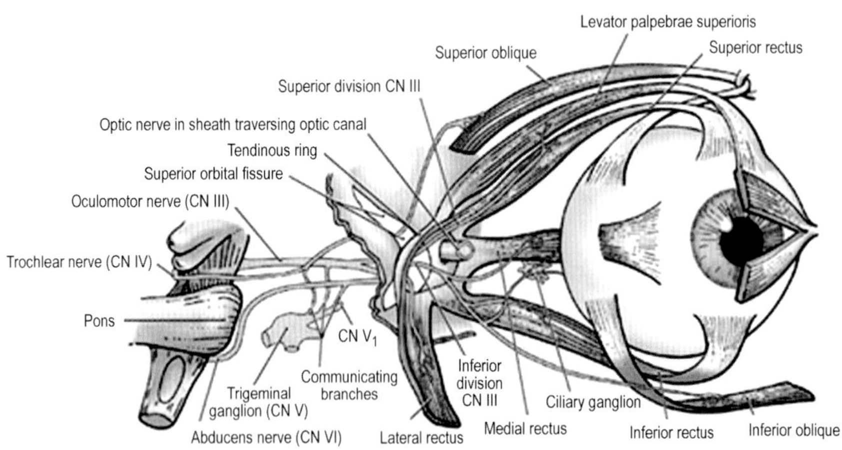

Figure 2.24. Distribution of the oculomotor, trochlear, and abducens nerves to the extraocular muscles.[1] CN = cranial nerve. Reprinted with permission from Wolters Kluwer (Agur AMR, Dalley AF II, eds. Grant's Atlas of Anatomy. 12th ed. Philadelphia, PA: Lippincott Williams & Wilkins; 2009:822). Copyright © 2009 Lippincott Williams & Wilkins.

the internal acoustic meatus. The facial canal initially runs forward (labyrinth part), then makes a sharp posterior turn at the point of the facial nerve's sensory geniculate ganglion to pass just deep to the medial wall of the tympanic cavity (tympanic part). The geniculate ganglion and facial canal create a bulge in the medial wall of the tympanic cavity (prominence of the facial canal). The facial nerve turns inferiorly (mastoid part) to exit the cranium through the stylomastoid foramen. In the face, it sends off a posterior auricular branch before terminating in the "parotid plexus," from which five motor branches arise to muscles of facial expression (Figure 2.25). While in the vertical,

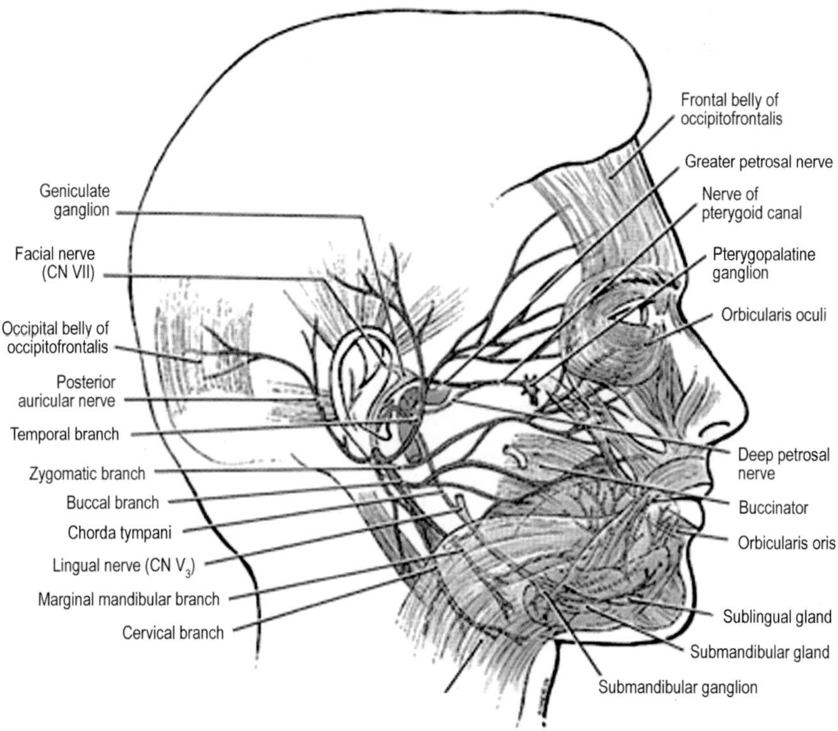

Figure 2.25. Distribution of the facial nerve within the facial canal and on the face (lateral view).[7] CN = cranial nerve. Reprinted with permission from Wolters Kluwer (Agur AMR, Dalley AF II, eds. Grant's Atlas of Anatomy. 12th edn. Philadelphia, PA: Lippincott Williams & Wilkins; 2009:830). Copyright © 2009 Lippincott Williams & Wilkins.

mastoid part of the facial canal, the nerve gives off the following three branches: greater petrosal nerve, nerve to stapedius, and the chorda tympani (Table 2.8).[5] The facial nerve can be tested by asking the patient to wrinkle the forehead, shut the eyes tightly, flare the nostrils, and open and close the lips.

The ***vestibulocochlear nerve*** (cranial nerve VIII), composed of axons of the spiral processes of bipolar neurons, carries sound and balance information from the inner ear to the brain. It emerges from the pontomedullary junction and enters the internal acoustic meatus of the petrous temporal bone, where it bifurcates into a cochlear and a vestibular division. The cochlear division carries auditory information from hair-cell receptors within the organ of Corti through the spiral ganglion, both of which are located in the cochlea of the inner ear. The vestibular division carries information through the vestibular ganglion about the position of the head from cristae in the three

Table 2.8. Distribution of Branches of the Facial Nerve.

Branch	Distribution
Greater petrosal nerve	Carries preganglionic parasympathetic fibers through the pterygoid canal to the pterygopalatine ganglion; zygomatic branches of the maxillary nerve distribute postganglionic fibers to the lacrimal gland
Nerve to stapedius	Passes from the facial canal into the tympanic cavity to supply the stapedius muscle with motor fibers
Chorda tympani	Also enters the tympanic cavity, then exits through the petrotympanic fissure to join the lingual branch of the mandibular nerve; carries taste information from the anterior two-thirds of the tongue and preganglionic parasympathetic fibers to the submandibular ganglion (through the lingual nerve)
Posterior auricular	Ascends between the mastoid process and external acoustic meatus to supply the occipitalis muscle and posterior auricular muscles
Temporal, zygomatic, buccal, mandibular, cervical	Terminal motor branches that arise in the parotid gland and supply muscles of the scalp and face that change facial expressions by pulling on the skin

semicircular canals and maculae in the utricle and saccule. A defect in the cochlear system from the brainstem nuclei to the cochlea itself results in sensorineural hearing loss. This can be tested for by placing a vibrating tuning fork at the apex of the patient's forehead and asking if it is heard equally in both ears (Weber's test). Conduction hearing loss is caused by blockage or defects of the external or middle ear and can be assessed by placing a vibrating tuning fork on the patient's mastoid process, then moving it adjacent to the external acoustic meatus. It should be louder in the latter position, as air conducts sound better than bone.[2]

The ***glossopharyngeal nerve*** (cranial nerve IX) carries both motor and sensory fibers to and from derivatives of the third branchial arch. It appears from the lateral medulla and exits the cranium through the jugular foramen just posterior to the ICA. Two thickenings of the nerve as it exits the foramen are the superior and inferior sensory ganglia, containing cell bodies of all afferent neurons. Upon exiting the skull, the nerve sends out a tympanic branch that carries preganglionic parasympathetic fibers from the inferior salivatory nucleus of the medulla to the tympanic plexus, from which the lesser petrosal nerve to the otic ganglion originates. The parasympathetic fibers synapse at the ganglion and travel to the parotid gland on the auriculotemporal branch of V_3. Several fibers containing cutaneous sensation from the auricle are also carried in the glossopharyngeal nerve to the spinal trigeminal nucleus of the fifth cranial nerve. The distal glossopharyngeal nerve courses along the inferior border of the stylopharyngeus muscle from the styloid process to the surface of the middle pharyngeal constrictor, contributing to the pharyngeal plexus here. It sends out motor branches originating in the nucleus ambiguus of the medulla to the stylopharyngeus muscle. Table 2.9 details the sensory distribution of the glossopharyngeal nerve, and all branches are illustrated in Figure 2.26. The glossopharyngeal nerve also sends special sensory branches to the posterior tongue that carry taste information to the inferior solitary nucleus of the medulla. The glossopharyngeal nerve is the afferent arm of the gag reflex, and an absent reflex may indicate a lesion of the nerve.[3]

Table 2.9. Sensory Distribution of the Glossopharyngeal Nerve.

Branch	Distribution
Tympanic	General sensation to the middle ear and eustachian tube
Carotid sinus	Visceral sensation from the carotid sinus baroreceptor and carotid body chemoreceptor
Pharyngeal	Contributes to pharyngeal plexus of vagus nerve, which provides motor and sensory fibers to most of the larynx and pharynx; afferent limb of the gag reflex
Tonsillar	General sensation to the palatine tonsils
Lingual	General sensation to the base and posterior one-third of the tongue; carries taste fibers from posterior tongue

The ***vagus nerve*** (cranial nerve X) is another complex cranial nerve that distributes motor, sensory, and autonomic fibers to the head, neck, thorax, and abdomen (Figure 2.27). Within the head and neck, the vagus nerve provides sensation to the inferior pharynx and larynx and motor fibers to the soft palate, pharynx, and larynx.[5] Central processes of sensory neurons terminate in the spinal trigeminal nucleus while those of motor fibers terminate in the ambiguous nucleus. Taste sensation from the base of the tongue and the epiglottis is also carried by the vagus nerve to the solitary nucleus. The superior and inferior ganglia containing cell bodies of vagal sensory neurons are found within the vagus nerve as it passes through the jugular foramen. Upon exiting the skull, the vagus nerve gives rise to auricular and meningeal branches. It then descends through the neck within the carotid sheath, giving rise to pharyngeal, laryngeal, superior cardiac, and recurrent laryngeal branches. The right and left vagus nerves meet at the esophagus, forming the posterior and anterior esophageal plexuses, respectively. Anterior and posterior vagal trunks descend from the plexuses through the esophageal hiatus in the diaphragm to supply viscera of the thorax and the gut from the esophagus to the splenic flexure of the colon (Table 2.10). Lesions of the vagus nerve may result in paralysis of pharyngeal and laryngeal muscles, resulting in dysphagia or dysphonia, respectively, as well as deviation of the uvula to the unaffected side. Lesions also may result

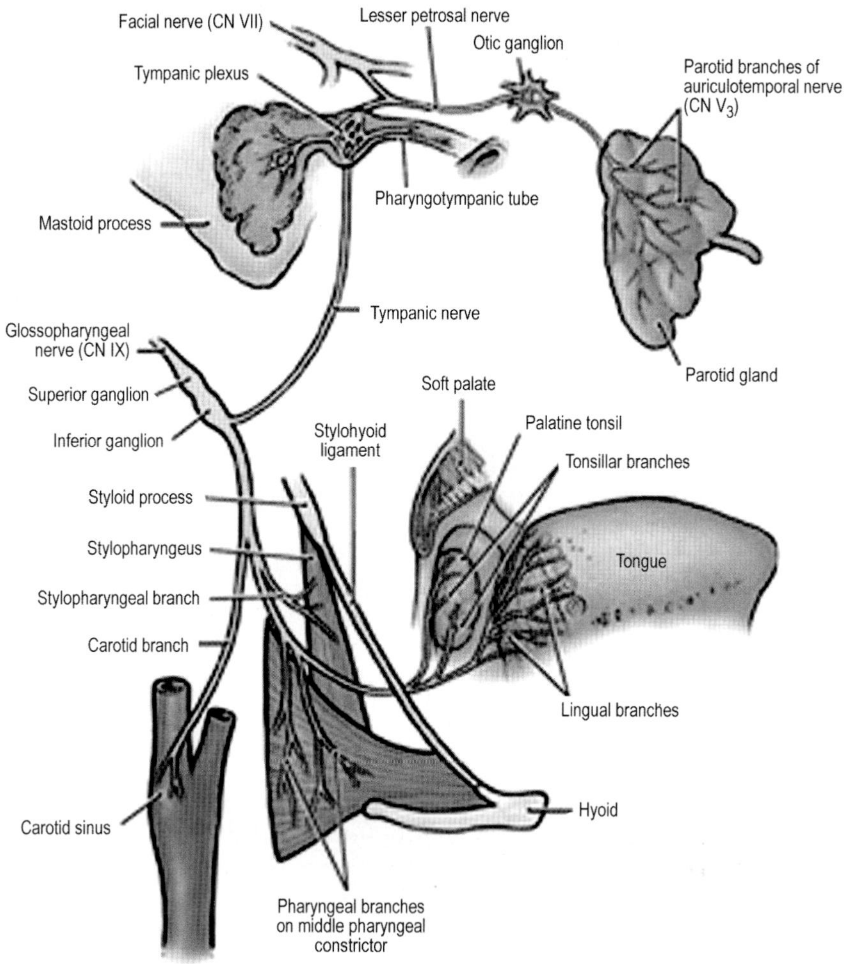

Figure 2.26. Distribution of the glossopharyngeal nerve includes secretomotor fibers to the parotid gland, visceral sensation from the carotid sinus, motor fibers to the stylopharyngeus, and sensory fibers from the pharynx and soft palate.[7] CN = cranial nerve. Reprinted with permission from Wolters Kluwer (Agur AMR, Dalley AF II, eds. Grant's Atlas of Anatomy. 12th ed. Philadelphia, PA: Lippincott Williams & Wilkins; 2009:835). Copyright © 2009 Lippincott Williams & Wilkins.

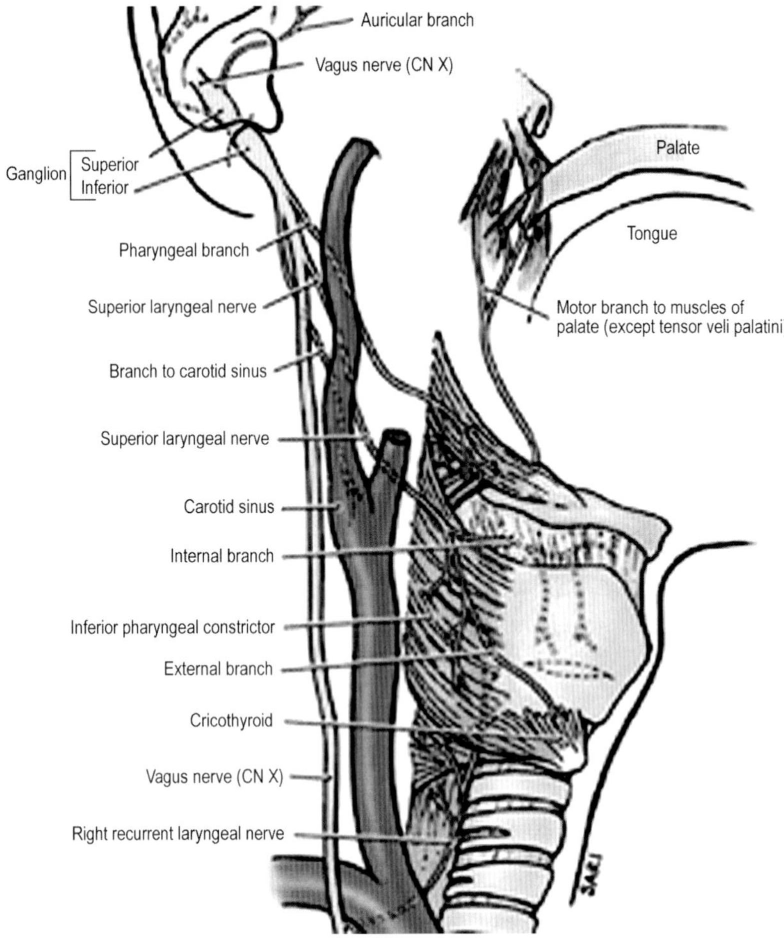

Figure 2.27. Distribution of the vagus nerve in the head and neck.[7] CN = cranial nerve. Reprinted with permission from Wolters Kluwer (Agur AMR, Dalley AF II, eds. Grant's Atlas of Anatomy. 12th ed. Philadelphia, PA: Lippincott Williams & Wilkins; 2009:837). Copyright © 2009 Lippincott Williams & Wilkins.

in the loss of the gag and cough reflexes, as the vagus nerve is involved in both.[3]

The ***accessory nerve*** (cranial nerve XI) is a motor nerve that supplies the sternocleidomastoid and trapezius muscles. Its nucleus is a column of motor neurons occupying the caudal medulla and the first five or six cervical segments of the spinal cord. It emerges from the

Table 2.10. Distribution of Branches of the Vagus Nerve.

Branch	Distribution
Auricular	Sensation from skin of the auricle and external acoustic meatus
Meningeal	Carries sensory fibers of the second cervical root to dura mater of the posterior cranial fossa
Pharyngeal	Courses to the surface of the middle pharyngeal constrictor muscle to form the pharyngeal plexus; this plexus sends motor fibers to the pharyngeal and palatine muscles (except stylopharyngeus and tensor veli palatini); efferent limb of the gag reflex
Superior laryngeal	Descends along the posterior aspect of the ICA and bifurcates into the internal and external laryngeal nerves
Internal laryngeal	Pierces the hypothyroid membrane to provide sensation to the larynx superior to the vocal folds, epiglottis, and base of the tongue (also carries taste information); afferent arm of the cough reflex
External laryngeal	Descends on the inferior pharyngeal constrictor, deep to the sternothyroid muscle, to supply the cricothyroid muscle
Recurrent laryngeal	Loops around the subclavian artery (right) and arch of aorta (left) to ascend on either side of the esophagus before running deep to the inferior pharyngeal constrictor muscle to supply muscles of the larynx (except for cricothyroid)

jugular foramen as two roots — the cranial root, which quickly joins the vagus nerve for distribution, and the spinal accessory nerve. The latter descends just anterior to the internal jugular vein before turning posterior to innervate the sternocleidomastoid muscle. The nerve appears from the posterior border of the muscle and passes through the posterior neck to the trapezius muscle. It runs along the deep surface of the trapezius, sending motor branches to the entire length of the muscle. The accessory nerve also receives sensory branches from the cervical plexus, allowing it to carry pain and proprioceptive information from the muscles it innervates. This cranial nerve can be tested by asking the patient to shrug his or her shoulders, an activity that requires the trapezius muscle.[5]

The ***hypoglossal nerve*** (cranial nerve XII) supplies the intrinsic and extrinsic muscles of the tongue with somatic motor fibers.[5] Motor neurons originate in the hypoglossal nucleus of the caudal medulla and emerge from the brainstem superior to the accessory nerve. The hypoglossal nerve exits the skull through the hypoglossal canal of the occipital bone and travels deep to the mandibular ramus, then anterior to reach the tongue. Motor and sensory fibers from the cervical plexus join the hypoglossal nerve briefly before exiting to form the inferior root of the ansa cervicalis and a meningeal branch. The former supplies muscles of the hyoid bone with motor fibers, and the latter supplies the dura mater of the posterior cranial fossa with sensation. The hypoglossal nerve terminates in lingual branches that splay out on the tongue muscles, providing motor fibers to the styloglossus, hyoglossus, genioglossus, and intrinsic muscles. Function of this nerve can be tested by asking the patient to protrude his or her tongue. Injury to the hypoglossal nerve will result in deviation of the tongue to the affected side.

References

1. **Gosain AK, Nacamuli R.** Embryology of the head and neck. In: Beasley RW, Aston SJ, Barlett SP, Gurtner GC, Spear SL, eds. *Grabb & Smith's Plastic Surgery.* 6th edn. Philadelphia, PA: Lippincott Williams & Wilkins; 2007:177–190.
2. **Cummings CW, Flint PW, Harker LA, et al**. *Cummings Otolaryngology: Head and Neck Surgery.* 4th edn. Philadelphia, PA: Mosby; 2004.
3. **Standring S.** *Gray's Anatomy.* 39th edn. New York, NY: Elsevier Churchill Livingstone; 2005.
4. **Sadler TW.** *Langman's Medical Embryology.* 10th edn. Philadelphia, PA: Lippincott Williams & Wilkins; 2006.
5. **Moore KL, Dalley AF II.** *Clinically Oriented Anatomy.* 5th edn. Philadelphia, PA: Lippincott Williams & Wilkins; 2006.
6. **Carlson BM**. *Human Embryology and Developmental Biology.* 3rd edn. Philadelphia, PA: Mosby; 2004.
7. **Agur AMR, Dalley AF II.** *Grant's Atlas of Anatomy.* 12th edn. Baltimore, MD: Lippincott Williams & Wilkins; 2009.
8. **Gray H**. *Anatomy of the Human Body.* Bartleby.com Web site. http://bartleby.com/107. Published May 2000. Accessed July 12, 2011.

FACIAL ANALYSIS 3

Ali Totonchi, MD; Bahman Guyuron, MD and Raja Mohan, MD

When considering surgery to correct craniofacial abnormalities in a patient, a thorough facial analysis is paramount before an operative plan is designed. Surgical intervention alongside orthodontic treatment helps achieve an optimal and predictable result.

3.1 History

First, the patient's perspective and desires should be discussed when performing the initial evaluation. Often, the patient's perceptions differ from those of the surgeon. In addition, a detailed history of the patient's current and previous medical problems should be gathered. Family history is also pertinent since siblings may have similar facial abnormalities. It is important to consider the history of speech problems or congenital craniofacial abnormalities.[1]

Comorbidities such as preexisting cardiac or renal dysfunction require consultation with a specialist to obtain advice for perioperative management. Patients with diabetes or those who are immunocompromised are at a greater risk for infection and may have complications with wound healing. Lastly, patients with bleeding tendencies or who bruise easily should be evaluated for any coagulation disorders such as Von Willebrand's disease.[2,3] Patients with coagulation disorders may not be aware of their condition and might require treatment intraoperatively for adequate hemostasis. Controlling blood pressure, whether it is high or low, is also key in preventing complications associated with bleeding, such as hematoma. As for any surgical procedure, patients should discontinue nonsteroidal anti-inflammatory medications and aspirin-containing products before the procedure.

3.2 Dental History and Examination

A detailed dental history is important in patients considering maxillofacial surgery. Any history of periodontal disease, tooth extractions, or previous dental procedures should be recorded; a current evaluation by a dentist is also essential. Patients who have had prolonged orthodontic treatment could have root resorption, which would render further orthodontic work imprudent.[4] Sometimes, patients undergo orthodontic treatment for what is in fact a skeletal problem and will actually require surgical treatment. The changes induced by the orthodontic treatments should be reversed before surgical intervention.[4]

The alignment of the teeth, location of the palatal vault, and shape of the arch should also be examined. Crowding indicates the inability of the dental arch to accommodate the teeth. Assessment of oral hygiene and periodontal disease are vital to the success of orthognathic surgery since their presence precludes orthodontic treatment, and surgery without orthodontic intervention should almost never be considered. One of the most important parts of the intraoral examination is assessing the patient's occlusion. Any overbite, overjet, or crossbite should be noted, and the angle classification should be determined. Details regarding angle classification and occlusion can be found in other sections of this book. Placing a tongue blade and asking the patient to bite down is a simple maneuver to assess the patient's occlusal canting and determine if there is any asymmetry.

Any history of temporomandibular joint (TMJ) dysfunction should be recorded. Patients with this condition may experience symptoms such as clicking, pain, locking, ear pain, bruxism, or headaches.

Preoperative imaging can assist with determining the presence and severity of the TMJ conditions. The masticatory function and tenderness of the muscles should be evaluated. The interincisal dimension, lateral excursion, and protrusive excursion should all be measured. A normal mandibular opening is 40 to 56 mm, and the normal range of lateral movement at 10 mm and protrusion is 9 to 13 mm.[5]

3.3 Psychological Assessment

Before the procedure, one must have a detailed discussion with the patient, parents, or legal guardians about the intended facial changes and potential risks and outcomes so that they understand the changes that can occur. Often, significant alterations in facial appearance are to be expected, and it may take time for the patient to adjust to these changes. The treatment plan and expected outcome should ultimately be based on the patient's desires. Even though the postoperative changes may be anatomically or "cephalometrically" correct, the patient may still be dissatisfied with the result. It is important to avert this scenario as much as possible.

3.4 Facial Analysis

A systematic approach to the face concentrating on the relationships of craniofacial, skeletal, and soft tissue components is suggested. The patient's skin is examined first to assess thickness, color, and consistency and is evaluated for its susceptibility to forming hypertrophic scars or keloids. Patients with red hair, light or freckled skin, and blue eyes are more susceptible to bleeding and developing hypertrophic scars.

The face may be divided into three different zones: upper, middle, and lower (Figure 3.1). The upper zone extends from the hairline to the glabella. The middle zone extends from the glabella to the subnasale. The third zone extends from the subnasale to the menton. The frontal view of the face can be split into five equal, vertical segments. Two segments are occupied by the eyes, extending from the lateral canthus to the medial canthus. One segment extends from one medial

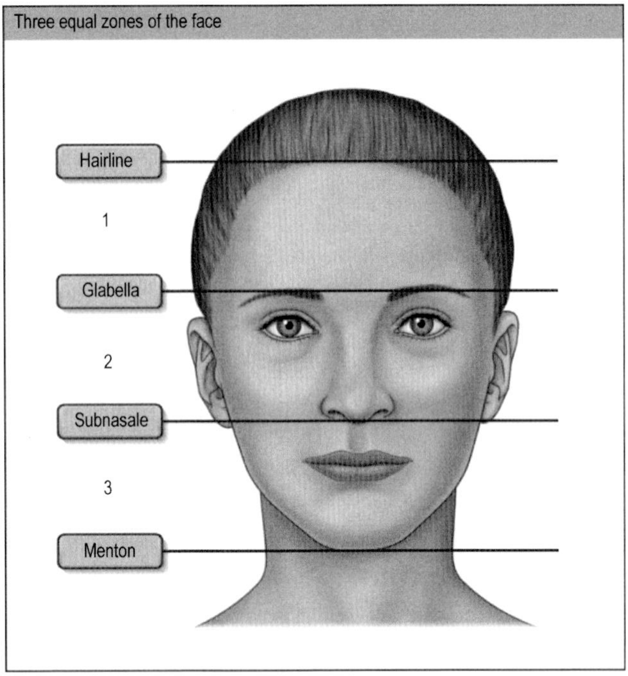

Figure 3.1. Lines passing through eyebrows and subnasale divide the face into three equal zones. Reprinted with permission from Elsevier (Guyuron B. Patient assessment. In: Guyuron B, Eriksson E, Persing JA. *Plastic Surgery: Indications and Practice*. Vol. 2. Philadelphia, PA: WB Saunders; 2009:1343–1351). Copyright © 2009 Elsevier.

canthus to the other and contains the nose, and the last two segments extend from the lateral canthi to the lateral border of the ipsilateral temple. Any asymmetry in these segments should be noted.

A top-down approach allows one to evaluate the entire face in a thorough manner. The forehead is examined for its length and width as well as for any irregularities. Wrinkles in the forehead are best assessed by asking the patient to close his or her eyes tightly and then gently open them.[6] This maneuver allows the forehead to relax. Vertical frown lines can be due to overactive corrugators and procerus muscles.[7] The eyebrows are examined for their symmetry and relationship to adjacent structures. The brows are arched with the peak located at the level of the lateral limbus. Ideally, the lateral ends of the brow are cephalad to the medial ends. The brow is usually 1 cm above the superior orbital rim in women and at the level of the rim in men. A vertical line should connect the medial brow to the ipsilateral alar base, while an oblique line drawn from the lateral canthus to the alar base should extend and connect to the lateral brow.[8]

When analyzing the middle zone of the face, the size and shapes of the eyes are checked (Figure 3.2) as well as their symmetry and position. Any exophthalmos warrants a workup for thyroid abnormalities. The lateral fissure of the eye should be approximately 2° cephalad to the medial fissure of the eye. The intercanthal distance and interpupillary distance are measured to assess the size and position of the eyes. Normal intercanthal distance is 28 to 32 mm, which should be equal to the orbital fissure distance from the medial to the lateral canthus.[9,10] An abnormally short intercanthal distance in conjunction with a suboptimal interpupillary distance is hypotelorism, whereas an increased distance is hypertelorism. The excessive intercanthal distance in the presence of normal interpupillary distance is termed telecanthus.

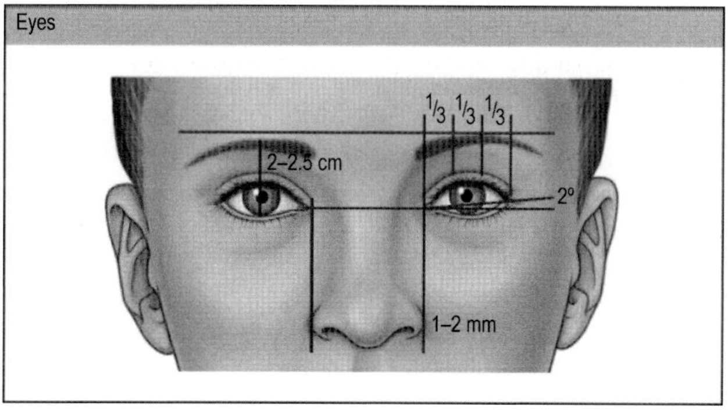

Figure 3.2. Width of the alar base is slightly wider than the intercanthal distance. The distance from eyelid to eyebrow and the position of the eyebrow arch in relation to the iris are shown. Reprinted with permission from Elsevier (Guyuron B. Patient assessment. In: Guyuron B, Eriksson E, Persing JA. *Plastic Surgery: Indications and Practice*. Vol. 2. Philadelphia, PA: WB Saunders; 2009:1343–1351). Copyright © 2009 Elsevier.

When examining the eye, the movement and position of the eyelids are also relevant. The upper eyelids cover 1 to 2 mm of the limbus. Any sclera that is visualized above the iris may indicate upper eyelid retraction or lid lag whereas too much overlapping may signify ptosis. Sclera visible below the iris demonstrates lower lid laxity, lower lid lag, or ectropion if there is also outward rotation of the lower lid margin. The eye has a vertical opening of 10 mm. The supratarsal fold is 3 to 4 mm above the lid margin in an eye that is open and 10 to 11 mm higher when the eyes are closed. Bell's phenomenon can be checked to determine if the patient is at risk of postoperative complications such as corneal dryness and ulceration. The patient is asked to close his or her eyes tightly, and the examiner opens the eyes to see if the globe rolls cephalad. A negative Bell's phenomenon means the globe does not rotate cephalad and the patient is at risk of corneal dryness (Figure 3.3).

Next, the nose is analyzed, and partitioning it into various aesthetic subunits allows better visualization of the abnormalities. The nasal bridge is checked for its width and prominence. Any additions to the radix or nasal bridge can cause the illusion of hypotelorism, whereas any reductions cause the illusion of hypertelorism.[11] The nasal tip is assessed for its prominence and size. The width of the

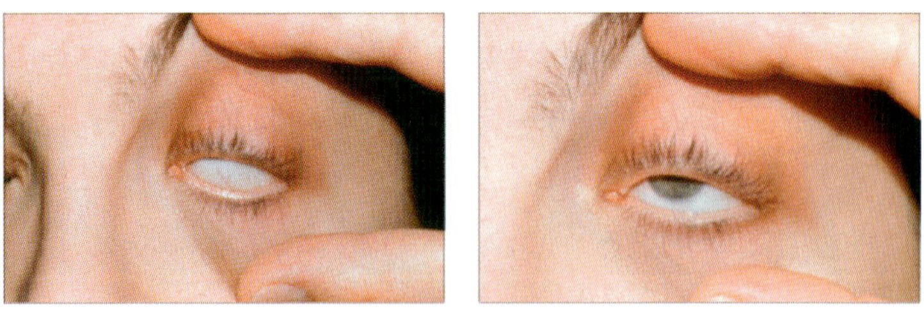

(A) (B)

Figure 3.3. (A) When the eyelids are separated against resistance, the globe rolls upward, demonstrating positive Bell's phenomenon. (B) After the eyelids are separated against resistance, and the globe does not rotate upward, this is negative Bell's phenomenon. Reprinted with permission from Elsevier (Guyuron B. Patient assessment. In: Guyuron B, Eriksson E, Persing JA. *Plastic Surgery: Indications and Practice*. Vol. 2. Philadelphia, PA: WB Saunders; 2009:1343–1351). Copyright © 2009 Elsevier.

lower lateral cartilages and alar domes is also measured. The alar bases and nostrils are reviewed for width and symmetry. The width of the alar base should be equivalent to or 1 to 2 mm greater than the intercanthal distance.[12] Inadequate nostril show can indicate a long nose or caudally positioned ala, while excessive show could indicate opposite conditions.

The ears can be checked for prominence, location, and symmetry from the frontal view. The antihelix is more noticeable than the helix. The helix projects 1 to 1.5 cm from the mastoid soft tissues. The length of the ear should equal the length of the nose, and the lower border of the earlobe should be at the same level as the subnasale. The ear is rotated 30° posteriorly relative to the vertical axis of the body.

The lower zone is examined next, and the lips are considered first for symmetry and shape. The upper lip (about 21 mm) from the subnasale to the stomion is usually one-half of the distance from the stomion to the menton. The distance from the subnasale to the stomion is also one-half of the length of the nose (Figure 3.4). Any length abnormality in the upper lip could be a skeletal abnormality. The direction of the oral commissure should be parallel to the ground and a line connecting the medial and lateral canthi. Any abnormality in direction could also be a skeletal abnormality. The length of the oral fissure is measured from commissure to commissure. Excessive oral commissure width is called *macrostomia*, and deficiency in this width is *microstomia*.

The chin is assessed for symmetry, shape, and position. A line drawn from the middle of the nasal bridge to the philtral dimple and chin should be straight.[13] The submental area is examined for any excess soft tissue or glandular hyperplasia.

The upper lip can be compared with the upper central incisors with the lips slightly open. In a face with normal occlusion and maxillary growth, up to 2 to 3 mm of central incisor show is acceptable. Greater central incisor show suggests vertical maxillary excess, and less show may indicate vertical maxillary deficiency. When the patient smiles fully, there should be minimal or no gum showing. If there is excessive gum showing, that could indicate maxillary excess or soft tissue deficiency.

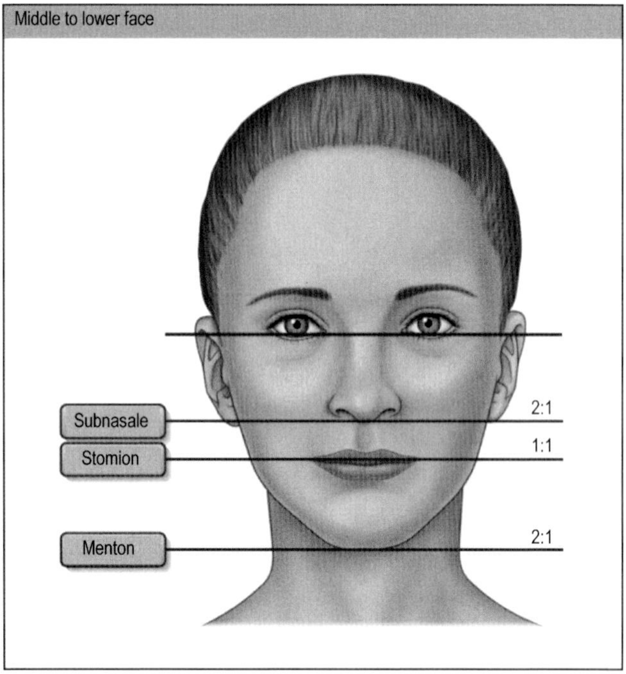

Figure 3.4. Proportions of the middle to lower facial areas. Reprinted with permission from Elsevier (Guyuron B. Patient assessment. In: Guyuron B, Eriksson E, Persing JA. *Plastic Surgery: Indications and Practice*. Vol. 2. Philadelphia, PA: WB Saunders; 2009:1343–1351). Copyright © 2009 Elsevier.

3.5 Profile Analysis

Similar to frontal analysis, the profile of the face is divided into three divisions of equal height: the upper, middle, and lower. The length of the forehead and any prominence is noted first. Next the supraorbital ridges and lateral orbital rims are compared with the position of the cornea. The supraorbital ridges project 8 to 10 mm anterior to the cornea, and the lateral orbital rims are 12 to 16 mm posterior.[14] The nasofrontal angle (the angle between forehead and nose) is usually 130° in men and 134° in women (Figure 3.5).[14] The forehead of the female is less inclined than that of the male. Masculine faces tend to have prominence of the supraorbital rim and glabella. Excessive frontal sinus pneumatization can cause a prominent glabella, which is also

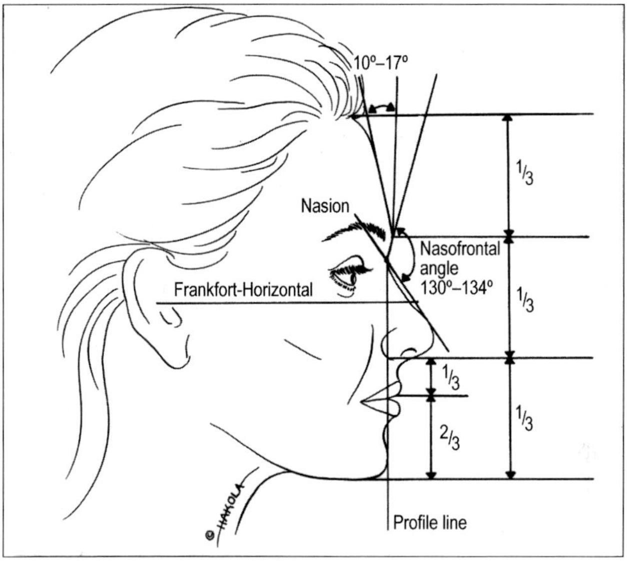

Figure 3.5. Profile of face showing anatomic relationships.[4]

known as *frontal bossing*.[6] The Frankfort-Horizontal is a line drawn from the upper margin of the opening of the external auditory canal to the low point on the lower margin of the orbit, used as a reference.

At this point, the dorsum of the nose is analyzed for any bony deformity. The nasal bridge is usually projected in a 34° angle for females and 36° for males in relation to the vertical facial plane. The nasion, or deepest part of the dorsum, should be located at the level of the upper lid margin and is 4 to 6 mm deep to the glabella. The nasolabial angle is approximately 100° for males and 105° to 108° for females. The columella is 4 mm caudal to the alar rim, and the alar base is 2 mm cephalad to the subnasale.[15] The appearance of the nasal spine should be compared with the location of the maxilla to determine if aesthetic abnormalities of the nasal spine are in fact due to maxillary abnormalities.

The profile of the lower division includes analysis of the length of the lips and their relationship to the chin. Reidel's plane, which is an imaginary line connecting the upper lip, lower lip, and chin, can assist

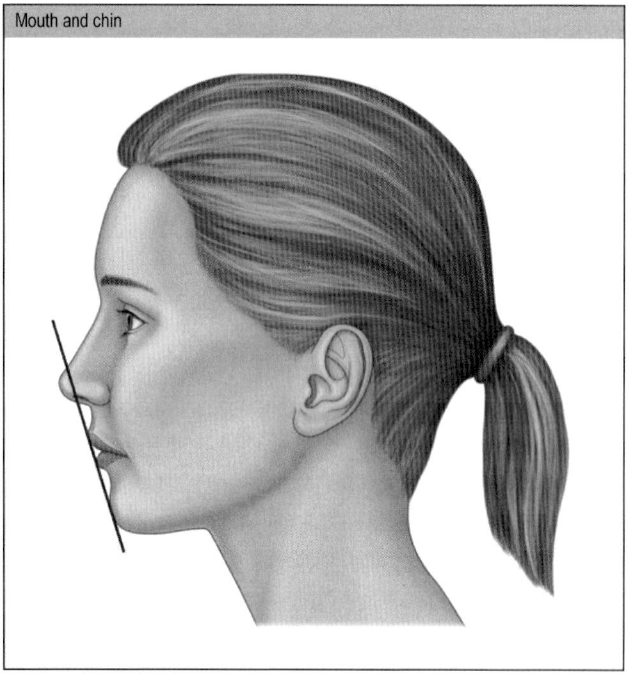

Figure 3.6. Reidel's plane of lip and chin line-up is a straight line connecting the most prominent portion of the upper lip to the lower lip. In pleasing profiles, the line usually contacts the most prominent portion of soft tissue chin. Reprinted with permission from Elsevier (Guyuron B. Patient assessment. In: Guyuron B, Eriksson E, Persing JA. *Plastic Surgery: Indications and Practice.* Vol. 2. Philadelphia, PA: WB Saunders; 2009:1343–1351). Copyright © 2009 Elsevier.

with analysis of this region for any abnormalities (Figure 3.6).[16] The upper lip is either anterior to or at the level of the lower lip. An upper lip that is posterior to the lower lip may signify maxillary deficiency or mandibular protrusion. Sometimes, a soft tissue deficiency can also produce this relationship. Significant deficiency of the lower lip may signify retrognathia, especially if the labiomental groove is deficient. The labiomental groove is 4 mm deep in females and 6 mm deep in males. Patients with a deep labiomental groove and retrognathia may need mandibular advancement as opposed to genioplasty. Akin to the frontal analysis, the submental area is assessed for soft tissue or glandular excess. Lip competence should also be observed. Any incompetence may be due to open bite, maxillary excess, or mandibular deficiency.

3.6 Photographic Analysis

An important part of the preoperative assessment is photographing the patient from a frontal, lateral, and oblique view. A digital camera or 35-mm single-lens reflex camera (with a 60- to 100-mm lens) along with dual lighting is recommended. A blue or black background should be used, and the patient should remove any jewelry, glasses, or makeup. The head should be in standard anatomic position and the patient should have a relaxed look. The photograph is taken from the top of the hair to the sternal notch, and a 1:1 reproduction ratio photo should be created.[17] Proper occlusal views should also be part of the planning and the patient's medical record.

3.7 Radiologic Examination

Lateral and anterior/posterior cephalogram and panoramic radiographs are ordered to screen for abnormalities. Traces of the cephalogram allow the surgeon to evaluate the bony and soft tissue anatomy, which help objectively determine the cephalometric relationships. A more detailed description of cephalometric analysis and imaging can be found in other portions of this book. Panoramic radiographs demonstrate pathology associated with the TMJs in addition to the dental anatomy.

3.8 Summary

Formulating an operative plan to reconstruct oral and maxillofacial defects requires a careful history and physical examination that includes a detailed facial analysis. The facial analysis provides the data needed to determine the optimal surgical management for any maxillofacial deformity.

References

1. **McCarthy JG, Coccaro PJ, Schwartz MD.** Velopharyngeal function following maxillary advancement. *Plast Reconstr Surg* 1979;64:180–189.
2. **Guyuron B, Zarandy S, Tirgan A.** Von Willebrand's disease and plastic surgery. *Ann Plast Surg* 1994;32:351–355.
3. **Totonchi A, Eshraghi Y, Beck D, McCrae K, Guyuron B.** von Willebrand disease: screening, diagnosis, and management. *Aesthet Surg J* 2008;28:189–194.
4. **Guyuron B, Cohen S.** Facial evaluation for orthognathic surgery. In: James Ferraro, ed. *Fundamentals of Maxillofacial Surgery.* New York, NY: Springer; 1997.
5. **Zide B.** The temporomandibular joint. In: McCarthy JG, ed. *Plastic Surgery.* Philadelphia, PA: WB Saunders; 1990:1475–1513.
6. **Guyuron B.** Patient assessment. In: *Plastic Surgery: Indications and Practice.* Philadelphia, PA: WB Saunders; 2008.
7. **Guyuron B.** Corrugator supercilii resection through blepharoplasty incision. *Plast Reconstr Surg* 2001;107:604–607.
8. **Ellenbogen R.** Transcoronal eyebrow lift with concomitant upper blepharoplasty. *Plast Reconstr Surg* 1983;71:490–499.
9. **Profitt WR, Epker BN, Ackerman JL.** Systematic description of dentofacial deformities: the database. In: Bell WH, Proffitt WR, White RP, eds. *Surgical Correction of Dentofacial Deformities.* Philadelphia, PA: WB Saunders; 1980.
10. **Whitaker LA.** Selective alteration of palpebral fissure form by lateral canthopexy. *Plast Reconstr Surg* 1984;74:611–619.
11. **Guyuron B.** Dynamics of rhinoplasty. *Plast Reconstr Surg* 1991;88:970–979.
12. **Farkas LG, Hreczko TA, Kolar JC, Munro IR.** Vertical and horizontal proportions of the face in young adult North American Caucasians: revision of neoclassical canons. *Plast Reconstr Surg* 1985;75:328–338.
13. **Gonzalez Ulloa M.** A quantum method for the appreciation of the morphology of the face. *Plast Reconstr Surg* 1964;34:241–246.
14. **Whitaker LA, Morales L Jr., Farkas LG.** Aesthetic surgery of the supraorbital ridge and forehead structures. *Plast Reconstr Surg* 1986;78:23–32.
15. **Powell N, Humphreys B.** *Proportions of the Aesthetic Face.* New York, NY: Thieme-Stratton; 1984.
16. **Reidel RA.** Analysis of dentofacial relationships. *Am J Orthod Dentofacial Orthop* 1957;43:103–119.
17. **Rohrich R, Muzaffar A.** Primary rhinoplasty. In: *Plastic Surgery: Indications, Operations, and Outcomes.* St. Louis, MO: Mosby; 2000.

FIXATION OF THE CRANIOFACIAL SKELETON 4

Gaby Doumit, MD, MSc and
Michael J. Yaremchuk, MD, FACS

4.1 Background

The need to immobilize fractured facial bones in anatomic apposition to effect healing has long been known. Hippocrates described[1] the closed reduction and external stabilization of mandibular fractures with the use of "bridal wire — a wire wrapped around two teeth on either side of the fracture." Open techniques of fracture reduction and immobilization were introduced in the 19th century. Gurdon Buck, in 1847, used interfragmentary wires to treat a fractured mandible.[2] Max Schede, in 1888, first described the use of steel plates and screws to treat mandible fractures.[3] It was not until corrosion-resistant materials were developed, such as stainless steel and the alloy Vitallium, that internal fixation for the facial skeleton became more common.[4]

Wire osteosynthesis has largely been replaced by more rigid fixation constructs that use miniaturized plates and screws. Plate-and-screw fixation allows skeletal positioning in three dimensions, often with sufficient stability to eliminate or reduce the need for jaw immobilization when occlusal bearing-bone segments are involved. This "rigid internal fixation" has become the gold standard for stabilization of the facial skeleton.[5]

4.2 Bone Healing

Healing of bone fractured by trauma or osteotomy requires stable apposition of the fracture surfaces. Gross movement or significant gaps between fractured bone segments lead to nonunion and fibrocartilaginous tissue formation. Bone heals by the following two mechanisms, which depend on the degree of bone-end apposition and movement.

4.2.1 *Primary bone healing*

When fracture segments are closely apposed (usually compressed) and sufficiently immobilized to eliminate any motion, the bone healing process is termed *primary*. Primary bone healing is characterized by the direct formation of bone. Under these conditions, the union of bone segments occurs without a preceding intermediary tissue type (i.e., a callus).

4.2.2 *Secondary bone healing*

A hematoma develops between the two bone segments after a fracture. The hematoma is then sequentially replaced by fibrous tissue, cartilage (in endochondral but not membranous bone), woven bone, and lamellar bone. As the tissues in the callus mature, stiffness is increased and strain is reduced across the bone segments. This process decreases motion at the fracture site. The result allows for bone formation and subsequent bone healing. This process is called *secondary* bone healing. It is the usual process occurring after facial skeletal rearrangement or repair, either because it is necessary to maintain small gaps between bone segments to create or maintain certain 3-dimensional relationships or because the scale of the fixation device required to eliminate any micromotion would be prohibitive.

4.3 Skeletal Reduction and Immobilization

Similar to long-bone fractures, facial bone fractures are treated by one of the two basic methods: closed reduction and external stabilization (or splinting), or open reduction and internal fixation.

4.3.1 *Closed reduction and external stabilization*

The three surgical procedures commonly used by craniofacial surgeons for closed reduction and external stabilization are maxillomandibular fixation (MMF), suspension wires plus MMF, and external fixators. Section 4.3.1.1 will discuss those procedures in detail.

4.3.1.1 *Maxillomandibular fixation*

MMF can be an effective way to reduce and immobilize certain simple fractures of the mandible. MMF requires an external device (Erich arch bars) to be applied to the upper and lower dental arches by wiring them to the teeth. Application of the arch bar to the lower teeth helps reduce tooth-bearing fracture segments. Occluding the fractured lower dental arch to the intact upper dental arch refines fracture reduction. Wiring the upper arch bar to the lower arch bar helps immobilize the fracture. Hence, MMF can be both a closed means of fracture reduction and a means of immobilization. By restoring occlusion, MMF is also used in more complex mandible fractures, or midface fractures, as a guide to accurate reduction (Figure 4.1).

MMF screws may be a time-saving alternative to Erich arch bars. MMF screws are self-drilling titanium screws designed to hold wires. They are inserted into the upper and lower dental arches. They may be used to maintain dental occlusion as a guide to midface fracture alignment when the upper and lower dental arches are intact (Figure 4.2).

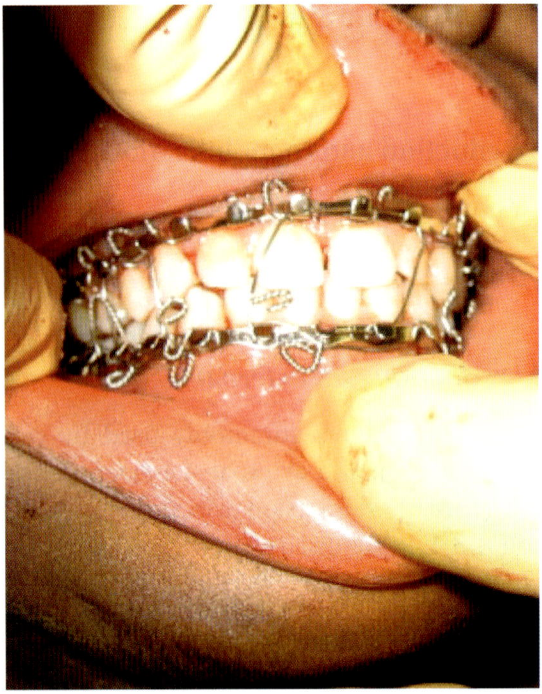

Figure 4.1. MMF with Erich arch bars.

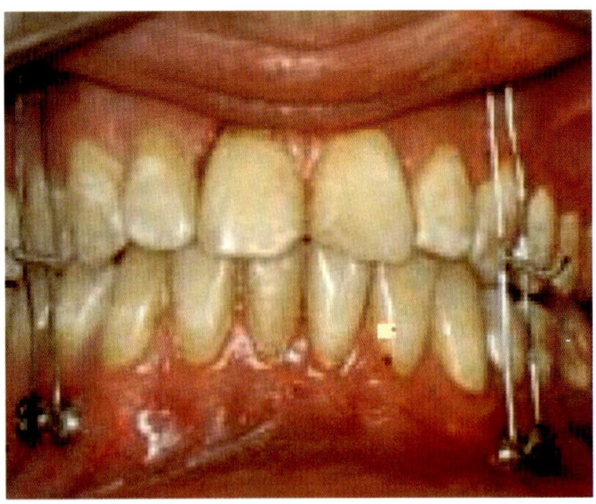

Figure 4.2. Maxillomandibular screws used for MMF.

4.3.1.2 *Suspension wires and MMF*

MMF can restore proper occlusal relationships between the upper and lower tooth-bearing segments, but it does not ensure the proper positioning of the teeth in relation to the rest of the facial skeleton.

Until the 1980s, midface fractures were reduced by restoring the occlusion with MMF and immobilizing the fracture using suspension wires. Wires were dropped down from the orbit, zygoma, or stable bone structures adjacent to or associated with the cranial base to suspend the occluded tooth-bearing segment. In certain cases, head frames were used to create a stable base for the suspension wires. Unfortunately, suspensory wires create only a vertical vector, which precludes control of sagittal positioning of the occluded segment — a major limitation. Suspension-wire tightening forces the midface toward the base of the cranium, resulting in a vertical foreshortening and retrusion of the midface (Figure 4.3).[6]

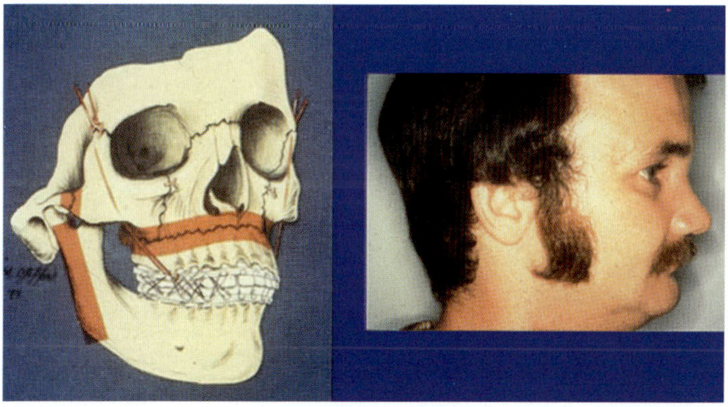

Figure 4.3. An example of subcondylar and Le Fort fractures treated with suspensory wires (left) and MMF causing vertical foreshortening and retrusion of the face (right). Reprinted with permission from Lippincott Williams & Wilkins (Manson PN, *et al.* Midface fractures: advantages of immediate extended open reduction and bone grafting. *Plast Reconstr Surg* 1985;76:1–10).

4.3.1.3 *External fixators*

External fixation is a method by which the bone segments are held in place by percutaneous wires attached to an external frame (Figure 4.4). In the past, it was frequently used to treat complex Le Fort fractures in an attempt to obtain 3-dimensional fracture positioning. Today, it is most often used in patients who have severe soft tissue injury, contamination, severe infection, or comminuted fractures of the mandible, often with bone loss. In addition, external fixators are practical for treating fractures in patients who are medically too unstable for major surgical procedures. They are usually used to provide temporary fixation and are replaced with internal fixation when the soft tissue envelope is repaired, infection is controlled, or the patient is medically stable. In some situations, external fixators are left in place until the fracture heals.

4.3.2 *Open reduction and internal fixation*

Open reduction and internal fixation techniques involve direct exposure of bone segments, their realignment, and immobilization.

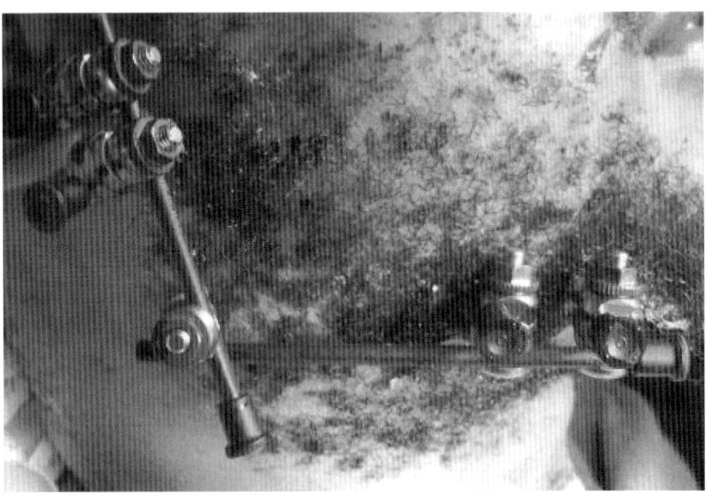

Figure 4.4. Clinical example of external fixator used to treat a severely comminuted mandibular fracture.

Surgical approaches have been borrowed from aesthetic and craniofacial surgery. They include the use of bicoronal, intraoral, and periorbital incisions. All fractures are exposed by surgical dissection in a subperiosteal plane.

4.3.2.1 *Interfragmentary wiring*

After fracture exposure and reduction, bone immobilization can be obtained by passing wire (usually 28 or 30 gauge) through drill holes placed on either side of the fracture. The ends of the wire are twisted to one another until a stable construct is obtained. Interfragmentary wiring can provide effective immobilization for simple fractures. However, the uniplanar nature of interfragmentary wiring limits its efficacy when immobilization needs become more complex. Interfragmentary wiring becomes less effective in restoring anatomy as the number of fracture segments or the 3-dimensionality of the construct to be restored increases, or both. The limitation of interfragmentary wiring is demonstrated in Figure 4.5.

With the advent of plate-and-screw fixation techniques that allow stable 3-dimensional reconstruction, interfragmentary wiring is most often used now for simple fractures or to help in temporary alignment of fractured segments before rigid fixation.

4.3.2.2 *Plate-and-screw fixation*

The use of miniaturized plates and screws, commonly referred to as *rigid fixation*, has revolutionized surgery of the craniofacial skeleton. The rigidity provided by these devices limits or eliminates motion between fracture segments, hence optimizing conditions for bone healing. The ability to bend plates in desired shapes allows precise, 3-dimensional bone positioning and therefore reconstruction (Figure 4.5).

For bones to heal in the desired position, the fixation devices must be strong enough to neutralize the force exerted by gravity, soft tissue deforming forces, or the muscles of mastication occurring at the

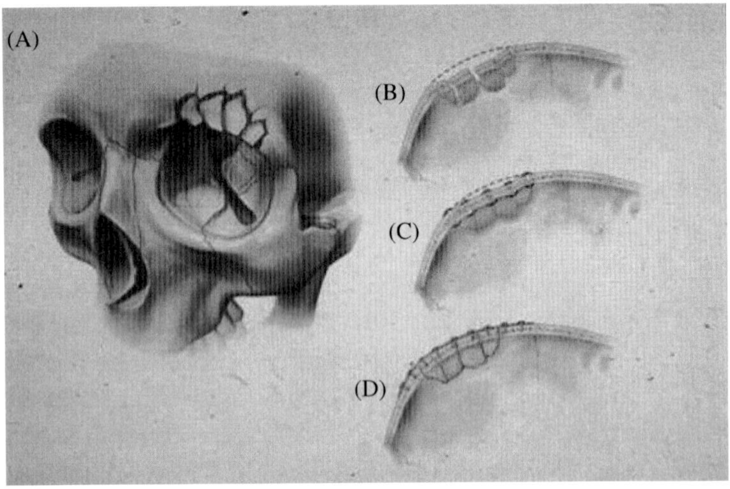

Figure 4.5. The difference in 3-dimensional result between wire and plate-and-screw fixation. (A) Comminuted supraorbital rim fracture. (B) Axial view shows loss of curvature. (C) Interfragmentary wiring collapses arch. The collapse is exaggerated by the inevitable bone loss occurring at the fracture sites. With increasing comminution, interfragmentary stabilization results in a uniplanar construct. (D) Plate-and-screw fixation allows restoration of preinjury curvature. The plate is bent to the desired shape, and the fracture segments are attached to it with screws.

fracture site. Since these distracting forces vary in different areas of the craniofacial skeleton, the design and scale of plates and screws vary accordingly. In general, larger, more rigid systems are used to counteract the muscles of mastication, and systems of lesser scale are used to counteract soft tissue deforming forces.

Plate-and-screw fixation techniques can provide desired skeletal configurations only if these devices are adapted to properly positioned bone segments. It is crucial to contour plates properly to the underlying bone since bone fragments adapt to the shape of the plate. Improper plate bending will result in bone malalignment (Figure 4.6). A malleable template will help to guide plate bending.

In the treatment of maxillary and mandibular fractures, it is essential to restore pretraumatic dental occlusion with MMF before reduction and fixation of the fractures.

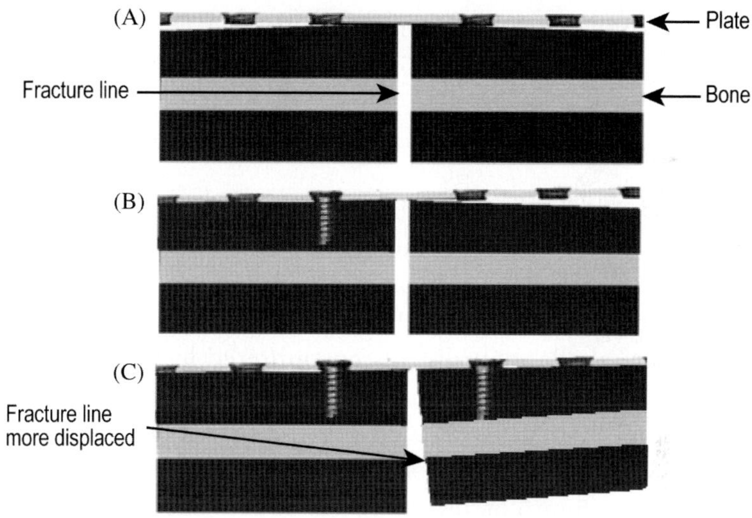

Figure 4.6. (A) The plate is not perfectly contoured to the bone. (B and C) As the screws are tightened, the bone adapts to the shape of the plate and the fracture becomes displaced.

In the treatment of facial fractures, plates should be placed in areas of adequately robust bone (i.e., buttresses).[7] In the face, there are four paired vertical buttresses; from anteromedial to posterolateral, they are the nasomaxillary, zygomaticomaxillary, pterygomaxillary, and mandibular ramus buttresses.[6] The vertical buttresses act as shock absorbers for vertically oriented impacts to the facial skeleton. Likewise, four horizontal buttresses — the frontal, zygomatic, maxillary, and mandibular arches — provide protection against horizontal forces. The mandibular ramus buttress establishes the posterior facial height while the horizontal buttresses allow precise restoration of facial projection and width.[6]

4.4 Implant Materials

The ideal implant material for fracture fixation should be biocompatible, resist corrosion, and be mechanically strong enough to maintain fracture reduction, yet be ductile to allow *in situ* plate-bone surface adaptation.[8] Implants are manufactured from metals and resorbable materials.

4.4.1 *Metals*

Stainless steel, Vitallium, and titanium are used in clinical practice.

Stainless steel typically consists of iron (62.5%), chromium (17.6%), nickel (14.5%), molybdenum (2.8%), and other components in minor amounts (2.8%).[8] Its nickel component accounts for 92% of the metal allergy problems encountered in humans. It does not create torque, displacement, or heating during magnetic resonance imaging. Stainless steel is strong and extremely rigid, making it difficult to adapt it to a bone surface; hence, it causes surface damage and resultant corrosion.[9] It has largely been removed from internal fixation devices in craniomaxillofacial fixation as it creates more radiologic scatter on computed tomography (CT) than does titanium.[10]

Vitallium consists of cobalt, chromium, and molybdenum. It has twice the tensile strength and hardness of other metals. In general, plates made from Vitallium have lower profiles than those from stainless steel or titanium. Vitallium usage has decreased because of difficulty adapting the plates to the bone surface of the craniofacial skeleton as a result of its rigidity and, more importantly, because of its higher radiologic scatter property.[5]

Commercially pure titanium consists of oxygen and titanium. Titanium has a high corrosion resistance. It produces no or minimal physiologic insult and it is inert *in vivo*. Commercially pure titanium has good strength, but it is less rigid than stainless steel and thus more easily adaptable to the bone surface than Vitallium or stainless steel. It has largely replaced stainless steel and Vitallium because of its lack of radiologic scatter.

4.4.2 *Resorbable materials*

Plating systems made of resorbable materials were developed to avoid the risk of growth restriction, i.e., transcranial and intracranial migration associated with the metal plates used in pediatric cranial vault reconstruction. Goldberg *et al.* reported a 14% incidence of transcranial migration and 7% incidence of intracranial plate migration with the use of metallic miniplates in infants.[11]

The resorbable plating systems most commonly used are composed of copolymers of high molecular alpha hydroxy acids, polyglycolic acid, and poly-L-lactic acid. In general, resorbable systems retain rigidity for 2 to 3 months and are resorbed completely in 1 to 2 years. Different manufacturers produce different products (Table 4.1).[5]

Table 4.1. Resorbable Rigid Fixation Systems for the Craniofacial Skeleton.

	Synthes Rapid (West Chester, PA)	**Stryker Inion CPS (Portage, MI)**	**Biomet lactoSorb SE (Jacksonville, FL)**	**KLS Martin Resorb (Jacksonville, FL)**
Composition	85:15 PLLA: Co-glycolide	PGA, PLLA, PDLLA, trimethylene carbonate	82:18 PLLA:PGA	PDLLA
Strength retention	8 weeks (85% strength)	Baby: 6–9 weeks Adult: 9–14 weeks	8 weeks (70% strength)	10 weeks
Resorption	1 year	Baby: 1–2 years Adult: 2–3 years	1 year	1–2 years
Set sizes	1.5, 2.0 mm	Baby: 1.5 mm Adult: 1.5, 2.0, 2.5 mm	1.5, 2.0 mm	1.6, 2.1 mm
Treatment of mandibular fracture	No	Yes, with IMF use	No	No

IMF = intermaxillary fixation; PDLLA = poly-D-L-lactic acid; PGA = polyglycolic acid; PLLA = poly-L-lactic acid.

The indications for resorbable plate usage in the fixation of the craniofacial skeleton have been expanded to include repair of mandibular fractures in the pediatric population and midface fractures in all age groups.[12–14]

The advantages of resorbable plates include ease of bone surface adaptation, absence of radiologic scatter, avoidance of subsequent surgery for plate removal, and reduced risk of stress shielding of the underlying bone. In general, resorbable implants have been well tolerated *in vivo*.

4.5 Plates

4.5.1 *Plate design and load*

Plate design and scale can be categorized by how they respond to mechanical forces.

Load-sharing plates share the load with the bone. They are not strong enough alone to support the applied forces across the fracture site. All cranial, midface, orthognathic, and most mandible plates are load-sharing plates. Over time, with healing, the implant is unloaded.

Load-bearing plates are used in the mandible. They are larger and thicker than load-sharing plates, and are used most often to treat severely comminuted mandible fractures or to immobilize the mandible with segmental bone defects.

Plates are characterized by their width, length, height, and profile. A plate's width and length are defined as the measures of its widest part and entire length, respectively. The height measures the plate's thickness. The profile measures the plate's thickness and the height of the screw above plate level.

Various plate configurations are available to stabilize specific anatomic areas or fracture configurations: box, star, Y shape, L shape, X shape, H shape, T shape, curved, mesh, straight, angle, and strut configurations are available (Figure 4.7).

Plates can be further categorized by the shape and features of their holes — round, oval, or threaded (Figure 4.8).

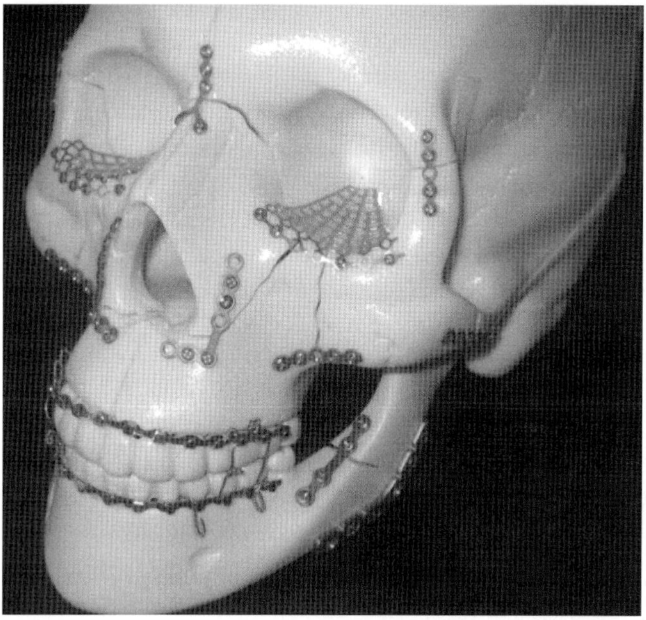

Figure 4.7. Example of different plate configurations that may be used for rigid fixation of the craniofacial skeleton.

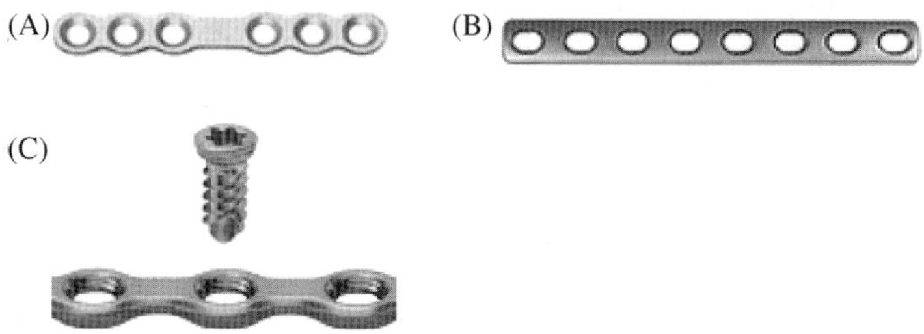

Figure 4.8. (A) Neutral plate (round holes); (B) compression plate (oval holes); (C) locking plate (threaded hole and screws).

(Images courtesy of Synthes Inc, West Chester, PA. 2009 Synthes, Inc).

4.5.2 *Neutral plates*

Most plates used to fixate the craniofacial skeleton are plates with round holes. They are referred to as neutral plates. Screws placed through the round holes immobilize the bone and protect the fracture site from rotation and bending.

4.5.3 *Compression plates*

Compression plates have unique oval holes with inclined edges. When screws are inserted eccentrically, the tapered, oval shape of the hole forces the screw head toward the center and compresses the fracture site (Figure 4.9). Compression plates are used for

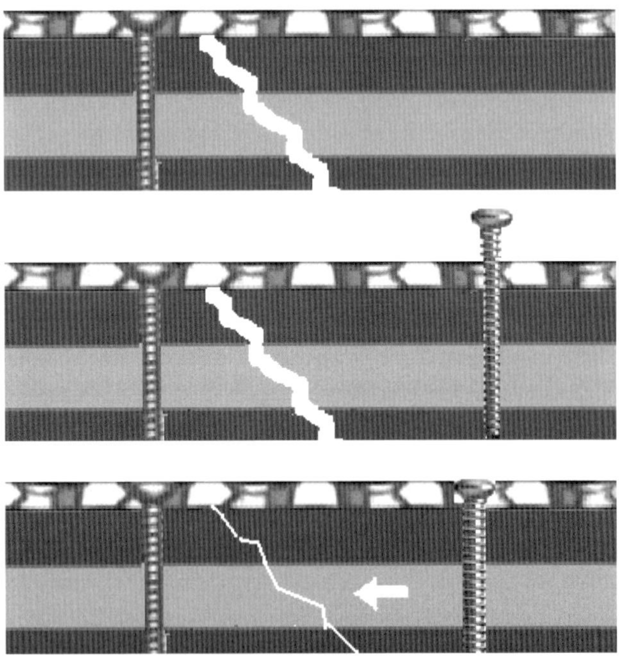

Figure 4.9. Compression plates. As the screws are inserted eccentrically, the oval shape of the hole forces the screw toward the center. This results in movement of the bone segment relative to the plate and leads to compression of the fracture segments.

simple mandible fractures that are stable when compressed and when fracture compression does not alter occlusion, both uncommon situations.

4.5.4 *Locking plates*

Locking plates have threaded holes to accept locking screws. Locking reconstruction plates and screws function as internal fixators; stability is attained by locking the screw to the plate. Loading forces are transmitted directly from the bone to the screws, then onto the plate, across the fracture, and again through the screws into the bone. The locking plate may ride slightly off the bone surface without jeopardizing rigid stability. Friction between plate and bone is not necessary for stability. This slight bony separation is actually advantageous. It allows blood to reach the bone beneath the plate. Locking reconstruction screws are also less likely to extrude.

4.6 Screws

Screws attach bone fragments to plates. They are characterized by their head configuration, drive mechanism, body, tip, length, outer diameter, thread, inner diameter, pitch, and flute (a design at the tip of the screw) (Table 4.2). A screw is named by the dimensions of its outer diameter.

A screw can be thread-forming, self-tapping, or self-drilling (Figure 4.10). Thread-forming screws, such as resorbable screws, have blunt tips. The surgeon must pre-drill and tap the hole prior to inserting the screw. Self-tapping screws possess two or three cutting flutes at their tip. They are inserted without tapping. Most screws used in craniomaxillofacial surgery are self-tapping and are in the range of 1.0 to 2.4 mm. Pretapping is recommended for screws 2.7 mm or longer.[15] Self-drilling screws have one or two cutting flutes for insertion without pre-drilling or tapping. IMF screws are examples of self-drilling, self-tapping screws with grooves under the heads to secure wires or elastics.

Table 4.2. Screw Characteristics.

Part of screw	Description	Image
Head	Contains the drive mechanism	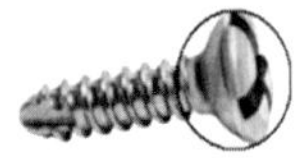
Drive mechanism	Design on the head that allows a driver to engage the screw and transfer torque	
Body	Located between the head and tip	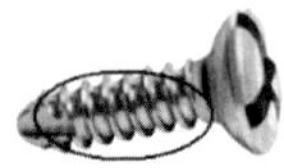
Tip	Parts of the screw that first pierce the bone	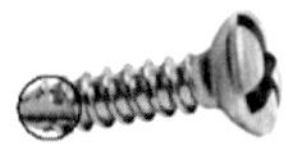
Length	Distance from head to tip	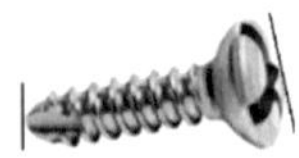
Thread	Projecting helical ridge that engages the bone	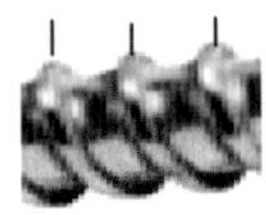
Pitch	Distance between adjacent screw threads	
Core diameter	Diameter at the base of the screw threads	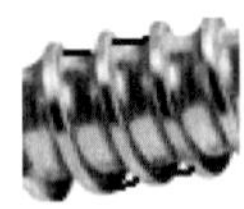
Outer diameter	Largest diameter of the threaded portion of the screw, giving the screw its name	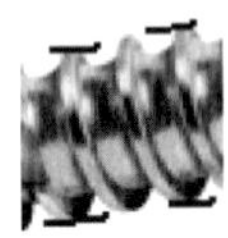
Flute	A design at the tip of the screw, allowing the threads to cut into bone	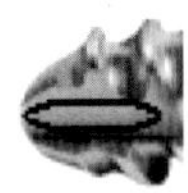

(Images courtesy of Synthes, Inc., West Chester, PA. 2009 Synthes, Inc.)

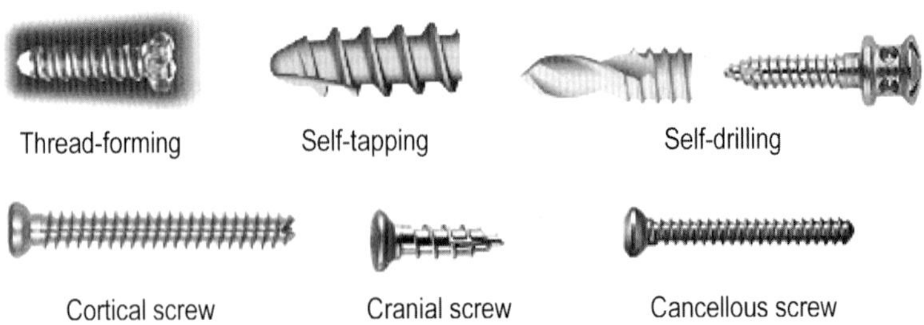

Figure 4.10. Screw types.

(Images courtesy of Synthes, Inc., West Chester, PA. 2009 Synthes, Inc.)

4.6.1 *Lag screw fixation*

A lag screw does not have a unique design characteristic. Lag screw fixation refers to the use of a screw to achieve interfragmental compression across a fracture site (Figure 4.11). Lag screws are placed perpendicular to the fracture site. The cortex adjacent to the screw head is overdrilled to the dimension of the outer diameter of the screw so that the threads do not gain purchase. The distal cortex is drilled to the core diameter. The screw passes freely through the proximal cortex up to the fracture line. The threads of the screw gain purchase only distal to the fracture line and mainly in the distal cortex. When the screw is tightened, the head pulls against the proximal cortex and the threads against the distal fragment, compressing the fracture line.

A second lag screw or a plate must be placed across the fracture site to neutralize rotational forces.

4.7 Fixation of Mandible Fractures

Mandibular fractures are treated with both rigid (load-bearing) and functionally stable (load-sharing) fixation (Table 4.3).[16]

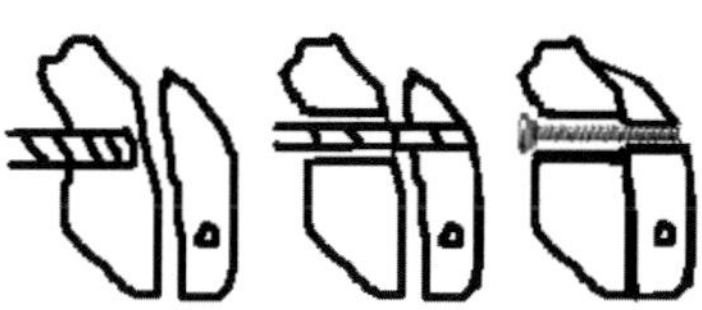

(A)

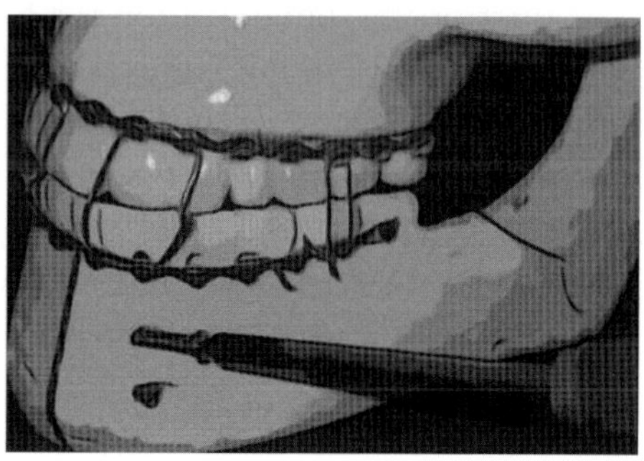

(B)

Figure 4.11. (A) Lag screw technique: proximal cortex is overdrilled to the outer diameter of the screw. The distal cortex is drilled to the core diameter of the screw. The threads of the screw gain purchase only distal to the fracture line, and they compress the fracture. (B) A second lag screw is being inserted perpendicular to the symphyseal fracture.

Table 4.3. Type of Fixation for Mandible Fractures.

Rigid fixation	Functionally stable fixation
One 2.4-mm compression plate (three screws on each side of the fracture)	One 2.4-mm compression plate (two screws on each side of the fracture)
Use of two plates over fracture site	One 2.0-mm miniplate + arch bar
Two lag screws across fracture	One lag screw + arch bar
Reconstruction plate (three screws on each side of the fracture)	One 2.0-mm miniplate without arch bar for angle fracture
One plate and one lag screw across fracture site	

Rigid fixation is defined as any form of internal fixation that eliminates interfragmentary micromotion at the fracture site under normal function. This form of fixation uses devices that are strong and large enough to withstand the full functional load with none of the load being borne across the fracture site. Its use is usually associated with primary healing unless the fracture segments are not in intimate, anatomic contact. A reconstruction plate with three screws on each side of a mandibular angle fracture is an example of rigid fixation.

Functionally stable fixation is a form of internal fixation that is not absolutely rigid. Functionally stable fixation uses stabilization implants that are small and of insufficient rigidity to endure the normal functional load applied across the fracture site. Instead, it relies on static or dynamic axial compression at the fracture site to increase interfragmentary friction, and it thus places a significant portion of the functional load needed for fracture immobilization on the bone rather than on the implant. Compression produced by a fixation device alone is static compression. Dynamic compression occurs when fixation devices are applied in such a way as to allow the muscle forces or weight of the body to produce additional compression. Load-sharing fixation is considered rigid when axial static compression is used, and it is considered nonrigid when dynamic, axial compression is used. Dynamic and rigid compression cannot be applied to all fractures. Fractures with bone loss and comminuted fractures cause the bone to become unstable in compression.

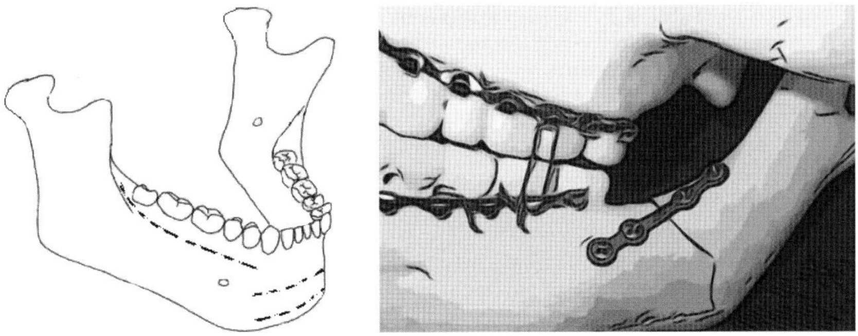

(A) (B)

Figure 4.12. (A) Champy's ideal line of osteosynthesis. (B) The proper position of a 2.0-mm miniplate for fixation of a mandible angle fracture.

Table 4.4. Factors Leading to Rigid Fixation of Mandibular Fracture.

Patient factors	Fracture factors
Atrophic mandible	Severely displaced fractures
Established infection	Multiple mandible fractures
Edentulous mandible	Comminuted fractures
History of radiation to the mandible	Fracture pattern

The Champy technique is an example of a functionally stable fixation that relies on dynamic compression. It uses a miniplate placed along the line of osteosynthesis — tension, compression, and torsion (Figure 4.12A). For example, for a simple fracture of the angle of the mandible, it uses a single 2.0-mm miniplate placed along the line of osteosynthesis (Figure 4.12B). Healing occurs by the formation of callus, which is secondary bone healing.

Patients and fracture factors dictate the surgeon's choice of internal fixation. In general, uncomplicated mandible fractures heal uneventfully with functionally stable constructs, relying on smaller plates and screws. MMF is most often unnecessary in the postoperative period. In contrast, complicated and infected mandible fractures will lead the surgeon to choose a more rigid fixation method (Table 4.4). Edentulous or

Table 4.5. Complications of Miniplating Systems.[17]

Complications	Incidence (%)
Infection	0–12
Pain	1.4–5.5
Implant palpability	1.6–3.3
Exposure	1.8–2.7
Osteomyelitis	2.2

noncompliant patients require rigid fixation. MMF is strongly encouraged in noncompliant patients.

4.8 Complications

Campbell and Lin reviewed the literature regarding complications associated with rigid internal fixation of the craniofacial skeleton.[17] They reported the range of complication rates associated with the use of miniplating systems (Table 4.5).

Overall, the incidence of plate removal after miniplate use varies from 3% to 18%.[17] Patients with multiple fractures require plate removal more frequently (14%) than patients with isolated fractures (6.5%).[18]

Campbell and Lin also reviewed the literature on complications of resorbable plates. Palpability of plates (4–9%), self-limited local inflammatory reactions (1–14%), infections (0–2%), and trauma-induced plate breaking (0–4%) were the most commonly reported.[17]

4.9 Summary

Fixation of the craniofacial skeleton has evolved significantly over the last 2 decades. In general, internal fixation with plates and screws is used to stabilize almost all osteotomies and fracture sites. In contrast, external fixators are reserved mainly for infected or severely comminuted fractures. In the present era, the material of choice for plates and screws in adults is titanium. In the pediatric population, resorbable plating systems have become more popular.

Lastly, the smallest fixation device that provides the necessary stabilization of bone segments should be used to stabilize fractures or osteotomies sites.

References

1. **Coletti D, Caccamese J. Jr.** Diagnosis and managment of mandible fractures. In: Fonseca RJ, Marciani RD, Turvey TA, eds. *Oral and Maxillofacial Surgery.* St. Louis, MO: Elsevier; 2009.
2. **Mukerji R, Mukerji G, McGurk M.** Mandibular fractures: historical perspective. *Br J Oral Maxillofac Surg* 2006;44:222–228.
3. **Dorrance GM, Bransfield JW, Mann JB, Ivy RH.** *The History of Treatment of Fractured Jaws.* Philadelphia, PA: Privately published; 1941.
4. **Bigelow H.** Vitallium bone screws and appliances for treatment of fracture of mandible. *J Oral Surg* 1943;1:131.
5. **Gilardino MS, Chen E, Bartlett SP.** Choice of internal rigid fixation materials in the treatment of facial features. *Craniomaxillofac Trauma Reconstr* 2009;2:49–60.
6. **Gruss JS, Phillips JH.** Complex facial trauma: the evolving role of rigid fixation and immediate bone graft reconstruction. *Clin Plast Surg* 1989;16:93–104.
7. **Manson PN, Hoopes JE, Su CT.** Structural pillars of the facial skeleton: an approach to the management of Le Fort fractures. *Plast Reconstr Surg* 1980;66:54–61.
8. **Prein J, Rahn B.** Scientific and technical backgrouund. In: Prein J, ed. *Manual of Internal Fixation in the Cranio-Facial Skeleton.* Berlin: Springer; 1998:Chapter 1.
9. **Steinemann S.** Metal for craniomaxillofacial internal fixation implants and its physiologic implications. In: Greenberg A, Prein J, eds. *Craniomaxillofacial Reconstructive and Corrective Bone Surgery.* New York, NY: Springer; 2006:107–112.
10. **Fiala TG, Novelline RA, Yaremchuk MJ.** Comparison of CT imaging artifacts from craniomaxillofacial internal fixation devices. *Plast Reconstr Surg* 1993;92:1227–1232.
11. **Goldberg DS, Bartlett S, Yu JC, Hunter JV, Whitaker LA.** Critical review of microfixation in pediatric craniofacial surgery. *J Craniofac Surg* 1995;6:301–308.
12. **Eppley BL.** Use of resorbable plates and screws in pediatric facial fractures. *J Oral Maxillofac Surg* 2005;63:385–391.
13. **Bell RB, Kindsfater CS.** The use of biodegradable plates and screws to stabilize facial fractures. *J Oral Maxillofac Surg* 2006;64:31–39.

14. **Laughlin RM, Block MS, Wilk R, Malloy RB, Kent JNJ.** Resorbable plates for the fixation of mandibular fractures: a prospective study. *J Oral Maxillofac Surg* 2007;65:89–96.
15. **Greenberg AM, Prein J.** *Craniomaxillofacial Reconstructive and Corrective Bone Surgery.* New York, NY: Springer; 2006.
16. **Hollier L, Kelly P.** Soft tissue and skeletal injuries of the face. In: Thorne CH, ed. *Grabb & Smith's Plastic Surgery.* 6th edn. Philadelphia, PA: Wolters Kluwer Health/Lippincott Williams & Wilkins; 2007:315–332.
17. **Campbell CA, Lin KY.** Complications of rigid internal fixation. *Craniomaxillofac Trauma Reconstr* 2009;2:41–47.
18. **Francel TJ, Birely BC, Ringelman PR, Manson PN.** The fate of plates and screws after facial fracture reconstruction. *Plast Reconstr Surg* 1992;90:568–573.

ORTHOGNATHIC SURGERY PART I: TERMINOLOGY AND SURGICAL TECHNIQUES 5

Mark Urata, MD, DDS; Jeffrey Hammoudeh, MD, DDS and Michael Lypka, MD, DMD

5.1 Introduction

Orthognathic surgery involves osteotomy, mobilization, and fixation of the maxilla, mandible, and/or chin in an effort to achieve a more anatomic relationship between the upper and lower jaws. The ultimate goal is not only to establish a normal dental relationship, but also, and perhaps more importantly, to achieve an esthetically pleasing facial soft tissue relationship. The diagnosis and treatment planning of all dentofacial deformities is complex and requires thorough knowledge of basic dental occlusion, cephalometric and facial analysis, and orthodontic principles.

5.2 Dental Analysis

Dental anatomy can be confusing initially as it seems to contradict with traditional anatomic terminology, especially with respect to the terms "proximal" and "distal." In dental anatomy, because the teeth are aligned in arches, the dental midline becomes the point of reference. Think of the dental arch stretched into a straight line to better understand the terminology. The back portion of a tooth would be distal (away from the midline), and the anterior portion of a fractured mandible would be termed the "distal segment."

- Dental terminology (Figure 5.1).
  - Mesial: Toward the midline.
  - Distal: Away from the midline.
  - Lingual: On the tongue side.
  - Palatal: On the palatal side.
  - Buccal: On the cheek side.

- Occlusion (how the teeth come together) (Figure 5.2).
  - Overjet: The horizontal overlap of the upper and lower incisors (normally 2 mm).
  - Overbite: The vertical overlap of the upper and lower incisors (normally 3 mm).
  - Openbite: Negative overbite.
  - Crossbite: The buccal surfaces of the maxillary teeth are lingual to the buccal surfaces of the mandibular teeth.

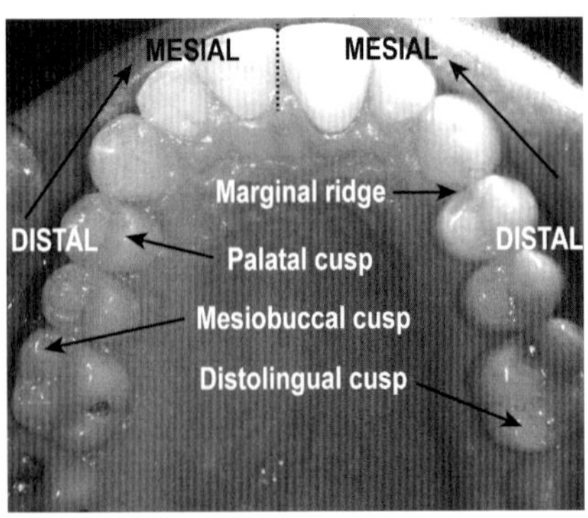

Figure 5.1.

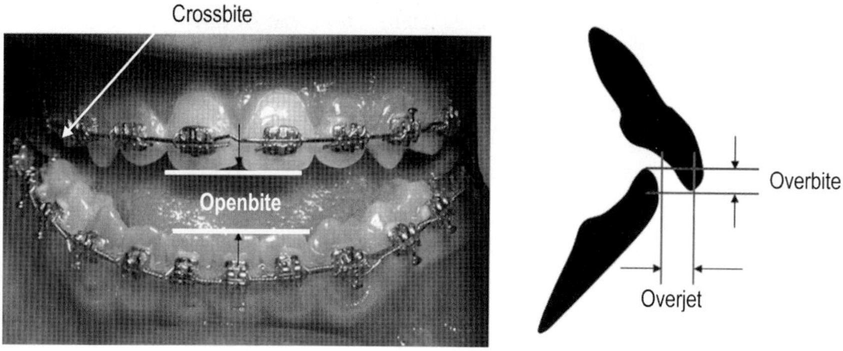

Figure 5.2.

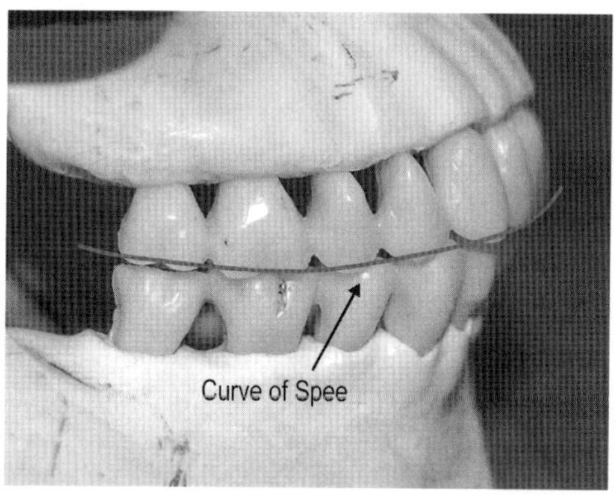

Figure 5.3.

- Curve of Spee: The natural curvature of the mandibular occlusal plane from incisor to molar teeth in the sagittal plane (Figure 5.3).
- Curve of Wilson: The natural curvature of the occlusal plane of the molar and premolar teeth in the coronal plane (Figure 5.4).
- Sphere of Monson: The 3-dimensional construct of the curves of Spee and Wilson (Figure 5.4).
  - *Note*: These terms have significance when orthodontic leveling of the arches is performed with arch wires; the curve of Spee is typically leveled (made flat) before orthognathic surgery.

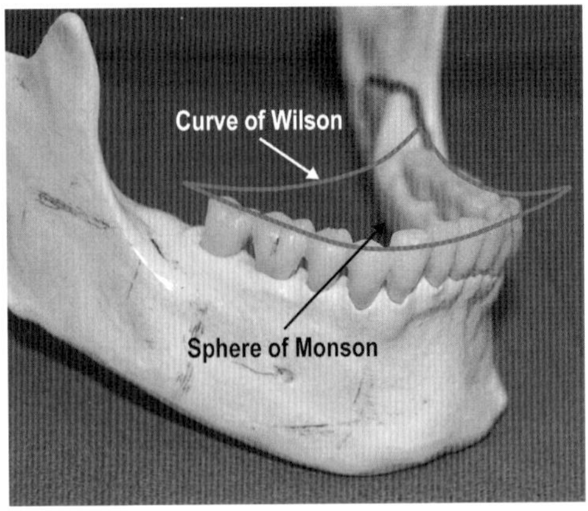

Figure 5.4.

- Described by Edward Angle, MD, DDS, in 1898, the ***Angle Classification of Occlusion*** describes the relationship of the upper first molar to the lower first molar (Figure 5.5):
  - Class 1: The mesiobuccal cusp of the maxillary first molar is in the buccal groove of the lower first molar.
  - Class 2: The distobuccal cusp of the maxillary first molar is in the buccal groove of the lower first molar.
    - Division 1: The maxillary incisors are proclined.
    - Division 2: The maxillary central incisors are retroclined and the lateral incisors are proclined.
  - Class 3: The mesiobuccal cusp of the maxillary first molar is in the distobuccal groove of the lower first molar:
    - *Note*: Keep in mind that the same patient may have different molar relationships on each side of the arch.

- Bolton analysis: This is a method to determine tooth size discrepancies between upper and lower arches (Figure 5.6). The added width of the anterior six teeth of the upper arch is slightly longer than the added width of the anterior six teeth of the lower arch by a constant ratio. If this ratio deviates, there is a tooth size

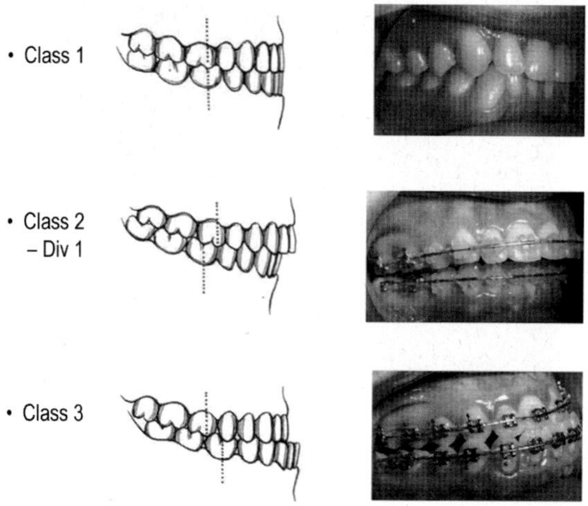

Figure 5.5.

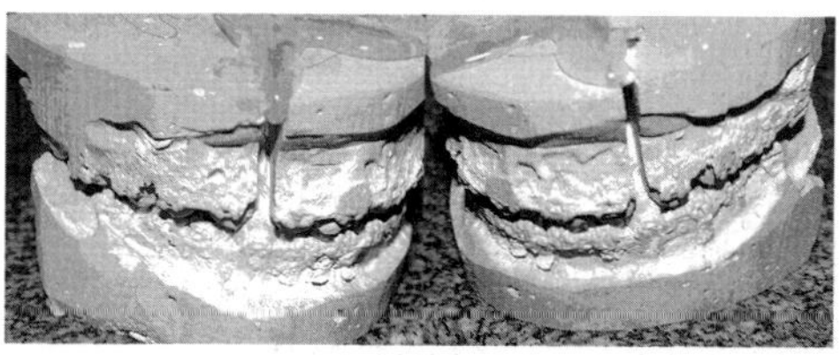

Figure 5.6. Segmental osteotomies between the lateral incisor and canine on both sides to increase upper arch length relative to the lower arch (Bolton discrepancy).

discrepancy; for example, a patient with peg (narrow) lateral incisors has an anterior upper arch width that is too small relative to the lower anterior teeth. This has significance when coordinating upper and lower arches for surgery. Spacing or filing of teeth (stripping) by the orthodontist might be necessary or segmental osteotomies might be needed at surgery.

- Dental compensations: Patients with skeletal disharmonies before surgical/orthodontic treatment have teeth that are abnormally angulated or positioned to make up for malaligned skeletal structures. The teeth are not aligned over the basal bone. These

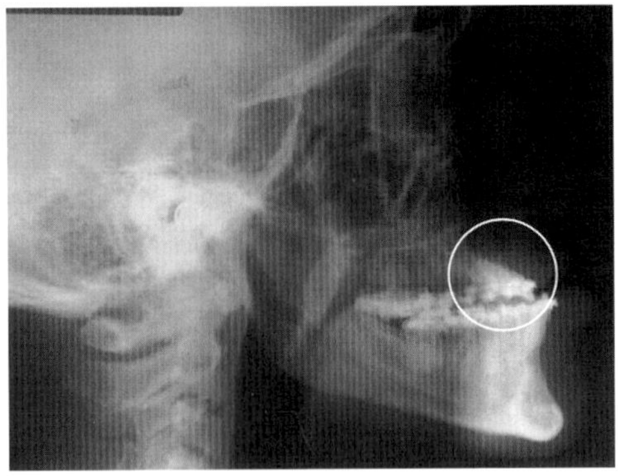

Figure 5.7. Cephalometric view. A class 3 skeletal patient with severely proclined upper incisors that will require orthodontic uprighting before orthognathic surgery. Extraction of upper premolars will be necessary to allow space for protraction of the upper teeth, making the patient's facial appearance and negative overjet worse.

abnormal positions need to be reversed before orthognathic surgery, often making the patient's facial esthetics worse just before surgery (Figure 5.7).

5.3 Facial Analysis

- Of critical importance in treatment planning in orthognathic surgery is the relationship of the upper incisor teeth to the upper lip. The patient should be assessed with the lips relaxed and in repose. It is in this position that treatment-planning decisions are made, not in the animated state (Figure 5.8).
  - Normally, 2–4 mm of upper incisor crowns should be visible below the upper lip at rest.
  - While smiling, 100% of the upper incisors should be visible, with some gingival display considered acceptable.
  - If excess upper incisor display is apparent at rest, either the maxilla is vertically long and/or the upper lip is short (Figure 5.9).

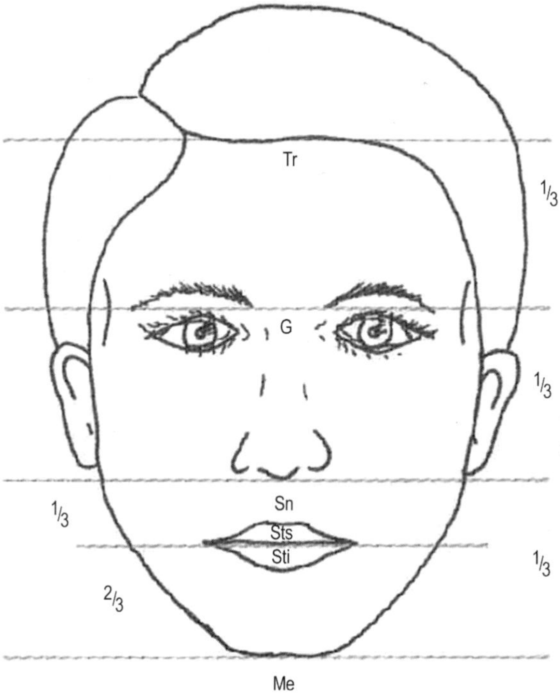

Figure 5.8. Facial thirds analysis is important in revealing facial disharmonies, such as vertical maxillary excess. Reprinted with permission from Quintessence Publishing Co., Inc (Ref. 1). Copyright © 2003 Quintessence Publishing Co., Inc.

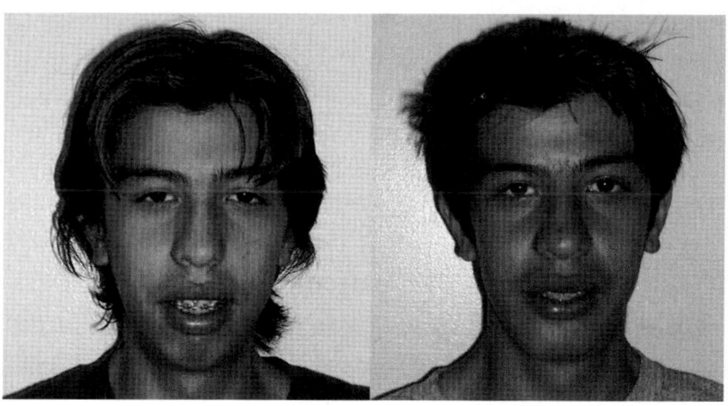

(A) (B)

Figure 5.9. Patient with (A) excessive incisor show at rest (vertical maxillary excess) before surgery and (B) with normalization after Le Fort I impaction.

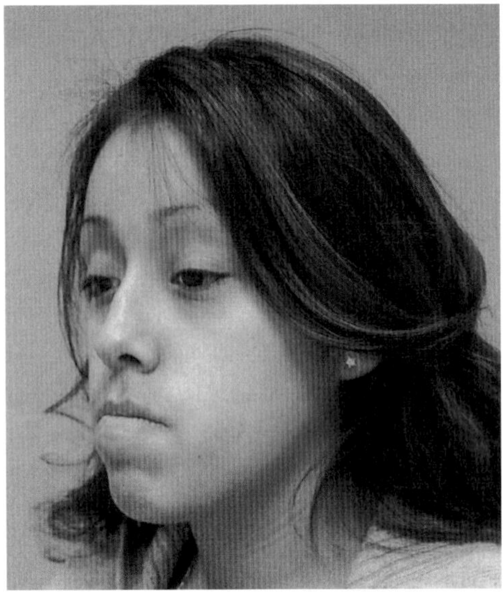

Figure 5.10. Patient exhibiting mentalis strain to obtain lip closure.

- Patients with vertical maxillary excess will often strain the mentalis muscle of the lower lip to facilitate lip closure (Figure 5.10).

- Upper and lower dental midlines should be compared with the facial midline.
- Asymmetries should be assessed with aid of a tongue blade (Figure 5.11).
- Although the angle classification describes occlusal relationships, the same terminology can be used to classify skeletal relationships in the sagittal plane (Figure 5.12):
  - Class 1 skeletal: normal relationship of the upper and lower jaws. (ANB angle: 0° to 4.5°. The ANB angle is the relationship of the maxilla to the mandible.)
  - Class 2 skeletal: the lower jaw is deficient (ANB angle $>4.5^\circ$).
  - Class 3 skeletal: the lower jaw is prognathic and/or the upper jaw is deficient (ANB angle $<0^\circ$).
  - *Note*: Skeletal and dental angle classifications do not always correlate. A patient may have a class 1 occlusion but a class 2 skeletal

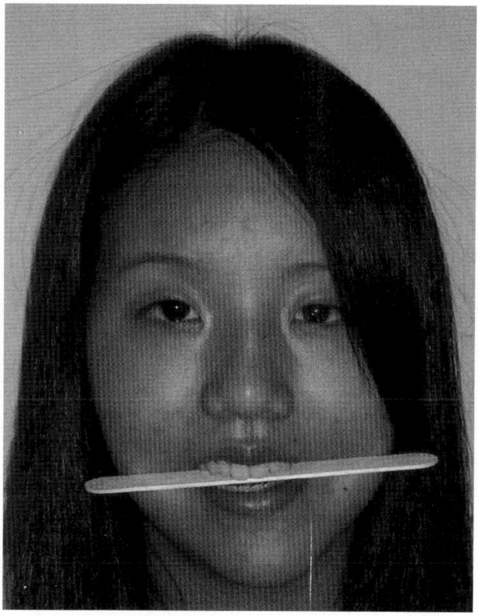

Figure 5.11. Biting on tongue blade reveals significant asymmetry and occlusal canting.

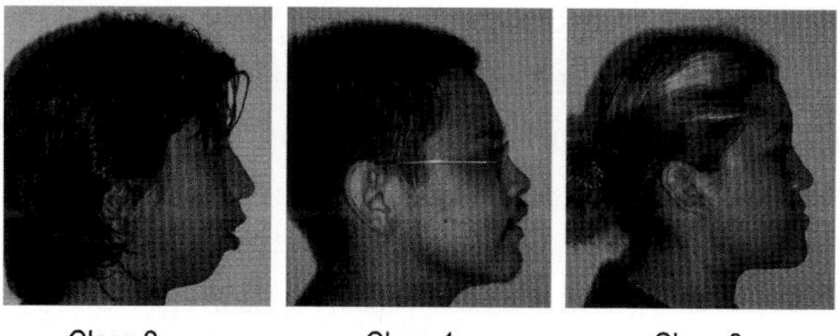

Figure 5.12.

relationship if he or she has had orthodontics to camouflage a class 2 malocclusion. This has relevance when planning for treatment of genioplasty: a class 1 occlusion does not necessarily mean the patient has a mandible of normal length and simply needs advancement genioplasty.

5.4 Cephalometrics

Cephalometric analysis, or the study of specific points and angles of the craniofacial skeleton on a standardized lateral or anterior/posterior (AP) skull film, should be considered an adjunct to the treatment planning of various dentofacial deformities. Cephalometric analyses are based on population norms; what may be considered normal for one patient may not be for the next. The ultimate ideal soft tissue appearance ("soft tissue paradigm") should be sought for each patient, not based on a numeric analysis aimed at "normalizing" a patient's radiograph. Below is a list of commonly plotted points on a lateral cephalogram (Figure 5.13):

- S = sella: center of sella turcica.
- N = nasion: intersection of the frontal and nasal bones.
- Ba = basion: anterior portion of foramen magnum.
- ANS = anterior nasal spine: most projecting point.
- PNS = posterior nasal spine: posterior point of hard palate.
- A = subnasale "A point": the most concave portion of the central anterior maxilla.
- B = supramentale "B point": the most concave portion of the anterior mandible.
- Pog = pogonion: the most projecting point of the chin.
- Me = menton: the most inferior point of the mandibular symphysis.
- Gn = gnathion: point halfway between Pog and Me.
- Go = gonion: angle of mandible formed by intersection of tangents from posterior border and lower border of the mandible.
- Or = orbitale: the lowest point of the inferior orbital rim.
- Po = porion: the most cephalic portion of the external auditory canal.
- Co = condylion: the most superior point of the condylar head.
- Ptm = pterygomaxillary fissure: base of the fissure.
- G = glabella: most projecting point of the frontal bone.
- Different reference planes and angles make up the various cephalometric analyses. Commonly used measurements are as follows (Figure 5.14):
  - SN = cranial base plane.

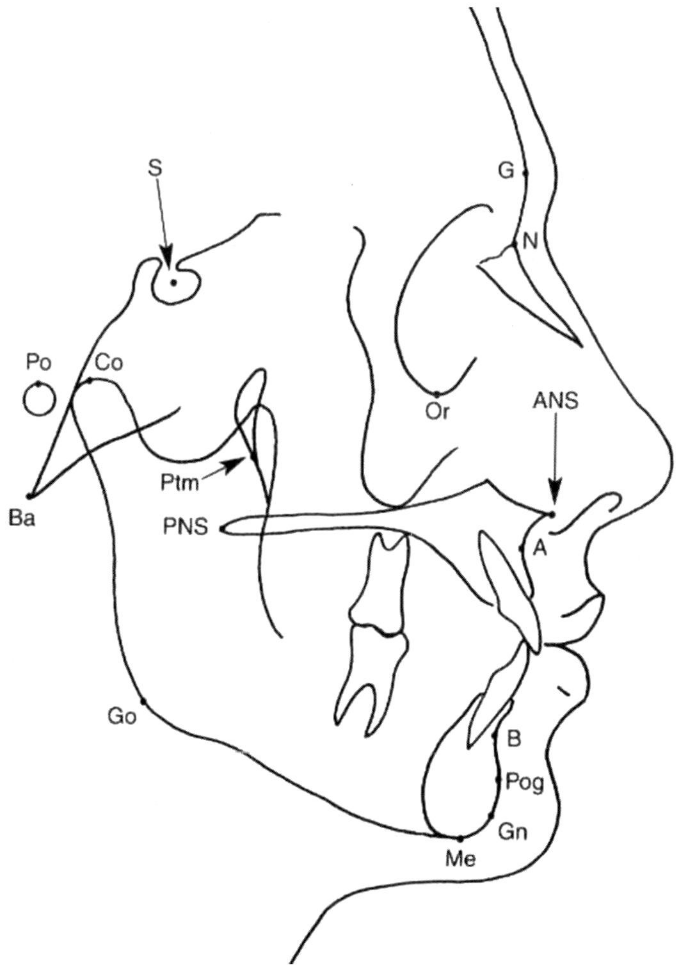

Figure 5.13. Reprinted with permission from Quintessence Publishing Co., Inc. (Ref. 1). Copyright © 2003 Quintessence Publishing Co., Inc.

- Or–Po = Frankfort horizontal plane. This plane parallels the floor in a standard lateral cephalogram.
    - *Note:* Many syndromic patients have an excessively angulated cranial base, thereby making any angle related to SN excessively abnormal. Normally, SN should be at a 6° angle to the Frankfort horizontal plane.

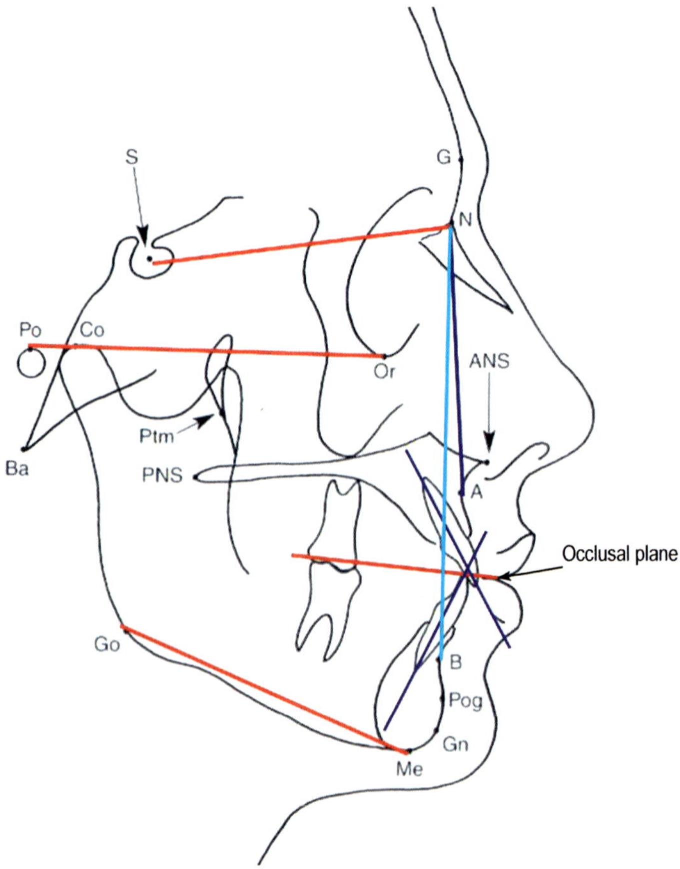

Figure 5.14. Reprinted with permission from Quintessence Publishing Co., Inc. (Ref. 1). Copyright © 2003 Quintessence Publishing Co., Inc.

- Occlusal plane = line bisecting the incisal overbite and molar contacts.
- SN–MP = mandibular plane angle, the angle between the cranial base and the lower border of the mandible (32°). A patient with Treacher Collins syndrome would have a high mandibular plane angle.
- SNA = relationship of the maxilla to the cranium (81°). A patient with a deficient maxilla would have an angle <81°.
- NA = relationship of the nasion to the subnasale A point, the most concave portion of the central anterior maxilla; subset of SNA.

- SNB = relationship of the mandible to the cranium (79°). A prognathic patient would have an SNB > 79°.
- NB = relationship of the nasion to the supramentale B point, the most concave portion of the anterior mandible; subset of SNB.
- SNPog = relationship of the chin to the cranium (80°).
- ANB = relationship of the maxilla to the mandible (0°–4.5°). A class 2 skeletal patient would have an ANB > 4.5°, whereas a class 3 skeletal patient would have an ANB < 0° (or a negative number).
- Maxillary incisor position = the maxillary incisor is related to NA both spatially and in angularity. The incisal edge should be 4 mm anterior to line NA, and the long axis should be angulated 22° relative to NA. These numbers provide information about incisor compensations in various dentofacial deformities. A class 3 skeletal patient may have proclined (> 22° and > 4 mm) upper incisors before orthodontic decompensation.
- Mandibular incisor position = the mandibular incisor is related to NB both spatially and in angularity. The incisal edge should be 4 mm anterior to NB, and the long axis should be angulated 25° relative to NB. Before orthodontic decompensation, a class 3 skeletal patient might have retroclined lower incisors (< 25° and < 4 mm), whereas a class 2 patient might have proclined incisors (> 25° and > 4 mm).

• Chin analysis: Although many analyses have been described including the E line, S line, Merrifield Z line, and Holdaway ratio, we prefer the *Ulloa-Gonzalez–Stevens line* (zero meridian line): a line dropped from the soft tissue nasion perpendicular to the Frankfort horizontal plane should meet soft tissue pogonion ± 2 mm (Figure 5.15).

5.5 Treatment Sequence

A new patient with a dentofacial deformity should be seen by both the orthodontist and surgeon before treatment is started. Both must

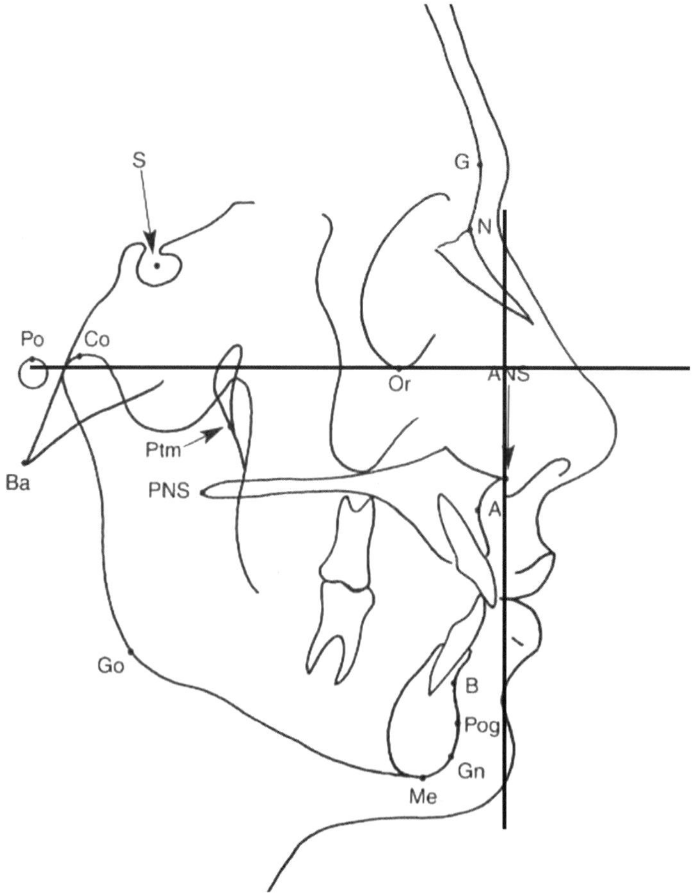

Figure 5.15. Reprinted with permission from Quintessence Publishing Co., Inc. (Ref. 1). Copyright © 2003 Quintessence Publishing Co., Inc.

agree on a treatment plan before surgery, as the orthodontic setup can be quite different depending on the planned surgery. Many times, a surgeon will be referred to a patient by an orthodontist who attempted orthodontic correction of a skeletal problem only to find that surgery was the only option to correct the problem. At this point in treatment, much dental compensation are present and the surgical plan is compromised.

- Phase 1 (6 months–2 years).
  - Surgical.
    - Possibly extract teeth (usually premolars) to relieve dental crowding and allow for arch alignment and leveling. Typical extraction patterns in a class 3 skeletal case with dental crowding are upper first and lower second premolars, and in a class 2 skeletal case, upper second and lower first premolars. These extraction patterns are completely opposite to those in a case that will be treated with orthodontics alone.
    - Remove wisdom teeth (this may also be done at the time of orthognathic surgery).
  - Orthodontic.
    - Level and align arches (eliminate curve of Spee and "straighten" teeth).
    - *Exception:* In an openbite case, it may be desirable to leave a step in the maxillary occlusal plane either between canine and lateral or canine and premolar teeth and level the occlusal plane surgically with a segmental osteotomy.
    - *Exception:* In a class 2 skeletal case with short lower anterior facial height, it is desirable to maintain the lower-arch curve of Spee such that as much vertical anterior height as possible is maintained. The arch can be leveled postoperatively.
    - Eliminate dental compensations.
    - Coordinate arches so that the upper and lower models occlude maximally.

- Phase 2.
  - Surgical (see below for specific surgical procedures).
    - At what age? At the end of facial growth (determined with serial cephalograms, hand film, or cervical-spine film). For girls, this is around the age of 15 years and for boys, around 18 years.

- Phase 3 (6 months–1 year).
  - Postsurgical orthodontics.

- *Note:* This is the most accepted and standard treatment sequence. Currently, after careful analysis, some perform surgery before orthodontics in an attempt to shorten treatment time.

5.6 Commonly Encountered Dentofacial Deformities

Although grouped separately here, the commonly encountered dentofacial deformities described below often coexist. It is difficult to discuss sagittal discrepancies (profile analysis) without also analyzing vertical relationships, as the following changes in the vertical position of the maxilla will affect mandibular position:

- Mandibular deficiency (class 2 skeletal) (Figure 5.16).
  - Approximately 10% of the population.
  - Features.
    - Everted lower lip with deep labiomental fold.
    - Increased overjet, class 2 malocclusion.
    - ANB angle > 4.5°.
  - Relative versus absolute mandibular deficiency: in a patient with a vertically long maxilla, the mandible (on its hinge axis) rotates downward and backward, giving the appearance of a deficient mandible (relative mandibular deficiency). Surgical correction by maxillary impaction allows upward and forward movement of the mandible, correcting the apparent mandibular deficiency.
  - Surgical treatment options (Figure 5.17).
    - Bilateral sagittal split osteotomy (BSSO) advancement.
    - Advancement genioplasty.

- Long face problems (vertical maxillary and/or mandibular excess).
  - Patient has the so-called smile (Figure 5.18).
  - Features.
    - Excessively long lower third of face.
    - Lip incompetence (with mentalis strain).
    - Tendency toward openbite.
    - Increased mandibular plane angle due to downward and posterior rotation of the mandible (Figure 5.19).

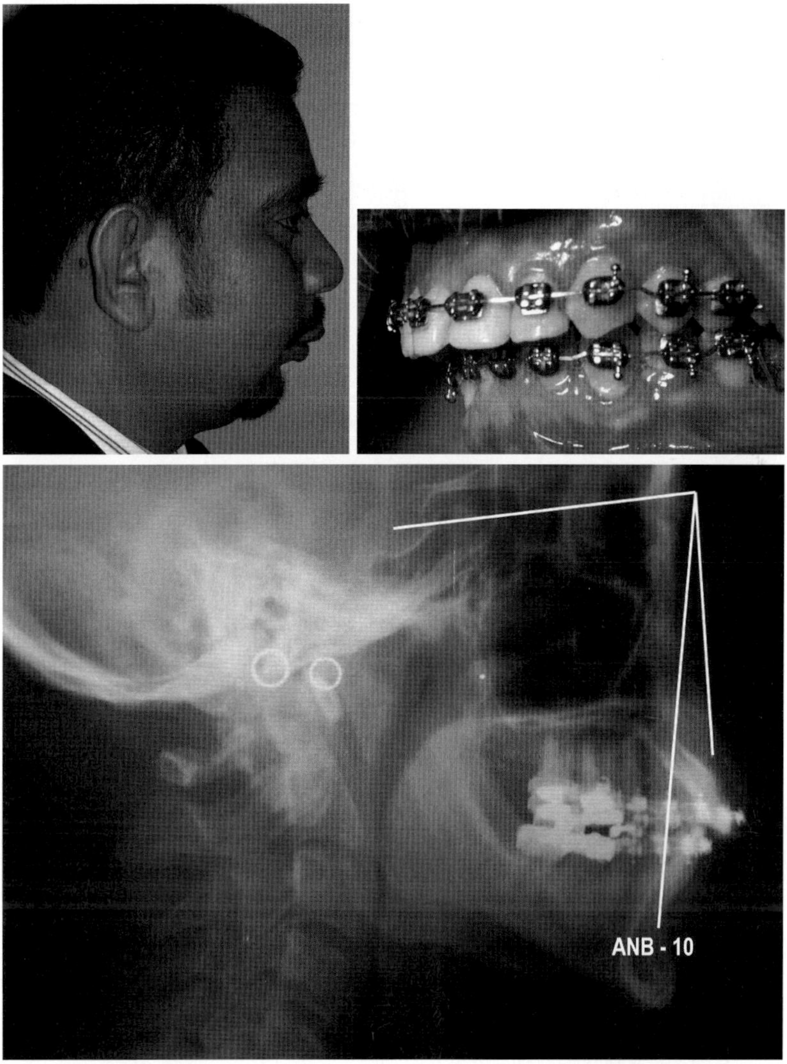

Figure 5.16. Typical facial, occlusal, and radiographic appearance of mandible-deficient case.

- *Note:* Although relative mandibular deficiency (described above) may exist in the patient with a long face, remember that mandibular excess is also possible; in that case, a normal-appearing mandible may actually be prognathic (excessively long) after the maxilla is affected and the mandible autorotates upward and forward.

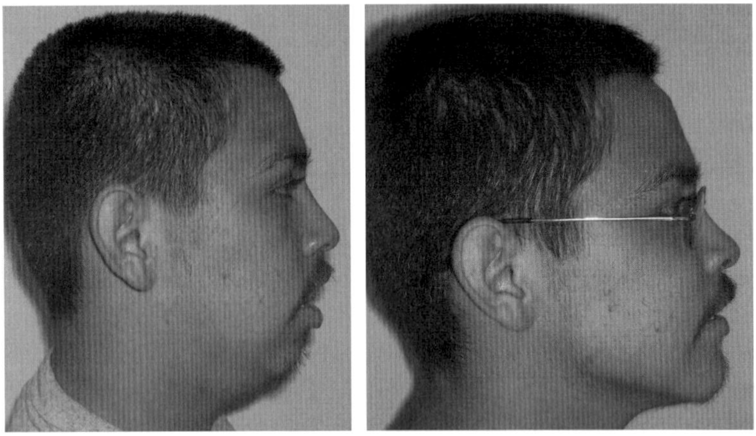

(A) (B)

Figure 5.17. Correction of (A) class 2 skeletal deformity with (B) BSSO advancement and genioplasty.

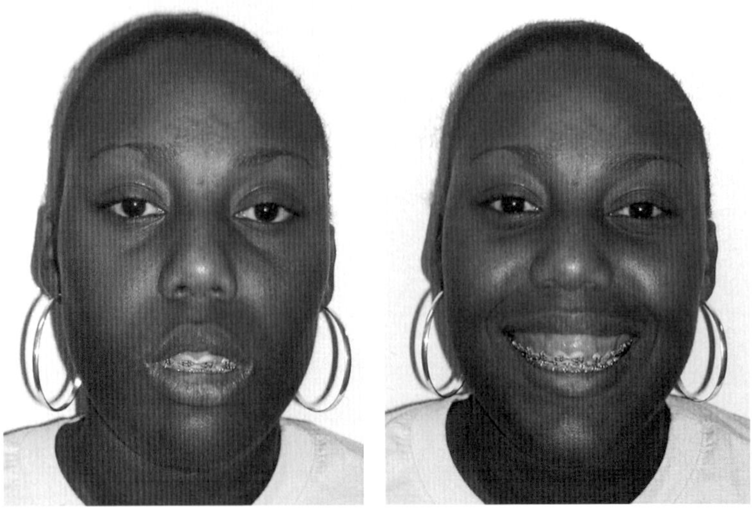

(A) (B)

Figure 5.18. Typical appearance of a long face patient exhibiting (A) lip incompetence at rest and (B) a "gummy" smile with animation.

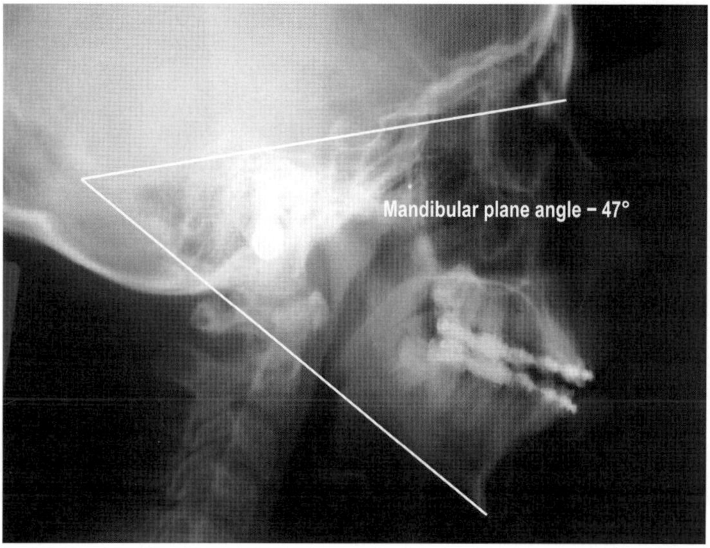

Figure 5.19. Vertically long maxilla causing downward and posterior rotation of the mandible with resultant high mandibular plane angle.

- The mandible may also contribute to the long face problem due to an excessively long anterior mandibular dental height (distance from lower incisor tip to inferior border of mandible; normal range is 40 mm to 44 mm).
- Surgical treatment options.
  - Le Fort I impaction with or without BSSO (maxillary excess) (Figure 5.20).
  - Vertical reduction genioplasty (vertical mandibular excess).

• Class 3 skeletal problems (Figure 5.21).
  - Often includes a varying combination of maxillary deficiency and mandibular excess, but maxillary deficiency is most commonly present.
  - Commonly seen in cleft patients, the craniofacial dysostosis syndromes, cleidocranial dysplasia, and Binder's syndrome.
  - Features.

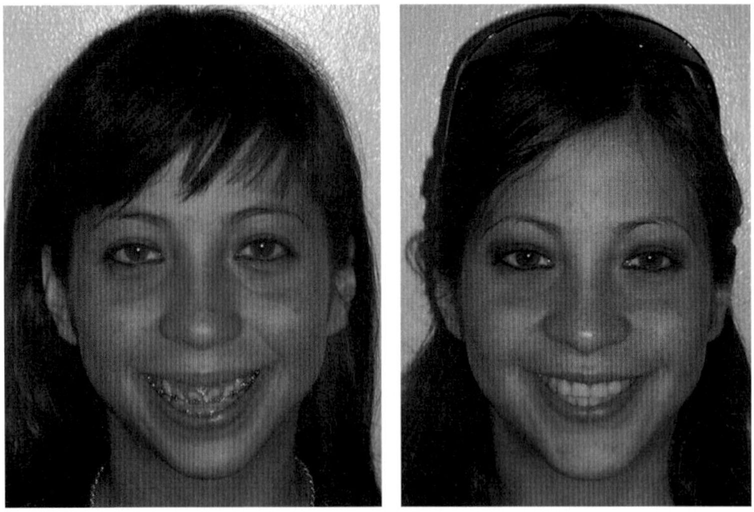

Figure 5.20. Patient with vertical maxillary excess treated with Le Fort I impaction and advancement genioplasty.

  - o Midface deficiency, sometimes including inferior orbital rims.
  - o Mandibular excess.
  - o Long chin-throat distance.
  - o Reduced labiomental fold.
  - o Negative overjet, class 3 malocclusion.
  - o Negative ANB angle.
- Relative versus absolute mandibular excess: in a patient with a vertically deficient maxilla (no tooth show at rest), the mandible (on its hinge axis) rotates upward and forward, giving the appearance of an excessively long mandible (relative mandibular excess). Surgical correction by maxillary downgraft allows downward and backward movement of the mandible, correcting the apparent mandibular excess.
- Surgical treatment options (Figure 5.22).
  - o Le Fort I advancement.
  - o BSSO setback.
  - o Vertical ramus osteotomy setback.
  - o Le Fort III advancement.

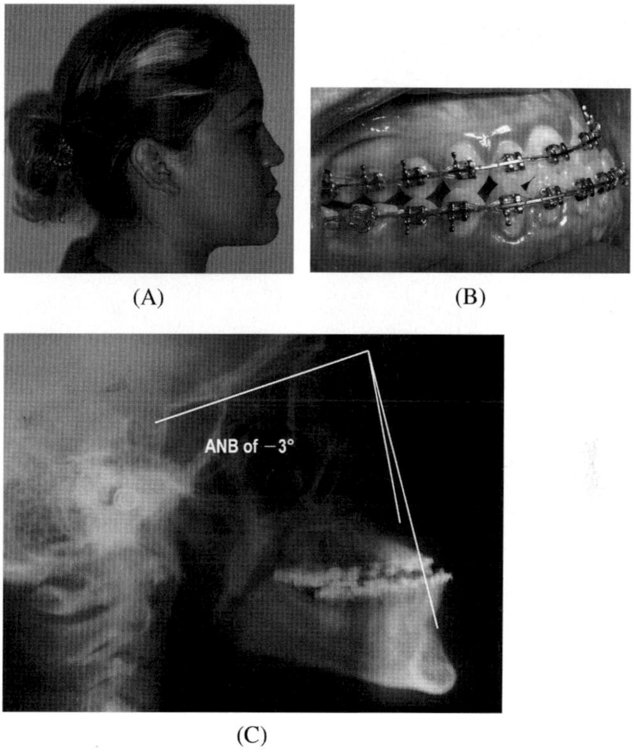

Figure 5.21. (A) Class 3 skeletal facial appearance and (B) class 3 malocclusion. (C) Cephalometric appearance of class 3 skeletal patient.

  - Le Fort II advancement.
  - Genioplasty.

- Asymmetry cases (Figure 5.23).
  - Perhaps the most challenging cases for achieving a good result. These are the cases where 3-dimensional computer-aided planning is especially useful.
  - Commonly seen in the patient with hemifacial microsomia.
  - Requires accurate treatment planning with the aid of an AP cephalogram. Horizontal planes reveal asymmetry (Figure 5.24):
    - Cranial base plane — assess orbital dystopia.
    - J plane — maxillary plane.

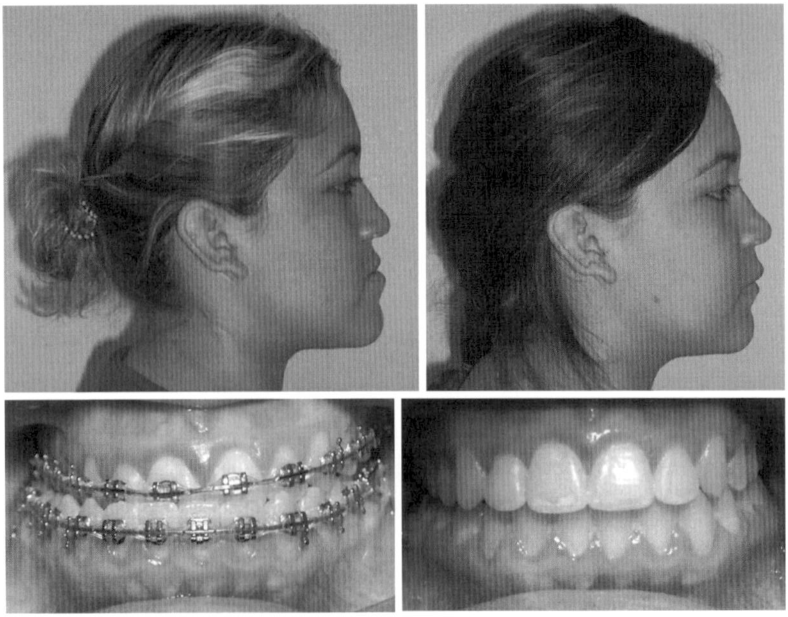

Figure 5.22. Correction of class 3 skeletal deformity with Le Fort I advancement and BSSO setback.

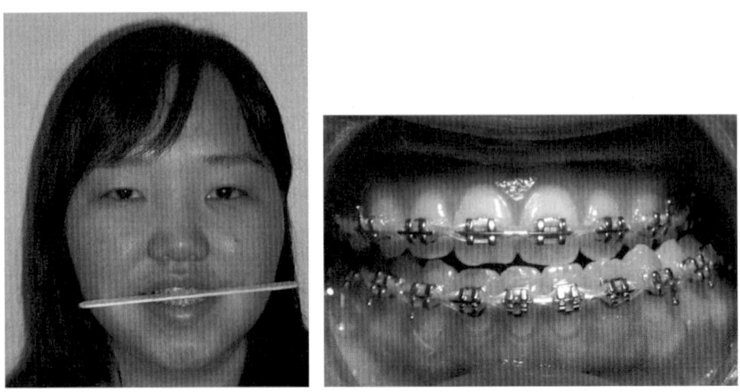

Figure 5.23. Asymmetric class 3 skeletal patient.

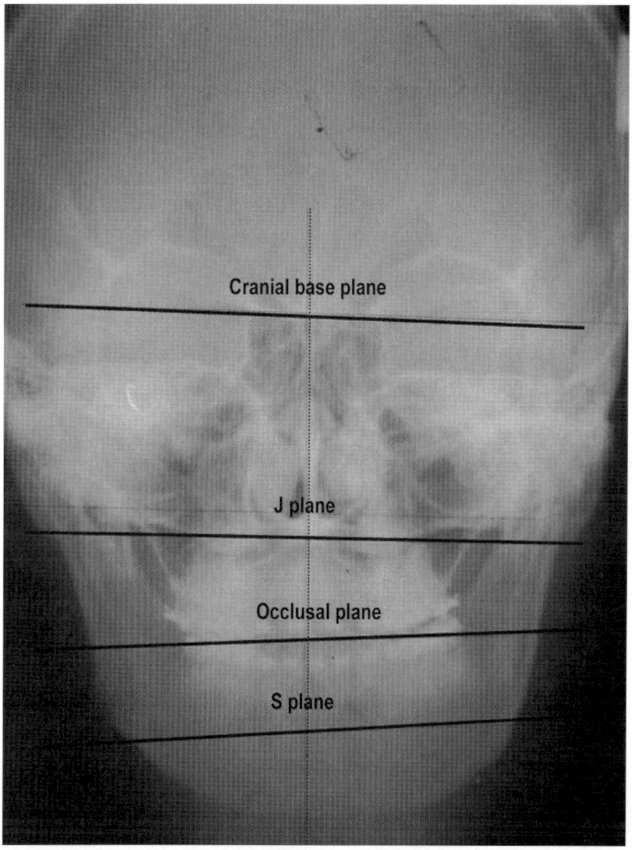

Figure 5.24. Anterior/posterior cephalogram. Horizontal planes help treatment plan surgical movements.

    - Occlusal plane.
    - S plane — mandibular plane.
  - Surgical treatment options.
    - Le Fort I osteotomy.
    - BSSO.
    - Genioplasty.
- Transverse discrepancies.
  - These are problems in the way the dental arches occlude in the coronal plane. An example would be in a patient with a posterior

crossbite. Most commonly, the maxilla is narrow and needs to be widened.

- In the growing patient, the maxilla can be expanded orthodontically with palatal expanders. Once the midline palatal suture fuses, however, surgical therapy is necessary to correct the deformity.
- Surgical treatment options (Figure 5.25).
  - Surgically assisted rapid palatal expansion (SARPE); also called surgically assisted maxillary expansion (SAME) — a form of distraction osteogenesis, this procedure is a Le Fort I osteotomy with a midline split, *without* down-fracture and with limited lateral nasal wall osteotomy.
  - Segmental Le Fort I osteotomy.
  - BSSO with midline split to narrow mandible.
  - *Note:* In general, for transverse discrepancies larger than 7 mm, a SARPE will be required before definitive orthognathic surgery, whereas lesser discrepancies can be corrected at the time of surgery with segmental osteotomies.

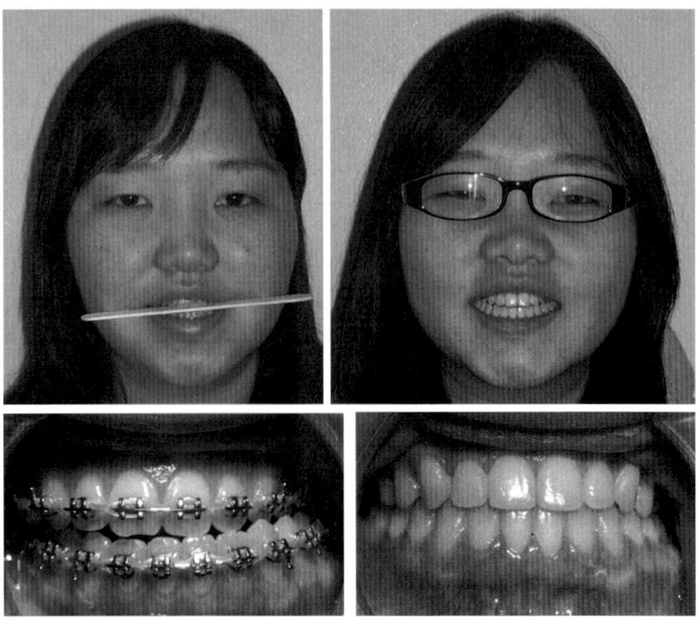

Figure 5.25. Correction of asymmetry case with Le Fort I, BSSO.

5.7 Preoperative Evaluation

Whether the traditional approach to orthognathic surgery or 3-dimensional computer-aided treatment planning is used, preoperative evaluation begins with precise presurgical records, thoughtful treatment planning, and accurate model surgery. A flaw in any of these steps will lead to a suboptimal result. Although computer-aided treatment planning and model surgery is now a reality, it has not reached the mainstream. We will discuss the traditional approach here.

- Presurgical records: The goal of taking records is to replicate the patient's anatomy on an articulator, a device that simulates a patient's jaw joint, so that model surgery can be performed. The following data must be collected:
  - Facial photographs: frontal (lips in repose, patient smiling, tongue blade for asymmetry cases), laterals (3 2), obliques (3 2).
  - Dental photographs: incisor and molar views (3 2).
  - Upper and lower dental arch impressions.
    - Alginate impressions are poured into stone.
  - Facebow transfer: This device references the upper jaw in space to the temporomandibular joint (TMJ) such that the upper cast can be mounted on the articulator (Figure 5.26).
    - *Note*: Pointers to reference the orbital rims may be added to the facebow to perform model surgery for Le Fort III osteotomies.
  - Bite record in centric relation (of utmost importance).
    - The relationship of the upper to the lower jaw is obtained with a bite record, using either wax or impression material, with the patient's condyles in a hinge position (also known as centric relation). The bite record is critical to the final surgery because all splints made are a direct result of correctly mounted models.
  - Radiographs: orthopantomogram, lateral and AP cephalograms, possibly periapical films if segmental osteotomies are planned.

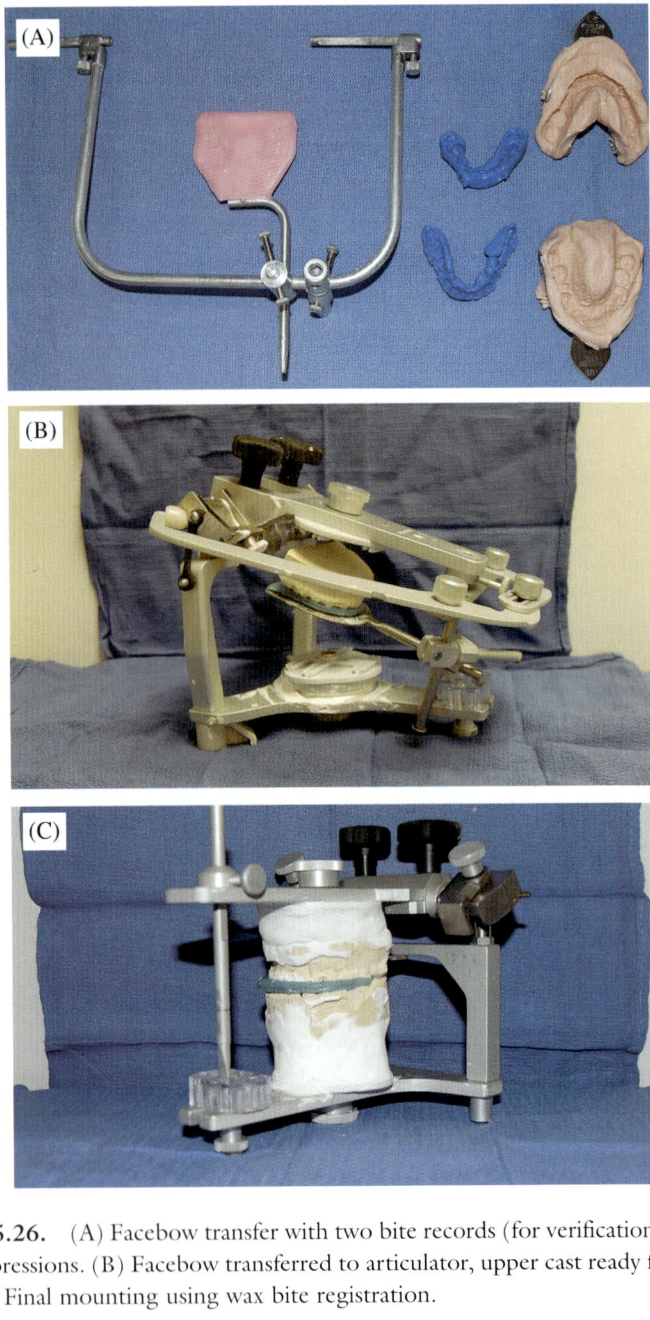

Figure 5.26. (A) Facebow transfer with two bite records (for verification) and alginate impressions. (B) Facebow transferred to articulator, upper cast ready for mounting. (C) Final mounting using wax bite registration.

- Treatment planning: Based on an analysis of the patient's photographs, models, and radiographs, a treatment plan can be constructed. A decision needs to be made as to whether the patient's problem can be corrected with a single-jaw surgery or whether the patient will need two-jaw surgery. Many factors go into this decision, including soft tissue esthetics, dental analysis, and severity of the deformity. Regardless of the plan, some concepts are important:
  - The most important determinant of maxillary position is the upper incisor position (discussed in Chapter 3, Facial Analysis).
    - For every millimeter the upper incisor is advanced, there is approximately a 60% increase in incisor show. Thus, if the maxilla is advanced 3 mm, there will be 2 mm of extra incisor show at rest.
    - The vertical movement of the upper incisor occurs in a 1:1 ratio; if the incisor is moved up 2 mm, there will be 2 mm less of incisor show.
  - With mandibular advancement, there is a 1:1 ratio of bony to soft tissue change at the pogonion. The labiomental fold becomes shallower. With setback, the opposite is true.
  - For chin position, bony to soft tissue relationship is approximately 1:1. If the chin is advanced 5 mm, the soft tissue projection should increase by the same amount.
- Model surgery: the purpose of model surgery is to make dental splints so that the mobilized jaws can be positioned at surgery according to the decided treatment plan. It is important to realize that dental splints reference the jaws in all dimensions except the vertical dimension, which must be measured at surgery with external or internal references. In single-jaw surgery, the model surgery is simplified greatly since the jaw not operated upon becomes the "positioner" for the mobilized jaw. A splint simply needs to be fabricated with the models in maximum intercuspation (centric occlusion). For two-jaw cases, the model surgery is more involved, requiring fabrication of two splints. Briefly, for two-jaw surgery (Figure 5.27):
  - Reference upper model with model block.

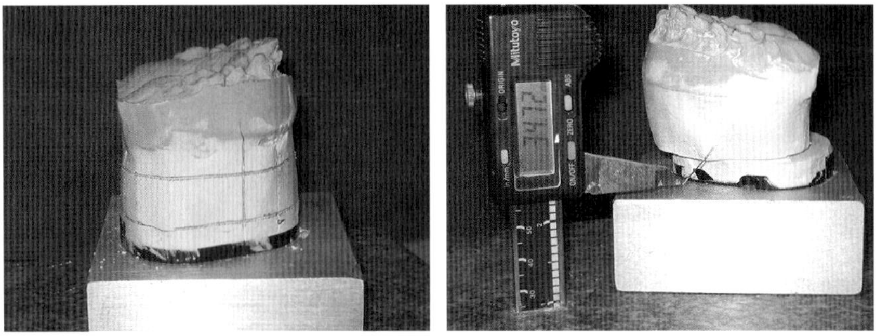

(A) (B)

Figure 5.27. (A) Upper cast on model block and (B) newly positioned maxilla after the model is sectioned from mounting base.

- Section upper cast from mounting base (simulating Le Fort I osteotomy).
- Perform segmentation of model if necessary to fit lower arch.
- Reposition upper cast on mounting base in planned new-treatment position (with aid of model block measurements).
- Fabricate intermediate splint (maxillary positioning splint) with original lower mounting and new maxillary mounting.
- Mount a duplicated lower cast in maximum intercuspation with the newly mounted upper model and fabricate final splint.
- If a "splint-in-splint" method is necessary because of a segmented upper jaw, make final splint before intermediate splint (Figure 5.28).

5.8 Preoperative Considerations

- Patients may auto-donate blood before the procedure.
- Immediately preoperatively, patients should receive intravenous antibiotics, either a first-generation cephalosporin or ampicillin/sublactam, and dexamethasone.
- The mouth should be rinsed with chlorhexidine 0.12%.
- Splints should be placed on the operating-room back table in chlorhexidine 0.12%.

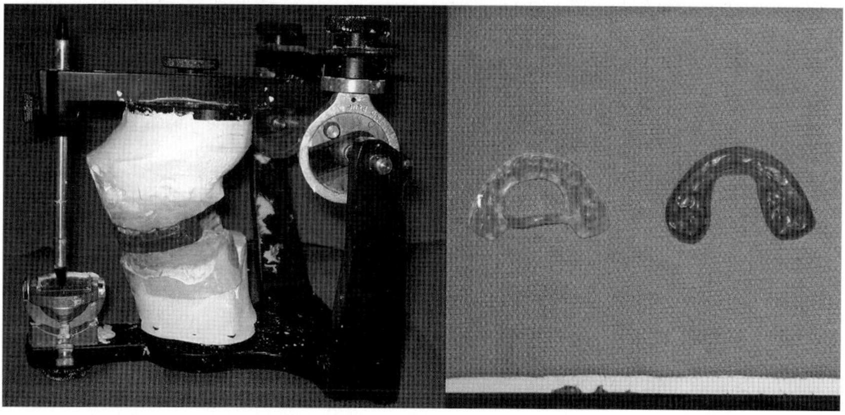

(A) (B)

Figure 5.28. (A) Final mounting for intermediate splint fabrication ("splint-in-splint" method) with (B) polished final and intermediate splints.

5.9 Surgical Techniques

- Le Fort I osteotomy (Figure 5.29).
  - This is a horizontal osteotomy above the apices of the teeth.
  - The procedure should be performed with hypotensive anesthesia with the patient in a slight reverse Trendelenburg position.
  - Infiltrate upper buccal vestibule with lidocaine with epinephrine.
  - Place vertical reference marker at nasion with a Kirschner wire.
  - After identifying the parotid ducts, make an incision down to bone in the depth of the upper vestibule from each maxillary buttress to the midline. Leave an adequate cuff of alveolar mucosa for later suturing.
  - Perform subperiosteal dissection of the AP surfaces of the maxilla, identifying the infraorbital nerve on both sides. The posterior extent of the dissection ends at the pterygomaxillary fissure. Carefully, without tearing, dissect the nasal mucosa from the lateral walls and floor of the nose.
  - If segmental osteotomies are planned, perform interdental cuts with chisel while the maxilla is stable.

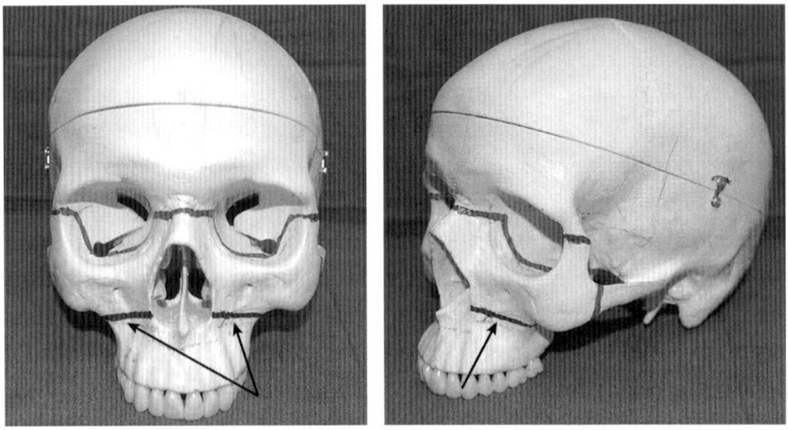

Figure 5.29. Le Fort I osteotomy.

- Use a reciprocating saw to perform osteotomies of the AP maxillary walls. The osteotomy begins at the lateral nasal wall at a point just above the floor of the piriform aperture and extends posteriorly below the zygomatic buttress through the posterior maxillary wall.
- Separate the septum from the maxillary crest with a safe-sided chisel. Complete lateral nasal wall and posterior maxillary wall osteotomies with a chisel.
- Last, perform pterygomaxillary dysjunction with a curved chisel by placing one finger on the pterygoid hamulus for tactile feedback (Figure 5.30). Angling the chisel inferiorly, away from the maxillary artery, perform the osteotomy. Some advocate use of an oscillating saw for this step.
- Down-fracture the maxilla with finger pressure. Laminer spreaders may be necessary to mobilize the scarred cleft maxilla. The maxilla should be freely mobile.
- Remove excess bone of the palatal aspect of the nasal septum, lateral nasal walls, and posterior maxillary walls.
- Apply splint to maxillary teeth, place the patient in intermaxillary fixation with wires or elastics, and rotate the maxillomandibular complex into place on the condylar hinge axis. Avoid exerting too much pressure anteriorly as this can unseat the

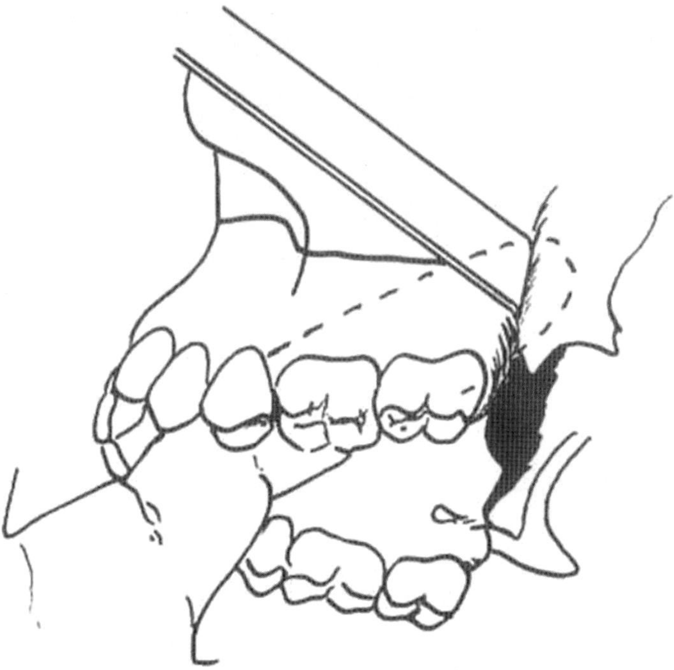

Figure 5.30. Pterygomaxillary dysjunction. Reprinted with permission from Quintessence Publishing Co., Inc. (Ref. 1). Copyright © 2003 Quintessence Publishing Co., Inc.

condyles, causing an anterior openbite when intermaxillary fixation is released.

- Trim bone as necessary to achieve the best bony contact and proper vertical relationship as measured with a vertical reference.
- Apply rigid fixation at the nasomaxillary and zygomaticomaxillary buttresses. Lindorf plates may also be used (Figure 5.31).
- Release intermaxillary fixation and check occlusion.
- Perform alar cinch suture to avoid excessive nasal base widening. Perform V-Y advancement of the upper lip mucosa to gain more upper lip fullness (Figure 5.32).
- Close mucosal incision with chromic gut or polyglactin 910 (Vicryl) sutures.

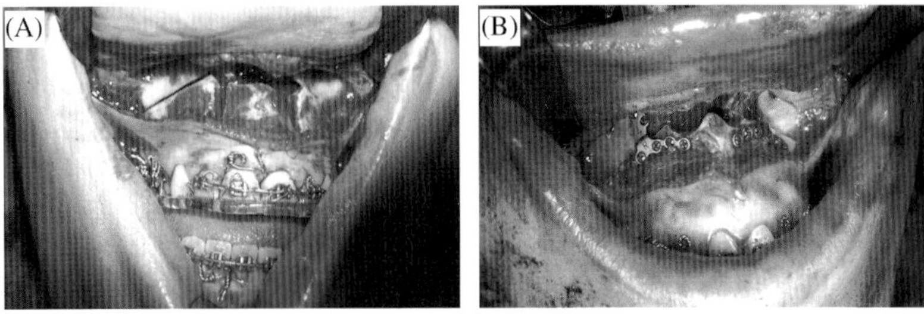

Figure 5.31. (A) Le Fort I segmental osteotomy and (B) example of fixation with Lindorf plates.

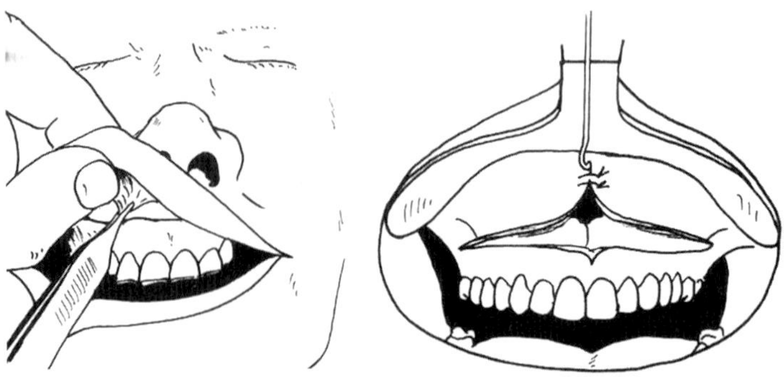

(A) (B)

Figure 5.32. (A) Alar cinch and (B) V-Y advancement. Reprinted with permission from Quintessence Publishing Co., Inc. (Ref. 1). Copyright © 2003 Quintessence Publishing Co., Inc.

- BSSO. This is a BSSO (Figure 5.33), or a separation of buccal and lingual cortices of the ramus of the mandible on both sides. Perform the following steps on both sides.
  - Inject local anesthetic with epinephrine into the soft tissues at the ramus.
  - Insert bite block and tongue (sweetheart) retractor.
  - Make incision through mucosa, buccinator muscle, and periosteum down to bone on a line paralleling the anterior ramus and external oblique ridge from midramus to approximately the lower first molar. Leave an adequate cuff of soft tissue to sew to

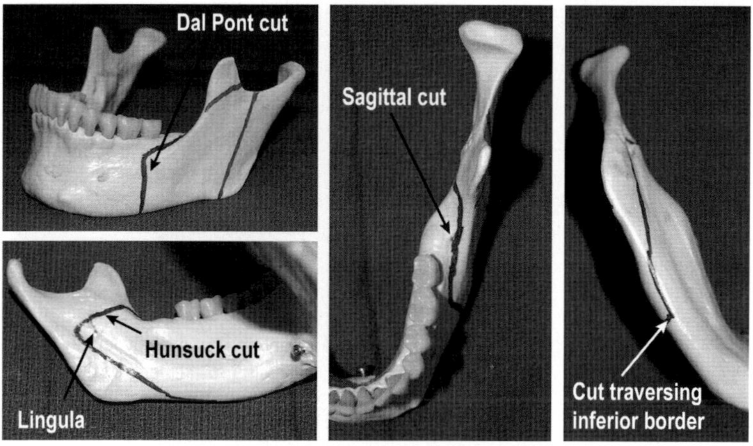

Figure 5.33. Sagittal split osteotomy.

at the conclusion of the procedure. Avoid entering the buccal fat pad.

- Perform subperiosteal dissection on the buccal side of the mandible down to the inferior border. Continue dissection to lingual side of ramus, taking care to remain subperiosteal and not to slip into the lingual soft tissues (Figure 5.34). Use coronoid stripper to elevate temporalis muscle attachments from the anterior ramus. Identify the lingula (where the inferior alveolar nerve enters the mandible).
- Perform medial corticotomy (Hunsuck cut) with reciprocating saw (some use a side-cutting bur) above the level of the lingula and stop it just posterior to the lingual, curving it into the sagittal osteotomy.
- The sagittal cut parallels the buccal surface of the mandible. Stop the sagittal cut at the first or second molar area. (The nerve is furthest from the buccal side of the mandible at the second/third molar.)
- Perform buccal vertical corticotomy (Dal Pont cut), being sure to perforate through the inferior border. Connect it with a sagittal cut with a smooth curve. Perform a second vertical cut

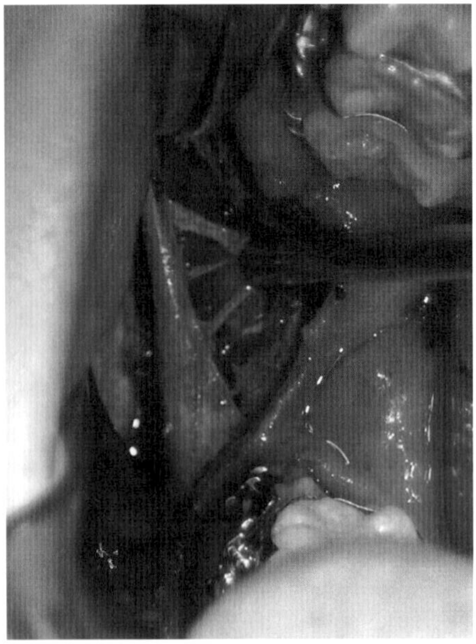

Figure 5.34. Surgical exposure of ramus.

posterior to this osteotomy if a setback is planned (according to the planned amount of setback).

- Splitting may be performed in many ways. Open the sagittal cut from above with a large chisel or elevator to identify the nerve (it should be in the distal segment). The nerve may need to be teased from the proximal segment. Once the nerve is identified, a chisel may be used to "split" the mandible. The osteotomy can be opened like a book, from anterior to posterior.
- Place the patient into intermaxillary fixation, trim necessary bone to achieve intimate bony contact, seat condyles, and fixate proximal and distal segments with either positional screws (with the aid of a trochar) or plates. Do not use lag screws, to avoid malpositioning of condyles. For advancement, "firmly" seat condyles into centric relation. For setback, "passively" seat condyles.
- Release intermaxillary fixation and check occlusion.
- Close incision with chromic gut.

- Genioplasty.
  - Infiltrate the anterior mandibular vestibule with local anesthetic with epinephrine.
  - Perform vestibular incision down to the bone, leaving a generous cuff of mucosa, from canine to canine.
  - Perform subperiosteal dissection of the chin, identifying mental foramina bilaterally. Avoid stripping the periosteum to the inferior border, thus maintaining the origin of the mentalis muscle.
  - Perform horizontal osteotomy with saw at least 5 mm below apices of mandibular incisors. Continue with lateral extension to inferior borders of mandible at least 5 mm below mental foramina. Be sure to be bicortical, especially in the inferior border region.
  - Position chin in desired location. May remove wedge of bone to reduce chin vertically (Figure 5.35).
  - Fixate chin with plates and screws (Figure 5.36).
  - Resuspend mentalis muscle with polyglactin 910 suture to prevent "witch's chin." Close mucosal incision with chromic gut.

- Vertical ramus osteotomy (Figure 5.37).
  - Alternative to BSSO setback.
  - Follow same incision design as for sagittal split osteotomy.
  - The buccal side of the entire ramus is exposed subperiosteally.

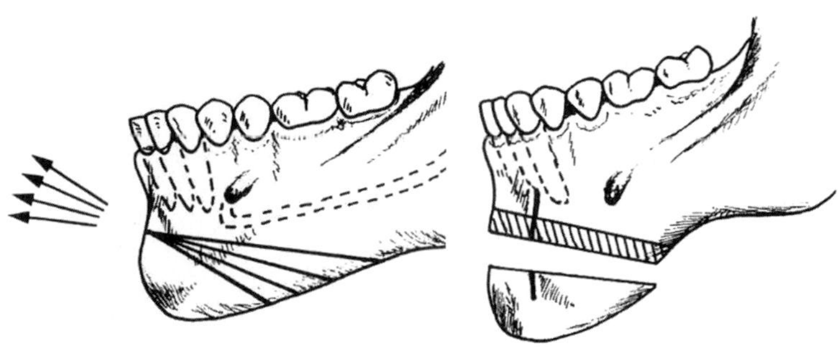

Figure 5.35. Possible osteotomy designs. Reprinted with permission from Quintessence Publishing Co., Inc. (Ref. 1). Copyright © 2003 Quintessence Publishing Co., Inc.

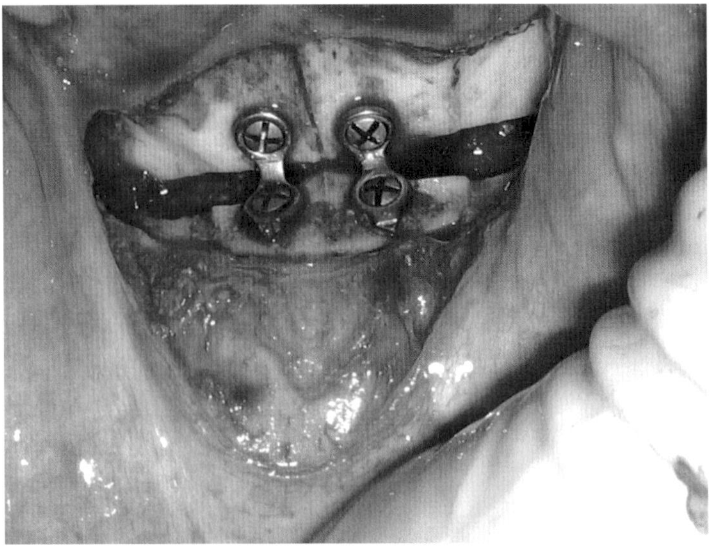

Figure 5.36. Preferred fixation of advancement genioplasty to prevent palpability of hardware.

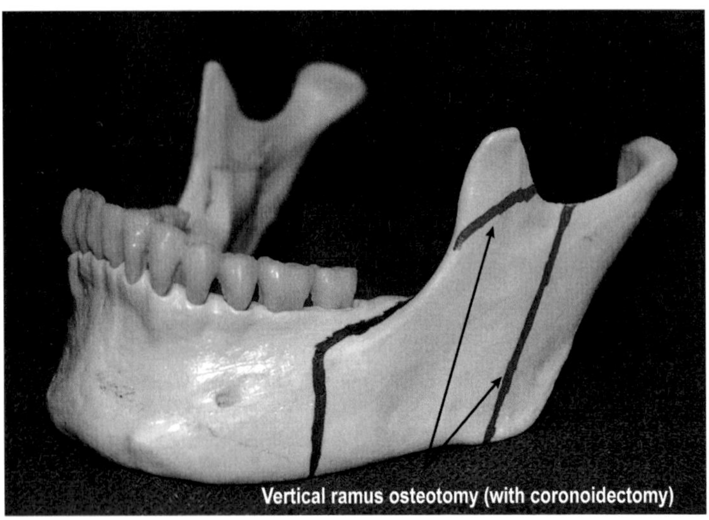

Figure 5.37.

- A vertical cut is made from the sigmoid notch to the inferior border, paralleling the posterior border of the ramus.
- The mandible is set back, and the patient is kept in intermaxillary fixation for 2 to 4 weeks. The osteotomies can also be rigidly fixated.

- Le Fort III osteotomy (Figure 5.38): the Le Fort III osteotomy is useful in cases where inferior orbital rim and nasal projection is needed. It may be safely combined with a Le Fort I osteotomy in the same procedure to achieve a better occlusion. The bony orbital rim position may be treatment-planned and referenced at surgery with a dental splint.
  - Draw coronal incision with zig-zag pattern in temporal regions.
  - Infiltrate local anesthetic with epinephrine into scalp and maxillary buccal vestibule.
  - Elevate the coronal flap in the subperiosteal plane, exposing zygomatic arches; medial, inferior, and lateral orbital walls; and

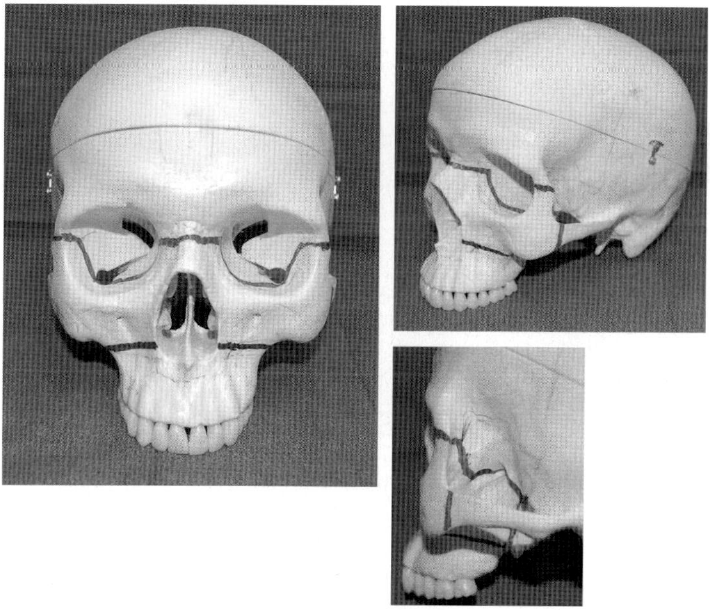

Figure 5.38. Le Fort III osteotomy.

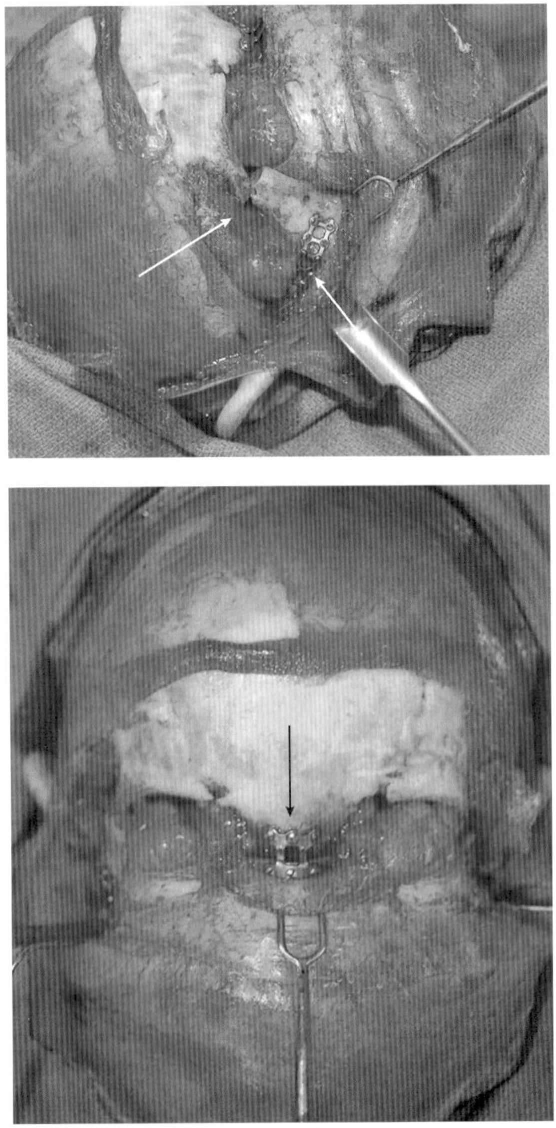

Figure 5.39. Coronal exposure with nasofrontal, zygomaticofrontal, and zygomatic arch osteotomies.

nasofrontal junction. Do not detach the medial canthal tendons (Figure 5.39).
- Osteotomize zygomatic arch at its most anterior aspect on both sides.
- Perform lateral orbital wall cut with reciprocating saw from inferior orbital fissure to zygomaticofrontal suture.
- Use chisel to perform orbital floor cut from inferior orbital fissure to medial wall, posterior to the posterior lacrimal crest.
- Identify anterior ethmoidal foramen of medial orbital wall (to mark the distinction between intracranial and extracranial), and make a nasofrontal cut with saw below this level.
- Perform medial wall osteotomy with chisel, connecting the nasofrontal cut with the floor osteotomy.
- Make maxillary vestibular incision if Le Fort I is planned or bilateral posterior incisions if an isolated Le Fort III osteotomy is planned.
- Perform pterygomaxillary dysjunction.
- Divide septum with curved Mayo scissors.
- Finally, from the coronal approach, separate the facial skeleton from the cranium in the midline with a chisel.
- Down-fracture the facial skeleton with the aid of Rowe disimpaction forceps. Mobilize completely.
- Apply splint and intermaxillary fixation.
- Place rigid fixation at arches and nasofrontal area. Bone-graft to fill large gaps.
- Close coronal incision in standard fashion.

5.10 Postoperative Considerations

- Dexamethasone should be continued for 24 h.
- Postoperative antibiotics may be considered.
- The patient should continue to rinse with chlorhexidine 0.12% three times a day. The patient can also start brushing teeth as soon as possible.
- Postoperative intermaxillary fixation and splint retention vary among practitioners.

  - Postoperative intermaxillary fixation does not prevent relapse but may help achieve a more stable occlusal result. In most cases, guiding elastics at the canines and molars are all that is necessary, allowing early range of motion.
  - The final splint may be removed immediately at surgery if the occlusion is very stable. More commonly, it is retained for 2 to 4 weeks, and in the case of segmental osteotomies, 4 to 6 weeks.
- Surgical stability: based on a review of patients followed longitudinally at the University of North Carolina, the relative stability of the various surgical procedures can be organized as follows (Figure 5.40)[2]:

- Postoperative sequelae.
  - After Le Fort I osteotomy:
    - Improved nasal breathing is expected due to widening of the alar base.
    - No more sinus disease than in the general population.
    - Return of sensory distribution of the infraorbital nerve is expected within 1 month.
    - Velopharyngeal insufficiency is rare after Le Fort I advancement and, when it occurs, usually resolves within 3 to 6 months. The cleft case with borderline velopharyngeal closure preoperatively may be more problematic.

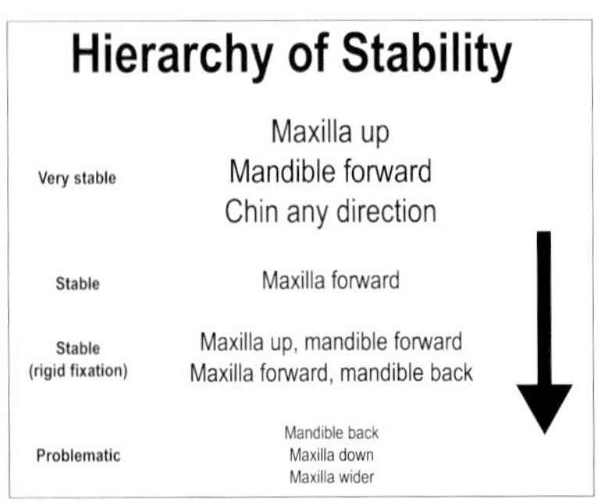

Figure 5.40.

- After BSSO:
  - Sensory loss in the distribution of the inferior alveolar nerve is almost universal immediately postoperatively, with return of function usually within 3 to 6 months. Little improvement is expected after 1 year.
  - Although a small percentage will have improvement and a small percentage will have worsening, most patients will have no change in TMJ symptoms.

5.11 Complications

- Preoperative.
  - Errors in treatment planning.
  - Poor orthodontic preparation.
- Intraoperative.
  - Unfavorable fracture or "bad splits" (Figure 5.41).
  - Hemorrhage.
  - Nerve transection.
- Postoperative.
  - Infection.
  - Failure of fixation.

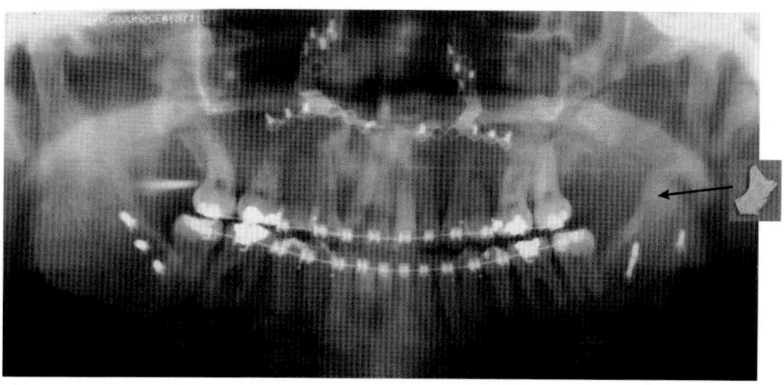

Figure 5.41. Buccal plate fracture of proximal segment after BSSO.

- Devitalization of teeth.
- Avascular necrosis.
- Persistent paresthesia/anesthesia.
- Temporomandibular disorder.
- Malocclusion.
- Nonunion/malunion.
- Condylar resorption.
- Vascular.
  - Secondary hemorrhage: usually occurs approximately 1 week after Le Fort I osteotomy. Requires initial treatment with nasal packing and, often, interventional embolization of maxillary artery.
  - Carotid cavernous fistula.
- Relapse.
- Unfavorable esthetic result.
- Epiphora.
  - Damage to nasolacrimal apparatus.
  - Corneal abrasion.
- Blindness.
- Facial nerve paralysis.

5.12 Conclusion

- Knowledge of dental anatomy and occlusion, facial and cephalometric analyses, and basic orthodontic principles is a prerequisite for the orthognathic surgeon (see Table 5.1).
- In addition to a good orthodontic setup, good results with orthognathic surgery begin with accurate patient records, and correct diagnosis and treatment planning (Figure 5.42).
- Vertical and transverse relationships must be carefully assessed, as correction of these discrepancies will have a profound effect on sagittal (profile view) relationships (Figure 5.43).
- Upper incisor position is the key to treatment planning in two-jaw cases.

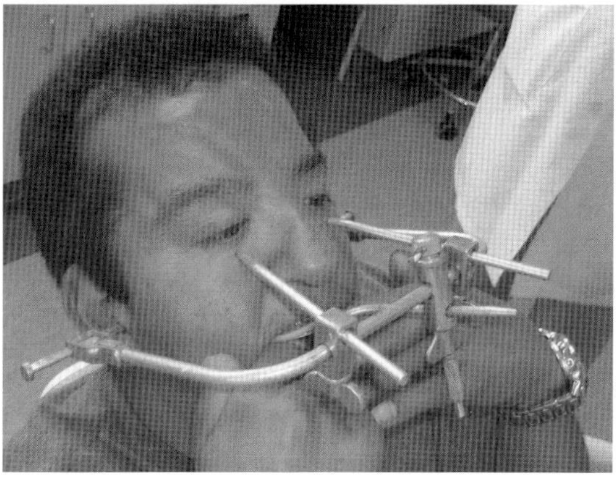

Figure 5.42. Facebow with infraorbital markers to reference inferior orbital rims to aid in model surgery.

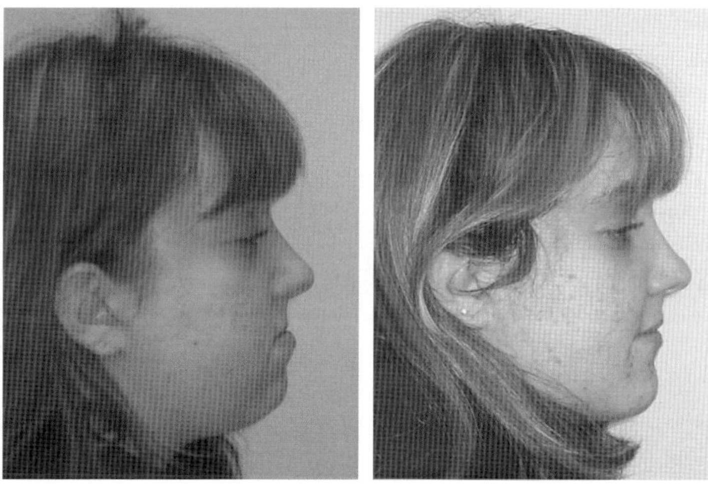

(A) (B)

Figure 5.43. Patient with Crouzon's disease (A) before and (B) after modified Le Fort III osteotomy and genioplasty.

- Cephalometric analysis should be considered an adjunct to orthognathic surgery treatment planning.
- Technical tips.
  - For Le Fort I osteotomy, make sure the condyles are well seated in the fossa when positioning the maxilla before fixation to avoid postoperative openbites.
  - For BSSO, make sure the buccal vertical osteotomy traverses the inferior border. Ensure neutral positioning of condyles, and trim segments accordingly before fixation.
  - For genioplasty, make sure cuts are made 5 mm below the apices of the teeth and mental foramina. Make sure osteotomy traverses the inferior border laterally.

Table 5.1. A Historical Timeline of Various Orthognathic Surgery Innovations and Techniques.

Contributor	Location	Year	Contribution
Simon Hullihen, MD	United States	1849	Described mandibular anterior subapical osteotomy
David Cheever, MD	United States	1867	First Le Fort I osteotomy for tumor resection (patient died)
Edward Angle, MD, DDS	United States	1898	Classification of occlusion that bears his name
Villa Blair, MD	United States	1906	Body ostectomy
		1907	Horizontal osteotomy of ascending ramus via extraoral approach with Gigli saw
Günther Cohn-Stock, MD, DMD	Germany	1921	First maxillary anterior segmental osteotomy
		1927	First to document Le Fort I osteotomy for correction of malocclusion
George Axhausen, MD, DMD	Germany	1934	Le Fort I osteotomy with postoperative elastic traction
Martin Wassmund, MD, DMD	Germany	1935	Maxillary anterior segmental osteotomy variant

(Continued)

Table 5.1. *(Continued)*

Contributor	Location	Year	Contribution
Varaztad Kazanjian, MD, DMD	United States	1937	Beveled mandibular horizontal osteotomy via extraoral approach
Karl Schuchardt, MD, DMD	Germany	1942	Described precursor variant of the sagittal split osteotomy via intraoral approach
		1942	Pterygomaxillary dysjunction for Le Fort I osteotomy
Sir Harold Gillies, MD	England	1942	Performed first Le Fort III osteotomy
Otto Hofer, MD, DMD	Germany	1944	Extraoral genioplasty
R. Trauner, MD, DMD	Switzerland	1955	Described sagittal split osteotomy; Obwegeser's teacher
Hugo Obwegeser, MD, DMD*	Switzerland	1957	Intraoral sliding genioplasty
G. Dal Pont, MD, DMD	Germany	1961	Placed buccal corticotomy of sagittal split osteotomy further anteriorly
S. Wunderer, MD, DMD	Germany	1962	Maxillary anterior segmental osteotomy variant
Hugo Obwegeser, MD, DMD*	Switzerland	1965	First two-jaw surgery
Hans Luhr, MD	Germany	1967	Introduced rigid fixation to the maxillofacial skeleton
Paul Tessier, MD	France	1967	Father of craniofacial surgery, refined the Le Fort III osteotomy
E. Hunsuck, MD, DMD	Germany	1968	Modified medial corticotomy of sagittal split osteotomy to end just posterior to the lingula instead of to posterior border

(Continued)

Table 5.1. *(Continued)*

Contributor	Location	Year	Contribution
William Bell, DDS	United States	1975	Presented biologic basis for maxillary and mandibular osteotomies
Chad Gordon, DO[10,11]	United States	2011	Introduction of orthognathic principles and practice to Le Fort-based facial transplantation

*Perhaps the most influential surgeon in the field of orthognathic surgery.

Reference

1. **Reyneke JP.** *Essentials of Orthognathic Surgery.* Chicago, IL: Quintessence Publishing Company, Inc; 2003.
2. **Bailey LJ, Cevidanes LHS, Proffit WR.** Stability and predictability of orthognathic surgery. *Am J Orthod Dentofacial Orthop* 2004;126:273–277.
3. **Betts NJ, Turvey TA.** *Oral and Maxillofacial Surgery: Orthognathic Surgery.* Vol. 2. Philadelphia, PA: WB Saunders; 2000.
4. **Fuller JL, Denehy GE.** Concise Dental Anatomy and Morphology. 2nd edn. St. Louis, MO: Mosby Year-book Inc; 1984.
5. **Posnick JC.** *Craniofacial and Maxillofacial Surgery in Children and Young Adults.* Philadelphia, PA: WB Saunders; 2000.
6. **Precious DS, Lanigan DT.** *Oral and Maxillofacial Surgery Clinics of North America: Risks and Benefits of Orthognathic Surgery.* Philadelphia, PA: WB Saunders; 1997.
7. **Proffit WR, White RP, Sarver DM.** *Contemporary Treatment of Dentofacial Deformity.* St. Louis, MO: Mosby; 2002.
8. **Vachiramon A et al.** A novel model surgery technique for Le Fort III advancement. *J Craniofac Surg* 2007;18:1230–1235.
9. **Xia JJ, Gateno J, Teichgraeber JF.** New clinical protocol to evaluate craniomaxillofacial deformity and plan surgical correction. *J Oral Maxillofac Surg* 2009;67:2093–2106.
10. **Gordon CR, Susarla S, Peacock Z, Cetrulo C, Zins J, Papay F, Kaban L, Yaremchuk MJ.** Osteocutaneous maxillofacial allotransplantation: Lessons learned from a novel cadaver study applying orthognathic principles and practice. *Plast Reconstr Surg* 2011;128(5):465–479.
11. **Gordon CR, Susarla S, Peacock Z, Kaban L, Yaremchuk MJ.** Lefort-based maxillofacial transplantation: Current state-of-the-art and refined technique. *J Craniofacial Surg* 2012;23(1):81–87.

ORTHOGNATHIC SURGERY PART II: COMMON PATTERNS OF DENTOFACIAL DEFORMITIES AND CASE STUDIES

6

Jeffrey C. Posnick, DMD, MD
and Neil Agnihotri, DMD, MD

6.1 Definition and Prevalence of Dentofacial Deformities

The term *dentofacial deformity* refers to significant deviations from normal proportions of the maxillomandibular complex that also have a negative impact on the interrelationship of maxillary and mandibular dentition. The affected individual will have varied degrees of compromise in head and neck functions, including breathing, swallowing, speech articulation, chewing, lip closure/posture, and facial aesthetics. Effects on the temporomandibular joints (TMJs), the periodontium, and the teeth themselves may also occur. The presenting facial dysmorphology will in general have at least some effect on psychosocial health.

Surgery to reposition the jaws (orthognathic procedures) as part of a team approach for the correction of dentofacial deformities is recommended to manage the skeletal, dental, and soft tissue dysmorphology. Speech therapy, dental work, orthodontics, or surgical procedures alone are inadequate as isolated treatment modalities. For the experienced surgeon and orthodontist, the accurate diagnosis of a dentofacial deformity will usually be clear after the initial examination and review of standard records.[1–7] The favorable correction through a combination of effective orthodontic alignment of the teeth combined with precise surgical repositioning of the jaw (or jaws) will be beneficial.

According to published epidemiologic studies in both the United States and the United Kingdom, it seems as though 5% of the population at a minimum will have a dentofacial deformity with a severe malocclusion requiring jaw surgery for full correction.[8–10] It is likely that as many as 20% of individuals presenting for orthodontic assessment would ideally require not just orthodontics but jaw straightening procedures.[8–10]

6.2 Heredity, Developmental Influences, and Other Etiologic Factors

Knowing the etiology of a dentofacial deformity can be important in the fundamental understanding of how and when to treat the problem. Knowledge of any associated conditions (e.g., hemifacial microsomia with cervical spine anomalies) is useful both to limit complications during treatment and for the family's planning issues. With an understanding of the natural history of the condition, occasionally an opportunity to prevent or at least lessen the deformity may arise. Knowing how the muscles within the neck and face affect the development of a dentofacial deformity as well as head and neck function is also important.[11,12] Factors that are known to both cause and alter dentofacial deformities can be subdivided as follows:

- Known syndromes and anomalies with dentofacial deformities;
  - deficiencies of midline structures
  - deficiencies/anomalies of neural crest origin
  - clefting of the lip and palate
  - achondroplasia

  - premature suture closure of the cranial vault and skull base
  - overgrowth syndrome or anomalies
- environmental and neuromotor effects on skeletal growth;
- muscle and soft tissue effects on skeletal growth;
- respiratory patterns and effects on skeletal growth;
- congenital myopathies and effects on skeletal growth;
- hereditary tendencies in the development of dentofacial deformities;
- effects of trauma on skeletal growth;
- effects of tumors/growths on skeletal growth.

6.3 Nasal Airway Considerations

At the time of orthognathic surgery, the surgeon has an opportunity to further contribute to the patient's quality of life by simultaneously addressing long-standing breathing and sinus drainage difficulties that may coexist with the jaw deformity. Preexisting breathing difficulties may range from isolated symptomatic nasal airway obstruction to obstructive sleep apnea (OSA), and should not be overlooked.[13–19] The frequency of combined nasal obstruction and maxillary deformity has been recognized and discussed in the published literature for more than 100 years.[20]

Nasal airway deformities (septal deviation, inferior turbinate enlargement, constricting pyriform apertures, and elevated nasal floor) commonly coexist with maxillary deformity.[17] Favorable access to the nasal septum, inferior turbinates, pyriform apertures, and nasal floor to correct these airway obstructions/deformities is possible through the Le Fort I (down-fracture) osteotomy commonly used in orthognathic surgery.[17] There is both animal experimental and human clinical research to support a link between oral (mouth) respiration, open-mouth posture, and the development of maxillomandibular disharmonies.[11,12,19,20] Using rhesus monkeys as an experimental model, Harvold *et al.* completely blocked the nares in newborn monkeys.[11,12] They observed consistent facial morphologic changes that gradually occur with growth in the presence of a constant open-mouth, protruding-tongue mandibular posture.[11,12] In human children who have significant nasal obstruction, clinical observational studies document a similar chronic downward and backward posture of the mandible.[19] Over several years, the affected children develop what we now recognize as a long face growth pattern.[21] This is documented by a measurable vertically long and horizontal retrusive maxillomandibular dysmorphic growth.[22]

Posnick *et al.* documented that, when indicated, simultaneous management of the maxillary jaw deformity (Le Fort I osteotomy) and intranasal pathology (septoplasty, reduction of inferior turbinates, widening the nasal aperture, and recontouring of the nasal floor) is effective for the symptomatic relief of nasal airway obstruction.[17] The complication rate for the intranasal procedures and Le Fort I osteotomy when completed simultaneously are minimal and not higher than expected when each procedure is carried out as an isolated event.[17]

6.4 Temporomandibular Disorders: Effects of Occlusion, Orthodontics, and Surgery

The prevalence of temporomandibular disorders (TMDs) in the general population as reported in the literature varies widely. It is estimated that an average of 32% of the population reports at least one symptom of TMD, and an average of 55% demonstrates at least one clinical sign.[22–24] TMD includes various symptoms and signs of the TMJ, masticatory muscles, and related structures. This may include a spectrum of referred head and neck pain, joint noise (popping, clicking, crepitus), reduced or altered mandibular movement (muscle spasm or disk displacement with or without reduction), condylar head erosion, and pain on direct palpation of either the TMJ or the masticatory muscles. Occlusal factors (degrees of malocclusion) are often claimed to be associated with TMD.[22–24] Interestingly, studies document that correcting a baseline jaw deformity with malocclusion through orthodontics and orthognathic surgery improves the presenting TMD in most treated patients, although a minority get worse.[25]

6.5 Psychosocial Considerations

Individuals presenting with a dentofacial deformity are not a monolithic group. They might arrive for evaluation in childhood, adolescence, or any time in adulthood. The etiology of the jaw deformity may be congenital, developmental, posttraumatic, or post-tumor resection with or without combined radiation therapy. A combination of orthodontic treatment and orthognathic (jaw straightening) surgery, often in conjunction with additional dental rehabilitation, may be required to correct the dysmorphology, improve head and neck function, enhance facial aesthetics, or restore the dentition.

The initial discussion concerning the need for orthognathic surgery may come as a shock to a patient and the family. They may have inaccurate preconceived ideas about the surgery and expected convalescence. The decision-making role of the parents and compliance (attitude) of the adolescent will also be important. Any dysfunctional family interactions at this moment of stress will also come into play. From the adolescent patient's point of view, social interactions with his or her peers and concerns about the interpretation (by others) of any change in their appearance as well as their evolving self-image and identity will also carry weight in ways that are ongoing and somewhat unpredictable.[26]

6.6 Treatment Planning: Achieving Form and Function and the Importance of the Direct Visual Examination

Clinicians who are asked to correct a dentofacial deformity must direct their attention to both form and function. As Buckminster Fuller stated, rarely are the two objectives (i.e, form and function) divergent. In the achievement of a harmonious face, attention must also be directed toward the practical objectives of improving the upper airway, occlusion, speech, and deglutination. Facial aesthetic perfection is not a specific millimeter distance or degree of angulation but a visual impression at conversational distance in 3-dimensional life. At the same time, neither "divine proportions" as described by Euclid nor biologic realities (circulation requirements for wound healing) nor the individual's personal preferences can be ignored in the process.[27–29]

At the time of the preoperative face-to-face planning examination of the patient by the operating surgeon, several evaluations will have already been carried out. Review of all relevant medical and dental records, photographic, radiographic, and dental studies and analysis should be fresh in mind. The patient is examined while upright and sitting in the natural head position (NHP). The teeth are in centric relation and the lips are relaxed. The NHP is considered the most rational, physiologic, and anatomic orientation for evaluating the face, jaws, and teeth.[28] The patient is also viewed by the surgeon from different perspectives during facial animation. In a patient with a dentofacial deformity, a global overview of the head and neck should include consideration of:

1. Symmetry and harmony of the upper facial skeleton (i.e, cranial vault, orbits, nasofrontal process, and zygomatic arches).
2. Quality of the overlying soft tissue envelope of the head and neck (i.e, hypoplasia, hyperplasia, effects of trauma and aging); recognition of distortions versus intrinsic anomalies of the soft tissues.
3. The unique facial aesthetic units (i.e, external nose, external ears, periorbital soft tissues).
4. Symmetry and harmony of the lower facial skeleton (maxilla, mandible, chin).
5. History of cervical spine symptoms and signs and current neck range of motion.
6. History of TMJ symptoms and signs (TMDs) and current mandibular range of motion.
7. Dental rehabilitative needs including but not limited to orthodontic progress.

6.7 Detailed Maxillomandibular Surgical Planning

Confirming that the upper facial skeleton and the soft tissue envelope of the head and neck do not require surgical attention and that the neck and mandibular range of motion are intact without significant limitations is essential before focusing on detailed maxillomandibular surgical planning. Qualitative decisions concerning which components of the maxillomandibular skeleton are asymmetric or disproportionate, or both, and thus require surgical repositioning, will have already been discussed with the patient/family and other treating clinicians but are now reconfirmed.

Assuming that both the maxilla and mandible are part of the dentofacial deformity that requires surgical reconstruction (two-jaw surgery), quantitative decisions (to the millimeter) of the preferred aesthetic and desired functional repositioning of the upper jaw (at the time of Le Fort I osteotomy) must first be made. When thinking through the details of maxillary (surgical) repositioning, it is understood that the upper jaw (in two-jaw surgery) will serve as the platform on which the mandible is to be placed. The outcome for the lower jaw will then depend entirely on the new (surgical) position of the maxilla and the orthodontic alignment of the teeth. Concerning the maxilla, the surgeon makes eight basic quantitative (to the millimeter) decisions (assessments):

1. Assess current and preferred horizontal position of the maxillary incisor crown.
2. Assess current and preferred vertical position of the maxillary incisor crown.
3. Reconfirm advantage of (need for) segmentation of the maxilla to achieve preferred arch form.
4. Assess current and preferred A-point to B-point relationship of the jaws. Determine the need to alter the posterior (vertical) maxillary height (maxillary plane change) to achieve objectives (pitch orientation).
5. Assess the baseline chin morphology. Anticipate location of pogonion after jaw repositioning. Consider advantages of genioplasty and the preferred horizontal and vertical position of the chin.
6. Assess the baseline pyriform rims/floor of the nose/anterior nasal spine morphology. Anticipate their location after maxillary repositioning and any advantages of recontouring the pyriform rims/floor of the nose/ANS to achieve objectives.

7. Assess the presence of any maxillary cant (role orientation) in comparison with the upper face. Determine the preferred upper jaw repositioning to correct a baseline cant.
8. Assess current and preferred position of the maxillary dental midline in comparison with the upper facial midline (yaw orientation). Anticipate any potential yaw effect of the new (surgical) maxillary position on the mandible and face.

6.8 Analytic Model Planning and Splint Construction

Orthognathic reconstruction, unlike most surgical procedures, involves precise preoperative dental and aesthetic preparation. The surgeon carries out a detailed face-to-face examination combined with a facial photographic and radiographic analysis. Immediate presurgical records include current and accurate dental impressions of the maxilla and mandibule, bite registration in centric relation, face bow registration for transfer to a semiadjustable articulator, and specific facial measurements. The dental models are placed on a semiadjustable articulator using the face bow and centric relation bite registrations. This information is used for further analysis and completion of the model planning. Acrylic splints are fabricated and used intraoperatively to further ensure the reliable execution of predetermined facial aesthetic and functional objectives. Although clinical decisions concerning the preferred aesthetic positioning of the jaws in the operating room remains both an art and a science, the technical aspect of model planning should be precise and consistent. Model planning with the use of prefabricated splints continues to be the standard of care for bimaxillary and segmental maxillary osteotomies.[30]

6.9 The Basic Orthognathic Procedures

Maxillofacial surgeons and orthodontists are the primary clinicians caring for individuals with jaw deformities/malocclusion and the associated facial dysmorphology. When orthognathic reconstruction is indicated, the surgeon generally uses a limited number of surgical techniques to facilitate the 3-dimensional repositioning of the skeletal units (maxilla, mandible, and chin) to achieve improvements in head and neck function and to enhance facial aesthetics.[31,32] By and large, these options include the Le Fort I (type) osteotomy with or without segmentation of the down-fractured maxilla, sagittal split osteotomies of the ramus of the mandible, and an oblique osteotomy of the chin. These three basic procedures and fixation techniques were described by Hugo Obwegeser and Hans Luhr respectively and have evolved gradually to their current usage.[31]

By understanding details for the safe execution of maxillary (Le Fort I), mandibular (sagittal splitting of the ramus), and chin (osteoplastic genioplasty) osteotomies, each skeletal unit may be precisely repositioned during one operation.[31,32] Other simultaneous adjunctive procedures, such as septoplasty, reduction of inferior turbinates, recontouring of the pyriform rims, removal of wisdom teeth, or neck soft tissue procedure (i.e, cervical flap elevation, neck deflattening, and platysma muscle placation), are routinely and safely performed when indicated to improve head and neck function (e.g., occlusion, chewing, speech articulation, swallowing, breathing, lip closure) and to achieve the desired facial refinements.[17,31,33,34] Special circumstances and unusual anatomy require variations in these techniques, but developing a standard surgical approach limits morbidity and increases the efficiency of treatment.[29,35]

6.10 Complications Associated with Orthognathic Surgery

An unavoidable fact of clinical practice is that no matter how accurate the diagnosis and how meticulous the surgeon, complications will occur after orthognathic procedures.[29,35,36] By understanding the nature of the presenting dentofacial deformity, the patient-specific risk factors, any associated conditions/malformations, unique psychosocial aspects, and any current head and neck dysfunction, complications can be minimized. The probability of perioperative problems can be understood and should be presented to the patient and family for consideration before treatment. In addition to executing precise orthognathic procedures, achieving informed consent and accomplishing patient education are also essential components of comprehensive care.

6.11 Malocclusion After Orthodontics and Orthognathic Surgery

There are inherent limitations to both orthodontic tooth movement and surgical repositioning of the jaws (and jaw segments) imposed by the alveolar bone and the soft tissue envelope surrounding the facial skeleton.[29,35] Malocclusion after orthognathic surgery and orthodontic treatment is one potential adverse consequence if the biologic boundaries are not respected. This includes mechanical/technical aspects of the tooth and bone repositioning, initial healing requirements, and difficulties associated with a long-term stability of the mechanically relocated teeth, jaws, and jaw segments. Adhering to basic biomechanical principles and with clinical experience, the frequent patterns of dentofacial deformities with malocclusion can be safely and reliably corrected and maintained in most cases. The vector changes of the jaws, jaw segments, and teeth that are more prone to relapse are known, and so are many of their reasons.[37,38] Each orthodontic tooth movement and maxillary and/or mandibular osteotomy and proposed vector change has unique nuances that may require special considerations (e.g., flap design, osteotomy design, flap mobilization, interpositional grafting needs, fixation requirements, splint management and retention options) to achieve and maintain the results. These and other considerations should be incorporated into the treatment plan from the outset.

6.12 Common Patterns of Dentofacial Deformities

6.12.1 *Primary mandibular deficiency growth pattern with or without arch-width discrepancy*

Mandibular deficiency is the most prevalent form of dentofacial deformity (Case study: Patient 1; Figure 6.1).[10] It is more common in whites than in blacks or Asians, suggesting that a hereditary component is a predominant part of the etiology. Mandibular deficiency frequently presents with a degree of maxillary constriction that will also require correction.[39] Functional aspects may include articulation errors in speech and swallowing difficulties resulting from the Angle class II excess overjet malocclusion. Difficulties with chewing during the day and upper airway

Case Study: Patient 1

A 33-year-old woman presented to the surgeon (J.C.P.) for evaluation of a long-standing dentofacial deformity with malocclusion. By the early teenage years, it was known that she had a jaw deformity characterized by mandibular deficiency with a class II excess overjet malocclusion. She was treated by an orthodontist with growth modification techniques (twin block) but without successful "stimulation" of the mandible. She then underwent camouflage orthodontics, including maxillary bicuspid extractions with retraction of the anterior dentition and proclination of the mandibular incisors to improve the overjet relationship. Despite several years of treatment, a molar class II excess overjet malocclusion remained.

She presented to an orthodontist for further correction of the occlusion and in the hope of achieving an improved profile. She was referred for surgical evaluation (J.C.P.) with a request for a "stronger profile" and relief of the double chin. Jaw, chin, and neck surgery in combination with lower bicuspid extractions and orthodontic decompensation was offered and accepted as a way to alleviate the symptoms and signs, and to enhance facial appearance. The surgery proposed and carried out included:

- bilateral sagittal split ramus osteotomies of the mandible,
- oblique osteotomy of the chin,
- neck liposuction.

The articulated dental casts of the model surgery planning indicate the vector changes planned and carried out:

- mandibular movements
  - 11-mm advancement at the incisors
- chin movements
  - horizontal advancement

Operative time was approximately 1.5 hours. No blood replacement was required. The patient was extubated in the operating room at the end of surgery. She remained in the hospital for 1

(*Continued*)

Case Study: Patient 1 (*Continued*)

night and was then discharged to the care of her husband. At the 2-week postoperative interval, she returned to work. At 5 weeks after surgery, she returned to a normal diet, physical activities (sports and gym), and her orthodontist's care. After orthodontic detailing, the appliances were removed (7 months postoperatively). She is shown before and 1 year after completion of treatment (Figure 6.1).

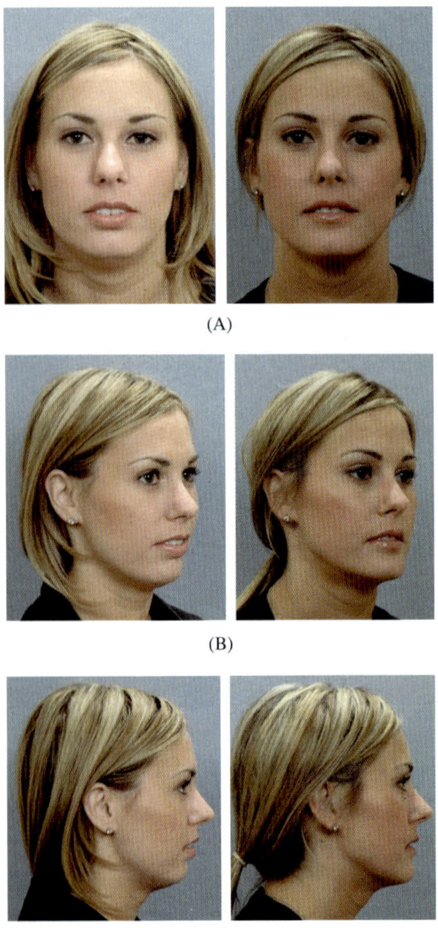

Figure 6.1. Patient 1. (A) Frontal facial views in repose before and after treatment. (B) Oblique facial views before and after treatment. (C) Profile facial views before and after treatment.

(D)

(E)

(F)

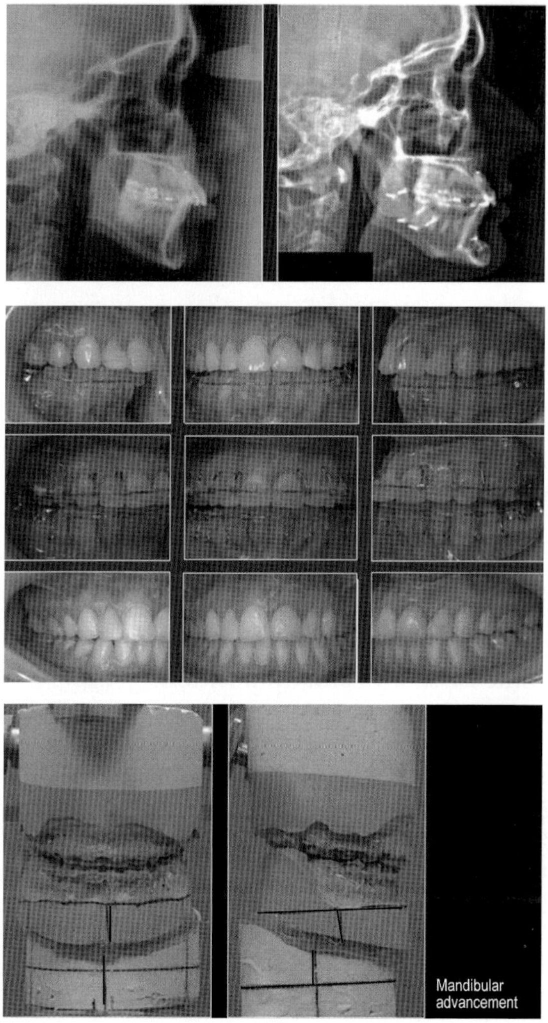

Figure 6.1. ***(Continued)*** (D) Lateral cephalometric views before and after treatment. (E) Occlusal views before redo orthodontics, immediately presurgery, and 1 year after completion of treatment. (F) Articulated dental casts of model surgery planning.

obstruction at night (retropositioned tongue) also occur.[13,14] A higher incidence of TMD resulting from the mandibular deficiency class II malocclusion is also common.[25] Clinical characteristics include a curled and everted lower lip with an accentuated labiomental fold. The angles of the mandible tend to be relatively square. There is a retruded weak chin with a convex profile. The deficient mandible gives the illusion of a large nose. There is a short chin-to-neck length and angle. This patient's clinical concerns tend to center on the unattractive lower lip contours and lack of prominence of the chin (weak profile).[39–41]

When a combined orthodontic and surgical approach is agreed to, the orthodontist removes dental compensations. Extraction of mandibular first bicuspids to create space for the correction of anterior crowding and avoidance of "flaring" (i.e, incisor procumbency) is frequently required. In addition to mandibular advancement, maxillary surgery is often required primarily to correct arch-width discrepancies.[39] Through the Le Fort I osteotomy, improvement in the upper lip–upper tooth relationship by alteration of the vertical height can be carried out simultaneously. Any deficiencies in the horizontal position of the maxilla can also be corrected. Intranasal procedures (septoplasty, inferior turbinate reduction) can be accomplished through the Le Fort I osteotomy if clinically indicated.[17] An oblique osteotomy of the chin with horizontal advancement is generally helpful to further improve profile aesthetics and lip position.[42]

6.12.2 *Asymmetric mandibular excess growth pattern*

The term *asymmetric mandibular excess* is useful for name recognition but falls short of explaining the cause and effects of this common pattern of jaw deformity.[43,44] It results in an uneven Angle class III malocclusion. The overall effect on mandibular morphology; the secondary deformities that it causes on the maxilla, chin, and teeth; and the distortions that are visually observed in the overlying soft tissue envelope are dependent on multiple factors. They include the intensity of the mandibular hyperactivity; the patient's age when the abnormal bone growth begins; any underlying hereditary dentofacial deformity tendency; and any treatment previously rendered (orthodontic, dental, or surgical) before the patient arrives to the maxillofacial surgeon for evaluation.

Obwegeser believes that this dentofacial deformity is caused by two different growth regulators.[44] The first one causes *hemimandibular hyperplasia.* This is a more rare form and is clinically characterized by an increasing volume of all parts of the affected side of the mandible but without resulting in a deviation of the midline of the chin to the opposite side. The second growth regulator causes the more common *hemimandibular elongation.* This dentofacial deformity is characterized by an elongation of all parts of the affected side of the mandible, often with widening at the gonial angle and with clear displacement of the midline of the chin and shifting of the mandibular midline to the opposite side of the face. In patients with asymmetric mandibular excess, skeletal scintigraphy (technetium Tc 99m bone scan) is a useful method to assess the state of residual mandibular excess growth.[45]

The perioperative orthodontic treatment should achieve the correct positioning of the teeth into the respective basal bone in each jaw. At the completion of presurgical orthodontic treatment, the position of the teeth and the alveolar bone should not hamper the ability of the surgeon to achieve maximum mirror-image skeletal symmetry, Euclidean facial proportions, and a preferred long-term stable condition.[1–7] In general, the presenting maxillomandibular deformities are best managed with classic orthognathic techniques carried out at skeletal maturity to improve both head and neck function and to enhance facial aesthetics.[31,45,46] This will include, at a minimum, sagittal split ramus osteotomies of the mandible. In general, the maxilla is secondarily deformed and will benefit from a Le Fort I osteotomy with 3-dimensional repositioning. An oblique osteotomy of the chin will likely further improve facial symmetry. The need for a high condylectomy remains limited and is considered only in the presence of significant, progressive, active disease at the time of diagnosis.[44]

6.12.3 *Long face growth pattern: Maxillary vertical excess with mandibular deformity*

The prevalence of long face growth patterns within a dentofacial deformity referral pattern is thought to be approximately 20 to 25% (Case study: Patient 2; Figures 6.2 and 6.3).[10] The diagnostic criteria for a long face growth pattern includes an excess anterior facial height

Case Study: Patient 2

A recent college graduate, aged 21 years, presented for evaluation of a long-standing dentofacial deformity with malocclusion and chronic obstructive nasal breathing. Since early childhood, she was known to have had difficulty breathing through her nose. Through her teenage years, a long face deformity with anterior open bite, significant overjet, and class II malocclusion developed. This was treated with camouflage orthodontics for 6 years (age 9–15), and included four bicuspid extractions in attempts to "close the open bite." No attention was paid to either the facial disproportion or her difficulty breathing through the nose. After removal of the orthodontic brackets and despite the use of retainers, the dental crowding and the anterior open bite recurred.

She presented for evaluation to the orthognathic surgeon (J.C.P.) with facial disproportion and head and neck dysfunctions including difficulty chewing, swallowing, speaking, breathing, and lip closure. There was a class II molar relationship, anterior open bite, excess positive overjet, and anterior dental crowding. Early periodontal and enamel deterioration was present. Physical examination also confirmed septal deviation and hypertrophic inferior turbinates with a tight nasal aperture, explaining the chronic obstructive nasal breathing symptoms. Jaw and intranasal surgery in combination with further orthodontic treatment was offered and accepted as a way to alleviate the symptoms and signs, and to enhance facial appearance. Single-stage simultaneous surgery proposed and carried out included:

- maxillary Le Fort I osteotomy in three segments;
- bilateral sagittal split ramus osteotomies of the mandible;
- oblique osteotomy of the chin;
- septoplasty;
- inferior turbinate reduction;
- recontouring of the nasal floor/rims/anterior nasal space.

(*Continued*)

Case Study: Patient 2 (*Continued*)

The articulated dental casts of the model surgery planning indicate the vector changes planned and carried out:

- maxillary movements
  - 5-mm advancement at the incisors
  - 5-mm vertical intrusion at the incisors
  - segmentation of the maxilla (three pieces) for arch expansion and correction of curve of Spee
  - 2-mm counterclockwise rotation of the maxillary plane
- mandibular movements
  - horizontal advancement
  - vertical shortening
  - counterclockwise rotation of the mandibular plane
- chin movements
  - vertical shortening
  - horizontal advancement

Surgery time was approximately 3 hours. No blood replacement was required. The patient was extubated in the operating room at the end of surgery. She remained in the hospital for 2 nights and was then discharged to the care of her parents. Two weeks after surgery, she returned to office-based work. At the 5-week postoperative interval, she returned to a normal diet, physical activities (sports and gym), and her orthodontist's care. After orthodontic detailing, the appliances were removed (6 months postoperatively). She is shown before and 4 years after completion of treatment (Figure 6.3).

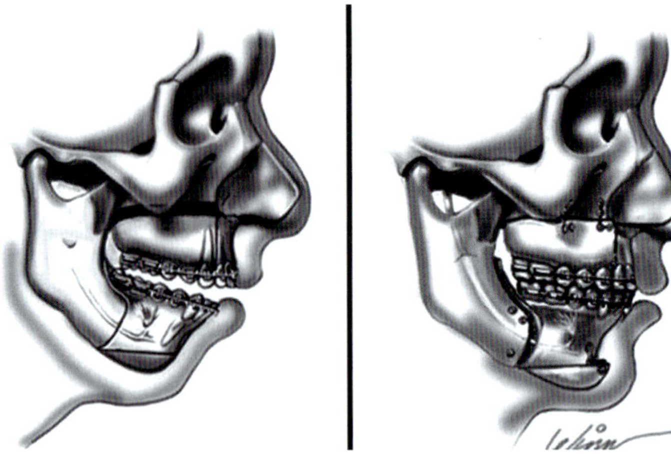

(A) (B)

Figure 6.2. llustrations, profile view, of long face growth pattern. (A) Indication of location of proposed osteotomies. (B) After completion of osteotomies and fixation. Reprinted with permission from Wolters Kluwer Health (Posnick JC, *et al.* Consequences and management of nasal airway obstruction in the dentofacial deformity patient. *Curr Opin Otolaryngol Head Neck Surg* 2010;18:323–331). Copyright © 2010 Wolters Kluwer Health Lippincott Williams & Wilkins.

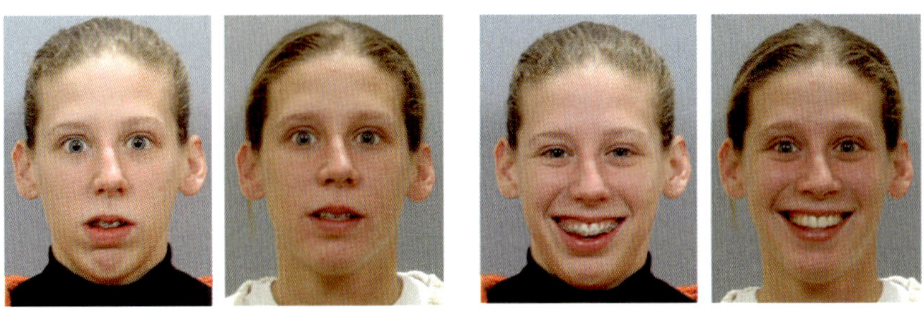

(A) (B)

Figure 6.3. Patient 2. (A) Frontal facial views in repose before and after treatment. (B) Frontal facial views with smile before and after treatment.

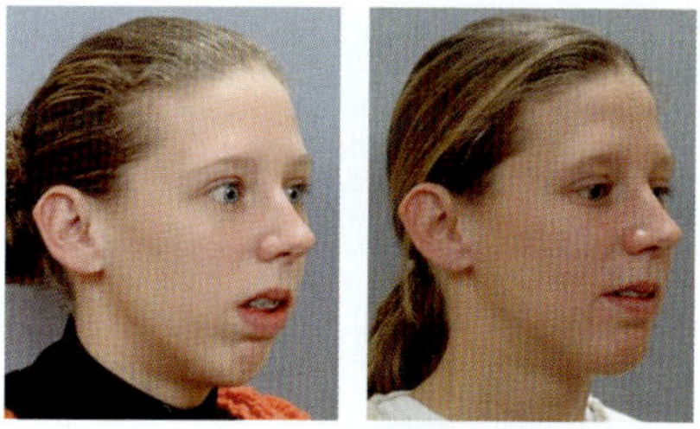

(C)

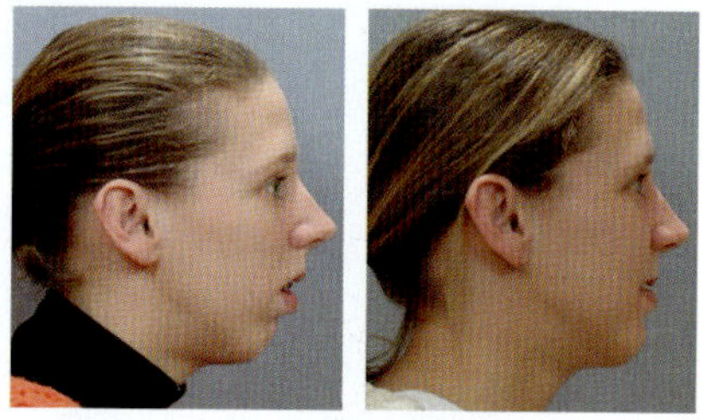

(D)

(E)

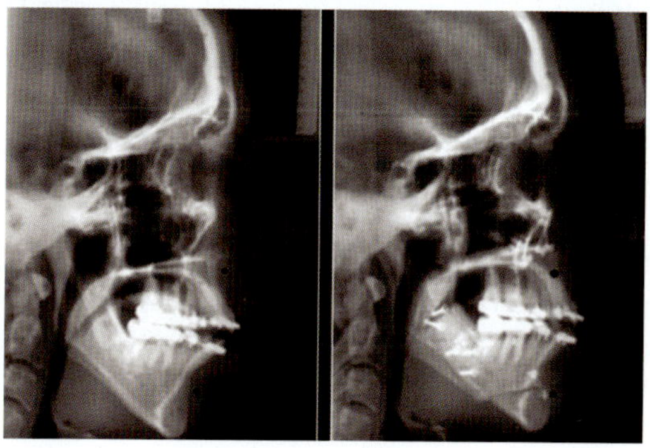

(F)

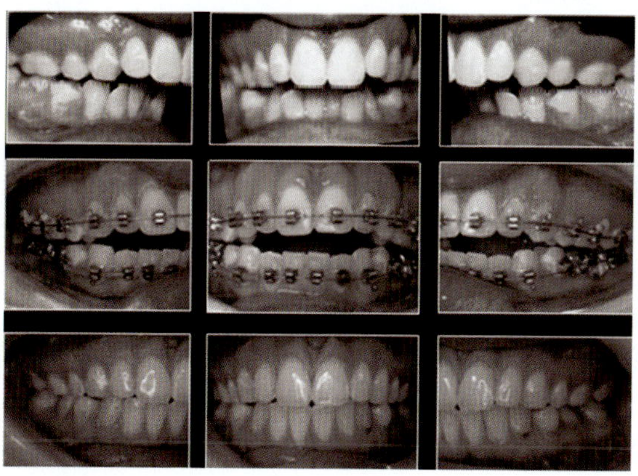

Figure 6.3. (***Continued***) (C) Oblique facial views before and after treatment. (D) Profile views before and after treatment. (E) Lateral cephalometric views indicating A-point and B-point position before and after treatment. (F) Occlusal views pre-redo orthodontics, immediately presurgery, and 4 years after completion of treatment.

(G)

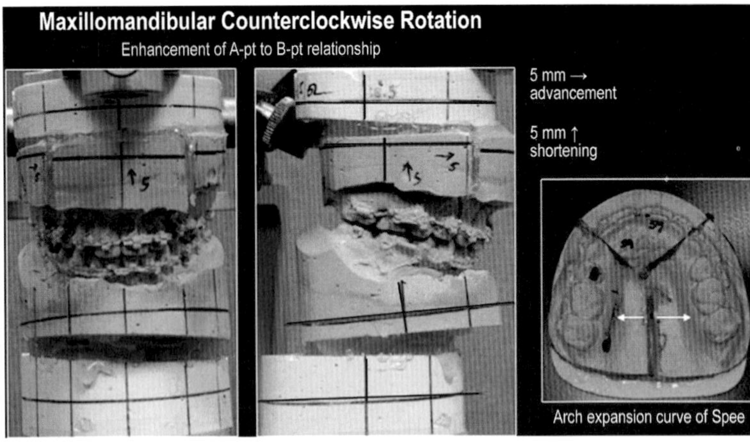

Figure 6.3. (***Continued***) (G) Articulated dental casts of model surgery planning. Reprinted with permission from Wolters Kluwer Health (Posnick JC, *et al.* Consequences and management of nasal airway obstruction in the dentofacial deformity patient. *Curr Opin Otolaryngol Head Neck Surg* 2010;18:323–331). Copyright © 2010 Wolters Kluwer Health — Lippincott Williams & Wilkins.

(primarily with elongation of the lower third) leading to disproportion between facial height and width.[21,46,47] This generally results from an excessive eruption of the posterior maxillary dentition. The increased lower facial height causes the mandible to rotate downward and backward. The excessive lower anterior facial height makes any baseline mandibular horizontal deficiency seem worse and any true mandibular excess seem better. Dental compensations result, and an anterior open bite is generally present. There is wide lip separation at rest, resulting in mentalis strain in attempts to achieve lip closure. Consistent radiographic findings in the long face condition include[21,46,47]:

- increased mandibular plane angle;
- increased total anterior facial height;
- decreased percentage of upper to lower facial height.

The perioperative orthodontic goals are to position the teeth solidly into alveolar housing within each arch. In the presence of arch-width constriction and excess curve of Spee, segmental orthodontics is preferred. This will be followed by effective segmental maxillary osteotomies.[38,47] The teeth will finally occlude appropriately only at the time of surgery. The surgical approach for the treatment of the classic long face deformity is best carried out through a combination of osteotomies including Le Fort I (often in segments), bilateral sagittal split ramus osteotomies of the mandible, and an oblique osteotomy of the chin.[45] If septoplasty, inferior turbinate reduction, and/or nasal floor recontouring is required to improve chronic obstructive nasal breathing, this is carried out simultaneously.[17] An important aspect of nasal aesthetics and airway management is to simultaneously recontour the floor of the nose, pyriform rims, and anterior nasal spine region through the exposure provided by the Le Fort I down-fracture. Anterior neck soft tissue procedures (i.e, cervical flap elevation, neck fact removal, and platysma placation) are carried out when indicated.[31]

The basic vector changes required in the maxilla to correct the long face growth pattern frequently include horizontal advancement, vertical shortening, transverse widening, and correction of the curve of Spee (to match the mandibular arch). Basic vector changes generally also incorporate counterclockwise rotation, especially of the mandibular plane as needed. This is to achieve a preferred A-point to B-point relationship when viewing the patient's profile in the NHP.[48,49] The immediate presurgical models will confirm details of any needed segmentation of the maxilla.

6.12.4 *Maxillary deficiency with relative mandibular excess (class III skeletal pattern)*

Class III skeletal problems are generally caused by a combination of maxillary deficiency and relative mandibular excess (Case study: Patient 3; Figure 6.4).[50–52] Through trial and error, it is now recognized that both growth modification in the preadolescent and camouflage treatment in a teenager or adult as methods of managing this

Case Study: Patient 3

A 20-year-old college student presented to the orthognathic surgeon (J.C.P.) for evaluation of a long-standing dentofacial deformity with malocclusion and chronic obstructive nasal breathing. Since the early teenage years, he was known to have a jaw deformity characterized by relative mandibular excess combined with maxillary deficiency. The occlusal consequence was a severe Angle class III negative overjet malocclusion. No previous orthodontic treatment had been carried out. At presentation, head and neck dysfunctions included difficulty with chewing, swallowing, speaking, breathing, and lip posture. Physical examination also confirmed septal deviation and hypertrophic inferior turbinates, explaining the chronic obstructive nasal breathing symptoms. Jaw and intranasal surgery in combination with perioperative orthodontics to remove dental compensations was offered and accepted as a way to alleviate the symptoms and signs and to enhance facial appearance. Single-stage simultaneous surgery proposed and carried out included:

- maxillary Le Fort I osteotomy;
- bilateral sagittal split osteotomies of the mandible;
- oblique osteotomy of the chin;
- septoplasty;
- inferior turbinate reduction;
- removal of impacted wisdom teeth.

The articulated dental casts of the model surgery planning indicate the vector changes planned and carried out:

- maxillary movements
  - 6-mm advancement at the incisors
  - 2-mm vertical lengthening at the incisors
  - 4-mm clockwise rotation of the maxillary plane
- mandibular movements
  - clockwise rotation of the mandibular plane

(*Continued*)

Case Study: Patient 3 (*Continued*)

- no change in horizontal position at the incisors
- chin movements
- vertical shortening

Operative time was approximately 3 hours. No blood replacement was required. The patient was extubated in the operating room at the end of surgery. He remained in the hospital for 2 nights and was then discharged to the care of his parents. He remained in the immediate area for 1 week before returning home (out of state). Two weeks after surgery he returned to school. At the end of the 5-week postoperative interval, he returned to a normal diet, physical activities (sports and gym), and his orthodontist's care. After orthodontic detailing, the appliances were removed 5 months postoperatively. He is shown before and 1 year after completion of treatment.

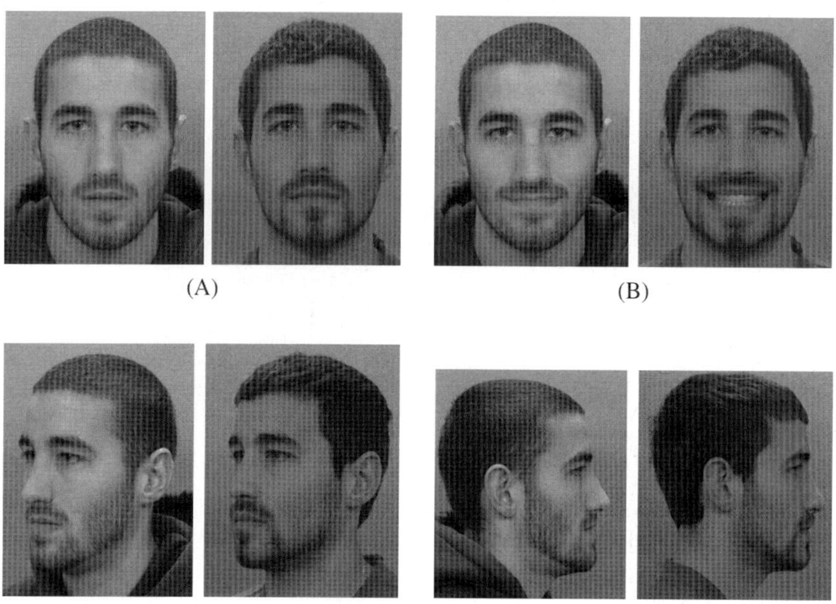

(A) (B) (C) (D)

Figure 6.4. Patient 3. (A) Frontal facial views in repose before and after treatment. (B) Frontal facial views with smile before and after treatment. (C) Oblique facial views before and after treatment. (D) Profile views before and after treatment.

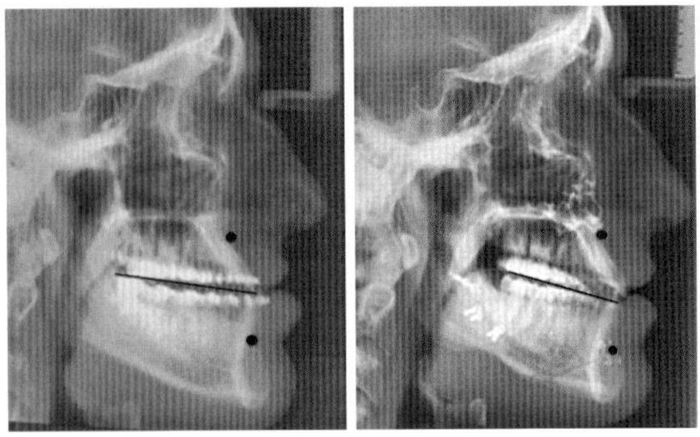

(E)

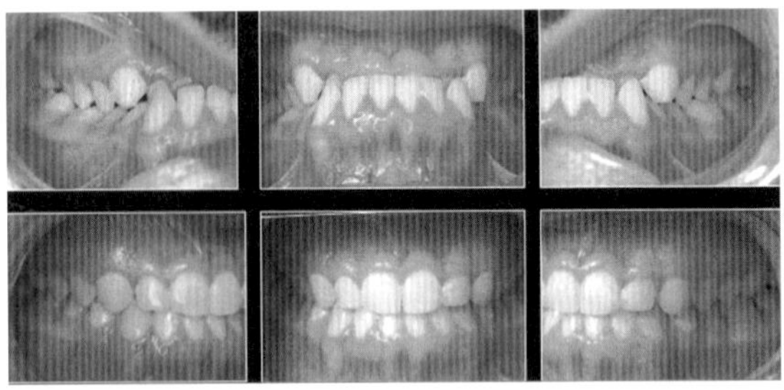

(F)

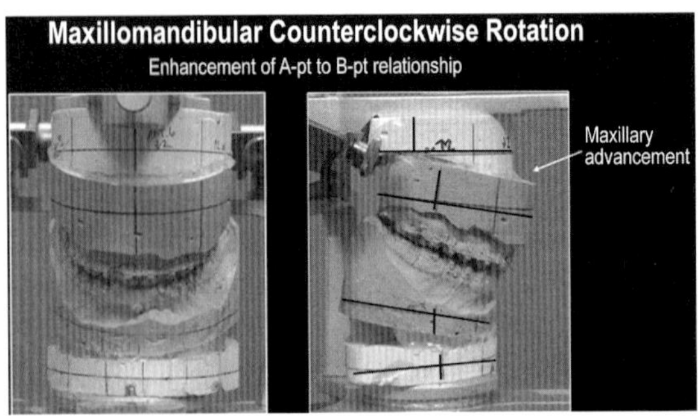

(G)

Figure 6.4. (*Continued*) (E) Lateral cephalometric views indicating A-point and B-point locations before and after treatments. (F) Occlusal views before treatment and 1 year after completion of treatment. (G) Articulated dental casts of model surgery planning. Reprinted with permission from Elsevier (Ref. 53). Copyright © 2006 American Association of Oral and Maxillofacial Surgeons. http://www.sciencedirect.com/science/journal/02782391.

type of dentofacial deformity are at best relatively ineffective.[35] In addition, even mild degrees of class III facial appearance are aesthetically noticeable as unattractive by the general population.

There is a strong family tendency for mandibular excess. The so-called Hapsburg jaw in the European Hapsburg royal family is well documented. Overall, the development of a class III jaw disharmony is multifactorial and complex. It may result from a combination of skeletal and dental features and from variations in magnitude, direction, and timing of facial growth. Individuals with this form of dentofacial deformity will frequently have functional impairments including articulation errors in speech, chronic obstructed nasal breathing, difficulty with swallowing and chewing, wide lip separation with excess effort required for lip seal, and detrimental long-term effects on the dentition and periodontium resulting from the malocclusion.

Classic clinical characteristics include long chin–neck length, protrusive chin with a prominent lower third of the face, reduced labiomental fold, sunken appearing midface and cheeks, and narrow alar base with paranasal flattening. Naturally occurring dental compensations often include mandibular incisors that are upright or lingually inclined, class III malocclusion, and a narrow maxillary arch with negative overjet. Radiographic findings are consistent with clinical observations and include maxillary horizontal deficiency, procumbent maxillary incisors, flat base of the nose, negative overjet, prognathic appearing mandible, and a dysmorphic bony chin.

The timing and sequencing of treatment is important. Actively growing individuals with mandibular excess can be expected to outgrow an early surgical correction and then require retreatment.[50] A reasonable method to assess growth maturation is through serial cephalometric tracings. Surgery is delayed until deceleration of growth can be documented. In most cases, this should *not* negate plans to complete treatment before graduation from high school.

Perioperative orthodontic objectives are to remove dental compensations. Bicuspid extractions in the maxillary arch may be indicated to provide necessary space to uncrowd and correct incisor inclination. Leveling of the mandibular arch is more straightforward. This classic dentofacial deformity will require at a minimum a Le Fort I osteotomy with horizontal advancement to achieve desirable facial aesthetics.[49,53] Typically, additional vector changes in the maxilla are preferred (e.g., transverse widening, vertical adjustment, clockwise maxillary plane rotation). Reconstruction is usually combined with sagittal split ramus osteotomies of the mandible to place the distal mandible into ideal occlusion consistent with the new maxillary location, and to achieve a preferred A-point to B-point position.[48,53] An osteotomy of the chin with horizontal or vertical change, or both, is also frequently desirable.[42] If chronic obstructive nasal breathing is present resulting from septal deviation or inferior turbinate hypertrophy, then these problems are simultaneously managed (septoplasty, inferior turbinate reduction) through the down-fracture Le Fort I osteotomy.[17] If the wisdom teeth are impacted and require removal for long-term dental health reasons, this can be carried out simultaneously.[33,34] The clinician's ability to communicate the potential risks, complications, alternative approaches, and benefits of the recommended treatment to the patient and family is essential.[29] When the patient and family are informed, shared responsibility for the treatment outcome is more likely.[26]

6.12.5 *Short face growth pattern: Maxillomandibular deficiency*

This dentofacial deformity has the common denominator of a significant degree of vertical and horizontal deficiency in the maxilla, mandible, and chin (Case study: Patient 4; Figure 6.5).[3,40] There is a decrease in the height of the lower face as measured from subnasion to menton. The ratio of the lower facial height compared with the upper facial height (subnasion-to-glabella) also confirms diminished lower anterior facial height. The aesthetic presentation is consistent and includes an apparent redundancy of the soft tissue drape of the lower face, creating "chubby cheeks" in the adolescent and an aged look later in life.

Clinical examination of the individual with a *short face growth pattern* includes a pseudo-prominence of the nose, acute nasolabial angle, measurable and visually apparent short lower facial height, and a disproportionate facial width-to-height ratio. Normally, there is a 1:2 relationship between the distance from the base of the nose to the

Case Study: Patient 4

A 35-year-old woman presented to the surgeon (J.C.P.) with concerns about having a "big nose and pointed chin." She specifically asked for a "reduction rhinoplasty and reduction genioplasty." Before graduation from high school, she underwent a full course of orthodontic treatment with achievement of a satisfactory occlusion. She is a college graduate and gainfully employed in the business sector.

Examination confirmed maxillomandibular deficiency (short face growth pattern) with a short lower anterior facial height and limited horizontal projection of the jaws. In repose, there was no dental show. With broad smile, only half of the maxillary incisor crowns showed. The bony chin was vertically short with a prominent pogonion. There was a deep-bite malocclusion.

Jaw surgery was offered and accepted as a way to correct the presenting facial disproportion and enhance aesthetics. Minimum orthodontic tooth movement was needed, but minor improvements in arch form could be accomplished simultaneously. Use of orthodontic brackets at the time of surgery and during postoperative recovery would also limit periodontal sequelae. The procedures proposed and carried out included:

- maxillary Le Fort I osteotomy;
- bilateral sagittal split osteotomies of the mandible;
- oblique osteotomy of the chin;
- neck liposuction.

The articulated dental casts of the model surgery planning indicate the vector changes planned and carried out:

- maxillary movements
  - 5-mm advancement at the incisors
  - 4-mm vertical lengthening at the incisors
  - 3-mm clockwise rotation of the maxillary plane

(*Continued*)

Case Study: Patient 4 (*Continued*)

- mandibular movements
  - horizontal advancement at the incisors
  - vertical lengthening at the incisors
  - clockwise rotation of the mandibular plane
- chin movements
  - vertical lengthening (interposition block hydroxyapatite graft)

Operative time was approximately 2.5 hours. No blood replacement was required. The patient was extubated in the operating room at the end of surgery. She remained in the hospital for 2 nights and was then discharged to the care of her companion. After the 2-week postoperative interval, she returned to work. At the 5-week postoperative interval, she returned to a normal diet, physical activities (sports and gym), and her orthodontist's care. After orthodontic maintenance and detailing, the appliances were removed 3 months postoperatively. She is shown before and 1 year after completion of treatment.

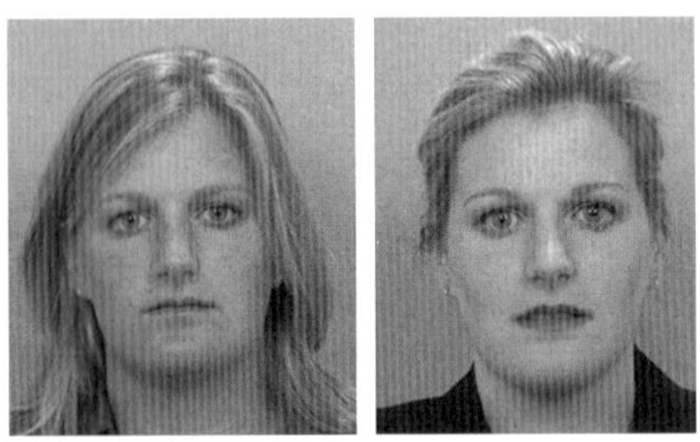

(A)

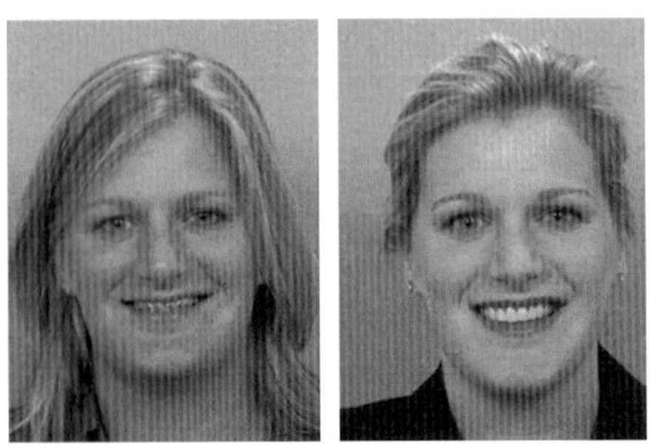

(B)

Figure 6.5. Patient 4. (A) Frontal facial views in repose before and after treatment. (B) Frontal facial views with smile before and after treatment.

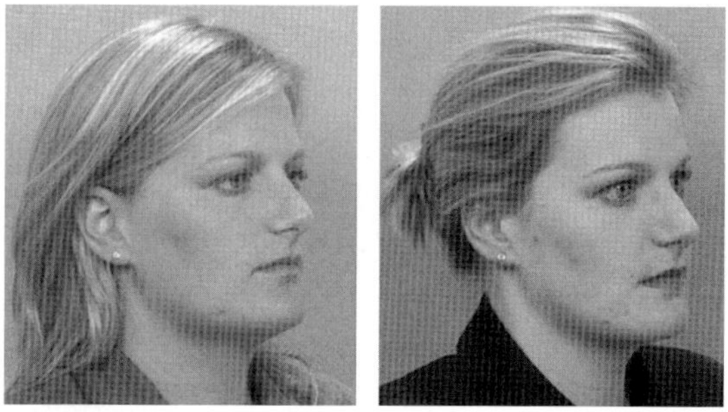

(C)

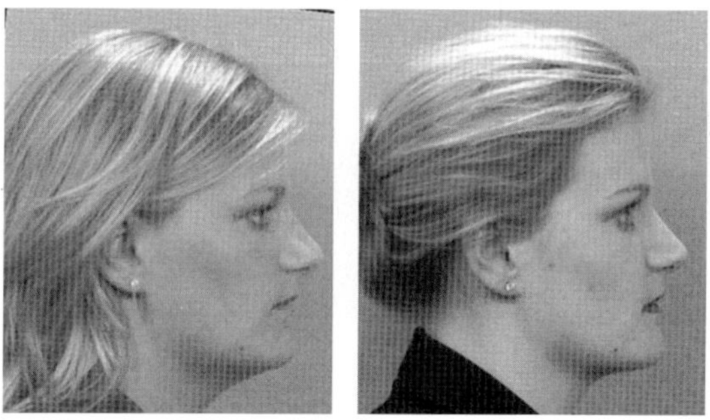

(D)

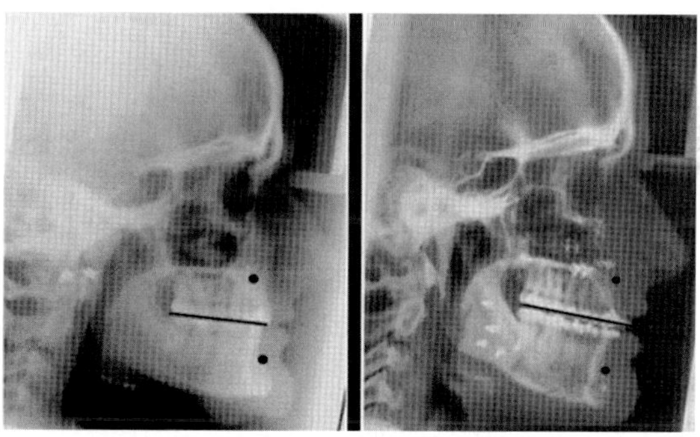

(E)

Figure 6.5. (*Continued*) (C) Oblique facial views before and after treatment. (D) Profile views before and after treatment. (E) Lateral cephalometric views indicate A-point to B-point relationship before and after treatment.

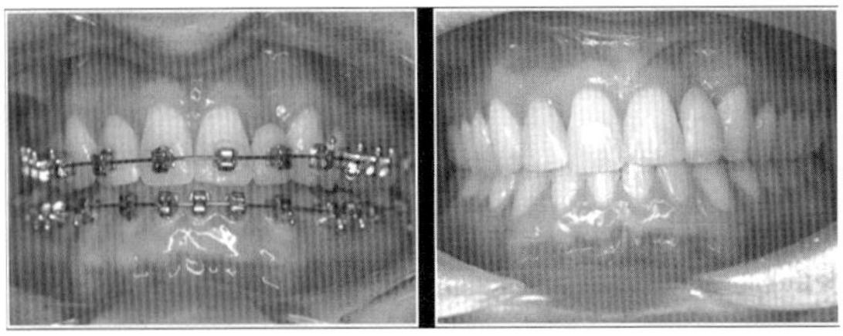

(F)

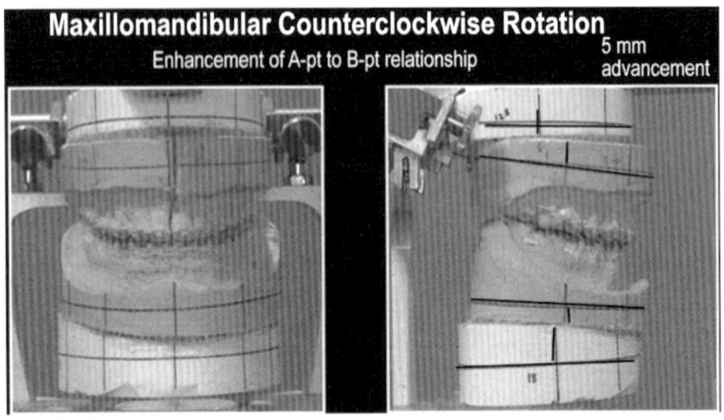

(G)

Figure 6.5. (*Continued*) (F) Occlusal views pre-orthodontics and 1 year after completion of treatment. (G) Articulated dental casts of model surgery planning. Reprinted with permission from Elsevier (Ref. 53). Copyright © 2006 American Association of Oral and Maxillofacial Surgeons. http://www.sciencedirect.com/science/journal/02782391.

upper lip and the distance from the lower lip to the chin. In the individual with a short face, the relationship is closer to 1:1. The labiomental sulcus is deep and the lower lip is everted further, confirming the degree of mandibular deficiency. The maxillary incisor teeth are often completely covered by the upper lip, creating an edentulous appearance with the lips in repose and an unattractive smile, with no gingiva showing. With the teeth in occlusion, the oral commissure appears wide and the lips project forward in front of procumbent incisors. Individuals are frequently described as having a sad or unhappy look in repose based on the wide and downturned oral commissures.[3] Not infrequently, articulation errors in speech and swallowing difficulties result from the Angle class II deep-bite malocclusion. Difficulties with chewing and with lateral and protrusive mandibular movement may also result from the class II deep-bite malocclusion. Upper airway obstruction in the short face growth pattern often exists and should be ruled out.[13,14,17] A higher incidence of TMD resulting from the jaw dysmorphology and presenting with malocclusion is to be expected.[24]

To restore facial proportions and preferred facial aesthetics, there must be both vertical and horizontal expansion of the maxillomandibular complex.[3,40] Accomplishing these objectives successfully eliminates soft tissue bunching and restores a pleasing soft tissue envelope. This changes the overall facial aesthetic appearance from sad and old to young and more attractive. While the indications for surgery in this condition may be to improve function, a compelling aspect is typically to enhance facial aesthetics. The aesthetic advantages of lengthening and projecting the preoperative short and retrusive lower face toward Euclidean proportions are immediately apparent visually and do not require quantification.

Surgical planning begins with a decision concerning the magnitude of vertical lengthening, horizontal advancement, and clockwise rotation required in the maxilla.[49] A common mistake is to err on the side of insufficient lengthening of the midface, believing that the short upper lip will not accommodate skeletal lengthening. Experience has shown that the upper lip that appears short and hypotonic will stretch as the maxilla lengthens. The old thinking was that vertical lengthening of the upper jaw was unstable and inadvisable. We now know that with mobilization of the down-fractured maxilla, vertical lengthening and horizontal advancement can be reliably carried out with reasonable occlusal stability and the routine achievement of improved aesthetics.[38] This requires well-designed and well-executed osteotomies, full mobilization of the upper jaw, stable plate and screw fixation, and the use of interpositional grafts. Bilateral sagittal split osteotomies of the mandible and a vertical lengthening genioplasty are also required components of the reconstruction.

6.12.6 *Bimaxillary dental protrusive growth pattern*

Bimaxillary dental protrusion can occur in any racial group, but facial divergence (convexity) and lip prominence is strongly influenced by race and ethnic characteristics.[10] Greater degrees of lip and incisor prominence occur in Asians and blacks than in whites. Etiologic factors favoring the pattern of dentofacial deformity include heredity, perioral habits (e.g., thumb sucking), and the effects of muscle forces (strong tongue and weak lip forces) during growth and development.

Peck and Peck set out to determine the public's concept of beauty as related to the Caucasian profile.[51] They found that the general public admires a more prominent face compared with the accepted cephalometric (normative data) and the orthodontic (clinical) standards of their day (e.g., four bicuspid extractions with orthodontic retraction). Review of the literature confirms that as a group, African Americans differ from Caucasian Americans in dental, skeletal, and soft tissue facial parameters. The question is, at what point does attractive fullness (convexity) of the profile become dysmorphic and unattractive?[50]

Abnormal growth of the maxillomandibular skeleton may produce a dentofacial deformity combined with *dentoalveolar protrusion*, resulting in both dental and facial disharmony. This growth pattern may be associated with class I, class II, and class III molar relationships but always with maxillary and mandibular incisor procumbency and anterior open-bite malocclusion. The affected individual will also have a varied degree of lip incompetence and mentalis strain at lip closure, excessive exposure of the anterior teeth in repose, excessive gingival show with smile, and often a retrusive chin and profile.

Correction of the anterior open-bite malocclusion associated with this growth pattern for most individuals entails extraction of first premolars followed by orthodontic retraction of the anterior teeth into the edentulous gaps.[54] This treatment also tends to retract the lips and reduce the facial convexity. To determine which patients will also benefit from jaw osteotomies, the clinician should assess pretreatment skeletal, dental, and soft tissue parameters.[54] The evaluation includes the maxillomandibular skeleton aspects (sagittal and vertical facial proportions), dental aspects (incisor inclination, spacing, crowding, curve of Spee, arch-width, and occlusion), and soft tissue aesthetics, including dynamic position of the lips (lip-to-tooth relationship in repose and smile, interdental gap, presence of mentalis strain with closure, nasolabial angle, and labiomental fold). There must be a compelling aesthetic and functional rationale for shortening the anterior vertical dimension of the face and altering the horizontal projection to proceed with a surgical approach.[41] Facial aesthetic disharmony associated with accentuated degrees of this condition include:

- Excessive separation of the lips at rest (lip incompetence); as a general rule, lip separation at rest should be less than 4 mm;
- excessive effort required to bring the lips into closure (lip strain/mentalis strain);
- excessive prominence of the lips when viewed in profile.

All three dysmorphic aspects should be present to confirm the diagnosis of a dentofacial deformity associated with dentoalveolar protrusion to the extent that it requires surgical correction.[3,55]

When surgical repositioning of the jaws (Le Fort I in segments combined with sagittal split ramus osteotomies) or just the anterior components of the jaws (anterior segmental osteotomies) is undertaken to resolve the dentofacial deformity (facial disharmony) and anterior open bite (occlusal disharmony), the surgical option should be selected according to patient-specific facial characteristics and dental findings.[54] When the presenting findings show significant excess of vertical or horizontal facial components or both, a Le Fort I osteotomy with segmentation combined with sagittal split ramus osteotomies of the mandible will be required. This approach provides the flexibility needed to alter the maxilla and mandible in all three dimensions (horizontal, vertical, and transverse); to simultaneously improve head and neck function (breathing, swallowing, chewing, and speech); and to enhance facial aesthetics. An osteotomy of the chin with horizontal advancement is also frequently carried out to further improve profile aesthetics and ease of lip closure.[42]

6.12.7 *Obstructive sleep apnea*

The National Sleep Foundation estimates that some form of snoring or OSA occurs in 90 million Americans.[15] About 50% of people older than 40 years snore. Among habitual snorers, the incidence of OSA is at least 17% in men and 15% in women. It is estimated that 18 million Americans have OSA but only 2 million of those have been diagnosed. OSA is a associated with higher risks of hypertension, coronary artery disease, stroke, congestive heart failure, atrial fibrillation, impotence, mortality, and behavioral and cognitive problems. Much of the excess mortality reported to be associated with OSA is due to accidental trauma related to daytime sleepiness (with a 10 times greater likelihood of dying in an automobile accident and a significant increase in accidents in the workplace, and so forth), but the increased incidence of cardiovascular disorders clearly plays a role.[15]

OSA is characterized by recurrent sleep-induced collapse of the pharyngeal airway leading to hypoxemia, hypercarbia, and fluctuations in intrathoracic pressure caused by increased respiratory effort, with arousal from sleep being required to reestablish airway patency.[15] Most evidence supports the concept that individuals with OSA have an anatomic predisposition to airway collapse.[13,14,18] Daytime (awake) protective mechanisms that increase activity of the pharyngeal dilator muscles fail during supine sleep with resulting collapse of the pharyngeal airway. The frequent locations of pharyngeal collapse include the velopharynx (behind the soft palate) and the oropharynx (behind the tongue), or both. An individual's unique (baseline) skeletal (jaw) anatomy will have a dramatic effect on the size of the upper airway (lumen diameter). This is in addition to the environmental causes (i.e, obesity) that thicken the pharyngeal/oral soft tissue volume (narrow the airway) and the forces that maintain and further open it up (pharyngeal dilator muscle contraction).

Prinsell has stated, "Maxillomandibular advancement (MMA) surgery for OSA is a highly successful and potentially definitive primary single-stage surgery that may result in a significant reduction in OSA-related health risks, as well as financial savings for the healthcare system."[13] Li *et al.* reached the same conclusion, stating, "Maxillomandibular advancement surgery is the most effective procedure for OSA."[14] Vicini *et al.* completed a prospective randomized controlled trial to assess the effectiveness of surgery versus ventilation in individuals with documented severe OSA (apnea–hypopnea index

[AHI] level >30).[18] Fifty consecutive subjects who had severe OSA were enrolled and randomized into a conservative (continuous autotitrated positive pressure) or surgical (MMA) treatment group. One year after MMA surgery or continuous autotitrated positive-pressure treatment, both groups showed a remarkable improvement of mean AHI and Epworth sleepiness scale levels.[18] The degree of improvement was not statistically different between the two groups. The MMA group (N =25) had a mean age of 49 years with a body mass index of 32.7 and a mean preoperative AHI of 56.8. After MMA surgery, the mean postoperative AHI dropped to 8.1. There were no fatal events, significant bleeding, or complications requiring surgical revision procedure. In conclusion, MMA proved to be a valuable alternative therapeutic tool in adults with severe OSA, with a success rate equivalent to that of therapeutic ventilation treatment.[18]

6.12.8 *Cleft-orthognathic surgery*

The successful reconstruction of congenital cleft lip and palate is inextricably connected with orthodontic care and skeletal surgery (Case study: Patient 5; Figures 6.6 and 6.7).[56–58] The unfortunate negative effects of surgical repair of cleft palate have been known to clinicians for more than 200 years.[19] Good *et al.* reviewed the Boston Children's Hospital long-term cleft lip and palate results.[59] The research concluded that 48% of their patients with a repaired unilateral cleft lip and palate (UCLP) and 76.5% of those with bilateral cleft lip and palate (BCLP) required and underwent jaw reconstruction. They believe that the need for orthognathic surgery depends on the severity of the cleft type as well as the number and extent of previous operative procedures that then predispose to maxillary hypoplasia. The Hospital for Sick Children (Toronto, Canada) found that 48.3% of their complete UCLP patients required or underwent cleft orthognathic surgery.[60] A full 59.4% of the patients with UCLP referred to their center after at least cleft lip repair required orthognathic surgery. They found that 65% of their BCLP patients required or underwent orthognathic surgery.[60] A full 70% of children with BCLP referred to their team sometime after cleft lip repair were found to require orthognathic surgery. Chen *et al.*

Case Study: Patient 5

This 17-year-old Asian girl was born with a left-sided complete UCLP. She underwent lip and palate repair earlier in life. She presented to the surgeon (J.C.P.) for evaluation in the adult dentition and was found to have maxillary deficiency to the extent that orthodontics alone could not correct the occlusion without introducing an unacceptable dental compensation. She was also found to have a residual labial and palatal fistula through the cleft site extending back to the incisive foramen. Bony defects extended throughout the cleft into the floor of the nose and hard palate. There was a cleft dental gap in the location of the congenitally missing lateral incisor. The right lateral incisor was hopelessly palatally displaced and out of occlusion. The left maxillary first bicuspid was congenitally absent. The mandible was well positioned with good symmetry. The chin was vertically long and flat.

She was referred to the surgeon (J.C.P.) for an orthognathic consultation. In addition to the above-mentioned findings, examination also confirmed a deviated septum and hypertrophic inferior turbinates with a tight nasal aperture explaining the chronic obstructive nasal breathing symptoms. A naso-endoscopic guided speech assessment confirmed adequate velopharyngeal closure. Jaw and intranasal surgery in combination with orthodontic treatment was offered and accepted as a way to alleviate the symptoms and signs and to enhance facial appearance. Orthodontic dental decompensation was to level and align the maxillary dentition in two segments and in the mandible according to standard techniques. Single-stage simultaneous surgery proposed and carried out included:

- maxillary Le Fort I osteotomy in two segments with differential repositioning;
- oblique osteotomy of the chin;
- septoplasty;
- inferior turbinate reduction;

(*Continued*)

Case Study: Patient 5 (*Continued*)

- anterior iliac crest graft for interpositional placement at the Le Fort I site;
- removal of wisdom teeth and extraction of retained lateral incisor.

The articulated dental casts of the model surgery planning indicate the vector changes planned and carried out:

- maxillary movements
  - 7-mm advancement at the incisors
  - 1-mm vertical lengthening at the incisors
  - segmentation of the maxilla (two segments) for:
    - closure of cleft dental gap (15-mm advancement of the lesser segment)
    - closure of dead space at cleft site
    - closure of oronasal fistula
- chin movements
  - vertical shortening
  - horizontal advancement

Operative time was approximately 4 hours. No blood replacement was required. The patient was extubated in the recovery room just after completion of surgery. She remained in the hospital for 2 nights and was then discharged to the care of her parents. Two weeks after surgery, she returned to sedentary activities (school work, computer work). At the 5-week postoperative interval, she returned to a normal diet, physical activities (sports and gym), and her orthodontist's care. After orthodontic maintenance and detailing, the appliances were removed 8 months postoperatively. She is shown before and 1 year after completion of treatment.

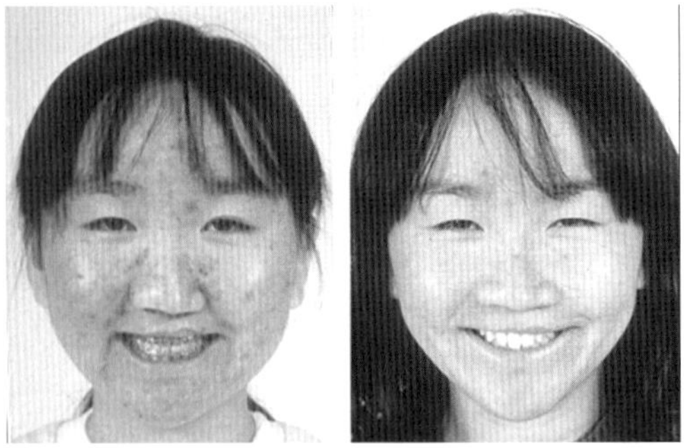

(A)

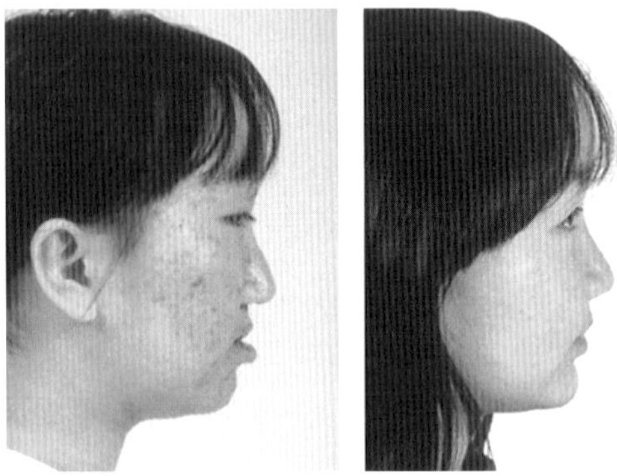

(B)

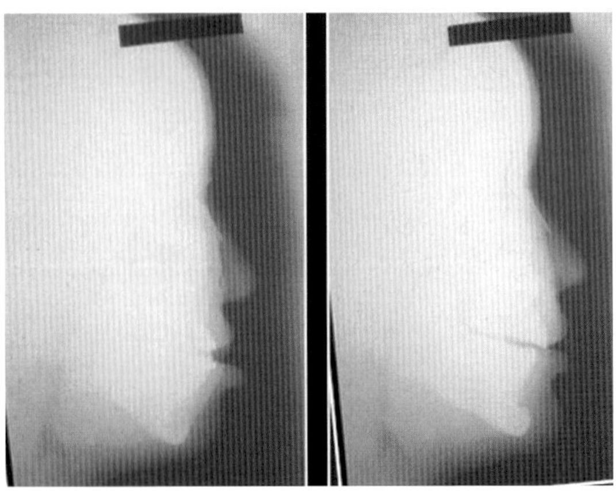

(C)

Figure 6.6. Patient 5. (A) Frontal facial views with smile before and after treatment. (B) Profile facial views before and after treatment. (C) Lateral cephalometric views before and after treatment.

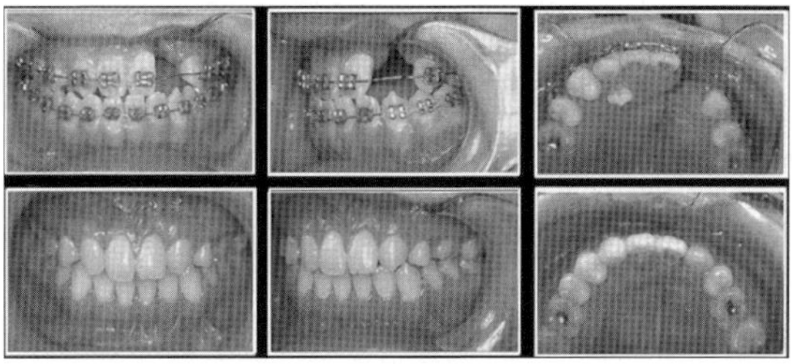

(D)

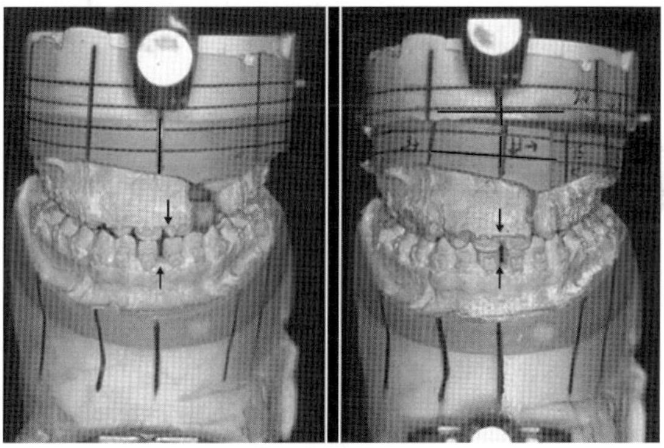

(E)

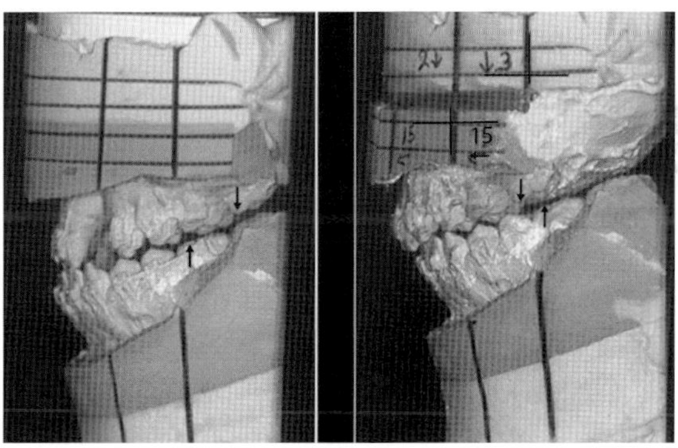

(F)

Figure 6.6. (*Continued*) Patient 5. (D) Occlusal views immediately presurgery and 1 year after completion of treatment. (E) Frontal views of articulated dental casts before and after model surgery planning. (F) Lateral views of articulated dental casts before and after model surgery planning.

(A)

(B)

(C)

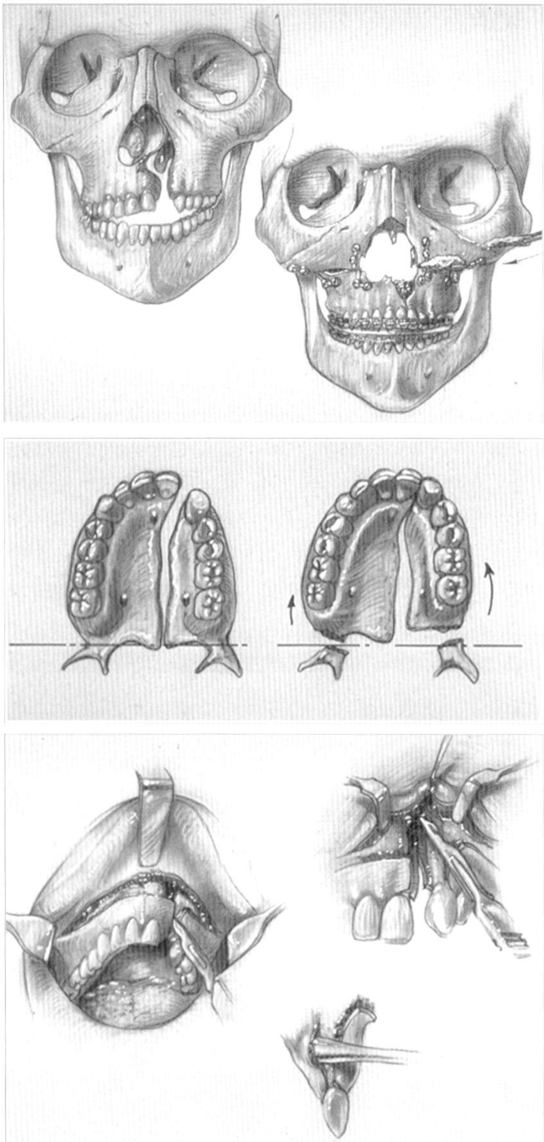

Figure 6.7. (A) Illustrated frontal view of bony skeleton before and just after fixation of Le Fort I osteotomy in two segments. The inferior turbinates have been reduced, and a submucous resection of the deviated septum has been performed. Iliac bone graft has been placed along the nasal floor. A miniplate is placed vertically along each zygomatic buttress and pyriform aperture region. (B) Palatal view of bony segments before and after repositioning. (C) Illustration of direct incisions for completion of osteotomies and fistula closure.

(D)

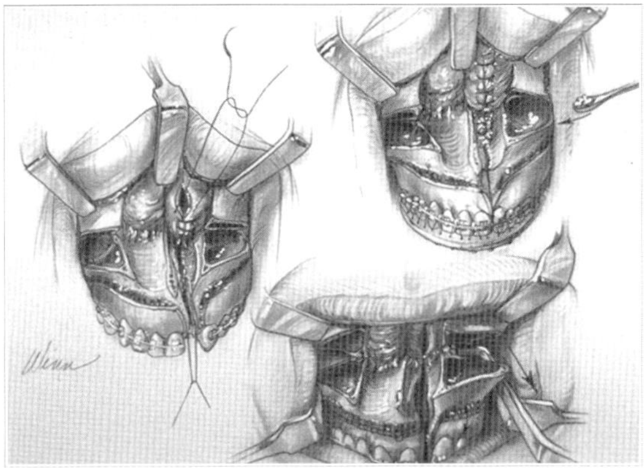

(E)

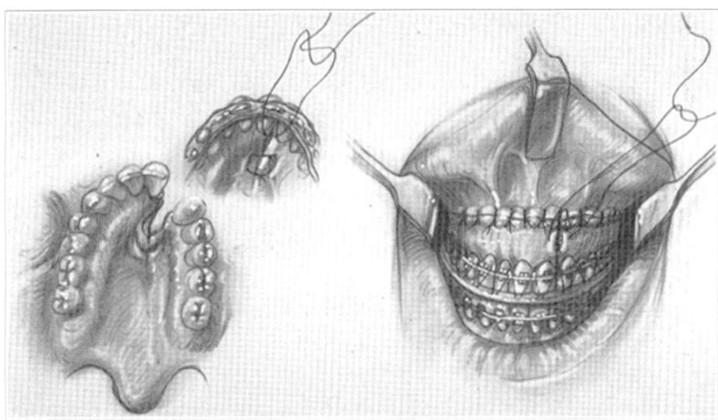

Figure 6.7. (*Continued*) (D) Illustration of down-fractured Le Fort I osteotomy in two segments after submucous resection of septum, reduction of inferior turbinates through the nasal mucosa opening, and watertight nasal side closure. (E) Illustration indicating oral side wound closure on both labial and palatal aspects after differential segmental repositioning. Reprinted with permission from Elsevier (Posnick JC. Modified Le Fort I performed in two segments in a patient with unilateral cleft lip. In: Russell RC, ed. *Instructional Courses, Plastic Surgery Education Foundation*. Vol. 4. St. Louis, MO: Mosby; 1992:129–157).

believe that the need for orthognathic surgery in the isolated cleft palate teenager of Asian ethnic background may approach 50%.[61]

The reconstruction of a cleft lip and palate is best delivered through collaborative care by appropriate medical and dental specialists.[56,57,62,63] It is not sufficient for individual practitioners, be they surgeons, orthodontists, restorative dentists, speech pathologists, or otolaryngologists, to carry out extensive treatment without informing the patient and family of the options and considering clinical input from the other specialists caring for the patient. Correction of the residual skeletal deformities in the adolescent with a cleft challenges the ingenuity and skill of the orthognathic surgeon and cleft team.[56–58,62–64] The central deformity is maxillary hypoplasia/dysplasia. This is frequently combined with residual oronasal fistula, bone defects, cleft dental gaps, intranasal sites of obstruction, soft tissue scarring, and velopharyngeal dysfunction. Secondary deformities of the nose, mandible, and chin are also common.[56,57,62,63] Methods are available to manage the presenting cleft jaw deformities, malocclusion, and associated defects.[58,64] Successful skeletal reconstruction provides a stable foundation on which final soft tissue lip and nose reconstruction may be carried out. The knowledge and expertise are currently available to enhance the quality of life and well-being of the patient with a cleft jaw deformity.

6.12.9 *Idiopathic condylar resorption*

In the condition of uncertain origin commonly referred to as *idiopathic condylar resorption*, the condyles of the mandible partially resorb, causing a loss of condylar height and secondary alteration of the maxillofacial morphology and occlusion. *Progressive condylar resorption* is the term used to describe conditions resulting in similar loss of condylar height, but with known associations (e.g., juvenile rheumatoid arthritis, systemic lupus erythematosus, Sjögren's syndrome, mandibular trauma, steroid effects).[65] In general, idiopathic condylar resorption has the following presentation:

- Most often affects females between 15 and 35 years old;
- generally results in bilateral and symmetric condylar involvement;
- results in progressive condylar resorption followed by stabilization without further loss of condylar height;
- has no consistent or proven inciting event or etiology;
- once quiescent, generally results in satisfactory painless TMJ function with satisfactory mouth opening.

Maxillofacial morphologic findings generally include:

- Change in shape of the condylar heads (e.g., flattening and thinning);
- decrease in condylar height;
- loss of posterior facial height;
- mandibular repositioning with clockwise rotation;
- Angle class II anterior open-bite malocclusion.

Orthognathic procedures, orthodontics, or restorative dentistry to correct the end-staged malocclusion and facial dysmorphology is more likely to be successful if condylar resorption has been stable for approximately 2 years (Case study: Patient 6; Figure 6.8).[65,66] Stability

Case Study: Patient 6

The patient is a systemically healthy young woman who at the age of 12 years experienced severe TMJ discomfort with limited and painful mouth-opening that lasted approximately 6 months. Mandibular retrusion with an anterior open bite progressively developed over the next 12 months. At the age of 13, the patient's orthodontist carried out a camouflage approach that included maxillary first bicuspid extractions. Over the next 2 years, a "neutralization" of the occlusion was accomplished.

At the age of 16 years, the parents consulted this surgeon (J.C.P.) with concerns about facial aesthetics, the upper airway, and long-term periodontal health. Review of radiographs showed partially resorbed condylar heads with cartilaginous caps and intact cortical rims. Clinically, there was satisfactory painless, vertical mouth-opening. No progression of condylar resorption had occurred in at least the previous 18 months. The diagnosis of idiopathic condylar resorption in remission was made. Physical examination confirmed septal deviation and hypertrophic inferior turbinates consistent with the chronic obstructive nasal airway breathing symptoms. The presence of OSA syndrome was suggested. The patient elected to

(*Continued*)

Case Study: Patient 6 (*Continued*)

undergo redo orthodontics, including mandibular bicuspid extractions and orthognathic and intranasal surgery. Single-stage simultaneous surgery proposed and carried out included:

- maxillary Le Fort I osteotomy;
- bilateral sagittal split osteotomies of the mandible;
- oblique osteotomy of the chin;
- septoplasty;
- inferior turbinate reduction;
- neck liposuction;
- extraction of wisdom teeth.

The articulated dental casts of the model surgery planning indicated the vector changes planned and carried out:

- maxillary movements
  - 4-mm advancement at the incisors
  - 1-mm vertical intrusion at the incisors
  - 1-mm counterclockwise rotation of the maxillary plane
  - 4-mm cant correction
  - 1-mm dental midline repositioning
- mandibular movements
  - horizontal advancement
  - counter clockwise rotation of the mandibular plane
- chin movement
  - horizontal advancement

Operative time was approximately 3 hours. No blood replacement was required. The patient was extubated in the operating room at the end of surgery. She remained in the hospital for 2 nights and was then discharged to the care of her parents. Two weeks after surgery, she returned to sedentary activities. At the 5-week postoperative interval, she returned to a normal diet, physical activities (sports and gym), and her orthodontist's care. After orthodontic detailing, the appliances were removed 5 months postoperatively. She is shown before and 1 year after completion of treatment.

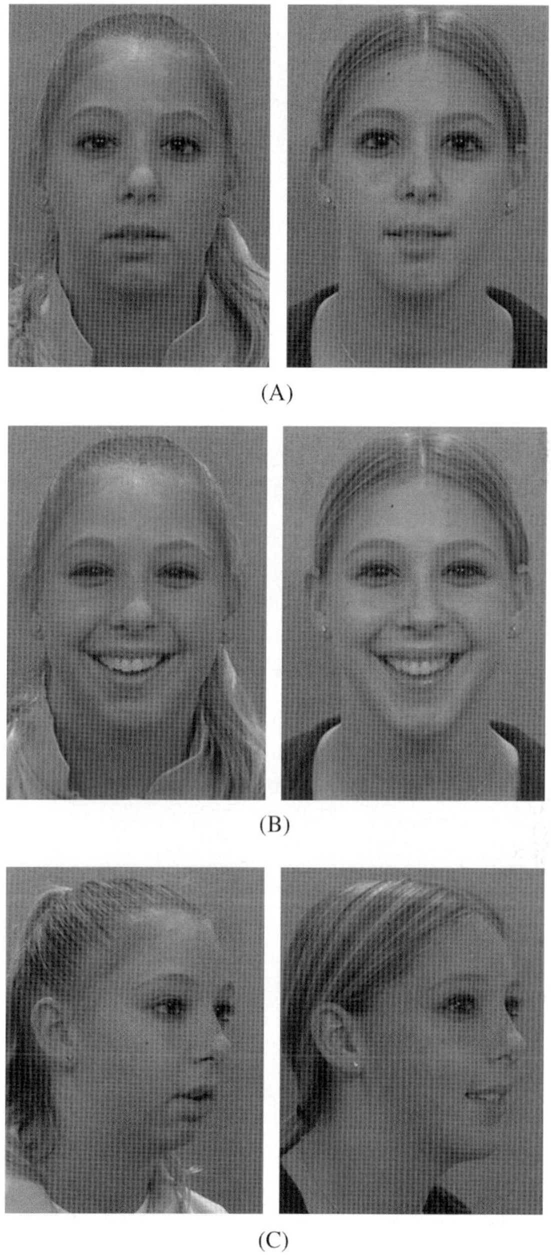

Figure 6.8. Patient 6. (A) Frontal facial views in repose before and after treatment. (B) Frontal facial views with smile before and after treatment. (C) Oblique facial views before and after treatment.

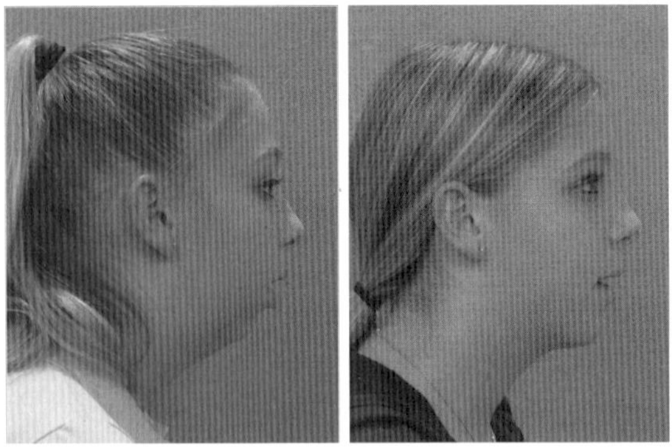

(D)

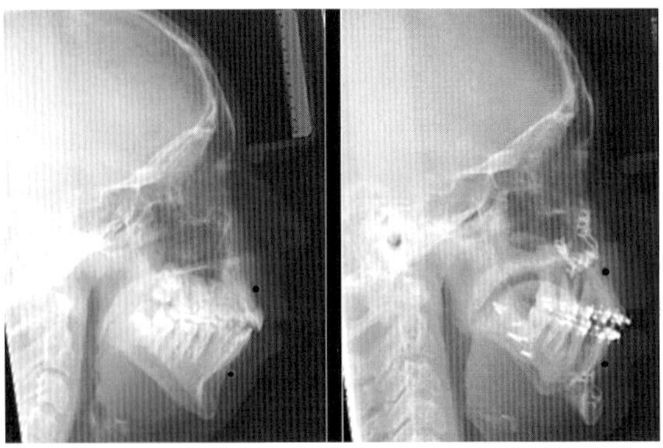

(E)

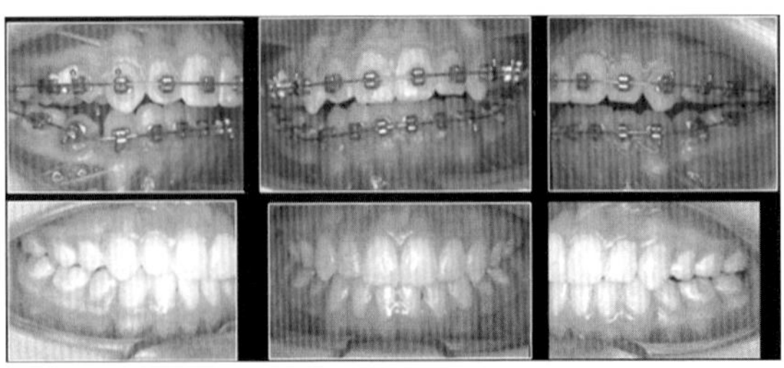

(F)

Figure 6.8. (***Continued***) Patient 6. (D) Profile facial views before and after treatment. (E) Lateral cephalometric views indicate A-point and B-point positions before and after treatment. (F) Occlusal views during orthodontic (dental) decompensation and 1 year after completion of treatment.

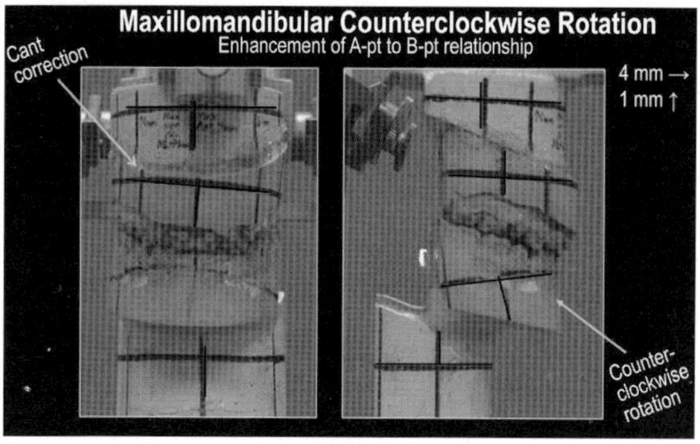

(G)

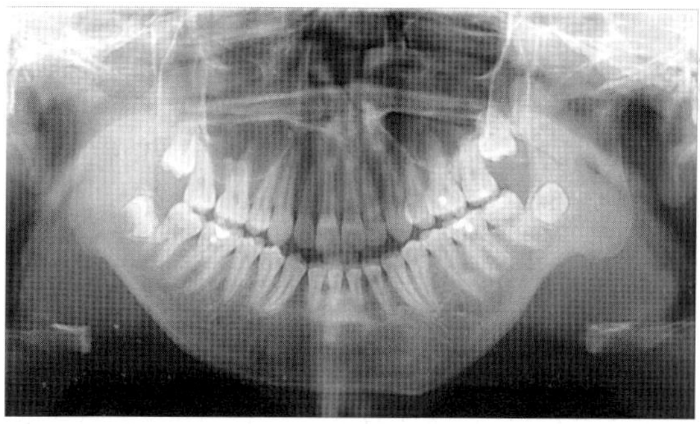

(H)

Figure 6.8. (***Continued***) (G) Articulated dental casts of model surgery planning. (H) Panorex radiograph before orthognathic surgery, indicating bilateral partial condylar head resorption. Reprinted with permission from Elsevier (Ref. 65). Copyright © 2007 American Association of Oral and Maxillofacial Surgeons. http://www.sciencedirect.com/science/journal/02782391.

can be documented by there being minimal further changes in occlusion, intact cartilaginous cap, and an underlying rim of cortical bone over the partially resorbed condyles. The use of technetium Tc 99m methylene diphonate quantitative condylar bone scintigraphy can be useful to assess whether condylysis is active.[45] To achieve favorable facial aesthetics and improvement in head and neck dysfunction (chewing, swallowing, breathing, speech), surgical repositioning of the maxilla (Le Fort I), mandible (ramus osteotomies), and chin (oblique osteotomy) is generally required.[63] Limiting the surgery to either the maxilla or mandible with the idea of achieving a more stable occlusal result is not substantiated in the literature and is likely to result in suboptimal facial aesthetics. The key to achieving a successful morphologic (aesthetic) outcome for most patients is to surgically accomplish horizontal advancement and counterclockwise rotation of the maxillomandibular complex.[49]

6.13 Conclusion

The term *dentofacial deformity* refers to significant deviations from normal proportions of the maxillomandibular complex that also have a negative impact on the interrelationship between maxillary and mandibular dentition. This condition affects at least 5% of the general population but as many as 20% of individuals who present for orthodontic evaluation. Affected persons have compromised functions of the head and neck that may include breathing, swallowing, speech articulation, chewing, lip closure/posture, and facial aesthetics. The favorable correction of the facial dysmorphology and presenting head and neck dysfunction, through a combination of effective orthodontic alignment of the teeth and precise surgical repositioning of the jaws and intranasal procedures, is predictable and long-lasting.

References

1. **Bell WH.** Section 1: Diagnosis and treatment planning. In: Bell WH, Profitt WR, White RP Jr., eds. *Surgical Correction of Dentofacial Deformities.* Vols. 1 and 2. Philadelphia, PA: WB Saunders; 1980:3–233.
2. **Sarver DM.** Facial analysis. In: Sarver DM, ed. *Esthetic Orthodontics and Orthognathic Surgery.* St. Louis, MO: Mosby; 1998:1–60.
3. **Rosen HM.** Principles, Part 1. In: Rosen HM, ed. *Aesthetic Perspectives in Jaw Surgery.* New York, NY: Springer; 1999:1–76.
4. **Profitt WR, White RP.** Diagnosis and treatment planning approaches, Part 2. In: Profitt WR, White RP, Sarver DM, eds. *Contemporary Treatment of Dentofacial Deformity.* St. Louis, MO: Mosby; 2003:91–268.
5. **Reyneke J.** Basic guidelines for the diagnosis and treatment in specific dentofacial deformities. In: Reyneke J, ed. *Essentials of Orthognathic Surgery. Quintessence*; 2003:151–246.

6. **Arnett W, Mclaughlin RP.** Facial treatment planning. In: Arnett W, Mclaughlin EP, eds. *Facial and Dental Planning for Orthodontists & Oral Surgeons.* Mosby; 2005:223–280.
7. **Profitt WR.** Diagnosis and treatment planning, Section 3. In: Profitt WR, Sarver DM, eds. *Contemporary Orthodontics.* 4th edn. Elsevier; 2006:145–294.
8. **Brook PH, Shaw WC.** The development of an index of orthodontic treatment priority. *Eur J Orthod* 1989;11:309–320.
9. **Richmond S, Roberts CT, Andrews M.** Use of the Index of Orthodontic Treatment Need (IOTN) in assessing the need for orthodontic treatment pre- and post-appliance therapy. *Br J Orthod* 1994;21:175–184.
10. **Profitt WR, Fields HW Jr, Moray LJ.** Prevalence of malocclusion and orthodontic treatment need in the United States: estimates from the NHANES III survey. *Int J Adult Orthodon Orthognath Surg* 1998;13:97–106.
11. **Harvold EP, Chierici G, Vargervik K.** Experiments on the development of dental malocclusions. *Am J Orthod* 1972;61:38–44.
12. **Harvold EP, Tomer BS, Vargervik K, Chierici G.** Primate experiments in oral respiration. *Am J Orthod* 1981;79:359–372.
13. **Prinsell JR.** Maxillomandibular advancement surgery in a site-specific treatment approach for obstructive sleep apnea in 50 consecutive patients. *Chest* 1999;116:1519–1529.
14. **Li KK, Powell NB, Riley RW, Zonato A, Gervacio L, Guilleminault C.** Morbidly obese patients with severe obstructive sleep apnea: is airway reconstructive surgery a viable option? *Laryngoscope* 2000;110:982–987.
15. **Young T, Peppard PE, Taheri S.** Excess weight and sleep-disordered breathing. *J Appl Physiol* 2005;99:1592–1599.
16. **Yaggi HK, Concato J, Kernan WN, Lichtman JH, Brass LM, Mohsenin V.** Obstructive sleep apnea as a risk factor for stroke and death. *N Engl J Med* 2005;353:2034–2041.
17. **Posnick JC, Fantuzzo JJ, Troost T.** Simultaneous intranasal procedures to improve chronic obstructive nasal breathing in patients undergoing maxillary (Le Fort I) osteotomy. *J Oral Maxillofac Surg* 2007;65:2273–2281.
18. **Vicini C, Dallan I, Campanini A, *et al.*** Surgery vs ventilation in adult severe obstructive sleep apnea syndrome. *Am J Otolaryngol* 2010;31:14–20.
19. **Linder-Aronson S, Woodside DG, Hellsing E, Emerson W.** Normalization of incisor position after adenoidectomy. *Am J Orthod Dentofacial Orthop* 1993;103:412–427.
20. **Angle EH.** *Malocclusion of the Teeth.* 7th edn. Philadelphia, PA: SS White; 1907.
21. **Schendel SA, Eisenfeld J, Bell WH, Epker BN, Mishelevich DJ.** The long face syndrome: vertical maxillary excess. *Am J Orthod* 1976;70:398–408.

22. **McNamara JA Jr., Türp JC.** Orthodontic treatment and temporomandibular disorders: is there a relationship? Part 1: clinical studies. *J Orofac Orthop* 1997; 58:74–89.
23. **Türp JC, McNamara JA Jr.** Orthodontic treatment and temporomandibular disorders: is there a relationship? Part 2: clinical implications. *J Orofac Orthop* 1997;58:136–143.
24. **Okeson JP.** Functional anatomy. In: Okeson JP, ed. *Management of Temporomandibular Joint Disorders and Occlusion.* 4th edn. St. Louis, MO: Mosby; 1998:1–148.
25. **Abrahamsson C, Ekberg E, Henrikson T, Bondemark L.** Alterations of temporomandibular disorders before and after orthognathic surgery: a systematic review. *Angle Orthod* 2007;77:729–734.
26. **Posnick JC, Wallace J.** Complex orthognathic surgery: assessment of patient satisfaction. *J Oral Maxillofac Surg* 2008;66:934–942.
27. **Livio M.** *The Golden Ratio: The Story of Phi, the World's Most Astonishing Number.* New York, NY: Broadway Books; 2002.
28. **Moorrees CFA, Kean MR.** Natural head position, a basic consideration in the interpretation of cephalometric radiographs. *Am J Phys Anthropol* 1958;16:213–214.
29. **Posnick JC.** Orthognathic surgery: general considerations; complications; and patient educational material. In: Posnick JC, ed. *Craniofacial and Maxillofacial Surgery in Children and Young Adults.* Philadelphia, PA: WB Saunders; 2000: 1103–1112.
30. **Ellis E III.** Bimaxillary surgery using an intermediate splint to position the maxilla. *J Oral Maxillofac Surg* 1999;57:53–56.
31. **Posnick JC.** Le Fort I, sagittal splits and genioplasty: historical perspective and step-by-step approach. In: Posnick JC, ed. *Craniofacial and Maxillofacial Surgery in Children and Young Adults.* Philadelphia, PA: WB Saunders; 2000: 1081–1102.
32. **Obwegeser HL.** Orthognathic surgery and a tale of how three procedures came to be: a letter to the next generations of surgeons. *Clin Plast Surg* 2007;34: 331–355.
33. **Precious DS, Lung KE, Pynn BR, Goodday RH.** Presence of impacted teeth as a determining factor of unfavorable splits in 1256 sagittal-split osteotomies. *Oral Surg Oral Med Oral Pathol Oral Radiol Endod* 1988;85:362–365.
34. **Precious DS.** Removal of third molars with sagittal split osteotomies: the case for. *J Oral Maxillofac Surg* 2004;62:1144–1146.
35. **O'Ryan F.** Complications with orthognathic surgery. In: Fonseca R, Turvey T, Marciani R, eds. *Oral & Maxillofacial Surgery.* 2nd edn. Vol. 3. WB Saunders; 2008:419–489.

36. **Posnick JC, Rabinovich A, Richardson DT.** Blood replacement practices for complex orthognathic surgery: a single surgeon's experience. *J Oral Maxillofac Surg* 2010;68:54–59.
37. **Profitt WR, Turvey TA, Phillips C.** Orthognathic surgery: a hierarchy of stability. *Int J Adult Orthodon Orthognath Surg* 1996;11:191–204.
38. **KretschmerWB, Baciut G, Baciut M, Zoder W, Wangerin K.** Stability of Le Fort I osteotomy in bimaxillary osteotomies: single-piece versus 3-piece maxilla. *J Oral Maxillofac Surg* 2010;68:372–380.
39. **Posnick JC.** Mandibular deficiency with or without maxillary deformity. In: Posnick JC, ed. *Craniofacial and Maxillofacial Surgery in Children and Young Adults.* Philadelphia, PA: WB Saunders; 2000:981–1003.
40. **Rosen H.** Facial skeletal expansion: treatment strategies and rationale. *Plast Reconstr Surg* 1992;89:798–808.
41. **Rosen H.** Aesthetics in facial skeletal surgery. *Perspect Plast Surg* 1993;6:1.
42. **Posnick JC.** Aesthetic alteration of the chin: evaluation and surgery. In: Posnick JC, ed. *Craniofacial and Maxillofacial Surgery in Children and Young Adults.* Philadelphia, PA: WB Saunders; 2000:1113–1124.
43. **Posnick JC.** Asymmetric mandibular prognathism with or without maxillary deformity. In: Posnick JC, ed. *Craniofacial and Maxillofacial Surgery in Children and Young Adults.* Philadelphia, PA: WB Saunders; 2000:1057–1080.
44. **Obwegeser HL.** Condylar hyperplasia, Part 2. In: Obwegeser HL, ed. *Mandibular Growth Anomalies.* Berlin: Springer; 2001:137–352.
45. **Cisneros GJ, Kaban LB.** Computerized skeletal scintigraphy for assessment of mandibular asymmetry. *J Oral Maxillofac Surg* 1984;42:513–520.
46. **Fields HW, Warren DW, Black K, Phillips CL.** Relationship between vertical dentofacial morphology and respiration in adolescents. *Am J Orthod Dentofacial Orthop* 1991;99:147–154.
47. **Posnick JC.** Maxillary excess with or without mandibular deficiency. In: Posnick JC, ed. *Craniofacial and Maxillofacial Surgery in Children and Young Adults.* Philadelphia, PA: WB Saunders; 2000:1025–1056.
48. **Rosen HM.** Occlusal plane rotation: aesthetic enhancement in mandibular micrognathia. *Plast Reconstr Surg* 1993;91:1231–1244.
49. **Rosen HM.** Maxillary advancement for mandibular prognathism: indications and rationale. *Plast Reconstr Surg* 1991;87:823–834.
50. **Alexander AE, McNamara JA Jr., Franchi L, Baccetti T.** Semilongitudinal cephalometric study of craniofacial growth in untreated class III malocclusion. *Am J Orthod Dentofacial Orthop* 2009;135:700.e1–700.e14.
51. **Peck H, Peck S.** A concept of facial esthetics. *Angle Orthod* 1970;40:284–318.

52. **Posnick JC.** Mandibular excess and maxillary deficiency. In: Posnick JC, ed. *Craniofacial and Maxillofacial Surgery in Children and Young Adults.* Philadelphia, PA: WB Saunders; 2000:1004–1024.
53. **Posnick JC, Fantuzzo JJ, Orchin JD.** Deliberate operative rotation of the maxillo-mandibular complex to alter the A-point to B-point relationship for enhanced facial esthetics. *J Oral Maxillofac Surg* 2006;64:1687–1695.
54. **Baek SH, Kim BH.** Determinants of successful treatment of bimaxillary protrusion: orthodontic treatment versus anterior segmental osteotomy. *J Craniofac Surg* 2005;16:234–246.
55. **Ricketts RM.** The biologic significance of the divine proportion and Fibonacci series. *Am J Orthod* 1982;81:351–370.
56. **Posnick JC.** Cleft-orthognathic surgery: the unilateral cleft lip and palate deformity. In: Posnick JC, ed. *Craniofacial and Maxillofacial Surgery in Children and Young Adults.* Philadelphia, PA: WB Saunders; 2000:860–907.
57. **Posnick JC.** Staging of cleft lip and palate reconstruction. In: Posnick JC, ed. *Craniofacial and Maxillofacial Surgery in Children and Young Adults.* Philadelphia, PA: WB Saunders; 2000:785–826.
58. **Posnick JC.** Orthognathic surgery in a cleft patient. In: Russell RC, ed. *Instructional Courses, Plastic Surgery Education Foundation.* Vol. 4. St. Louis, MO: Mosby; 1992:129–157.
59. **Good PM, Mulliken JB, Padwa BL.** Frequency of Le Fort I osteotomy after repaired cleft lip and palate or cleft palate. *Cleft Palate Craniofac J* 2007; 44:396–401.
60. **Daskalogiannakis J, Mehta M.** The need for orthognathic surgery in patients with repaired complete unilateral and complete bilateral cleft lip and palate. *Cleft Palate Craniofac J* 2009;46:498–502.
61. **Chen ZQ, Qian YF, Wang GM, Shen G.** Sagittal maxillary growth in patients with unoperated isolated cleft palate. *Cleft Palate Craniofac J* 2009;46: 664–667.
62. **Posnick JC.** Cleft-orthognathic surgery: the bilateral cleft lip and palate deformity. In: Posnick JC, ed. *Craniofacial and Maxillofacial Surgery in Children and Young Adults.* Philadelphia, PA: WB Saunders; 2000:908–950.
63. **Posnick JC.** Cleft-orthognathic surgery: the isolated cleft palate deformity. In: Posnick JC, ed. *Craniofacial and Maxillofacial Surgery in Children and Young Adults.* Philadelphia, PA: WB Saunders; 2000:951–978.
64. **Posnick JC, Tompson B.** Cleft-orthognathic surgery: complications and long-term results. *Plast Reconstr Surg* 1995;96:255–266.
65. **Posnick JC, Fantuzzo JJ.** Idiopathic condylar resorption: current clinical perspectives. *J Oral Maxillofac Surg* 2007;65:1617–1623.
66. **Troulis MJ, Tayebaty FT, Papadaki M, Williams WB, Kaban LB.** Condylectomy and costochondral graft reconstruction for treatment of active idiopathic condylar resorption. *J Oral Maxillofac Surg* 2008;66:65–72.

PRINCIPLES AND PRACTICE OF MANDIBULAR DISTRACTION OSTEOGENESIS

7

Edward J. Caterson, MD, PhD and
Joseph G. McCarthy, MD

7.1 Principle

The biology of regeneration harnesses highly regulated and complex signaling pathways to direct both recruited and resident cells to secrete and maintain mineralized extracellular matrix.

7.2 Introduction

Distraction has become part of the fabric of craniofacial surgery. It is a tissue engineering concept. The practice of distraction preceded the realization of tissue engineering as a discipline, but for the craniofacial surgeon it is an example of surgically harnessing the body for regenerative medicine. The concept and practice of craniofacial distraction evolved from the need for greater quantities of quality bone during reconstructive procedures. This as a driving force resulted in the development of bony distraction rather than the continued pillage of ribs, iliac crest tibia, or the radius for bone-building blocks.

Bone distraction had its roots in the treatment of extremity fractures after keen observation of bone/callus formation and the use of gradual and continuous traction for fracture reduction. Ilizarov is credited with popularizing bony distraction in the extremities using external fixators for limb lengthening.[1] As the Tessier skeletal advancement techniques were refined in the craniofacial skeleton, it became obvious that there was a need to generate bone without disrupting the bone/soft-tissue interface.[2,3]

Distraction was first applied in craniofacial animal models and introduced in the clinical arena in the late 1980s, when McCarthy and colleagues at New York University initiated clinical studies to demonstrate the efficacy of human mandibular distraction.[4–6] Since these initial reports, the treatment concept has been extended to other regions of the craniofacial skeleton. The patient population eligible for distraction is large, involving patients with congenital, developmental, post-traumatic, and postablative reconstruction needs. It is a real-time tissue engineering of bone and the associated soft tissue by harnessing the intrinsic processes involved in healing and regeneration. Within this clinical application are a few underlying principles that allow the healing system to serve as a bone factory for the craniofacial surgeon.

There are three types of distraction osteogenesis: unifocal, bifocal, and trifocal (Figure 7.1). These types have in common an osteotomy, specific directions of force, and the creation of potential space for a mineralized matrix to be generated. *Unifocal* distraction consists of a single osteotomy with distraction forces applied on either side of the osteotomy (Figure 7.1). *Bifocal* distraction involves a single osteotomy separated by a transport segment (Figure 7.1). The transport segment is a piece of bone that will be distracted into the defect with new bone formation filling the defect behind the transport segment. The transport segment is delivered into the skeletal defect by forces applied by the spanning distraction device. The leading edge of the transport segment has a fibrocartilage cap that must be replaced with a bone graft after the transport segment has been "docked" finally.[7] *Trifocal* distraction uses two osteotomies and two transport segments to fill a skeletal defect bidirectionally (Figure 7.1).

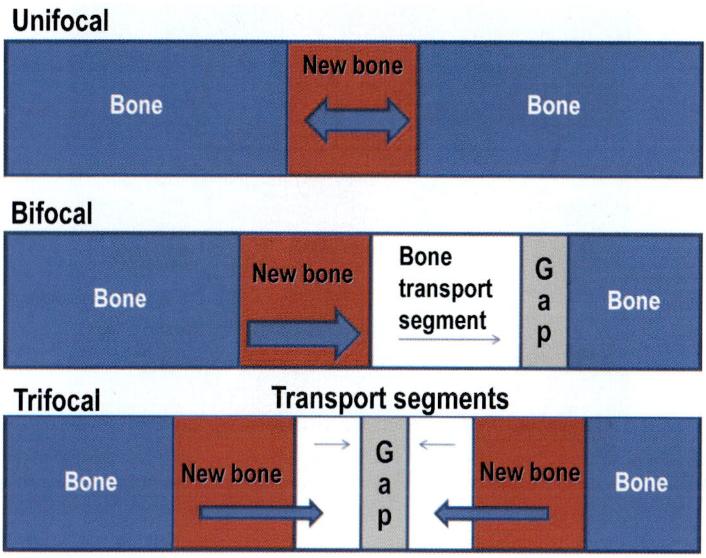

Figure 7.1. The three types of distraction osteogenesis are unifocal, bifocal, and trifocal. The solid red area represents the newly generated bone formed after distraction of the osteotomy/corticotomy site. The arrows designate the direction of the distraction forces. Transport distraction can be bifocal or trifocal, and is used when there exist a bony gap that needs to be closed. The transport segments are native bone (white) and are used as leading edges of bone to close a gap in the bone.

7.3 Biology of Distraction

Biomechanical forces are the inciting signals that initiate elongation of the callus at the osteotomy site. There is an extensive body of literature to characterize the histologic events associated with distraction.[8,9] Study of the distraction zone allows for greater understanding of the biologic events and gives insight into how to exert greater control over the biologic process. Extending from the osteotomy site are discrete zones that are staged in the process of forming mature bone: the zone of fibrous tissue, the zone of extending bone formation, the zone of bone remodeling, and the zone of mature bone (Figure 7.2).[4]

After a corticotomy has been performed and during the active distraction phase there are discrete zones of activity that have been characterized.

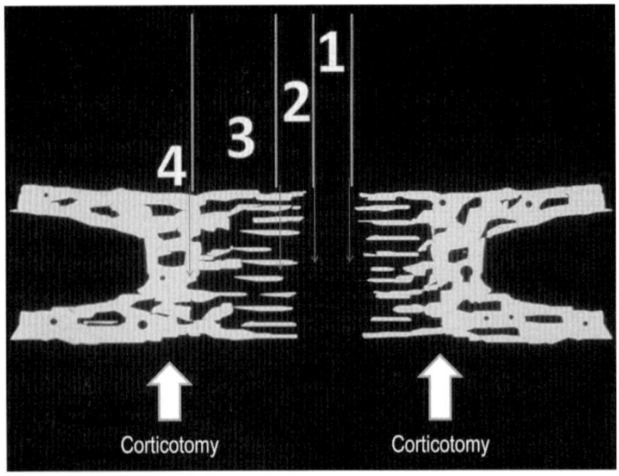

Figure 7.2. Zones of distraction. *Zone 1: Zone of fibrous tissue* is an area of longitudinally oriented parallel strands of collagen with mesenchymal progenitor cells located throughout the matrix. *Zone 2: Zone of extending bone formation* is an area where mesenchymal precursor cells are in direct contact with maturing osteoblasts on small mineralized spicules of calcified extracellular matrix. The osteoblasts assume a longitudinal orientation in the direction of distraction. *Zone 3: Zone of bone remodeling* consists of advancing bone resorption, osteoclast cutting cones, and greater bony apposition. There are more osteoclasts in this zone than in other regions of the bony generate. *Zone 4: Zone of mature bone* is the area containing early compact cortical bone located adjacent to the mature bone in the bony generate. Reprinted with permission from Lippincott Williams & Wilkins (Ref. 8).

Zone 1: Zone of fibrous tissue is an area of longitudinally oriented parallel strands of collagen with mesenchymal progenitor cells located throughout the matrix and inflammatory cells serving to secrete the raw material for calcified extracellular matrix formation. The parallel fibers of collagen serve as the raw material and scaffold for calcified extracellular matrix secretion.

Zone 2: Zone of extending bone formation is an area where mesenchymal precursor cells are in direct contact with maturing osteoblasts on small mineralized spicules of calcified extracellular matrix. The osteoblasts assume a longitudinal orientation in the direction of distraction. The osteoblasts have differentiated from the mesenchymal progenitor cell population and help to secrete extracellular matrix within the collagen bundles. This zone is found to have marked increases in alkaline phosphatase, pyruvic acid, and lactic acid throughout the activation period of distraction. It is an area with relative ischemia. This area, the bone generate, serves to signal progenitor cell homing.[1,10] The spatial and temporal patterns of transforming growth factor (TGF)-β1 mRNA expression and protein construction coincide with osteoblast migration, differentiation, and extracellular matrix synthesis. In addition, vasculogenesis and osteocalcin gene expression coincide with the TGF-β1-directed mineralization.[11]

Zone 3: Zone of bone remodeling is an area consisting of advancing bone resorption, osteoclast cutting cones, and greater bony constitution within the generate. There are more osteoclasts in this zone than in other regions of the bony generate.

Zone 4: Zone of mature bone is the area containing early compact cortical bone located adjacent to the mature bone in the bony generate. The bone is further characterized as having spicules of much larger size, and the spicules are less longitudinally oriented but instead are approaching the architecture of mature lacunar canalicular systems.

7.4 Practice

The application of the principles of regeneration has not only led to new avenues of study within the biology of craniofacial distraction but has also guided the application of distraction to the biology of reparative bone formation.

In the clinical scenario, distraction is compartmentalized into several phases of clinician/patient interaction based on the underlying biology: the latency phase, the activation phase, and the consolidation phase. A *latency phase* is suggested by experimental evidence to be the optimal interval of time before initiation of mechanical distraction. The latency phase can vary in different clinical scenarios and can range from as short as 24 hours, as in the infant, to upward of a week. In practice, it is known that the presence of mesenchymal cells and angiogenic mechanisms are critical to adequate bony generation. Therefore, with respect to the biology, the latency phase allows for the inflammatory signals within the osteotomy to recruit mesenchymal precursors to orchestrate the complex events that create mature bone. The latency phase also acts as a period of time for critical inosculation of blood vessels that will serve as the supply lines for cellular recruitment and homing. As stated above, the clinical scenario can dictate in part the latency phase, as some authors have suggested in animal models that there is no significant difference in immediate and delayed distraction as far as final bone formation is concerned.[12]

However, the underlying principles must be that an adequate vascular soft-tissue envelope must be present and that there must be an adequate number of precursor cells recruited from remote and surrounding locations. Obvious to this scenario is the fact that the osteotomized bone segments must be in apposition or close proximity before the onset of activation, because this allows for the secretion of extracellular matrix across the fracture site gap. The secreted extracellular matrix will later undergo mineralization in a time-dependent fashion. In the New York University protocol, we typically wait for 5 days (latency period) before initiating mandibular activation. In the infant, distraction is initiated as early as 1 day after the osteotomy.

The *activation phase* of distraction is associated with several variables regarding rate and frequency of distraction. In most models of craniofacial distraction, a rate of 1 to 2 mm/day of activation results in adequate bony generation.[8,13] It has also been demonstrated that dividing the daily distractions into small, more frequent distraction intervals accelerates bone formation.[1] This has been validated by experimental models that assay for biochemical markers of osteoblast formation and maturation.[11] It has yet to be determined scientifically what frequency is optimal or whether continuous distraction is optimal. However, there are practical issues of patient care in selecting a frequency that is likely to be implemented by the caregivers, especially in the case of pediatric distraction. It is also important to recognize and respect the underlying biologic principle that the activation phase must not outstretch the ability of mesenchymal precursor migration or bony inosculation. In the New York University protocol, we routinely distract at a rate of 1 mm/day with a frequency of twice-daily activation (0.5-mm increments).

The *consolidation phase* is the final phase of distraction before the removal of the distraction devices. Consolidation is the time period required for mineralization of the secreted extracellular matrix. In general, the mineralization process proceeds from the peripheral zones, closest to the osteotomy sites, to the central regions that are further away from the osteotomy sites.[9,14] The total time of consolidation is usually between 6 and 12 weeks. It should be noted that the consolidation phase may be lengthened depending on the clinical situation. It may be prudent in the face of a history of radiation, infection, prior attempts at distraction, or a compromised vascular envelope to extend the consolidation phase. As a general rule, the consolidation phase should be at least four times as long as the activation phase of distraction; usually 8 weeks is adequate. It is preferable to have radiographic evidence of mineralization of the bony generate, as in mandibular distraction.

7.5 Blood Supply and Device Stability

The success of distraction is, in part, directly related to the bone–blood supply as well as the soft-tissue envelope. Events that decrease blood flow to the distracted segments have been shown to negatively affect the regenerate.[15] Therefore, conditions such as radiation, the type of surgical technique, and decreased regional blood flow can affect the quality of bone generated. This is likely related to the observation that blood vessels must be in close proximity to the osteocyte, creating a functional lacunar system. Experimental evidence suggests that nutrient vessels must be at least 100 μm away from the healing callus to have adequate calcified extracellular matrix deposition.[16] Experimental data suggest that the distraction zone becomes relatively ischemic for a prescribed period of time during activation, and that endothelial and mesenchymal progenitor cells home to the ischemic generate site during activation and remain present throughout consolidation.[10] In unsuccessful distraction, it is evident that persistent ischemia may prevent mesenchymal progenitors from differentiating. Ischemia leads to the production of fibrous tissue or scar, lacking osteocytes and endothelial cells.[17]

Stable fixation of the osteotomized bone segments is a critical factor for successful distraction; distraction in the face of skeletal instability is futile. In a stable environment, bone formation is created directly throughout the distraction zone without a cartilaginous intermediate. Motion at the osteotomy site results in a mixture of unorganized cartilage and fibrous tissue deposition, that become interposed within the distraction zone. The effect of stable fixation on generate bone formation is thought to be multifactorial, but it is clear that motion can affect vasculogenesis through shear and by inducing granulation tissue.[9,18] In clinical terms, ischemia-induced fibrous tissue interposed within the distraction site leads to fibrous union and pseudoarthrosis.

7.6 Patient Selection

Distraction osteogenesis has been applied clinically to the mandible in every age group and has included patients with congenital mandibular hypoplasias as well as developmental, posttraumatic, and postoncologic ablation deficits. It is important to recognize that distraction can be accomplished in the face of soft-tissue deficiencies because, by its nature, elongation of the bone similarly elongates the associated soft tissue, a phenomenon termed *distraction histiogenesis.* It is the gradual accommodation of the soft tissue that prevents relapse and has in part made distraction preferable to conventional techniques, especially when there is associated soft-tissue deficiency. With conventional techniques requiring advancement of > 10 mm, the soft tissue imposes considerable stress because it has not been "distracted"; thus, the skeletal movement is more prone to relapse because the soft tissue has not expanded concomitantly.

Age is also a consideration in formulating a plan for mandibular distraction. In general, we reserve distraction for children older than 2 years unless there is airway compromise. Airway compromise can be improved if there are identifiable structural deficiencies in the form of hypoplastic mandibles (with glossoptosis), as in severe Treacher Collins syndrome, Pierre Robin syndrome, or craniofacial microsomia. In the neonate, mandibular distraction is indicated in severe cases of micrognathia, especially in those with upper airway obstruction, and may prevent the need for tracheotomy. This type of tongue-based airway obstruction can be diagnosed through a combination of computed tomography, direct laryngoscopy, flexible fiberoptic bronchoscopy, and sleep studies. If tracheotomy is already present, distraction can be used to expedite decannulation of the tracheotomy. In young children, mandibular distraction can remedy upper airway obstruction that coincides with obstructive sleep apnea by pulling the posterior tongue base forward from the posterior pharyngeal wall.

Distraction in our unit is used frequently as an early component of a comprehensive treatment plan for patients with severe craniofacial microsomia. It is useful in craniofacial microsomia, both unilateral and bilateral, because of its ability to expand the associated soft-tissue deficiency. During the phase of mixed dentition, from age 6 to adolescence, the patients generally undergo orthodontic treatment to promote dentoalveolar growth. Mandibular distraction is performed, during the mixed dentition phase, only in patients with airway compromise or in those with significant dysmorphism who have not previously received any prior intervention. After skeletal maturity (age 17–18 years), in patients with minimal mandibular occlusal deformities, classic orthognathic procedures are used instead of distraction. In the case of the mandible, this translates to various combinations of osseous genioplasty and bilateral sagittal split osteotomies to correct mandibular deficiencies. However, many patients with congenital conditions have already undergone multiple procedures and thus have an increased scar burden in the operative area. This scar burden can lead to increased relapse and restriction of movement with the classic orthognathic techniques.[19] Also, with classic orthognathic techniques, movements of >10 mm often encounter soft-tissue resistance, with inevitable relapse. With distraction osteogenesis, there is an associated soft-tissue histiogenesis with a gradual soft-tissue response to the incremental bony movement.[20] This unique property of distraction allows for orthognathic movements of greater magnitude and stability by circumventing the inherent soft-tissue envelope resistance.

The modified Pruzansky classification system for bilateral and unilateral mandibular hypoplasia is useful in guiding the planned

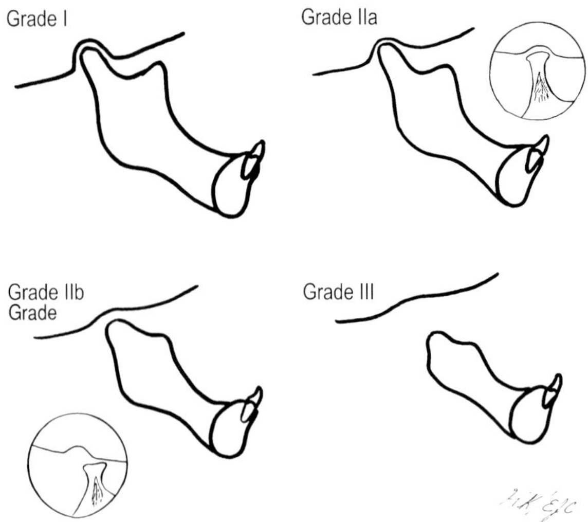

Figure 7.3. The Pruzansky classification system for bilateral and unilateral mandibular hypoplasia as modified by Mulliken and Kaban. Grade I mandibles are of normal shape but are reduced in size. Grade II mandibles demonstrate hypoplasia as well as shape change of the coronoid and condyle. Grade II is subdivided: Grade IIa mandibles maintain condylar head/glenoid fossa spatial relationship in the sagittal plane (top right insert); Grade IIb mandibles demonstrate displacement of the malformed condyle medially outside the sagittal plane of the TMJ (bottom left insert). Grade III mandibles have no condyle, ramus, or coronoid.

mandibular distraction (Figure 7.3).[21,22] Grade I mandibles are of normal shape but are reduced in size. Grade II demonstrates hypoplasia as well as stunting of the coronoid and condyle. Grade II mandibles were subdivided from the original Pruzansky classification by Mulliken and Kaban.[21] Grade IIa maintains the stunted coronoid and condyle with maintenance of the condylar head/glenoid fossa spatial relationship in the sagittal plane. These malformed condyles can still be used in the mandibular reconstruction because the position of the glenoid condyle is preserved. Grade IIb mandibles are hypoplastic with aberration of the coronoid and the condyle, but the malformed condyle is displaced medially outside the sagittal plane of the temporomandibular joint (TMJ). It is this lack of a functional joint position that portends poor joint function. Grade III mandibles have no condyle, ramus, or coronoid, and distraction is not possible with this type of osseus architecture. Grade III mandibles require autologous bone reconstruction of the condyle/ramus deficit. With different pathologic and congenital states, the preoperative plan needs to be amended for each clinical scenario.

7.7 Vector Selection

Surgical planning is of the utmost importance for optimal results. The first step in planning the mandibular distraction is to define the skeletal hypoplasia. The bony deficiency can predominate in one anatomic area such as the ramus or the body, or the entire mandible can be deficient. After defining the anatomic region to be distracted, the selection of the appropriate vector of distraction is one of the most important decisions for facilitating a successful treatment plan. Distraction can occur in the vertical, horizontal, or oblique plane in relation to the maxillary occlusal plane. The maxillary occlusal plane is a guide upon which the mandible translates through the distraction process.[23] This plane also serves as the anatomic reference to define the vector of distraction (Figure 7.4).

A horizontal vector forms an angle with the maxillary occlusal plane of < 30°. An oblique vector of distraction forms an angle with the maxillary occlusal plane between 30° and 45°. Likely the most commonly used vector of distraction is the vertical vector that forms an angle with the occlusal plane that is between 45° and 90°.

A vertical vector of distraction is preferred for lengthening a deficient ramus (as in Treacher Collins patients) in the vertical direction.[9] The vertical vector also results in greater counterclockwise symphyseal rotation, leading to horizontal projection of the mandible and greater closure of the anterior open bite.[24] The vertical vector lengthens the ramus unit and has the advantageous effect of symphyseal uprighting. However, one of its most important contributions is that it produces horizontal projection of the mandible and greater closure of the anterior open bite through counterclockwise rotation of the mandible (Figure 7.5). In bilateral mandibular distraction, using a vertical vector increases the posterior facial height and serves to remove the

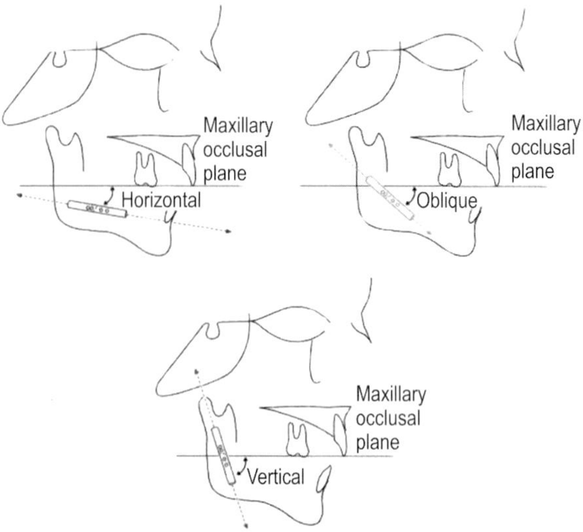

Figure 7.4. Defining the vector of distraction. The maxillary occlusal plane is the guide on which the mandibular distraction translates and the vector of distraction is defined in relation to this plane. A horizontal vector forms an angle with the maxillary occlusal plane of $< 30°$. An oblique vector forms an angle with the maxillary occlusal plane between 30° and 45°. The vertical vector forms an angle with the occlusal plane that is between 45° and 90°. Reprinted with permission from Wolters Kluwer Health (Ref. 24). Copyright © 2008 American Society of Plastic Surgeons.

posterior dentition from occlusion (posterior open bite). Disocclusion of the posterior dentition allows the mandible to autorotate until dental occlusion is reestablished anteriorly (Figure 7.6). In some instances, the location of the osteotomy and fixation of the distraction device may be technically challenging, especially in the face of inadequate bone stock. In this case, it may become necessary to compromise by placing the distraction device in an oblique plane. Also, in clinical practice, the vertical vector of distraction seems to be associated with more pain during the activation phase of distraction. We hypothesize that this may be related to the condyle's being loaded during activation, causing some discomfort in the TMJ.

The horizontal vector of distraction along the long axis of the mandible in a plane with the body is chosen to lengthen the mandible

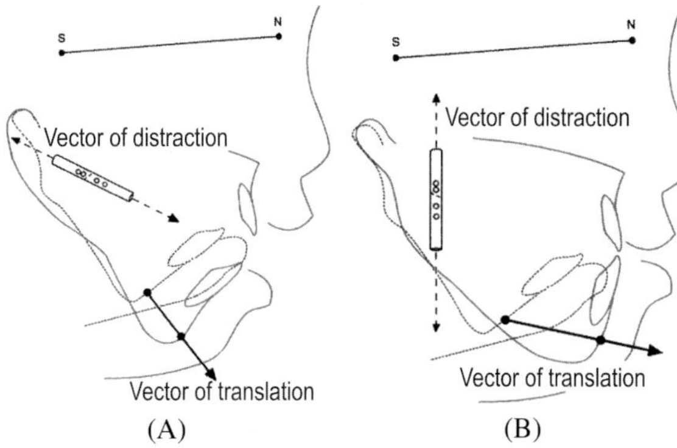

Figure 7.5. Result of vector selection in bilateral mandibular distraction. (A) A horizontal vector of distraction results in symphyseal flattening, downward vertical translation of the mandible, and limited closure of the anterior open bite. (B) A vertical vector of distraction lengthens the ramus unit and therefore has the effect of symphyseal uprighting, horizontal projection of the mandible, and greater closure of the anterior open bite through counterclockwise rotation of the mandible. Reprinted with permission from Wolters Kluwer Health (Ref. 24). Copyright © 2008 American Society of Plastic Surgeons.

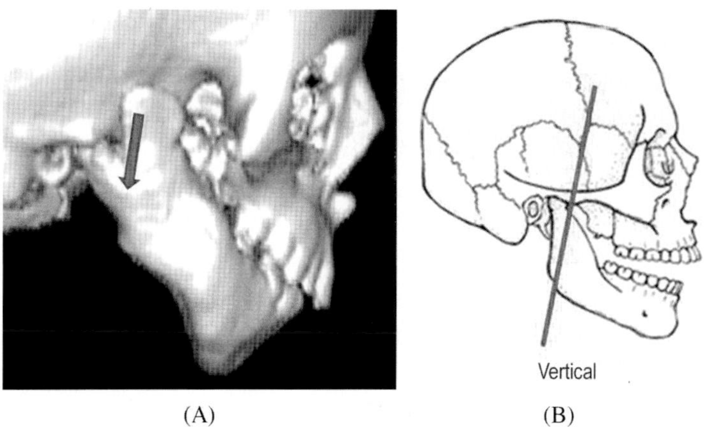

Figure 7.6. (A) Reformatted computed tomogram of a patient with Treacher Collins syndrome. The deficiency is more pronounced in the mandibular ramus (arrow). (B) A vertical vector of distraction is optimal to correct this deficiency. The vertical vector is useful in the elongation of the ramus when it is important to close an anterior open bite and initiate counterclockwise autorotation of the mandible.

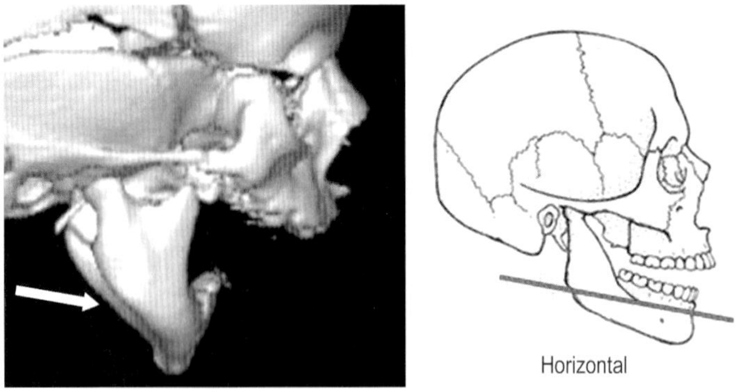

(A) (B)

Figure 7.7. The horizontal vector of distraction. (A) Reformatted computed tomogram of a patient with Pierre Robin syndrome with predominant deficiency in the mandibular body (arrow). (B) A horizontal vector of distraction can be selected to correct the deficiency. The horizontal vector extends new bone formation in the horizontal plane of the mandible. It is indicated in conditions in which the mandibular body is deficient.

in the purely horizontal plane, as in patients with Pierre Robin syndrome who are unresponsive to conservative management (Figure 7.7). In unilateral distraction, the horizontal vector of distraction produces a marked mandibular midline shift but minimal elongation of the affected ramus.[25] In bilateral horizontal distraction, the body of the mandible moves horizontally against the maxillary occlusal plane. This movement is acceptable in patients with a flat maxillary occlusal plane. However, in conditions with a steep maxillary occlusal plane, distraction with a horizontal vector fails to elicit posterior disocclusion of the dentition, and therefore there is little if any counterclockwise rotation. Without this posterior open bite disocclusion and mandibular autorotation, the symphyseal plane remains flat and the pogonion moves in a downward instead of anterior direction (Figure 7.5).[24] The horizontal vector of distraction and the osteotomy are perpendicular to the pull of the masseter muscle. Without stable fixation there is a theoretical risk that the masseter muscle contraction can induce torsion on the distal segment of the mandible. However, the horizontal vector of distraction may present the least technical challenge to the surgeon in terms of exposure, osteotomy, and device placement. With horizontal placement of a distraction device, the activation arm, in the internal distraction device, may be placed within the oral cavity. This allows the surgeon greater flexibility with the placement of the distraction device in the horizontal plane through an extraoral (Risdon) incision, or through an intraoral approach.

The oblique vector is the compromise between the horizontal and vertical vectors of distraction. The oblique vector of distraction serves both to lengthen the body of the mandible and to vertically elongate the ramus of the mandible. It is often used when there is not enough bone stock in the ramus to place the device in a purely vertical vector. The oblique vector also tends to avoid the discomfort associated with activation in the vertical direction, from presumed condyle loading.[26]

Surgical outcome often depends on accurate preoperative planning and prediction. It is possible to predict the mandibular response to distraction and to use the appropriate vector to achieve the desired response. In general, a more vertical vector is preferred because it closes the anterior open bite and provides horizontal projection of the mandible at the chin point. However, the mandibular response is affected by more than the vector of distraction, and careful consideration needs to be given to the bony and soft-tissue deficits, dental anatomy, and pathogenesis of the mandibular deficiency. In all mandibular distraction cases, the patient must be carefully monitored during all phases of distraction. During the activation phase, progress is monitored until the clinical end point is reached. During the consolidation phase, the generated bone can still be manipulated through a number of molding techniques (see Section 7.9) to allow the mandibular dentition to be brought into the proper occlusion with the maxillary dentition.

7.8 Surgical Technique

Preoperative preparation for mandibular distraction involves deciding between an external and internal distraction device as well as planning the vector of distraction. External devices were the first devices available; they are relatively easy to place and can be removed without the need for another surgical procedure. They are especially indicated when there is limited bone stock. These devices are sometimes cumbersome, being remote from the moment arm of distraction, and they can be dislodged in the active pediatric population. In addition, the external device requires pin care, and scarring results from pin migration during the activation phase. Internal devices can be more challenging to place, especially when the bone stock is inadequate for device placement. With internal devices there are more limitations with bony purchase, and there is more stripping of the periosteum; the latter, theoretically, has the deleterious effect of decreasing bone–blood supply. In clinical practice, no difference has been noted with bone healing using either an external or an internal device. Most mandibular distractions performed in our unit are with a semiburied internal distraction device placed through a modified Risdon incision (Figure 7.8). The semiburied internal device allows for greater flexibility

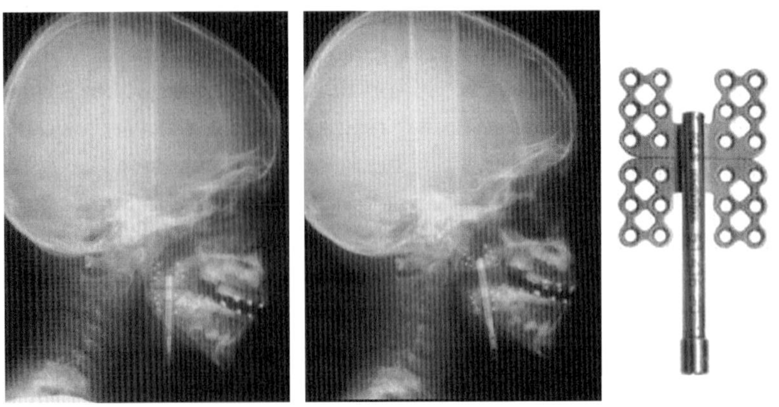

(A) (B) (C)

Figure 7.8. The semiburied device. (A) Cephalogram of a patient with the semiburied device placed in a vertical vector before activation of distraction. (B) At the end of the activation phase, awaiting ossification of the generated bone. (C) A close-up of the device itself. The use of the semiburied device allows for greater flexibility of vector selection, especially when a vertical vector is preferred, as in this mild case of craniofacial microsomia for lengthening of the ramus in the vertical dimension.

in the vector of distraction selection; it is especially indicated for the vertical vector. Internal devices also do not have the associated scarring with pin migration during the activation process.

In most cases, nasal intubation is preferred, but anesthesia can be administered with either an oral or a nasal intubation. It is prudent to outline the mandibular border with a skin marker. With the extraoral approach, care must be taken not to damage the soft tissues that may be sites for further reconstructive surgery, especially in patients with microtia. A 2- to 4-cm skin incision is made below the border of the mandible; the dissection is extended toward the mandible to the level of the platysma. The platysma is incised, and the dissection is performed by spreading with a blunt instrument within the tissues deep to the platysma until the inferior border or attachment of the masseter muscle is reached. Care is taken to identify and avoid injury of the marginal mandibular nerve; after the nerve is localized, it can be retracted superiorly for protection. The dissection continues through the periosteum, and the subperiosteal plane is exposed broadly to provide access to the mandible for device placement. A combination of burring, reciprocating saw, and osteotomies are used to perform the mandibular corticotomy. The device is rigidly secured, and the corticotomy is then converted to an osteotomy. Finally, the device is tested in position, and the activation arm is placed through the incision or through a separate stab incision. The wound is closed in layers with absorbable sutures.

Depending on the amount of distraction required, after an appropriate latency phase, activation occurs until there is a slight overcorrection. Overcorrection is evidenced by the mandibular midline shift to the side opposite to distraction in unilateral cases and the development of a posterior open bite on the affected side. In the growing child, the amount of overcorrection must take into account the amount of predicted growth potential. The overcorrection is used because the distracted mandible maintains some of its inherent growth potential but at a lower rate than normal.[27] Clinical examination incorporates multiple points of evaluation throughout the activation phase of the distraction process. To stop the activation phase, the position of the chin point, oral commissure, occlusion, mandibular inferior border, ramus height, and associated soft tissue must be monitored clinically and radiographically.

7.9 Molding the Generate

In some patients who have undergone mandibular distraction before completion of skeletal maturity, malocclusions have developed from continued normal or asymmetric mandibular growth. Experience in the laboratory with animal models demonstrates that the generated bone can be distracted in multiple dimensions.[28–30] From these observations and from clinical experience, appeared the concept that the mandible could be gradually or acutely molded into the desired occlusal relationship by manipulating the zone of bony generate.[31] Long-term studies have shown that the generated bone can be molded during the period of bony consolidation.[32] Molding can be exerted on the generated bone by translational forces applied from either the distraction device itself or from the dentoalveolus. The application of forces through the device is related to the engineering of the device and the degrees of freedom associated with the device. Some devices are designed as curvilinear distraction devices or multidimensional devices that mold the generate along fixed planes. Most commonly, in our unit, the generated bone is molded though translational forces at the dentoalveolar level. In part, this is done because the clinical end point is a functional occlusal relationship with closure of an anterior open bite (Figure 7.9). The generate can often be molded with guiding elastics secured to plates or screws.

In applying molding forces, one must be careful to avoid excessive force on the dentition, as excessive tooth extrusion can result with molding. In our unit, we prefer that intermaxillary traction and mandibular molding are applied from skeletal anchorage points with orthodontic temporary anchorage devices or with partially buried 1.5- or 2.0-mm plates that have screw holes cut (Figure 7.10) to accept guiding elastics, as well as acrylic splints with "molding hooks" bonded to the upper and lower dental arch.[31] Intermaxillary elastic traction can then be applied to the splint and directly to the bone to distribute the molding forces of the generate over the entire dental

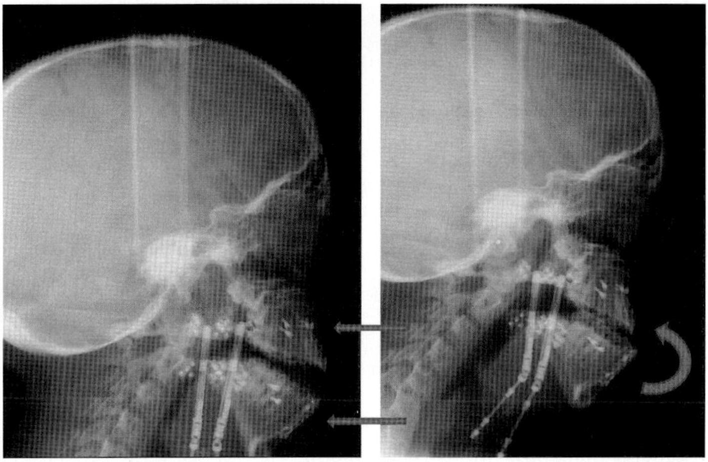

(A) (B)

Figure 7.9. Molding the generate in bilateral mandibular distraction. (A) Cephalogram of a patient after the completion of the activation phase of distraction. Note the vertical vectors and the anterior open bite. (B) After the generate is molded, the anterior open bite is closed (curved arrow), allowing for a more functional occlusion and opening of the posterior airspace with counterclockwise rotation of the mandible. Note that in the anterior maxilla and anterior mandible, small plates were placed at the time of distraction-device placement. These plates (straight arrows) provide points of fixation from which to mold the generated bone with guiding elastics.

arch and thus reduce the extrusion risk on individual teeth. Molding can be initiated during the latter aspect of the activation phase and can continue into the early consolidation phase. It should be noted that the fixation devices, i.e., the screws and pins that secure the distraction device, can actually migrate through the bone during the molding process. The craniofacial bone adheres to the piezoelectric theory of bone deposition, and thus forces applied to the generated bone can create bone deposition in regions of interest by exploiting the intrinsic properties of bone development.[33] On a clinical level, this allows the craniofacial orthodontist to make movements during the activation and consolidation phases of distraction to achieve an optimal occlusal relationship.

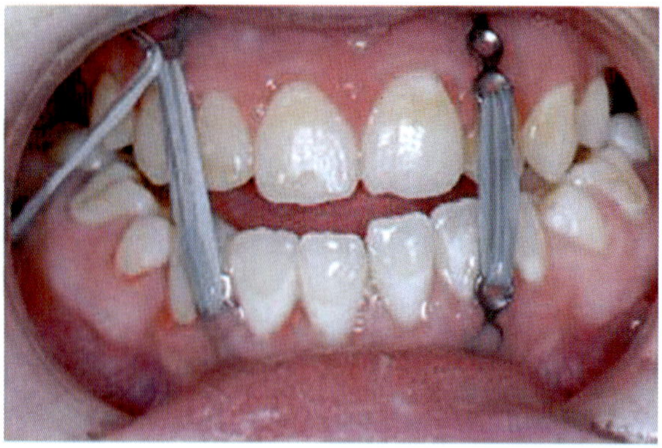

Figure 7.10. Intraoral elastics for generate molding. Intraoral view of a patient with Treacher Collins syndrome. The guiding elastics are molding the generated bone. Note that the plates are anchored to the bone in an effort to distribute the forces across the anterior aspect of the dentoalveolar arch.

7.10 Conclusions

The combined role of the surgeon and orthodontist working together is critical for a successful treatment outcome and extends from the preoperative period to well beyond the removal of the distraction devices. The need for molding of the generate with postactivation orthodontics and prosthodontic therapy must be conceived during the preoperative evaluation to achieve the optimal skeletal and occlusal relationship. Distraction osteogenesis is a form of tissue engineering, and understanding the basic mechanisms can allow one to investigate ways to accelerate the process of bone healing and consolidation. Mandibular distraction is of particular use when there are clinical indications for large orthognathic movements, especially in the face of a restrictive soft-tissue envelope. Distraction techniques also have a direct compensatory effect on the surrounding soft tissue (distraction histiogenesis). In unilateral distraction, the treatment goal is overcorrection of the affected side in the growing child. In the bilateral condition, the treatment goal is closing of the anterior open bite and the creation of an anterior crossbite. New indications will continue to evolve for mandibular distraction, and the application of the principles of distraction will continue to improve. Essential to improvement is careful preoperative planning, with measured and documented assessments of the clinical results.

References

1. **Ilizarov GA.** Clinical application of the tension-stress effect for limb lengthening. *Clin Orthop Relat Res* 1990;250:8–26.
2. **Tessier P.** The definitive plastic surgical treatment of the severe facial deformities of craniofacial dysostosis: Crouzon's and Apert's diseases. *Plast Reconstr Surg* 1971;48:419–442.
3. **Tessier P**. Relationship of craniostenoses to craniofacial dysostoses, and to faciostenoses: a study with therapeutic implications. *Plast Reconstr Surg* 1971;48:224–237.
4. **Karp NS, Thorne CH, McCarthy JG, Sissons HA.** Bone lengthening in the craniofacial skeleton. *Ann Plast Surg* 1990;24:231–237.
5. **McCarthy JG, Schreiber J, Karp N, Thorne CH, Grayson BH.** Lengthening the human mandible by gradual distraction. *Plast Reconstr Surg* 1992;89:1–10.
6. **Molina F, Ortiz Monasterio F.** Mandibular elongation and remodeling by distraction: a farewell to major osteotomies. *Plast Reconstr Surg* 1995;96:825–842.
7. **McCarthy JG.** Principles of craniofacial distraction. In: Thorne CH, ed. *Grabb and Smith's Plastic Surgery*. 6th edn. Philadelphia, PA: Lippincott Williams & Wilkins; 2007:96–102.
8. **Karp NS, McCarthy JG, Schreiber JS, Sissons HA, Thorne CH.** Membranous bone lengthening: a serial histological study. *Ann Plast Surg* 1992;29:2–7.
9. **McCarthy JG, Stelnicki EJ, Mehrara BJ, Longaker MT.** Distraction osteogenesis of the craniofacial skeleton. *Plast Reconstr Surg* 2001;107:1812–1827.
10. **Cetrulo CL Jr., Knox KR, Brown DJ, *et al.*** Stem cells and distraction osteogenesis: endothelial progenitor cells home to the ischemic generate in activation and consolidation. *Plast Reconstr Surg* 2005;116:1053–1067.
11. **Mehrara BJ, Rowe NM, Steinbrech DS.** Rat mandibular distraction osteogenesis: II. Molecular analysis of transforming growth factor beta-1 and osteocalcin gene expression. *Plast Reconstr Surg* 1999;103:536–547.
12. **Karaharju-Suvanto T, Karaharju EO, Ranta R.** Mandibular distraction: an experimental study on sheep. *J Craniomaxillofac Surg* 1990;18:280–283.
13. **Izadi K, Yellon R, Mandell DL, *et al.*** Correction of upper airway obstruction in the newborn with internal mandibular distraction osteogenesis. *J Craniofac Surg* 2003;14:493–499.

14. **Staffenberg DA, Wood RJ, McCarthy JG, Grayson BH, Glasberg SB.** Midface distraction advancement in the canine without osteotomies. *Ann Plast Surg* 1995;34:512–517.
15. **Stelnicki EJ, Stucki-McCormick SU, Rowe N, McCarthy JG.** Remodeling of the temporomandibular joint following mandibular distraction osteogenesis in the transverse dimension. *Plast Reconstr Surg* 2001;107:647–658.
16. **Ham AW.** Some histophysiological problems peculiar to calcified tissues. *J Bone Joint Surg Am* 1952;24-A-3:701–728.
17. **Klotch DW, Ganey TM, Slater-Haase A, Sasse J.** Assessment of bone formation during osteoneogenesis: a canine model. *Otolaryngol Head Neck Surg* 1995;112:291–302.
18. **Aronson J, Harrison B, Boyd CM, Cannon DJ, Lubansky HJ.** Mechanical induction of osteogenesis: the importance of pin rigidity. *J Pediatr Orthop* 1988;8:396–401.
19. **Munro IR.** Combining facial osteotomies for esthetic and occlusal change. *Clin Plast Surg* 1982;9:457–477.
20. **Aronson J.** Experimental and clinical experience with distraction osteogenesis. Cleft Palate *Craniofac J* 1994;31:473–482.
21. **Mulliken JB, Kaban LB.** Analysis and treatment of hemifacial microsomia in childhood. *Clin Plast Surg* 1987;14:91–100.
22. **Figueroa AA, Pruzansky S.** The external ear, mandible and other components of hemifacial microsomia. *J Maxillofac Surg* 1982;10:200–211.
23. **Grayson BH, McCormick S, Santiago PE, McCarthy JG.** Vector of device placement and trajectory of mandibular distraction. *J Craniofac Surg* 1997;8:473–482.
24. **Vendittelli BL, Dec W, Warren SM, Garfinkle JS, Grayson BH, McCarthy JG.** The importance of vector selection in preoperative planning of bilateral mandibular distraction. *Plast Reconstr Surg* 2008;122:1144–1153.
25. **Dec W, Peltomaki T, Warren SM, Garfinkle JS, Grayson BH, McCarthy JG.** The importance of vector selection in preoperative planning of unilateral mandibular distraction. *Plast Reconstr Surg* 2008;121:2084–2094.
26. **Shetye PR, Warren SM, Brown D, Garfinkle JS, Grayson BH, McCarthy JG.** Documentation of the incidents associated with mandibular distraction: introduction of a new stratification system. *Plast Reconstr Surg* 2009;123:627–634.
27. **Shetye PR, Grayson BH, Mackool RJ, McCarthy JG.** Long-term stability and growth following unilateral mandibular distraction in growing children with craniofacial microsomia. *Plast Reconstr Surg* 2006;118:985–995.
28. **Hollier LH, Rowe NM, Mackool RJ, *et al.*** Controlled multiplanar distraction of the mandible. Part III: Laboratory studies of sagittal (anteroposterior) and horizontal (mediolateral) movements. *J Craniofac Surg* 2000;11:83–95.

29. **Williams JK, Rowe NM, Mackool RJ, *et al.*** Controlled multiplanar distraction of the mandible. Part II: Laboratory studies of sagittal (anteroposterior) and vertical (superoinferior) movements. *J Craniofac Surg* 1998;9:504–513.
30. **McCarthy JG, Williams JK, Grayson BH, Crombie JS.** Controlled multiplanar distraction of the mandible: device development and clinical application. *J Craniofac Surg* 1998;9:322–329.
31. **McCarthy JG, Hopper RA, Hollier LH Jr, Peltomaki T, Katzen T, Grayson BH.** Molding of the regenerate in mandibular distraction: clinical experience. *Plast Reconstr Surg* 2003;112:1239–1246.
32. **Luchs JS, Stelnicki EJ, Rowe NM, Naijher NS, Grayson BH, McCarthy JG.** Molding of the regenerate in mandibular distraction. Part 1: Laboratory study. *J Craniofac Surg* 2002;13:205–211.
33. **Marino AA, Gross BD.** Piezoelectricity in cementum, dentine and bone. *Arch Oral Biol* 1989;34:507–509.

CRANIOFACIAL DISTRACTION OF THE MAXILLA 8

Scott P. Bartlett MD; Russell R. Reid, MD, PhD and Ivona Percec, MD, PhD

8.1 Introduction

Distraction osteogenesis of the midface is performed to correct bony and soft tissue deficits of the maxilla, zygoma, or fronto-orbital regions. To address specific anomalous midface morphologic relationships, distraction can be performed at one of four levels: Le Fort I, Le Fort II, Le Fort III, and the fronto-orbital and midface level, also known as the monobloc advancement. Midface advancement with distraction osteogenesis confers several advantages over conventional midface advancement, including avoidance of bone grafts, plates and screws; decreased surgical time; decreased blood loss; decreased hospitalization time; and improved aesthetics. The most important advantage conferred by distraction, however, is its ability to advance tissues over a greater distance in one procedure, thereby potentially obviating the need for a secondary advancement. Following traditional steps are required for distraction osteogenesis of the midface: (1) osteotomy, (2) latency period (3 to 7 days), (3) distraction (~1 mm/day), (4) consolidation (mineralization) period (3 to 6 weeks), and (5) removal of the distractor.

Distraction of the midface is most commonly performed for maxillary hypoplasia, typically resulting from impaired maxillary growth in patients who have undergone cleft lip and palate repair. Scar-tissue formation resulting from these repairs, in addition to primary maxillary growth deficits, can produce severe maxillary hypoplasia that requires very large bony advancements for full correction. Such patients can benefit from Le Fort I-type distraction osteogenesis. Midface dysplasia secondary to midface underdevelopment is also seen in a spectrum of craniofacial syndromes, collectively termed *craniofacial dysostoses*, including Apert's, Treacher Collins', Crouzon's, and Pfeiffer's syndromes, among others. Those patients with severe midface hypoplasia who have not yet completed facial growth may benefit from distraction osteogenesis at the Le Fort II or III level. The monobloc, or fronto-orbital and midface distraction, is typically performed for patients with syndromal midface growth deformity who also require advancement of the forehead and orbits at one stage. In this patient population, monobloc distraction significantly reduces complications when compared with traditional monobloc advancement because extradural dead space is avoided. Finally, the smallest group of patients requiring distraction osteogenesis are those with acquired anomalies. Among these are patients with posttraumatic midface retrusion, atrophy of edentulous zones, and defects resulting from oncologic or dysplastic processes.

8.2 Preoperative Planning

When operative intervention is indicated, the craniofacial surgeon completes the preoperative workup, obtaining any additional studies necessary for planning and completing the procedure. The preoperative evaluation can often be extensive and requires close collaboration between multiple medical specialists, most notably the orthodontist and craniofacial surgeon, to optimize the initial surgical outcome and the patient's long-term result. Preoperative testing and planning modalities are used in concert with physical examination findings to aid the surgeon in planning the operative approach in detail, including the total desired advancement as well as distraction vectors. Typically, preoperative 3-dimensional dental occlusion models and imaging studies are obtained, including frontal and lateral cephalograms, panoramic (Panorex) radiographs, and maxillofacial computed tomography (CT) with 3-dimensional reconstructions. It is important to consider any asymmetry including that affecting the mandibular and occlusal planes. Occlusal relations (anterior–posterior, transverse, open bite) should also be well delineated preoperatively. All these parameters must be examined to establish the correct distraction vector and distractor device placement. When planning a midface advancement procedure, one must also consider parameters such as the severity of exorbitism, the nature of anterior–posterior deficiency within the midface bony structures, and the position of the midface relative to the cranial base and mandible.[1] The surgeon typically calculates the expected total distraction distance in relation to anatomic deficits, as based upon the physical examination, CT imaging, and cephalometric analysis. Concurrently, he or she estimates the expected latency period (typically, 3–7 days), the speed and frequency with which distraction is to be conducted (typically, 1 mm/day) and the consolidation time, while taking into account the patient's age, prior surgery and scarring, and overall bone quality. Additionally, one must consider the patient's age with respect to the potential for growth and hence, whether overcorrection is necessary, to allow for anticipated secondary growth deficiency of the distracted segment.

The surgeon must subsequently determine whether the patient would benefit most from an internal or external distraction device. Internal distraction devices that are buried within the soft tissue exiting through the skin or mucosa are less obtrusive, resulting in diminished scar formation, but require a second procedure for removal and do not permit vector adjustment during the distraction process. In contrast, external distraction devices, while sometimes resulting in significant scarring, provide increased distraction flexibility through movement and alteration of the vector during distraction. Furthermore, external devices are easily removed. If either type of device can readily correct the anatomic defect, the decision is typically deferred to the families, although external halo-type devices are more commonly used overall.

Contraindications to distraction osteogenesis, though few, can cause significant morbidity in these patients if not appreciated. First, inadequate bone stock or very young age can result in distraction failure and severe damage to manipulated regions of bone. In addition, noncompliance with distraction regimens can result in distraction asymmetry, premature union, fibrous nonunion, or infection of the operative sites.

8.3 Le Fort I Maxillary Distraction

Isolated maxillary advancement, or Le Fort I maxillary distraction, is performed primarily on patients with midfacial retrusion secondary to cleft deformity (Figure 8.1, A–C).[2–5] In approximately 25% to 50% of patients with complete unilateral cleft lip and palate,[6,7] the class III malocclusion is sufficiently severe to warrant surgical intervention.[8] A subset of these patients requires advancements greater than can be obtained by traditional Le Fort I osteotomy and advancement. Because advancements up to 40 mm may be achieved with maxillary distraction, Le Fort I distraction (LF I DO) is considered the gold-standard treatment for these patients. LF I DO is typically performed on patients who are in the mixed dentition phase (ages 6–12) (Figure 8.1, D–H). Oral intubation may be used during these procedures, as there is no need for mandibulomaxillary fixation. After maxillary exposure by upper buccal sulcus incision, the osteotomy is made at the conventional Le Fort I lines on the maxilla: the lateral wall, medial sinus wall, nasal septum, and pterygomaxillary junction. Internal reference marks may be used to avoid injury to the root apices. The osteotomy line is horizontal and made parallel to the occlusal plane. A reciprocating saw is typically used to section the lateral wall of the maxilla in a posterior-to-anterior direction, although the sequence of cuts can vary based on the surgeon's preference. Importantly, plate-and-screw fixation is not necessary during this procedure. Consequently, the Le Fort I osteotomy can be made at a very high level, just inferior to the infraorbital foramen, thereby avoiding

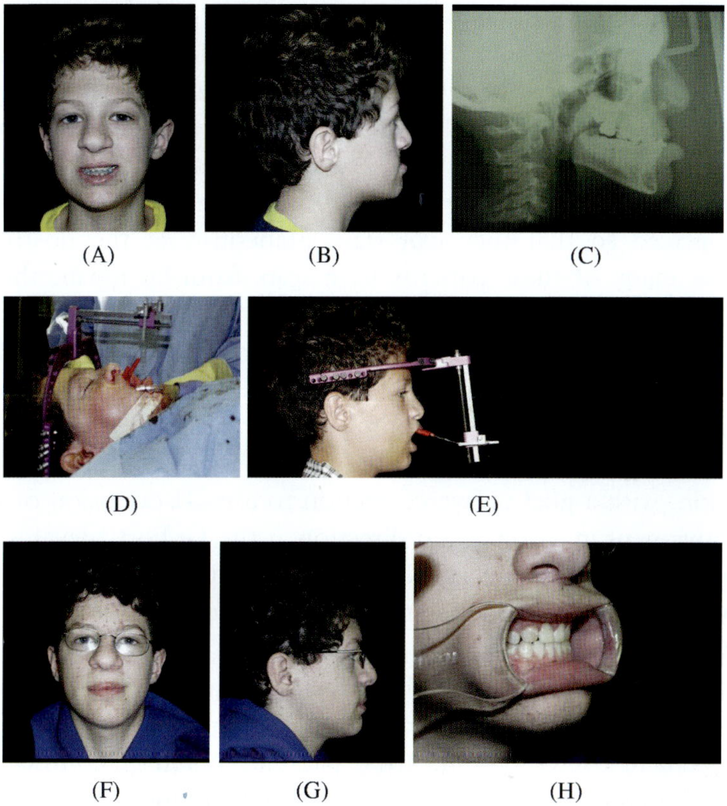

Figure 8.1. Le Fort I maxillary distraction for class III malocclusion: a 12-year-old boy with dentofacial skeletal abnormality secondary to complete cleft lip and palate deformity. (A and B) Severe maxillary retrusion evident on frontal and lateral photographs. (C) Lateral cephalogram. (D and E) Placement of distraction pins on the distal osteotomized segment, exiting below the upper lip. Postdistraction facial (F and G) and occlusal (H) views demonstrate excellent class I relations.

damage to the permanent tooth follicles. Alternatively, incomplete osteotomies can be made in order to protect the permanent teeth in these children, which may still be located high in the maxilla.

Several types of maxillary distractors are available. The rigid external distractor or similar external devices are particularly stable and permit modification of the distraction vector during activation. A variety of internal distractors are also available. Most centers prefer a halo-type external distraction system since they consider the Le Fort I internal device too cumbersome in these children. Initially, the exit pins were often placed below the upper lip, where they were attached to wires protected by a red rubber catheter over which the lip was draped (Figure 8.1, D–E). This proved uncomfortable for patients and continued to cause lip erosion. Accordingly, the pins are now often placed so that they exit transcutaneously at the nostril sill. Because many of these patients have scars from lip repair, the exit point can frequently be through the lip scar. As an alternative, a dentally mounted device can be used; however, it is difficult to obtain such custom-made devices that fit well and are not bulky. Percutaneous pins not only provide greater purchase but are also less awkward to place. The vector is usually selected in a forward and/or downward direction, with a goal of overcorrection to class II occlusion or overjet. Movement in a downward direction at the Le Fort I level is typically limited only by facial aesthetics, and this must be balanced against the need to close the anterior open bite.

Although it is widely known that children often partially outgrow the correction achieved with LF I DO, it continues to be the standard approach to severe midfacial retrusion. While LF I DO is typically completed to overcorrection, these patients should be counseled on the potential need for a second maxillary advancement with standard orthognathic surgery once they reach craniofacial maturity at age 17 or 18. The risks for LF I DO are the same as those for other midface distraction procedures and include hemorrhage (especially if the osteotomy cut is carried into the pterygomaxillary fissure), infection, poor bony healing, compound cranial fractures in the setting of minor trauma and, extremely rarely, blindness.

8.4 Le Fort II and III Midface Distraction

Le Fort II or III distraction, or complete midfacial advancement, is typically performed for children in the active growth phase who present with severe midface hypoplastic deficits resulting from syndromic disorders such as Apert's and Crouzon's syndromes.[9–12] Le Fort II distraction, though rarely performed, is indicated when the malar region is satisfactory but the entire pyramidal central face (nasomaxillary region) requires advancement. This infrequent morphology is typically observed only in cleft patients. Candidates for Le Fort III distraction characteristically demonstrate severe midface retrusion, exorbitism, malocclusion, sleep apnea, and difficulty with mastication. Unlike distraction at the Le Fort I or II level, the Le Fort III distraction is not an orthognathic procedure, but rather one whose goal is to reposition the malar eminences as well as the nasomaxillary region.

Le Fort III distraction procedures are frequently performed in the middle years (ages 5–10) before facial growth is completed. The Le Fort III osteotomies are made at the conventional Le Fort III lines after exposure through a coronal incision. The initial osteotomy is conducted vertically through the zygomatic arch with a reciprocating saw. After the frontozygomatic suture is identified, an osteotomy is used to separate the lateral orbital wall inferiorly to the infraorbital fissure, and the floor of the orbit is separated from the infraorbital fissure using a small fissure burr. The oral cavity is entered and the posterior wall of the maxilla and pterygoid plates are sectioned, with the final osteotomy being the separation of the vomer. The optimal distraction vector is determined by the orbito–ocular relations rather than by dental occlusion. Attempting to close an anterior open bite at the Le Fort III level can result in excessive vertical orbital distance. The end goal of Le Fort III distraction in the growing child is maximal zygomatic advancement and, ideally, overcorrection to a class II occlusion and overjet. There can be a degree of relapse and/or mandibular growth that gradually leads to relative retrodisplacement of the midface. Overadvancement may obviate the need for a second Le Fort III procedure later in life, allowing final occlusal adjustment at maturity with the simpler Le Fort I procedure.

Le Fort III distraction can be performed with bilateral submersible midface-distraction devices or with hemihalo-type external devices. The external distractor is the more adjustable of the two options, permitting change in the distraction vector after initial placement, unlike the internal device. Furthermore, because the internal devices tend to push, rather than pull, the face forward, syndromic patients with hypoplastic zygoma may suffer a fracture at the zygomaticomaxillary suture. This would cause the central midface to be left behind as the zygoma continues to be advanced. This scenario more commonly occurs if the osteotomies are incomplete, especially in the septal or retromaxillary region. The external device, in contrast, pulls the central midface forward, and is less likely to fracture at the zygomaticomaxillary suture, thereby resulting in a more convex profile.[13] Nevertheless, the final choice of using an internal versus external device is typically left to the craniofacial surgeon's and the family's preferences.

8.5 Frontal Facial Advancement: Monobloc Distraction

The monobloc, or fronto-orbital and midface advancement, is typically performed for patients with severe fronto-orbital retrusion, midface hypoplasia, and class III malocclusion resulting from syndromic disorders such as Apert's and Crouzon's syndromes.[14–16] These patients may also suffer from increased intracranial pressure, requiring expansion of the anterior cranial vault. The choice between conducting a Le Fort III versus a monobloc advancement depends almost completely on the patient's frontal and midface proportions.[17] In the setting of a midface retrusion, if the supraorbital position is satisfactory, as is common in patients who have undergone previous fronto-orbital advancement, a subcranial Le Fort III procedure is indicated. If there is significant exorbitism and fronto-orbital retrusion, then a monobloc procedure is indicated. During discussions with the families of patients who are candidates for monobloc advancement, it is explained that these defects could be corrected either by a single monobloc procedure or by forehead reshaping followed by midface distraction at a later date. Monobloc distraction is indicated when the forehead, orbits, and midface all need to be moved equivalent distances. When the upper orbit, forehead, and midface need to be moved differentially, the procedures are sequenced: a fronto-orbital advancement is done separately from a Le Fort III advancement by distraction.

During a conventional monobloc procedure, the forehead and midface are separated from the skull base and repositioned 3-dimensionally to correct the frontofacial disproportions. The frontal component of the procedure addresses the anterior cranial vault, releasing any intracranial hypertension affecting patients with bicoronal synostosis as well as improving the contour of the forehead. The orbital advancement repositions the entire functional orbit to correct exorbitism and enophthalmos in these patients. In addition, the nasal structures are advanced, improving not only aesthetics but also the nasal airway. Finally, advancement of the entire midface, including palate, maxilla, and zygoma, addresses functional problems with the oral airway, permitting improvements in speech and articulation as well as optimization of midface cosmesis.

Like other midface distraction procedures, monobloc distraction is frequently performed in the middle years (ages 5–10), before facial growth is complete. The osteotomies are made after exposure with coronal and upper buccal sulcus incisions. Because there is an intracranial component to this approach, the procedure is typically performed in collaboration with a neurosurgeon who executes the craniotomy of the forehead bone flap. Osteotomies are then performed bilaterally in the anterior zygomatic arch, lateral orbital wall, orbital roof, medial orbital wall, orbital floor, and pterygomaxillary buttresses.

Monobloc midface distraction can be accomplished with external or internal distraction devices. Many centers prefer the external device, which is positioned with two points of fixation to the frontal bone and two points of fixation to the maxillary dental splint; this permits rotational and vertical changes to the vector as distraction proceeds. Other centers prefer bilateral buried midface distractors. Certain surgeons have modified the internal distraction approach from using four separate distractors (two on the zygoma and two on the lateral orbits) that often eroded through the delicate skin of young patients, to using only two distractors on the zygoma. This approach, when carefully planned, can be equally effective for advancement while reducing postoperative complications such as infection.

Although historically, the monobloc osteotomy and advancement was considered one of the most risky of all craniofacial osteotomies due to a high rate of infection, the application of distraction osteogenesis to the monobloc procedure has markedly reduced the dreaded risk of infection, presumably secondary to the minimal dead space produced at the time of the osteotomy. Traditional monobloc advancement procedures create a bony gap between the anterior cranial base and the mobilized monobloc, creating the potential for contamination from the paranasal sinuses. Since monobloc distraction creates an osteotomy only and no such gap, the risk of bacterial contamination into the extradural area is minimized. Nevertheless, the risk of meningitis and leakage of cerebrospinal fluid should be stressed during family discussions. The other major risks for the monobloc advancement are similar to the risks of other midface distraction approaches, including hemorrhage, fractures, and poor bony healing.

8.6 Outcomes

Surgical outcomes in the relatively new field of craniofacial distraction have drastically improved over the past decade, making distraction osteogenesis procedures overwhelmingly safe and well tolerated.[18] Complications such as infection, bleeding, suboptimal scarring, aberrant bone healing (premature consolidation or fibrous malunion), dental injury, asymmetry, and technical failure of distractors have drastically decreased.[19,20] Very rarely, a postoperative complication such as hemorrhage or severe infection requires urgent reoperation. Yet, even patients who undergo reoperations for serious complications tend to do quite well once the problem is corrected. Typically, most complications are treated conservatively on an outpatient basis.

In part, this progress is due to developments in the safety of anesthesia. Improved communication between craniofacial surgeons and pediatric anesthesiologists has led to a greater understanding of the unique intraoperative needs of craniofacial patients. Further improvements came with new generations of distraction devices and craniofacial surgical sets that enabled greater flexibility and facility with device placement. Advances in the field of osteogenesis research have not only improved our understanding of distraction osteogenesis physiology but have also improved surgical outcomes through their clinical application. Furthermore, the optimization of antibiotic protocols has led to reduction in the rate of infections. Likewise, improvements in the quality of screening of banked blood products have enabled safe administration of these agents with minimal side-effect profiles. Finally, the evaluation and treatment of craniofacial patients by multidisciplinary teams that included pediatric orthodontists has been especially invaluable at improving outcomes by placing a given patient's craniofacial surgical needs into the greater context of his or her developmental and medical profiles.

The benefits of midface distraction osteogenesis over conventional midface advancement and bone grafting cannot be sufficiently emphasized. When distraction is performed in the middle years and overcorrection is achieved, there is a reasonably high likelihood that a second advancement procedure will not be required later in life. In contrast, when one performs a traditional Le Fort I, II, III, or monobloc advancement in the middle years, there is a very high likelihood that a second advancement procedure will be required at skeletal maturity. The avoidance of a second major craniofacial procedure is of inestimable value for the physical and emotional well-being of the patient and family.

8.7 Future Directions

Given the relatively recent birth of craniofacial distraction, numerous modifications, applications, and advances are emerging. Refinements to the existing process of distraction lie in three basic areas: (1) device technology, (2) device application, and (3) cotherapeutics.[21–23] Advances in the first two areas target the main disadvantage of distraction osteogenesis, which is the need for device removal after consolidation, which is especially difficult in a buried device. Along these lines, the use of biodegradable materials would eliminate the need for two-stage procedures and would therefore be an ideal substrate for this application. Modifications in material science and internal device technology will further popularize one-stage internal distraction and make the period of wearing the device (during latency, activation, and consolidation phases) easier for both patient and family. To this end, motorized systems driven by miniature microprocessors, which obviate outpatient device activation by family members, are a focus of future development. Enhancing our understanding of the basic molecular biology of distraction and its phases will lead to further vital co- and adjunct therapies. Yet even without these new directions for research, distraction osteogenesis has easily become the procedure of choice in the treatment of many craniofacial conditions. These techniques not only lower morbidity but also provide results that, in most instances, are superior to those obtained by conventional techniques.

References

1. **Alonso N, Munhoz AM, Fogaça W, Ferreira MC.** Midfacial advancement by bone distraction for treatment of craniofacial deformities. *J Craniofac Surg* 1998;9:114–122.
2. **Polley JW, Figueroa AA.** Management of severe maxillary deficiency in childhood and adolescence through distraction osteogenesis with an external, adjustable, rigid distraction device. *J Craniofac Surg* 1997;8:181–186.
3. **Molina F, Ortiz Monasterio F, de la Paz Aquila M, Barrera J.** Maxillary distraction: aesthetic and functional benefits in cleft lip-palate and prognathic patients during mixed dentition. *Plast Reconstr Surg* 1998;101:951–963.
4. **Toth BA, Kim JW, Chin M, Cedars M.** Distraction osteogenesis and its application to the midface and bony orbit in craniosynostosis syndromes. *J Craniofac Surg* 1998;9:100–113, 119–122.
5. **Figueroa AA, Polley JW.** Management of severe cleft maxillary deficiency with distraction osteogenesis: procedures and results. *Am J Orthod Dentofacial Orthop* 1999;115:1–12.
6. **Good PM, Mulliken JB, Padwa BL.** Frequency of Le Fort I osteotomy after repaired cleft lip and palate or cleft palate. *Cleft Palate Craniofac J* 2007;44: 396–401.
7. **Daskalogiannakis J, Mehta M.** The need for orthognathic surgery in patients with repaired complete unilateral and complete bilateral cleft lip and palate [published online ahead of print February 28, 2009]. *Cleft Palate Craniofac J* 2009;46:498–502. doi:10.1597108–176.1

8. **Linton JL.** Comparative study of diagnostic measures in borderline surgical cases of unilateral cleft lip and palate and noncleft class III malocclusions. *Am J Orthod Dentofacial Orthop* 1998;113:526–537.
9. **Chin M, Toth BA.** Le Fort III advancement with gradual distraction using internal devices. *Plast Reconstr Surg* 1997;100:819–832.
10. **Meling TR, Tveten S, Due-Tonnessen BJ, Skjelbred P, Helseth E.** Monobloc and midface distraction osteogenesis in pediatric patients with severe syndromal craniosynostosis. *Pediatr Neurosurg* 2000;33:89–94.
11. **Fearon JA.** The Le Fort III osteotomy: to distract or not to distract? *Plast Reconstr Surg* 2001;107:1091–1106.
12. **Fearon JA.** Halo distraction of the Le Fort III in syndromic craniosynostosis: a long-term assessment. *Plast Reconstr Surg* 2005;115:1524–1536.
13. **Gosain AK, Santoro TD, Havlik RJ, Cohen SR, Holmes RE.** Midface distraction following Le Fort III and monobloc osteotomies: problems and solutions. *Plast Reconstr Surg* 2002;109:1797–1808.
14. **Havlik RJ, Bartlett SP.** The treatment of "malignant" exorbitism with an extended supraorbital advancement. *Plast Reconstr Surg* 1995;95:1094–1097.
15. **Fukuta K, Saito K, Potparić Z.** A comparison of single-stage versus gradual fronto-parietal advancement in terms of extradural dead space and bone deposition. *Br J Plast Surg* 1998;51:169–175.
16. **Hirabayashi S, Sugawara Y, Sakurai A, Tachi M, Harii K, Sato S.** Fronto-orbital advancement by distraction: the latest modification. *Ann Plast Surg* 2002;49:447–451.
17. **Fearon JA, Whitaker LA.** Complications with facial advancement: a comparison between the Le Fort III and monobloc advancements. *Plast Reconstr Surg* 1993;91:990–995.
18. **Ortiz Monasterio F.** Craniofacial distraction: the first decade. Paper presented at the 81st Annual Meeting of the American Association of Plastic Surgeons; April 26–29, 2002; Seattle, WA.
19. **Fearon JA, Yu J, Bartlett SP, Munro IR, Chir B, Whitaker L.** Infections in craniofacial surgery: a combined report of 567 procedures from two centers. *Plast Reconstr Surg* 1997;100:862–868.
20. **Baker SB, Weinzweig J, Bartlett SP, Whitaker LA.** Brain abscess as a complication of orthognathic surgery: diagnosis, management, and pathophysiology. *Plast Reconstr Surg* 1999;104:480–483.
21. **Cohen SR.** Craniofacial distraction with a modular internal distraction system: evolution of design and surgical techniques. *Plast Reconstr Surg* 1999;103: 1592–1607.

22. **Cohen SR, Simms C, Burstein FD.** Mandibular distraction osteogenesis in the treatment of upper airway obstruction in children with craniofacial deformities. *Plast Reconstr Surg* 1998;101:312–318.
23. **Weinzweig J, Baker SB, Mackay GJ, Whitaker LA, Bartlett SP.** Immediate versus delayed midface distraction in a primate model using a new intraoral internal device. *Plast Reconstr Surg* 2002;109:1600–1610.

MONOBLOC ADVANCEMENT 9

James P. Bradley, MD and Henry Kawamoto, MD, DDS

9.1 Introduction

A *monobloc advancement* is a craniofacial procedure that involves moving the frontal bone region, orbits, and midface forward as a single unit. It is typically used in the reconstruction of craniosynostotic syndromes such as Apert's, Crouzon's, or Pfeiffer's syndromes (Figure 9.1).[1,2] In addition to improving the dysmorphology of these craniofacial dysostosis syndromes, a monobloc advancement may alleviate upper airway obstruction (obstructive sleep apnea or tracheostomy dependence), improve ocular exposure problems from severe proptosis, or correct elevated intracranial hypertension.

9.2 History

In 1950, Gillies first described a midface advancement technique.[3] However, this procedure was abandoned because of the perceived difficulty and the risk of morbidity and mortality. Twenty years later, Tessier performed an advancement of the midface with osteotomies that followed the fracture pattern at the Le Fort III level.[1] After extensive anatomic studies on cadavers and careful planning, this

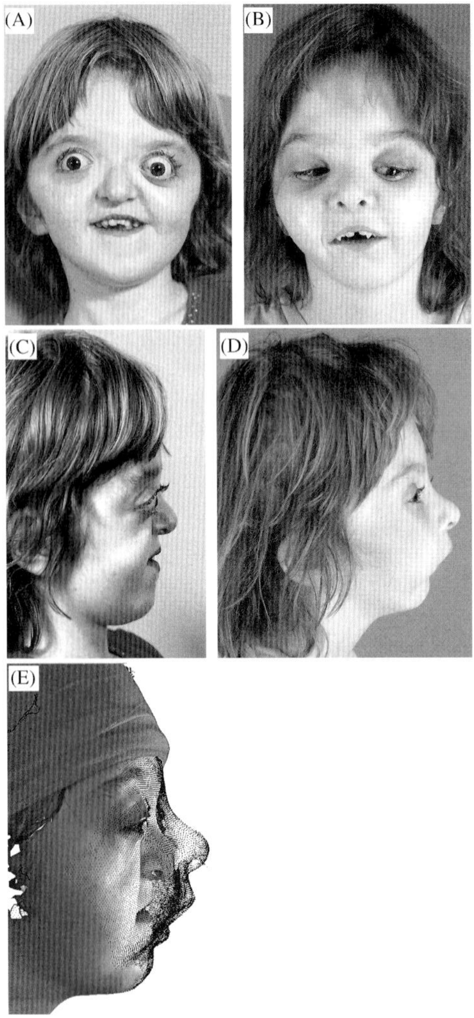

Figure 9.1. Patient with Apert's syndrome before (with hypertelorism and midface hypoplasia) and after (with correction by facial bipartition and monobloc distraction with Roman arch, keystone fixation modification). (A) Frontal preoperative view. (B) Frontal postoperative view. (C) Lateral preoperative view. (D) Lateral postoperative view. (E) Lateral view demonstrating preoperative image and postoperative wire mesh midface and forehead volume increase. Panels A–D reprinted with permission from Wolters Kluwer Health (Ref. 12). Copyright © 2008 by the American Society of Plastic Surgeons. Panel E reprinted with permission from Wolters Kluwer Health. (Chan FC, *et al.* Soft-tissue volumetric changes following monobloc distraction procedure: analysis using digital three-dimensional photogrammetry system [3dMD]. *J Craniofac Surg* 2013;24:416–420). Copyright © by Mutaz B. Habal, MD.

procedure was successfully performed in Paris and was then repeated as a demonstration in London.

Ortiz-Monasterio *et al.* are credited with performing one of the first monobloc procedures.[4] The Le Fort III procedure repositioned the midface alone, but the monobloc was unique in advancing the forehead, orbits, and midface as one unit. They reported performing the technique in a series of patients with Crouzon's syndrome. Among the seven cases they describe, the only complication was partial resorption of the frontal bone. Despite initial enthusiasm for the procedure, the communication of the nasal cavities and ethmoid sinuses with the intracranial space was thought to potentially contribute to serious infectious complications. Several authors questioned whether the risk of infection was too high to warrant its use.[5,6] Other anticipated complications were the need for prolonged ventilatory support, leakage of cerebrospinal fluid (CSF), major blood loss, and frontal bone necrosis. Some institutions banned the procedure; however, many surgeons continued to perform the monobloc advancement.

Van der Meulen applied the monobloc technique to the correction of orbital hypertelorism in a patient with a midline craniofacial cleft.[7] To correct the Apert's midface dysplasia and associated orbital hypertelorism, Tessier refined the vertical splitting and reshaping of the monobloc segment, thus correcting the midface deformity in three dimensions in a procedure now known as facial bipartition.[8] In 1983, Muhlbauer *et al.* reported performing monobloc advancement in an infant, but advocated its use only in cases of severe functional impairment.[9] Excellent results were reported by Kawamoto for monobloc and facial bipartition in patients with Apert's and Crouzon's syndromes.[10] However, he noted an exceedingly high complication rate in a subset of patients with ventriculoperitoneal shunts, possibly because the brain failed to fill the extradural space after the advancement.

More recently, it has been shown that gradual advancement by distraction osteogenesis after a monobloc osteotomy lowers the risk of complications.[11,12] With the distraction procedure and a delayed advancement (4- to 7-day latency), remucosalization of the nasofrontal area takes place before advancement. In addition, the traditional

Table 9.1. Indications for Monobloc Advancement Surgery.

1. Midfacial and forehead retrusive deformities
2. Upper airway obstruction
— Obstructive sleep apnea
— Tracheostomy dependence
3. Exorbitism
— Ocular keratitis
— Corneal ulcers
— Globe herniation
— Blindness
4. Intracranial hypertension

procedure requires bone grafting and rigid fixation, whereas the monobloc distraction procedure does not.

9.3 Indications

A monobloc advancement procedure is used in craniofacial dysostosis patients to correct (1) midfacial and forehead retrusive deformities, (2) upper airway obstruction (such as obstructive sleep apnea or tracheostomy dependence), (3) exorbitism (such as ocular keratitis, corneal ulcers, globe herniation, or blindness), and (4) intracranial hypertension (Table 9.1). In addition, a monobloc osteotomy may be used to facilitate a facial bipartition and correct either horizontal or vertical orbital dystopia.

9.4 Advantages and Disadvantages

The monobloc advancement procedure is advantageous because it avoids a second major procedure. In just one operation, both the forehead and midface deformities are corrected and functional improvement may be seen. The main disadvantage to a monobloc advancement is the risk of serious complications (e.g., meningitis, CSF leak, or complete frontal bone loss). In the past, this risk was considered too high for many institutions to advocate its use. The risk of infection may be caused by the large nasofrontal dead space and communication between epidural and ethmoidal sinus tissues left after the acute advancement of the facial–forehead unit. Now that monobloc distraction has been shown to be safer than anacute monobloc advancement, some institutions have been using monobloc distraction as their preferred treatment for craniofacial dysostotic patients with the operative indications listed above.

9.5 Alternative Treatment

There are treatment alternatives for craniofacial dysostosis patients with forehead retrusion and significant midface hypoplasia. Correction may involve either (1) staged procedures with fronto-orbital advancement followed by Le Fort III advancement or (2) a monobloc (one-unit) advancement. Sometimes the initial fronto-orbital advancement procedure performed in infancy maintains its correction so that only midface retrusion remains by midchildhood. In these patients, only Le Fort III advancement is necessary.

The first comparison of the monobloc procedure to the two-stage fronto-orbital advancement with subsequent Le Fort III procedure was reported by Fearon and Whitaker in 1993.[13] In their study, 29 patients (30 procedures) who had various craniofacial dysostoses were followed for a mean of 4 years after surgery. About 10 patients had undergone monobloc advancement and 20 patients had undergone the two-stage procedure. All five infectious complications occurred in the monobloc group despite the use of a galeofrontalis flap. The aesthetic result was deemed equivalent between the two groups and was improved if the procedure was done at an older age. Although the monobloc distraction has decreased morbidity, comparison with the staged fronto-orbital advancement with subsequent Le Fort III procedure has not been studied.

9.6 Timing

Patients with craniofacial dysostosis syndromes have cranial vault and midface deformities with common features and similar growth disturbances. Some surgical strategies, including timing and techniques, may thus be generalized for these syndromes. Optimal care, however, should be tailored to each individual diagnosis and each individual patient. The overall goals of the reconstructive surgical plan should be to minimize the number of operations, maximize the results, and achieve a predictable outcome. Typically, a monobloc advancement is necessary in midchildhood, at approximately age 8 to 12 years. At times, functional considerations (e.g., airway obstruction, ocular exposure, or intracranial hypertension) may push a surgeon to operate at a younger age. If the procedure is undertaken at too young an age, less than 8 years, then a subsequent monobloc advancement may be necessary because of growth or relapse. Temporizing therapies, like tarsorrhaphy suturing for ocular exposure or a continuous positive airway pressure mask for obstructive sleep apnea, may help delay a monobloc advancement until an appropriate age.

Recent case reports for severe craniofacial dysostotic patients have shown success with early, infant monobloc distraction using transfacial pins at the time of fronto-orbital advancement.[14,15] However, this new methodology has not been studied in detail.

Currently, for those severe cases, infant fronto-orbital advancement with a tracheostomy is most commonly performed in our institution.

9.7 Preoperative Planning

In preparing for a monobloc advancement, a CT with 3-dimensional reconstruction may be used as a "road map." In addition, we used 3-dimensional photographic imaging for preoperative, postoperative, and follow-up comparison of facial volumetric changes (Figure 9.1E). Other functional studies should be obtained if relevant to the case. These functional evaluations are often necessary for airway obstruction, ophthalmologic issues, and intracranial pathology. A sleep study will determine the degree of obstructive apnea and rule out a mixed component of central apnea. Ophthalmic evaluation should look for associated problems with visual acuity, strabismus, or optic disc changes from intracranial hypertension. In addition to ophthalmologic evaluation for signs of intracranial hypertension, symptoms (headaches, seizures, uncontrolled nausea and vomiting, or sudden personality changes) and CT changes should be considered. A preoperative orthodontic evaluation with full records (dental models, films, intraoral photographs) is also important. The procedural goals of monobloc advancement in midchildhood involve more orbital and forehead correction than occlusal correction; however, starting with a proper arch form and the benefit of guiding elastics during the distraction phase of an advancement are important for success.

9.8 External vs Internal Devices

The principles and use of distraction osteogenesis in the craniofacial skeleton have been well described by McCarthy and others.[16] Distraction osteogenesis was first described in conjunction with the monobloc procedure with an external device by Polley *et al.* in 1995.[17] Subsequently, Cohen *et al.* used an internal distraction device to advance the monobloc segment, claiming that the devices were less invasive and resulted in less blood loss, allowed for less relapse as a result of the gradual skin expansion, and resulted in overcorrection of the deformity and perhaps a lower rate of reoperation.[18,19] The external devices may be cumbersome, may require multiple adjustments, and often limit the consolidation period. With external devices, consolidation times may be as short as 3 weeks.[20] Patients with internal devices are more tolerant of the device, which allows for a longer consolidation period and possibly more stable bone formation. The newer internal devices may be removed without the need for a coronal flap turndown (Figure 9.2).

9.9 Surgical Technique

In our institution, we use zigzag coronal incision and subperiosteal dissection. The temporalis muscle is left down (to avoid temporal hollowing postoperatively) by dissecting just above the superficial layer of the deep temporal fascia (a plane just below the frontal branch of the facial nerve). Osteotomy sites are exposed with subperiosteal dissection around the circumferential orbit, down to the nasofrontal suture and to the zygomatic body. A small subperiosteal tunnel is

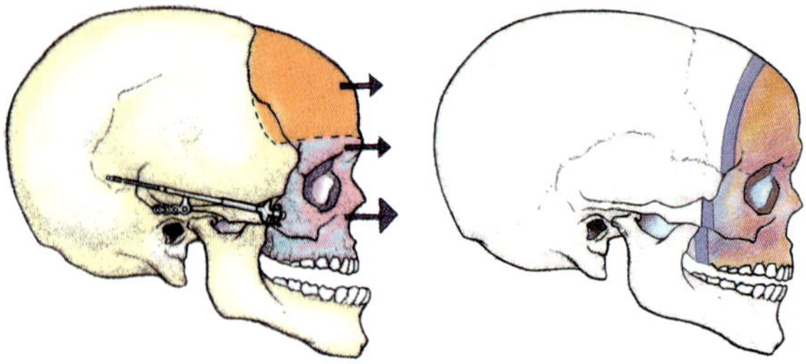
(A) (B)

Figure 9.2. (A) Illustration of right lateral skull with monobloc osteotomy before monobloc advancement. Midface and forehead retrusion is seen with internal distraction devices placed. (B) After advancement, consolidation and removal of distraction device. Shaded area depicts the area of advancement and generate bone formation with monobloc segment in an improved position. Reprinted with permission from Wolters Kluwer Health (Ref. 12). Copyright © 2008 by the American Society of Plastic Surgeons.

made under the temporalis muscle for the lateral-wall osteotomy. Intraoral exposure is used for the pterygomaxillary osteotomy. Craniotomy of the forehead bone flap is performed and, with retraction of the dura, the orbital roofs are exposed and dissection is completed back to the crista galli.

Osteotomies are to be performed bilaterally in the anterior zygomatic arch, lateral orbital wall, orbital roof, medial orbital wall, orbital floor, pterygomaxillary buttresses, and septum (after the midface down-fracture has started). Specifically, the lateral orbital wall osteotomy is made with a reciprocating saw passing underneath the temporalis muscle and directed toward the inferior orbital fissure. The lateral orbital wall osteotomy is carried up to the orbital roof through the sphenoid bone, then along the roof and across the cranial base anterior to the cribiform plate at the midline. A contralateral and symmetric osteotomy is made and connected to this midline osteotomy. Next, a small (4 mm) osteotome is used for the orbital floor between 1 and 2 cm posterior to the orbital rim and behind the lacrimal crest. The same osteotome is used for the medial wall osteotomy behind the medial canthus to complete the “doughnut osteotomy” around the globes. The Kawamoto osteotome is used for the pterygomaxillary osteotomies bilaterally.

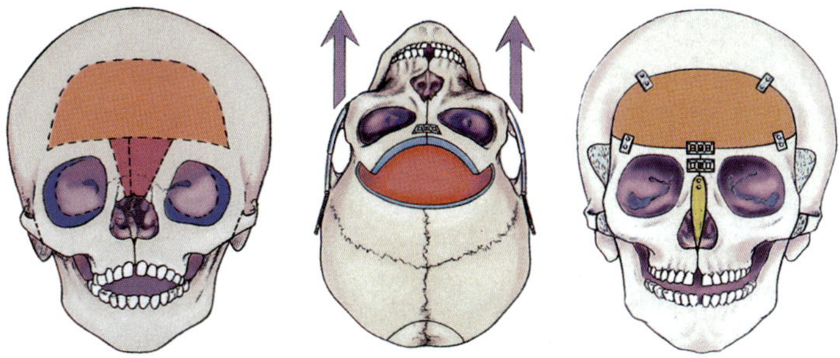

Figure 9.3. Illustration of facial bipartition osteotomy lines. (A) Frontal view shows craniotomy, midline asymmetric V-wedge excision of fronto-nasoethmoidal bone and midface buttresses (zygomatic arch, circumferential orbital walls, and pterygomaxillary). (B) Bird's-eye view demonstrates supraorbital bar, "Roman arch" curvature, anterior midline fixation, and Kawamoto midface distraction devices. (C) Frontal view after movement of facial bipartition segments with rigid fixation using midline keystone box and nasal bone graft. Reprinted with permission from Wolters Kluwer Health (Ref. 12). Copyright © 2008 by the American Society of Plastic Surgeons.

At this point, if correction of orbital dystopia using a facial bipartition is required, the following steps are performed (Figure 9.3). Just before the monobloc down-fracture, the intradacryon distance is measured with an orbital caliper. After completion of the dissection all the way down the nasal bones, a V excision is marked between the orbits in order to leave 16 to 20 mm of bone between the medial canthi region. This V includes the midportion of the supraorbital rim, the radix, and the central portion of the nasal bone. The V is planned so that there is a rotation point centered just above the nasal spine. At times, an asymmetric V wedge excision is used to correct any vertical orbital dystopia. Next, a midline 2-cm gingivobuccal sulcus incision is made intraorally, and subperiosteal dissection is performed to split the palate.

Next, the monobloc down-fracture is performed with the Rowe disimpaction forceps. During the down-fracture, the double-pronged septal osteotome is introduced within the nasofrontal separation and is directed toward the hard/soft palate interface to cut the perpendicular plate. (For a high-arched palate, an acrylic splint is used to avoid fracturing or uncontrolled splitting of the palate.) For complete side-to-side mobilization, the Rowe forceps are used to stretch the midface from side to side while the Kawamoto osteotome provides anterior traction in the pterygomaxillary osteotomy site.

Again, if a facial bipartition is being performed, the previously marked midline V is excised with the reciprocating saw. (It is important to remove bone above and behind the medial canthus to allow the greatest correction; however, a stable medial canthal attachment to bone is crucial.) The V is then removed with a Kocher clamp. At this point, any previously made dural injuries in this region are repaired while appropriate exposure exists. Through the previously dissected midline gingivobuccal sulcus incision, the hard palate is split with a reciprocating saw. A fine osteotome is used to complete the midline osteotomy between the central incisors. The bipartitioned halves are then brought together by rotating them to the midline. (Both horizontal and vertical correction may be done at this time if symmetric or asymmetric hypertelorism exists.) A convexity to the supraorbital region, or Roman arch, is created, and the correction of the intradacryon distance is confirmed with an orbital caliper (Figure 9.3C).[12] Midline rigid fixation is performed with an appropriately bent 1.0 titanium box plate and 5-mm screws.

If an acute advancement is planned, then the monobloc segment is positioned to achieve optimal orbital correction. (This may leave the patient with a class II malocclusion.) Cranial bone grafts are fixed within the advancement gap (in the anterior zygomatic arch region) using miniplates and screws. If gradual advancement is to be performed by monobloc distraction, an internal or external device is then secured. An internal distraction device is secured anteriorly to the zygomatic body just in front of the osteotomy site. Posteriorly, it is fixed to the temporal bone just behind the zygomatic root and above the external auditory canal (Figure 9.2). Distractors are tested and then returned to the start, or zero, position. An external (halo) device requires bolt fixation to the temporal skull and perialar/zygomatic skeletal wire fixation. An occlusal splint may also be used as a means of fixation for advancement.

A pericranial flap (10–34 cm) is sutured into the midline defect to separate the nasal sinus cavities from the epidural dead space. Fibrin glue is then used over the flap. If a facial bipartition is performed, excess midline skin may be dealt with by internal soft-tissue excision and a K-stitch.[21] This will allow the soft tissues to gradually contract. All incisions are then closed over drains. With a monobloc distraction, since no advancement is performed at the time of the operation, temporary, bilateral lateral tarsorrhaphies are performed to provide postoperative corneal protection. Again, for either an acute or gradual advancement, the end point of correction is planned to correct orbital and forehead deformities. Therefore, optimal occlusion is not the primary goal of the procedure.

Distraction is not started until postoperative day 7 (latency = 7 days). Distraction is not begun for a full week after monobloc osteotomy to allow for mucosal healing between the nasal (dirty) and the subdural frontal (clean) regions. In doing so, the dead space of the nasofrontal area created by the advancing monobloc segment is sealed off, possibly preventing infectious migration. Distraction is performed with an advancement of 0.5 mm twice daily for a total advancement of 1 mm per day (rate = 1 mm/day; rhythm = 23/day). Turning arms are removed when distraction is complete. Elastic rubber bands may be placed on maxillomandibular fixation screws or on brackets to guide the distraction segment and avoid an anterior open bite.

After the distraction phase is complete, the patients undergo a consolidation phase of 3 months. Internal distraction devices are then removed in the operating room through a 4-cm portion of the old incision and a percutaneous cheek incision. Coronal incision and flap turndown are not necessary for device removal.

9.10 Complications

There are risks involved with any facial advancement procedure (e.g., bleeding, dental injuries, blindness, malocclusion, nonunion). There are risks involved with any procedure with a craniotomy (e.g., bleeding, dural injuries, CSF leak, bone flap loss). The main concerns of a monobloc advancement are infectious complications. With a monobloc acute advancement, which separates the cranial base, there are increased risks of infection (meningitis), CSF leak, and frontal bone flap loss. With a monobloc advancement, there is direct communication of the epidural space (clean) and nasopharyngeal space (dirty), and there is a dead space created by the advancement. Important ways of minimizing the risks include (1) using a pericranial flap and fibrin glue, (2) not performing the procedure on patients who have a ventriculoperitoneal shunt, or (3) using distraction for a gradual advancement after several days of healing.

9.11 Summary

Patients with craniofacial dysostosis syndromes require cranial vault correction in infancy. By midchildhood, these same patients may require correction for midface hypoplasia and also correction for hypertelorism. Besides correction of facial deformities, indications for these procedures include upper airway obstruction, obstructive sleep apnea, tracheostomy dependency, and ocular problems (such as ocular keratitis, corneal ulcers, globe herniation, or blindness). Surgical correction may involve both forehead and midface advancement, and at times a facial bipartition. Traditionally, these procedures were done sequentially to reduce morbidity and involved acute advancement with bone grafting and rigid fixation.

Distraction osteogenesis techniques offer an alternative that is considered safer and has greater ability for simultaneous advancement. The reduced morbidity with monobloc distraction compared with acute advancement after monobloc osteotomy has been shown to include less infection (meningitis), CSF leakage, and frontal bone flap loss.[18] It is thought that monobloc distraction has the advantage of sealing off the region between the subdural space and nasal sinuses by allowing for healing of the mucosa for 1 week, before gradual advancement. In addition, less relapse has been noted compared with traditional techniques.[20] Also, monobloc distraction may be combined with a facial bipartition to correct hypertelorism. However, there is still a role for a monobloc osteotomy and acute advancement in the skeletally mature patient who requires a smaller advancement. (If a facial bipartition is necessary at skeletal maturity, then a hemi-Le Fort I is also performed to achieve proper occlusion.)

9.12 Pearls: Points of Emphasis

- Operative correction using monobloc advancement should be done at approximately 8 to 12 years of age unless functional problems arise earlier (e.g., obstructive sleep apnea, tracheostomy removal, ocular problems, or intracranial hypertension).
- Monobloc distraction decreases infectious complications by allowing for healing and decreasing the dead space between the subdural and nasopharyngeal spaces.
- Internal devices are better tolerated and allow for longer consolidation times; external devices allow for better vector control.
- Temporalis muscle preservation during monobloc osteotomies results in less temporal hollowing.
- The goal or end point of monobloc advancement during growth is orbit correction, not optimal occlusion.

References

1. **Tessier P.** The definitive plastic surgical treatment of the severe facial deformities of craniofacial dysostosis: Crouzon's and Apert's diseases. *Plast Reconstr Surg* 1971;48:419–442.
2. **Murray JE, Swanson LT.** Mid-face osteotomy and advancement for craniosynostosis. *Plast Reconstr Surg* 1968;41:299–306.
3. **Gillies H, Harrison SH.** Operative correction by osteotomy of recessed malar maxillary compound in a case of oxycephaly. *Br J Plast Surg* 1950;3:123–127.
4. **Ortiz-Monasterio F, del Campo AF, Carrillo A.** Advancement of the orbits and the midface in one piece, combined with frontal repositioning, for the correction of Crouzon's deformities. *Plast Reconstr Surg* 1978;61:507–516.
5. **Wolfe SA, Morrison G, Page LK, Berkowitz S.** The monobloc frontofacial advancement: do the pluses outweigh the minuses? *Plast Reconstr Surg* 1993; 91:977–989.
6. **Marchac D, Reiner D.** Early monobloc frontofacial advancement. In: Marchac D, ed. *Craniofacial Surgery.* New York, NY: Springer-Verlag; 1987:130–136.
7. **van der Meulen JC.** Medial faciotomy. *Br J Plast Surg* 1979;32:339–342.
8. **Tessier PL.** Apert's syndrome: acrocephalosyndactyly type I. In: Caronni EP, ed. *Craniofacial Surgery.* Boston, MA: Little Brown; 1985:280–303.

9. **Muhlbauer W, Anderl M, Marchac D.** Complete frontofacial advancement in infants with craniofacial dysostosis [abstract]. In: *Transactions of the Eighth International Congress of Plastic and Reconstructive Surgeons.* Montreal: Springer-Verlag; 1983:318.
10. **Kawamoto HK.** Complications associated with the monobloc frontofacial advancement. Paper presented at: American Association of Plastic Surgeons; May 3, 1988; Palm Beach, FL.
11. **Bradley JP, Gabbay JS, Taub PJ,** *et al.* Monobloc advancement by distraction osteogenesis decreases morbidity and relapse. *Plast Reconstr Surg* 2006;118: 1585–1597.
12. **Bradley JP, Levitt A, Nguyen J,** *et al.* Roman arch, keystone fixation for facial bipartition with monobloc distraction. *Plast Reconstr Surg* 2008;122: 1514–1523.
13. **Fearon JA, Whitaker LA.** Complications with facial advancement: a comparison between the Le Fort III and monobloc advancements. *Plast Reconstr Surg* 1993;91:990–995.
14. **Pellerin P.** Midface distraction with transfacial pin and external devices. Presented at: International Congress of ISCFS; September 27, 2009; Oxford, UK.
15. **Araund E, DiRocco F, Meyer P, Renier D.** Combined distraction, traction and contraction in extreme faciocraniosynostotic infants. Presented at: International Congress of ISCFS; September 30, 2009; Oxford, UK.
16. **McCarthy JG, Stelnicki EJ; Mehrara BJ, Longaker MT.** Distraction osteogenesis of the craniofacial skeleton. *Plast Reconstr Surg* 2001;107:1812–1827.
17. **Polley JW, Figueroa AA, Charbel FT, Berkowitz R, Reisberg D, Cohen M.** Monobloc craniomaxillofacial distraction osteogenesis in a newborn with severe craniofacial synostosis: a preliminary report. *J Craniofac Surg* 1995;6:421–423.
18. **Cohen SR, Boydston W, Hudgins R, Burstein FD.** Monobloc and facial bipartition distraction with internal devices. *J Craniofac Surg* 1999;10: 244–251.
19. **Cohen SR, Boydston W, Burstein FD, Hudgins R.** Monobloc distraction osteogenesis during infancy: report of a case and presentation of a new device. *Plast Reconstr Surg* 1998;101:1919–1924.
20. **Nishimoto S, Oyama T, Shimizu F,** *et al.* Fronto-facial monobloc advancement with rigid external distraction (RED-II) system. *J Craniofac Surg* 2004; 15:54–59.
21. **Urrego AF, Garri JI, O'Hara CM, Kawamoto HK, Bradley JP.** The K stitch for hypertelorbitism: improved soft tissue correction with glabellar width reduction. *J Craniofac Surg* 2005;16:855–859.

CRANIOFACIAL TRAUMA 10

Gerhard S. Mundinger, MD; Eduardo D. Rodriguez, MD, DDS and Paul N. Manson, MD

10.1 Introduction

The face is vitally important for communication, nutrition, perception, and interpersonal relationships. Aesthetic attractiveness and facial expression influence personality and success. Appropriate management of craniofacial trauma is thus crucial to maintaining livelihood and identity. Every facial injury results in damage to soft tissue, with many involving injury to both soft tissue and bone. Craniofacial trauma may present as an isolated injury or may be a component of multiple injuries to several organ systems.[1,2] Multidisciplinary cooperation between trauma surgeons, orthopedists, neurosurgeons, and plastic surgeons can facilitate a prompt reconstruction. Although there are a few true facial emergencies, the literature has historically underemphasized the advantages and superior aesthetic results of prompt, definitive anatomic reconstruction of facial bone and soft tissue injuries.[3–8] This chapter provides an overview of the evaluation and treatment of the most common craniofacial injuries.

10.2 Evaluation and Initial Treatment

Once the initial trauma evaluation is complete and life-threatening trauma has been adequately addressed, management can focus on clinical examination, computed tomography (CT) imaging, and initial treatment.[9–11]

10.2.1 *Physical examination*

Most facial injuries are accurately assessed by thorough clinical inspection; thus, methodical examination of all facial structures is essential. Examination proceeds from top to bottom (or bottom to top), and lateral to medial in each of the following facial regions: forehead, orbits, nose, maxilla, and mandible. Palpation of all bony surfaces should note tenderness and deformity. Discoloration, pain, localized tenderness, numbness or paralysis, malocclusion, crepitus, "step-off" margins of facial bones, double vision, decreased visual acuity, facial asymmetry, gross deformity, facial contour changes, and eye malposition are all symptoms that suggest deeper structural trauma. The search for occult lacerations must include the eyelids, ear canal, mouth, floor of the mouth, pharynx, and nose.

Frontal or basilar skull fractures may lacerate the dura, leading to pneumocephalus or cerebrospinal fluid (CSF) leak. CSF may exit from the nose (rhinorrhea) or ear (otorrhea), implying a communication between the subdural space and the external environment and raising the possibility of meningitis. CSF rhinorrhea or otorrhea is often obscured by the presence of blood mixed with draining CSF, making the confirmation of a CSF leak difficult. A "double ring sign" may be visible when draining blood and CSF are absorbed using a paper towel. In the presence of displaced fractures, intracranial repair of the dura is indicated. Definitive operative treatment is accompanied by the administration of prophylactic antibiotics. Therefore, rhinorrhea or otorrhea in the setting of craniofacial trauma should be evaluated thoroughly for the presence of CSF, and warrants detailed CT evaluation of the cranial base. Conversely, the presence of pneumocephalus on CT imaging raises high suspicion for a CSF leak.

The eye and visual function must be specifically evaluated. The symmetry of the pupil, speed of pupillary reaction, extraocular motion, and presence of hyphema are all noted. The presence of periorbital or subconjunctival ecchymoses implies the possibility of an orbital fracture or globe injury. In particular, one should palpate the superior and inferior orbital rims, zygomatic arches, and malar prominences. Visual acuity must be promptly evaluated, noting the presence of field defects, diplopia, or decreased light perception. Lacerations of the eyelid suggest the possibility of globe rupture, and the globe must be examined for integrity in these situations. Lacerations occurring in the medial third of the lower or upper eyelids suggest the possibility of lacrimal system injury, and the puncta and lacrimal duct should be thoroughly examined with a lacrimal probe when these lacerations are present.

Nasal examination is greatly facilitated by use of a nasal speculum. Pain and pressure sensation, including complete anesthesia or hypoesthesia, should be documented in the supraorbital, corneal, infraorbital, and mental nerve distributions. A neurologic facial examination must be completed and documented before administration of any local anesthesia or nerve blocks. Lacerations of major sensory or motor nerve branches and lacerations of the parotid duct should be managed in the operating room by direct repair with fine suture under magnification. Lacerations of the parotid duct are almost invariably accompanied by buccal facial nerve-branch laceration because the two structures travel next to one another.

An intraoral examination with direct palpation of the maxillary and mandibular dental arches and teeth is followed by an examination of the horizontal and vertical portions of the mandible. The movement of the jaw, its relation to the maxilla, and the occlusal relation of the maxillary and mandibular dental arches should be noted. If lucid and cooperative, the patient should be asked if the teeth meet together normally. The excursion of the mandible while palpating the temporomandibular joint (TMJ) should also be evaluated. The presence of step-off deformities in the dentition, bleeding, loose teeth, and intraoral lacerations suggest areas of deeper bony involvement.

10.2.2 *Radiographic examination*

All patients with significant facial injuries must have a CT of the face, cervical spine, and head.[12,13] Thin-cut, multiplanar CT imaging is currently the gold standard for bony injury. Plain roentgenograms provide little value. Images should include the frontal bone, frontal sinus, orbital and nasal regions, midface, and mandible, including the TMJs. If there is tooth involvement in any fracture identified on CT, a panoramic (Panorex) image can be obtained to assess tooth and tooth-root injury. In most cases, CT evaluation supplements and confirms the findings of a thorough clinical examination.

10.2.3 *Initial soft tissue and fracture management*

Lacerations are thoroughly inspected and accessed for depth and direction. Any foreign bodies are identified, the level of wound contamination is assessed, and damage to deeper structures, such as muscles, nerves, and bone, is identified.

Cleansing of soft tissue lacerations is accompanied by sharp debridement of the immediate contused tissue edge if possible, and scrubbing or pressure irrigation of the involved tissue. Thorough tissue irrigation helps to decrease contamination and remove foreign material. Areas where debridement should be conservative or avoided include the vermilion border, lips, eyelids, eyebrow, nostril rims, and distal nose. Scar formation is minimized by irrigation and sharp debridement that achieves a minimally contaminated, flat wound surface. Antibiotic use is required when the wound cannot be made "clean" by surgical debridement or in the presence of high-level contamination, such as animal or human bites. Direct primary closure of facial wounds is generally preferred, although open management is considered in special circumstances.

Any localized facial hematoma should be drained by direct incision over the fullest point. A small suction tip can then be inserted to aspirate the hematoma, or the hematoma cavity can be evacuated with sequential manual pressure. After evacuation, the cavity should be irrigated to remove any remaining clot and assess for recurrent bleeding. A soft, lubricated compression dressing is then applied.

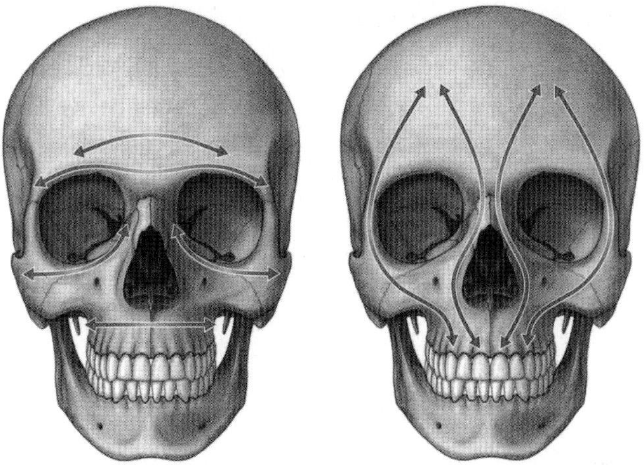

(A) (B)

Figure 10.1. (A) Horizontal and (B) vertical facial buttresses. The facial buttresses are the support pillars of the face and overlying soft tissues. Buttresses adjacent to fracture sites serve as anchor points for fixation hardware. Disrupted buttresses must be reduced and reconstructed to achieve optimal results. Reprinted with permission from Elsevier (Guyuron B, Eriksson E, Persing JA. *Plastic Surgery: Indications and Practice*. Vol. 1. 2009:633). Copyright © 2009 Elsevier.

After complete physical examination, evaluation of CT imaging, and initial soft tissue injury management, grossly displaced tissues and fractures can be manually repositioned. Intermaxillary fixation (IMF) can be applied to the jaws to temporarily stabilize fractures involving occlusal segments. The management of facial fractures therefore first requires identification of fractures in each anatomic region as visualized on CT. The fracture pattern in each anatomic region is then classified, and management options for the regional fracture pattern weighed by anatomic region, complexity, and peripheral facial buttresses (Figure 10.1). Regions are then considered in combination to generate a logical, graded, operative treatment sequence.

10.3 Frontal and Supraorbital Fractures

The frontal sinus generally consists of two asymmetric cavities separated by a bony partition (Figure 10.2). Signs of frontal sinus

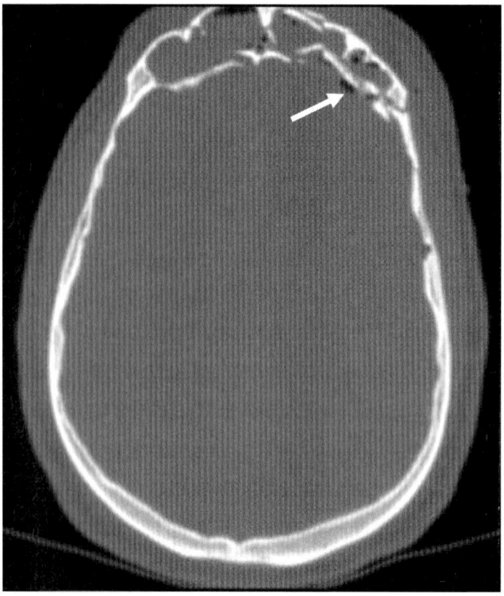

Figure 10.2. Comminuted frontal sinus fracture with compromise of the anterior and posterior walls. Associated pneumocephalus (white arrow).

fractures include nasal bleeding, external lacerations, or contusions in the forehead area.[14] In cases with significant displacement, a depression may be visualized in the skin overlying the frontal bone, sinus, or orbital rim. A CSF leak or subcutaneous emphysema may be present. Posterior wall fractures imply the possibility of a dural laceration, especially when the depth of displacement exceeds the thickness of the posterior table. Displaced posterior wall fractures generally require intracranial surgical exploration and dural repair.

Any fracture blocking the nasofrontal duct is treated by obliteration or cranialization of the sinus cavity to minimize the possibility of intracranial infection and mucocele development (Figure 10.3).[15,16] In these procedures, the frontal sinus mucous lining is stripped in its entirety, and a bur is used to lightly abrade the sinus walls. This eliminates mucosal invaginations (foramina of Breschet) and prevents mucosal regrowth. In sinus obliteration, the nasal frontal ducts are plugged and the remainder of the sinus is obliterated with bone graft. This eventually converts the sinus into a portion of the bony skull.

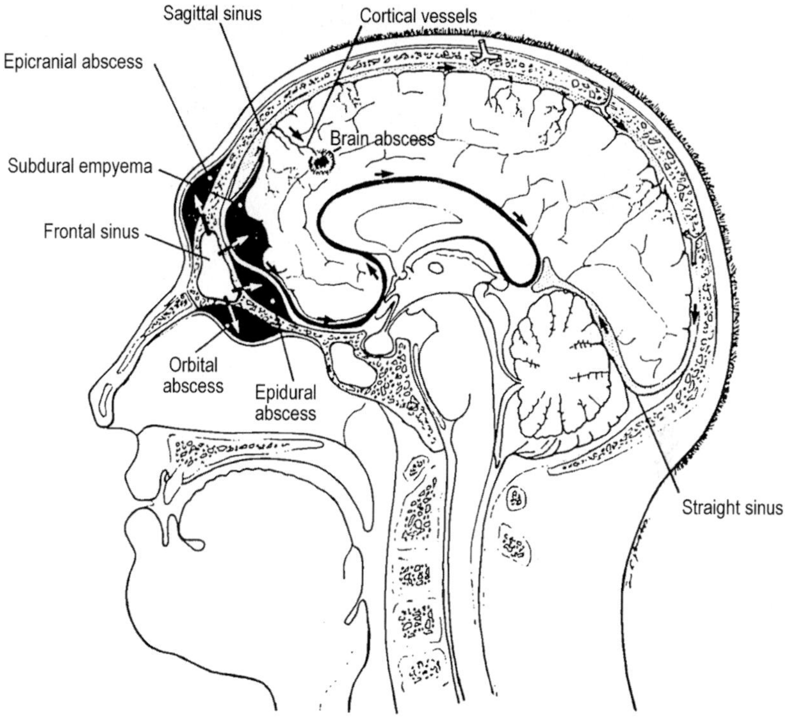

Figure 10.3. Sagittal section through the frontal sinus depicting potential routes for the spread of infection from the frontal sinus throughout the face and cranium. Reprinted with permission from John Wiley and Sons (Mohr RM, Nelson LR. Frontal sinus ablation for frontal osteomyelitis. *Laryngoscope* 1982;92:1006–1015). Copyright © 1982 John Wiley and Sons.

Alternatively, the sinus can be cranialized. After mucosal stripping and abrasion, the posterior wall of the frontal sinus is removed, and the brain and dura are allowed to rest on the remaining sinus floor and anterior wall (Figure 10.4). This effectively incorporates the sinus into the intracranial space.

The supraorbital rim of the frontal bone constitutes a sturdy prominence protecting the eye socket. Lacerations and bruises commonly occur in this area with fractures, which usually produce easily palpable step-off deformities. Numbness may occur in the distribution of the supraorbital or supratrochlear nerves. Supraorbital fractures typically produce smaller, isolated bony segments that are

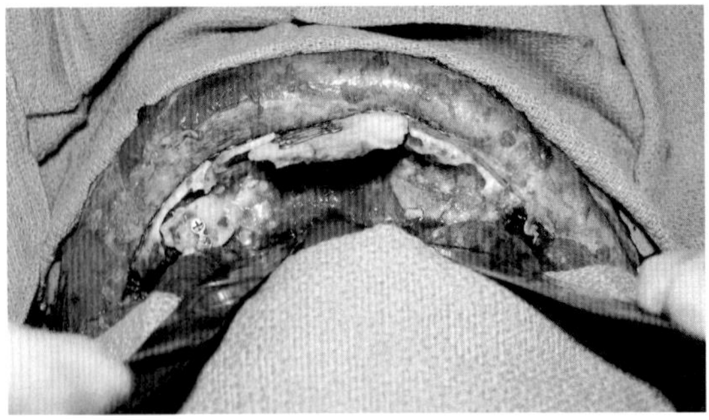

Figure 10.4. Intraoperative photo of reconstruction/frontal sinus cranialization of the case shown in Figure 10.2. The fracture was approached through a coronal incision.

depressed posteriorly and inferiorly. This results in an inferior and forward protrusion of the globe, lid ptosis, and possibly superior orbital fissure/orbital apex syndrome, or a superior gaze paresis that may mimic inferior rectus entrapment. Supraorbital fractures are preferably accessed through a coronal incision, but may be exposed through a suitable laceration overlying the fracture site.[17]

10.4 Nasal Fractures

Because of its prominence, fractures of the nose are the most common facial bone injury. The nose may be nondisplaced, or dislocated with both lateral and posterior displacement in frontal-impact injuries. The diagnosis of nasal fracture is suggested by epistaxis, bruising, laceration and swelling over the nose, and distortion of the appearance of the nose with lateral deviation or flattening. Intranasal inspection may reveal septal deviation or septal lacerations. Periorbital hematomas accompanying nasal fractures are diffuse and are not confined by the orbital septum to the boundaries of the orbital rim as with internal orbital fractures. At least one-third of nasal injuries have a small laceration over the nasal bridge. CT imaging delineates the exact anatomy of the displacement of all fracture segments, directing efforts at a closed reduction.

Nasal fractures are generally treated by closed reduction of the septum and nasal pyramid. General anesthesia, as opposed to an external nasal field block, facilitates an accurate closed reduction. Nasal fractures are first completed by thoroughly mobilizing the nasal pyramid in both lateral directions with Asch forceps. The septum is then restabilized at the facial midline. After completion and restabilization, the septum should be supported by Doyle splints and the nasal pyramid supported by an external nasal splint. Acute open reductions of the septum are discouraged, as they are associated with a higher incidence of septal perforation.

10.5 Orbital Fractures

Orbital fractures are commonly associated with combined periorbital and subjunctival hematomas.[18] Anesthesia is routinely present along the distribution of the infraorbital nerve, producing numbness in the ipsilateral nose, cheek, upper lip, and anterior maxillary teeth. Diplopia may be present with superior and inferior gaze owing to contusion or, less commonly, entrapment of the fascial suspensory system of the inferior rectus and inferior oblique extraocular muscles. A forced duction examination may be performed if extraocular muscle entrapment is suspected. Resistance or total blockage of rotational movement implies frank incarceration of the muscle or ligament system, or hemorrhage adjacent to the extraocular muscle system.

Fractures of the orbit are accompanied by globe injury in 10% of cases.[19] Corneal abrasions are most common, but globe laceration and rupture must always be suspected. A visual screening examination is mandatory for every orbital fracture, and consists of visual acuity, pupillary reaction, examination of the anterior and posterior chambers, and intraocular pressure. Injury to the optic nerve must also be evaluated; the most subtle sign is a pupil sluggishly reactive to light (Marcus Gunn pupil).

Classically, orbital floor fractures involve the inferomedial portion of the orbit (Figure 10.5). The pupil is displaced inferiorly, medially, and posteriorly. Orbital emphysema may or may not be present along with palpable crepitus. Ipsilateral epistaxis is almost invariably present.

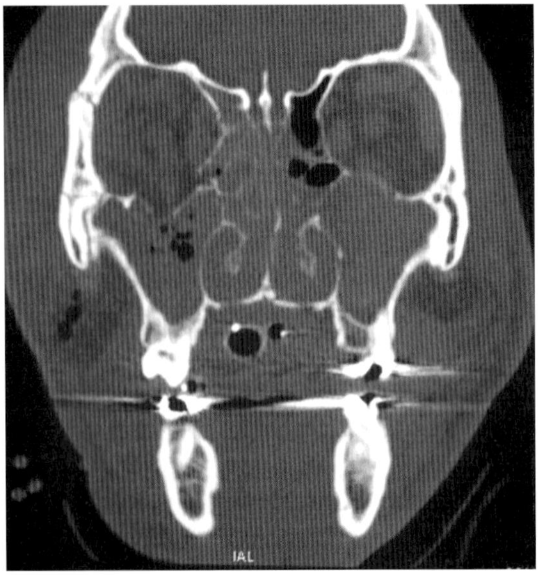

Figure 10.5. Coronal view of a right orbital fracture involving the medial, inferior, and lateral orbital walls. Note the opacity of the maxillary sinus, inferior displacement of orbital contents into the maxillary sinus, and subcutaneous emphysema.

Exophthalmos is a common initial finding and the result of intraorbital swelling or hemorrhage. As swelling and hemorrhage subside, the globe sinks into an orbit that has been enlarged by the fracture, eventually resulting in enophthalmos and globe retrusion. The radiographic examination of orbital fractures consists of axial, coronal, and sagittal CT views with both bone and soft tissue windows.

Absolute indications for surgery are significant enophthalmos or muscle entrapment, as confirmed by forced duction and CT. With gross displacement of floor and medial wall fractures, operative repair is indicated to prevent late enophthalmos.[20] Fractures of the inferior orbital rim, especially those involving the infraorbital foramen, are generally reduced to decompress the infraorbital nerve.

Fractures isolated to the orbital floor and medial wall may be approached by a midlid, infraorbital, subciliary, conjunctival, or coronal incision (Figure 10.6).[21] Subciliary incisions, while usually providing the best exposure, have the highest incidence of ectropion.[22] The

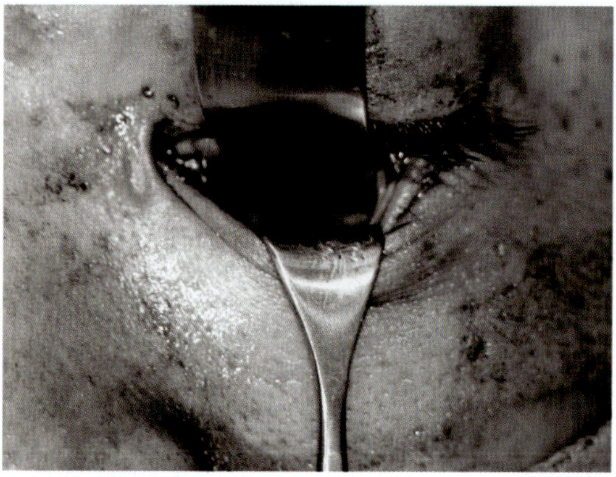

Figure 10.6. Orbital floor fractures are commonly approached via transconjunctival incisions. In this case, the maxillary sinus was readily visible through the orbital floor fracture gap.

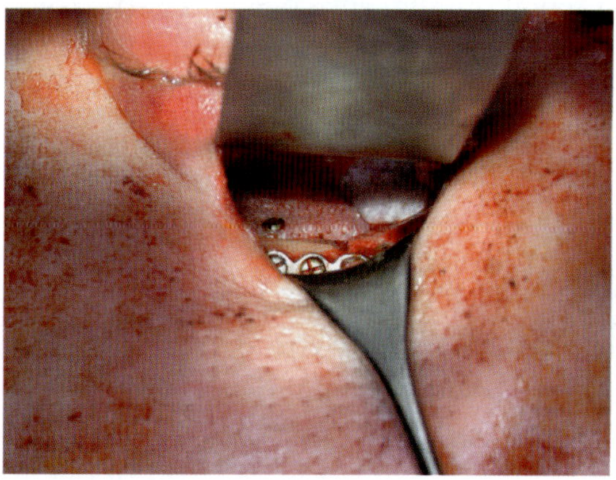

Figure 10.7. Intraoperative view of an inferior orbital floor fracture approached through an infraorbital incision, demonstrating rigid fixation of the infraorbital rim and alloplast reconstruction of the orbital floor.

exposure afforded with conjunctival incision can be increased with lower lid division or lateral canthotomy. The edges of the orbital floor or medial wall fracture are defined, and a suitably sized bone graft or alloplast (i.e., Medpor) is obtained and curved to the wall diameter (Figure 10.7).[23,24] The bone graft or alloplast is then stabilized by fixation to the orbital rim.

10.6 Nasal–Orbito–Ethmoidal Fractures

Nasal–orbito–ethmoidal (NOE) fractures involve the nose and medial orbital rim, producing an isolated fracture segment that includes the lower two-thirds of the medial orbital rim with the medial canthal ligament. This configuration allows for the potential migration of the medial canthal ligament, and must therefore be surgically corrected.

NOE fractures usually present with bilateral periorbital and subconjunctival hematomas and characteristic nasal dorsal depression/foreshortening from the accompanying frontal-impact nasal fracture.[25] Pain and tenderness are present with direct finger pressure over the medial canthal ligament, and palpation deeply in this area may produce a "click" as the bone is displaced. Unilateral or bilateral eyelid-spectacle hematomas may be present. Nasal lacerations, signs of septal trauma, epistaxis, and nasal airway obstruction are common. On palpation of the nose, bony crepitus may be detected. CSF leak, orbital emphysema, and pneumocephalus may all be present. Traumatic telecanthus (widening of the intercanthal distance) is present due to lateral displacement of one or both canthal ligament attachments, disrupting the usual 1:1 relationship between palpebral fissure length and distance between the medial canthi.

Clinical expertise is necessary to detect the difference between a significant nasal fracture and a minimally displaced NOE fracture. Bimanual intranasal/extranasal examination can aid greatly in this determination. In this examination, the pad of one index finger is placed externally on the side of the nose over the canthal ligament. A clamp is then placed intranasally directly under the ethmoid at the site of attachment of the medial canthal ligament. Movement of the medial orbital rim segment confirms the presence of a NOE fracture. NOE fractures are classically divided into three categories that determine appropriate treatment (Figure 10.8).[26] In Type I NOE fractures, there is significant displacement at the infraorbital rim and piriform aperture but minimal displacement at the internal angular process of the frontal bone. Type I fractures can be

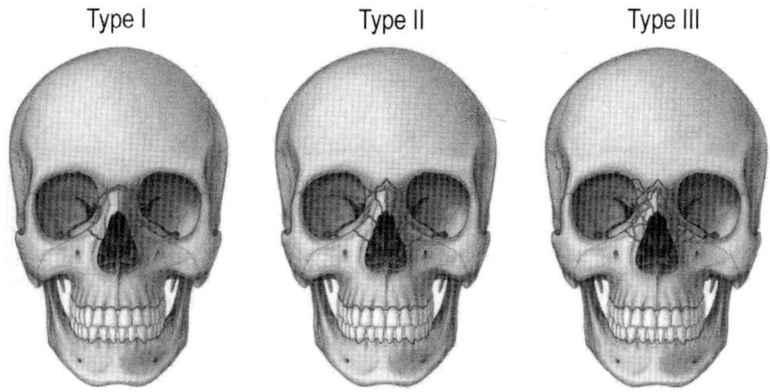

Figure 10.8. NOE fracture classification. Type I fractures are noncomminuted, and the medial canthus remains attached to its bony insertion. Type II fractures display comminution with retention of the medial canthus. In Type III fractures, comminution is present, and the medial canthus has been avulsed from its point of bony insertion. Reprinted with permission from Elsevier (Guyuron B, Eriksson E, Persing JA. *Plastic Surgery: Indications and Practice.* Vol. 1. 2009:632). Copyright © 2009 Elsevier.

addressed with gingival buccal sulcus and lower eyelid incisions alone.

In Type II NOE fractures, the central fracture segment bearing the medial canthal ligament is completely dislocated (Figure 10.9). Potentially, these fractures require full exposure with coronal, bilateral lower-eyelid, and gingival buccal sulcus incisions. All edges of the fracture are visualized and reduced transnasally. The canthal tendon-bearing bone segment is secured to ensure accurate medial canthus positioning.

In Type III NOE fractures, the medial canthus has been detached from its bony insertion and the structural integrity of the NOE buttresses completely compromised. Occasionally in comminuted fractures, the medial canthus must be operatively stripped from its site of attachment in order to perform accurate fracture reduction. In either case, the canthal ligament must be reattached with transnasal canthopexy (Figure 10.10). Two sets of transnasal wires are therefore necessary: one for the canthal attachment on each side, and one for internal bone reduction/fixation.

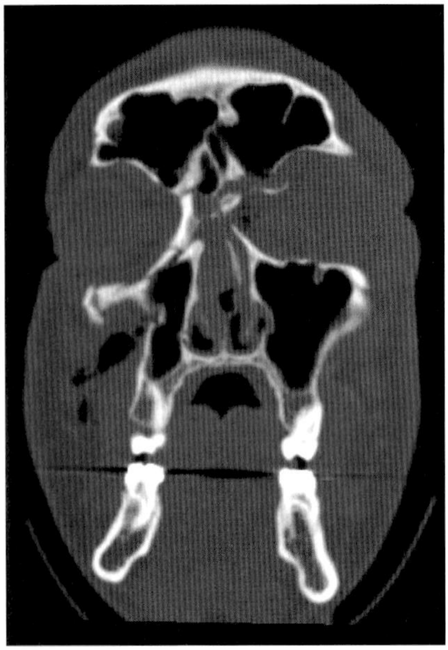

Figure 10.9. Coronal computed tomogram of a Type II NOE fracture.

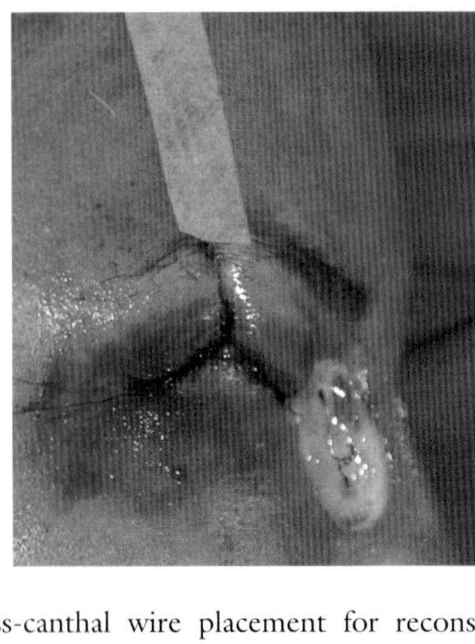

Figure 10.10. Cross-canthal wire placement for reconstruction of the medial canthus in a Type III NOE fracture.

10.7 Zygoma and Zygomaticomaxillary Complex Fractures

The zygoma constitutes the malar prominence and inferolateral portion of the orbital rim. It has five attachments to adjacent bone: (1) laterally to the temporal bone, (2) superiorly to the frontal bone, (3) medially to the maxilla, (4) inferiorly to the maxillary alveolus, and (5) laterally and posteriorly in the orbit to the greater wing of the sphenoid.

As with orbital fractures, zygomatic fractures are suggested by the combination of a periorbital and subconjunctival hematoma.[27] Invariably, unilateral nasal epistaxis due to hemorrhage within the maxillary sinus exiting through the ipsilateral nasal fracture is present. Depression of the malar eminence posteriorly or inferiorly and depression of the inferior orbital rim are common symptoms. When the zygoma is completely dislocated at the zygomaticofrontal suture, the lateral canthus may be inferiorly displaced since its attachment to Whitnall's tubercle is just inside the inferior surface of the lateral orbital rim (Figure 10.11). The lower lid follows the inferiorly

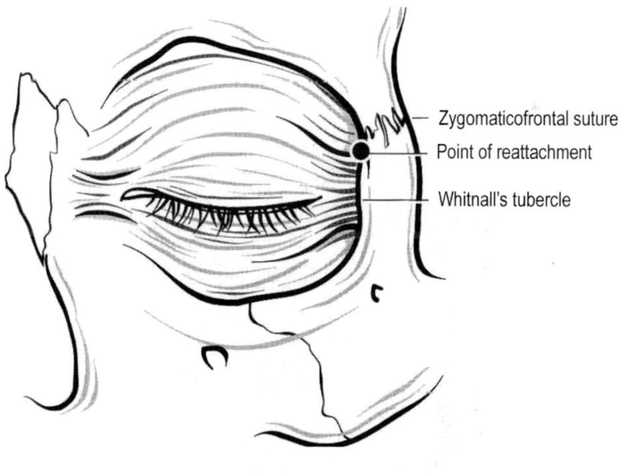

Figure 10.11. Laterally, Whitnall's ligament attaches to the zygoma at Whitnall's tubercle. Displaced zygoma fractures can therefore result in displacement of the lateral canthus. Reprinted with permission from Elsevier (Booth PW, Schendel SA, Hausamen JE. *Maxillofacial Surgery*. 2nd edn. Vol. 1. 2007:126). Copyright © 2007 Churchill Livingstone Elsevier.

displaced infraorbital rim. As the zygoma is displaced inferiorly and the orbit is enlarged, dystopia of the ocular globe and enophthalmos are evident. A step-off is frequently palpated at the inferior orbital rim and may occasionally be palpated at the zygomaticofrontal suture. Intraorally, irregularity of the maxillary buttress may be palpated or may be obscured by an upper buccal sulcus hematoma. When the body of the zygoma is posteriorly dislocated, or the arch medially dislocated, the bone may impinge on the coronoid process of the mandible, resulting in trismus or a lateral open bite.

Indications for surgery include interference with the coronoid process of the mandible, flattening of the malar eminence/loss of malar prominence, enophthalmos, diplopia, vertical malposition of the globe or lateral canthus, or anesthesia of the infraorbital nerve.

Isolated fractures of the zygomatic arch are treated by elevation through Gillies (temporal) or Lothrop (intraoral) approach. In the Gillies approach (named after Sir Harold Delf Gillies [1882–1960]), an incision in the temporal hair-bearing scalp permits insertion of an elevator under the deep temporal fascia to elevate the zygomatic arch. The same procedure may be accomplished intraorally (Figure 10.12). Because of periosteal continuity, isolated arch fractures are generally stable after this closed reduction, and a palpable click is

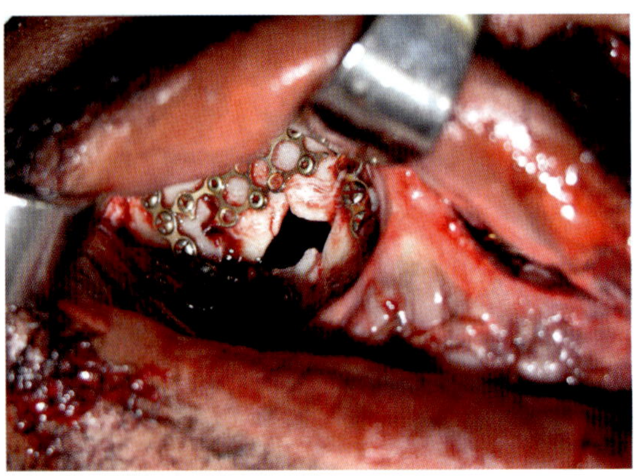

Figure 10.12. Reconstruction of a comminuted zygoma fracture accessed via a gingivobuccal sulcus incision.

often noticed when the segment is properly reduced. Fractures that are nondisplaced at the zygomaticofrontal suture may be approached with an intraoral incision.

More commonly, zygoma fractures are displaced at the zygomaticofrontal suture, inferior orbital rim, and zygomaticomaxillary buttress: hence the name zygomaticomaxillary complex fractures.[28] In this fracture pattern, accompanying zygomatic arch fractures are usually displaced medially. To achieve adequate visualization and accurate fixation at all the zygoma's buttresses, zygomaticomaxillary complex fractures require a three-incision approach.[29] The zygomaticofrontal suture is exposed through the lateral aspect of an upper-lid blepharoplasty incision. This is a 1-cm incision directly over the zygomaticofrontal suture as identified by palpation, and is completely within eyelid skin. A gingivobuccal sulcus incision and lower eyelid incision, as described previously, complete exposure of the zygoma at the zygomaticomaxillary buttress and inferior orbital rim. The zygomaticofrontal suture is stabilized with a loosely secured plate. Reduction is sequentially achieved at the zygomaticomaxillary buttress through a gingivobuccal sulcus incision and at the inferior orbital rim through a lower eyelid incision. Fixation at each site is stabilized loosely before being tightened once complete reduction is achieved at all sites.

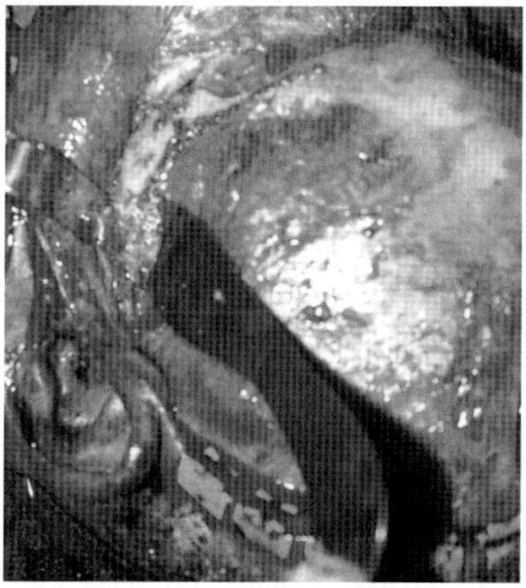

Figure 10.13. Coronal incisions provide excellent exposure for upper and midface trauma. Here a coronal incision is used to reconstruct a displaced zygoma fracture.

Rarely, extreme posterior displacement of the zygoma or lateral displacement of the zygomatic arch the zygomaticofrontal suture is best treated with open reduction by a three-incision procedure using a coronal incision in place of an upper lid blepharoplasty incision (Figure 10.13). The three-incision open reduction technique for zygomaticomaxillary complex fractures provides exposure of all major zygoma buttresses, and allows for precise alignment of the orbital process of the zygoma with the greater wing of the sphenoid in the lateral orbit.

10.8 Midface Fractures

Maxillary fractures are classified according to patterns described by René Le Fort in 1901 (Figure 10.14).[30] Le Fort fractures are usually multiple and generally more extensive on one side than the other. For instance, a Le Fort III superior-level fracture may be present on one side with a Le Fort II superior-level fracture on the other.

On physical examination, Le Fort fractures are suggested by mobility and malocclusion of the fracture segments.[31] To detect this mobility, the head is stabilized with one hand and upper maxillary alveolus mobility is confirmed with the other. Le Fort fractures generally produce facial elongation and midface retrusion. Fractures may be greensticked or impacted and therefore not display this characteristic mobility. Impacted or incomplete fractures may have only a slight occlusal disturbance, and are thus easily missed on physical examination. Physical signs of zygomatic, orbital, nasal, and/or nasoethmoidal fractures may be present as well, depending on the extent of the injury and level of the fracture. Le Fort fractures are invariably accompanied by bleeding from the nose, which may be profuse. Pneumocephalus, CSF leak, and orbital emphysema may occur in high fractures. Bilateral periorbital hematomas suggest the possibility of Le Fort II or III fractures. Generally, fluid is seen in both maxillary sinuses on CT, which should prompt a thorough investigation for the presence of midface fractures. About 10 to 15% of Le Fort fractures are accompanied by simultaneous fractures of the palate and maxillary alveolus.[32,33]

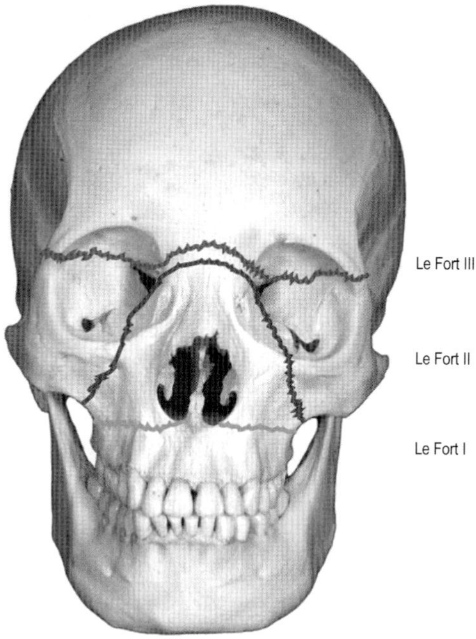

Figure 10.14. Frontal view of the skull illustrating the classic Le Fort I, II, and III fracture patterns. Reprinted with permission from Elsevier (*Mosby's Dental Dictionary*. 2nd edn). Copyright © 2008 Elsevier.

With the rare exception in the case of nondisplaced Le Fort I and II fractures, which can be treated with closed reduction and IMF in selected cases, Le Fort fractures are treated with IMF, open fracture reduction, and rigid fixation of the four anterior maxillary buttresses (the medial and lateral buttresses) through gingival buccal incisions (Figure 10.15).[34–37] If accurate rigid fixation is obtained, IMF may be released and light elastic traction used. If the bone segments are highly comminuted and fixation is not as stable or accurate, IMF is maintained for 3 to 4 weeks. The patient is subsequently observed for another 4 weeks in light elastic traction to ensure complete bone healing and stable occlusion.

Le Fort II fractures require gingival buccal and lower eyelid exposure (Figure 10.16). Occasionally, a coronal incision is required to

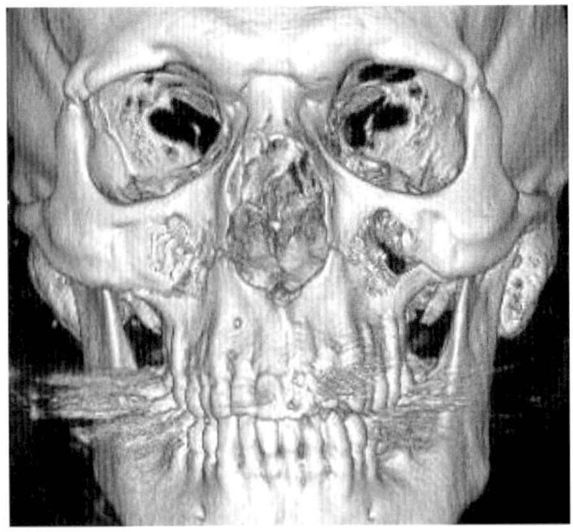

Figure 10.15. Composite 3-dimensional computed tomogram of a Le Fort I injury. Transmaxillary Le Fort I injuries generate a floating midface segment containing the lower maxilla and maxillary teeth.

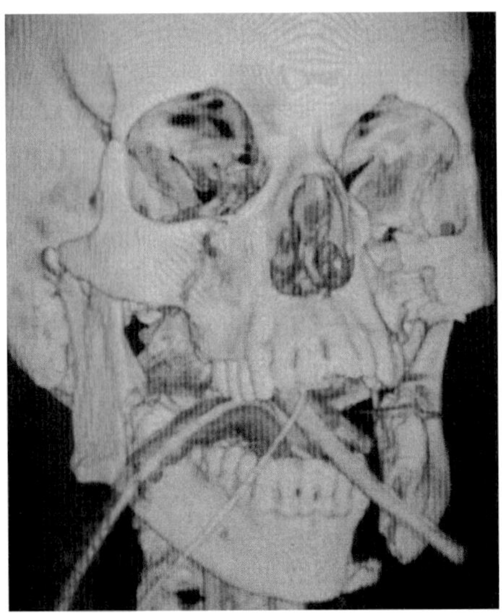

Figure 10.16. Le Fort II fractures generate a pyramidal midface fracture segment.

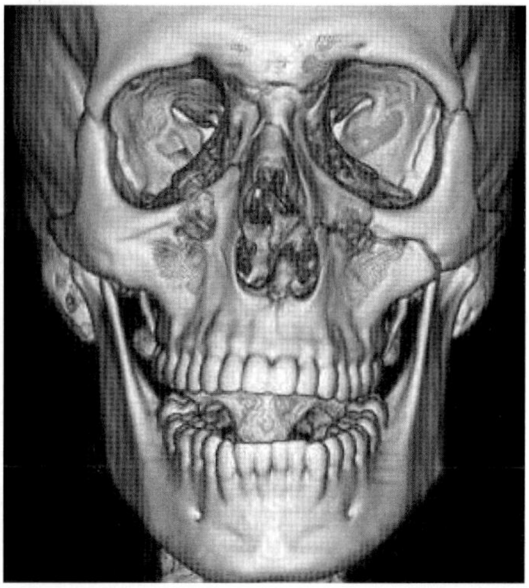

Figure 10.17. Le Fort III fractures generate a fracture segment containing the entire midface (craniofacial dissociation).

expose and treat nasal-frontal dissociation at the internal angular process of the frontal bone.

Le Fort III fractures generally involve a zygomatic component and a Le Fort I or II fracture component, or both. Therefore, treatment of the zygomatic component and its accompanying Le Fort I or II fractures are performed simultaneously (Figure 10.17). Fractures involving the internal orbit require internal orbital fracture reconstruction as previously described.

10.9 Mandible Fractures and TMJ Injury

Mandibular fractures are among the most frequent facial injuries; they appear in predictable patterns and are commonly missed on initial examination (Figure 10.18).[38] The symptoms of a mandibular fracture include pain, swelling, and abnormal occlusal relationships. Generally, patients will notice the slightest malocclusion from fractures of the tooth-bearing segments, or deviation of the mandible caused by fracture sites outside the tooth-bearing segments. There may be numbness in the distribution of the inferior alveolar nerve or

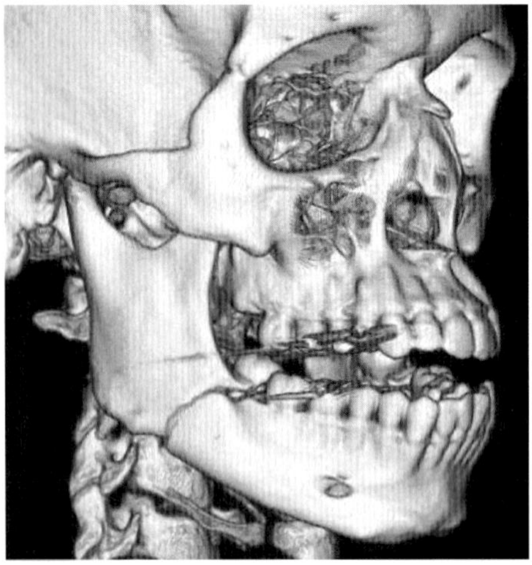

Figure 10.18. Right mandibular angle fracture.

its distal mental nerve branches. Swelling, gingival lacerations, floor-of-mouth ecchymosis, and bleeding or hematoma at the inferior jaw border are common. The patient invariably has some trismus or pain on moving the jaw and may be unable to bring the teeth into occlusion. Classically, subcondylar fractures are associated with a contralateral anterior open bite. On examination of the dental arch, there may be visible malalignment and level discrepancies. Palpation of the mandible may reveal a tender segment with loose, partially avulsed, or missing teeth. Alveolar fractures may result in mobile segments of dentition that may be separated from other mandibular fragments. Dental trauma that frequently accompanies mandibular fractures requires additional dental treatment and stabilization to minimize infection and provide proper dental alignment.

Assessment of these signs by visual inspection and bimanual palpation of all areas of the mandible, including the TMJ, is crucial.[39] Mandible fractures can lead to a painful locked TMJ, which results from subluxation of the condylar head or disk anterior to the glenoid fossa. This dislocation can be corrected with downward pressure on the posterior teeth of the affected side after appropriate sedation.[40]

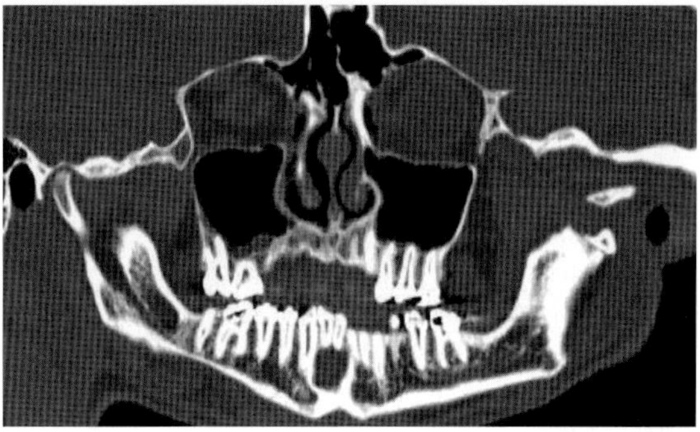

Figure 10.19. Computed tomogram panoramic (Panorex) image illustrating a fracture of the left mandibular condyle.

The identification of a single mandible fracture should prompt a thorough examination for additional mandible fractures. Common fracture combinations include angle/parasymphysis, subcondylar/symphysis, and subcondylar/parasymphysis. Frequently, fractures in the horizontal portion of the mandible are compounded into the mouth. Less commonly, they are open to the external skin.

Mandible films consist of CT imaging and a panoramic examination (Figure 10.19). Panoramic imaging alone of the mandible will miss symphyseal/parasymphyseal fractures. CT imaging provides a definite plan for operative intervention since it always confirms the length and type of necessary fixation.

If there is no malocclusion, the patient is able to function, and occlusal relationships are acceptable (i.e., favorable fracture), a soft diet is all that is required (Figure 10.20).[41] In other cases, the use of Ernst ligatures, Ivy loops, arch bars, and IMF may be required to restore and maintain normal occlusion. Fractures involving the dentition generally benefit from open reduction.[42] Upper and lower mandibular border fixation is advisable to guarantee stability of the reconstruction. Upper border fixation is usually unicortical to avoid tooth root injury.

Intraoral exposures are preferred for the anterior portion of the horizontal segment of the mandible, especially in the symphyseal and parasymphyseal area. Lag screws can be placed for fixation of

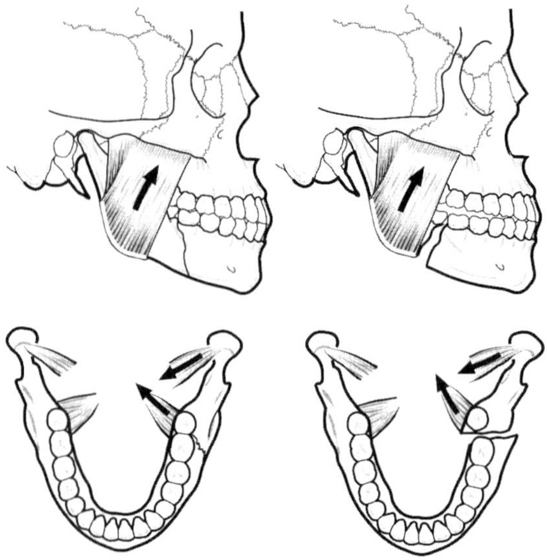

Figure 10.20. In favorable mandible fractures, muscle pull reduces the fracture (left images). In unfavorable fractures (right images), muscle pull distracts the fracture, necessitating fixation. Reprinted with permission from Elsevier (Booth PW, Schendel SA, Hausamen JE. *Maxillofacial Surgery.* 2nd edn. Vol. 1. 2007:38). Copyright © 2007 Churchill Livingstone Elsevier.

symphyseal fractures (Figure 10.21).[43] If a low subcondylar fracture requires open reduction, a Risdon or retromandibular incision is appropriate.[44] Higher fractures, such as condylar head dislocations, may require a combined periauricular and retromandibular approach, occasionally with exposure of the facial nerve.

Fractures of the edentulous mandible should be managed with open reduction procedures when possible.[45] However, when bone height and quality do not permit plate-and-screw fixation, these fractures may be effectively fixed with circumferential wires, splints, or acrylic saddles.

The duration of IMF depends on reduction stability, degree of fracture comminution, and patient cooperation. Patients who are mobile, cooperative, and able to maintain oral hygiene and nutrition, and who can make weekly clinic visits, are generally maintained in IMF for 4 to 6 weeks postoperatively. The patient who is placed in

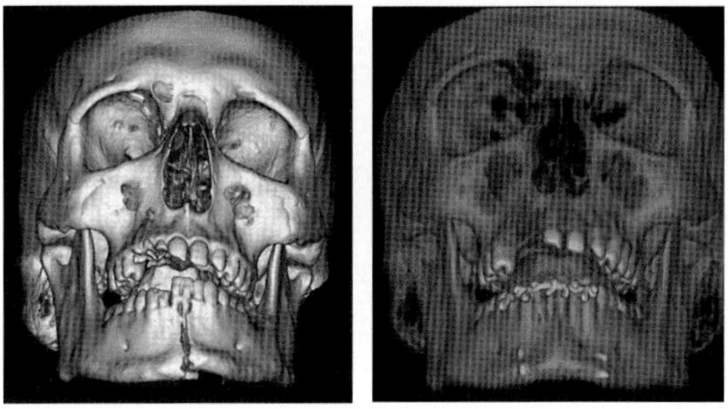

(A) (B)

Figure 10.21. Lag screw placement for fixation of a symphyseal fracture. (A) Preoperative image. (B) Postoperative image.

IMF will frequently lose 15 to 20 pounds over this period of treatment despite a blenderized diet. Careful observation of the occlusion with weekly clinic visits while patients are in IMF is essential.

10.10 Complex (Panfacial) Fractures and Gunshot Wounds

Panfacial refers to concomitant combinations of midface and mandibular and upper face fractures.[46] Often, these injuries are the result of massive blunt trauma or high-velocity gunshot wounds.[47] Whereas low-velocity gunshot wounds may be managed as closed injuries, high-velocity gunshot wounds or avulsive high-energy facial injuries produce extensive tissue damage and tissue loss. The soft tissues are cleaned, debrided, and closed over associated fractures without fracture fixation. The patient is then returned to the operating room every 48 hours for inspection, debridement of any further devitalized tissue, drainage, and irrigation. These serial "second-look" procedures prevent further tissue damage and minimize the damage caused by infection. Once no more soft tissue necrosis is seen, the missing bone and soft tissue can be reconstructed either serially or simultaneously.

In reconstructing complex craniofacial trauma, one must begin in a portion of the face and work sequentially through the various fractures.[48] Dividing the face into two conceptual units relative to the Le

Fort I level provides a framework for reconstruction. In this schematic division, the "lower face" refers to the mandible and the maxilla up to the Le Fort I level. The "upper face" refers to the zygoma, nose, nasoethmoidal region, and the frontal bone. Stabilization of the vertical and horizontal portions of the mandible with open reduction and internal fixation is crucial for accurate fixation of the lower face. Similarly, the frontal bone and cranial base are stabilized and serve as the main site of support for fixation of the upper face. Reconstruction begins inferiorly and proceeds superiorly. Initially, the maxilla is aligned with the mandible and stabilized at the dental arches through IMF. This provides an inferior platform for reconstruction and assures accurate maintenance of the occlusal relationship between the maxilla and mandible. The upper face is then stabilized to the lower face at the Le Fort I level. Once gross stabilization of the lower and upper face has been achieved with accurate occlusion, sequential treatment of associated fractures proceeds as previously described.

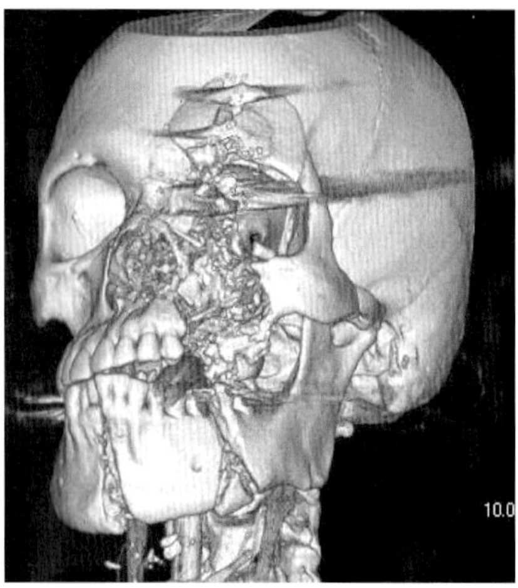

Figure 10.22. The force required to generate panfacial trauma is massive, as illustrated here in a composite 3-dimensional computed tomogram of a self-inflicted gunshot wound. Severe injury to associated soft tissue is common, necessitating complex reconstructive procedures, including microsurgical free-tissue transfer.

With complex fractures and high-velocity gunshot wounds, distant tissue is frequently required (Figure 10.22). Although microsurgical free-tissue transfer for the reconstruction of craniofacial trauma is well beyond the scope of this chapter, individual flaps of bone or soft tissue can be transferred to the area, or composite free-tissue transfer can achieve multiple reconstructive aims in a single stage.[49,50] Bony gaps are maintained by rigid fixation until these defects can be filled with vascularized bone harvested outside the zone of injury. Once the free-tissue transfer has completely healed, the patient's own cutaneous tissue can often be advanced over the transferred tissue. This achieves a more accurate color, contour, and hair match, producing a better overall aesthetic result.

References

1. **Murphy RX Jr., Birmingham KL, Okunski WJ, Wasser T.** The influence of airbag and restraining devices on the patterns of facial trauma in motor vehicle collisions. *Plast Reconstr Surg* 2000;105:516–520.
2. **Mithani SK, St-Hilaire H, Brooke BS, *et al.*** Predictable patterns of intracranial and cervical spine injury in craniomaxillofacial trauma: analysis of 4,786 patients. *Plast Reconstr Surg* 2009;123:1293–1301.
3. **Gruss JS, Antonyshyn O, Phillips JH.** Early definitive bone and soft-tissue reconstruction of major gunshot wounds of the face. *Plast Reconstr Surg* 1991;87:436–450.
4. **Girotto JA, MacKenzie E, Fowler C, Redett R, Robertson B, Manson PN.** Long-term physical impairment and functional outcomes after complex facial fractures. *Plast Reconstr Surg* 2001;108:312–327.
5. **Luce EA, Tubb TD, Moore AM.** Review of 1,000 major facial fractures and associated injuries. Plast Reconstr *Surg* 1979;63:26–30.
6. **Manson PN.** Re-operative facial fracture surgery. In: Grotting J, ed. *Re-operative Plastic Surgery.* St. Louis, MO: Quality Medical Publishing; 1995.
7. **Manson PN.** Re-operative facial fracture repair. In: Grotting J, ed. *Re-operative Aesthetic and Reconstructive Plastic Surgery.* St. Louis, MO: Quality Medical Publishing; 2007.
8. **Gruss JS.** Craniofacial osteotomies and rigid fixation in the correction of post-traumatic craniofacial deformities. *Scand J Plast Reconstr Surg Hand Surg Suppl* 1995;27:83–95.

9. **Manson P.** Facial injuries. In: Mathes SJ, ed. *Plastic Surgery*. 2nd edn. Philadelphia, PA: Elsevier; 2006.
10. **Suuronen R, Paatsama JK, Lindqvist C.** Establishing a clinical diagnosis and treatment plan. In: Booth PW, Schendel SA, Hausamen JE, eds. *Maxillofacial Surgery*. 2nd edn. St. Louis, MO: Churchill Livingston Elsevier; 2007:22–47.
11. **Manson P, Dufresne C.** Pediatric facial injuries. In: Mathes SJ, ed. *Plastic Surgery*. 2nd edn. Philadelphia, PA: Elsevier; 2006:381–462.
12. **Manson PN.** Dimensional analysis of the facial skeleton: avoiding complications in the management of facial fractures by improving organization of treatment based on CT scans. *Prob in Plast and Reconstr Surg* 1991;1:213–237.
13. **Manson PN, Markowitz B, Mirvis S, Dunham M, Yaremchuk M.** Toward CT-based facial fracture treatment. *Plast Reconstr Surg* 1990;85:202–214.
14. **Burstein F, Cohen S, Hudgins R, Boydston W.** Frontal basilar trauma: classification and treatment. *Plast Reconstr Surg* 1997;99:1314–1323.
15. **Rodriguez ED, Stanwix MG, Nam AJ, *et al.*** Twenty-six-year experience treating frontal sinus fractures: a novel algorithm based on anatomical fracture pattern and failure of conventional techniques. *Plast Reconstr Surg* 2008;122:1850–1866.
16. **Bell RB.** Management of frontal sinus fractures. *Oral Maxillofac Surg Clin North Am* 2009;21:227–242.
17. **Lacey M, Antonyshyn O, MacGregor JH.** Temporal contour deformity after coronal flap elevation: an anatomical study. *J Craniofac Surg* 1994;5:223–227.
18. **Stassen LFA, Kerawala CJ.** Periorbital and intraorbital trauma and orbital reconstruction. In: Booth PW, Schendel SA, Hausamen JE, eds. *Maxillofacial Surgery*. 2nd edn. St. Louis, MO: Churchill Livingston Elsevier; 2007:205–222.
19. **Brown MS, Ky W, Lisman RD.** Concomitant ocular injuries with orbital fractures. *J Craniomaxillofac Trauma* 1999;5:41–48.
20. **Manson PN, Clifford CM, Su CT, Iliff NT, Morgan R.** Mechanisms of global support and posttraumatic enophthalmos: I. The anatomy of the ligament sling and its relation to intramuscular cone orbital fat. *Plast Reconstr Surg* 1986;77:193–202.
21. **Manson PN, Iliff N.** Management of blow-out fractures of the orbital floor. II. Early repair for selected injuries. *Surv Ophthalmol* 1991;35:280–292.
22. **Phillips JH, Gruss JS, Wells MD, Chollet A.** Periosteal suspension of the lower eyelid and cheek following subciliary exposure of facial fractures. *Plast Reconstr Surg* 1991;88:145–148.

23. **Antonyshyn O, Gruss JS, Galbraith DJ, Hurwitz JJ.** Complex orbital fractures: a critical analysis of immediate bone graft reconstruction. *Ann Plast Surg* 1989;22:220–233.
24. **Glassman RD, Manson PN, Vanderkolk CA,** *et al.* Rigid fixation of internal orbital fractures. *Plast Reconstr Surg* 1990;86:1103–1111.
25. **Evans GR, Clark N, Manson PN.** Identification and management of minimally displaced nasoethmoidal orbital fractures. *Ann Plast Surg* 1995;35:469–473.
26. **Markovitz BL, Manson PN, Sargent L,** *et al.* Management of the medial canthal tendon in nasoethmoid orbital fractures: the importance of the central fragment in classification and treatment. *Plast Reconstr Surg* 1991;87:843–853.
27. **Manson PN.** Fractures of the zygoma. In: Booth PW, Schendel SA, Hausamen JE, eds. *Maxillofacial Surgery.* 2nd edn. St. Louis, MO: Churchill Livingston Elsevier; 2007:120–154.
28. **Stanley RB Jr.** The zygomatic arch as a guide to reconstruction of comminuted malar fractures. *Arch Otolaryngol Head Neck Surg* 1989;115:1459–1462.
29. **Gruss JS, Van Wyck L, Phillips JH, Antonyshyn O.** The importance of the zygomatic arch in complex midfacial fracture repair and correction of posttraumatic orbitozygomatic deformities. *Plast Reconstr Surg* 1990;85:878–890.
30. **Le Fort R.** Étude expérimentale sur les fractures de la machoire supérieure. *Rev Chir Paris* 1901;23:208–227, 360–379, 479–507.
31. **Manson P.** Midface fractures. In: McCarthy J, Boutros S, Galiano R, eds. *Current Therapy in Plastic Surgery.* Philadelphia, PA: Elsevier; 2006:236–251.
32. **Hendrickson M, Clark N, Manson PN,** *et al.* Palatal fractures: classification, patterns, and treatment with rigid internal fixation. *Plast Reconstr Surg* 1998;101:319–332.
33. **Rimell F, Marentette LJ.** Injuries of the hard palate and the horizontal buttress of the midface. *Otolaryngol Head Neck Surg* 1993;109:499–505.
34. **Manson PN, Clark N, Robertson B,** *et al.* Subunit principles in midface fractures: the importance of sagittal buttresses, soft-tissue reductions, and sequencing treatment of segmental fractures. *Plast Reconstr Surg* 1999;103:1287–1306.
35. **Baker NJ, Evans BT, Lang DA,** *et al.* Management of craniofacial, nasoethmoid, and grossly comminuted midface fractures. In: Booth PW, Schendel SA, Hausamen JE, eds. *Maxillofacial Surgery.* 2nd edn. St. Louis, MO: Churchill Livingston Elsevier; 2007:155–204.
36. **Crawley WA, Azman P, Clark N,** *et al.* The edentulous Le Fort fracture. *J raniofac Surg* 1997;8:298–307.

37. **Phillips J, Forrest C.** LeFort fractures. In: Prein J, ed. *A-O Manual of Internal Fixation in the Cranio-Facial Skeleton: Techniques Recommended by the AO/ASIF Maxillofacial Group*. New York, NY: Springer-Verlag; 1998.
38. **Luyk NH, Ferguson JW.** The diagnosis and initial management of the fractured mandible. *Am J Emerg Med* 1991;9:352–359.
39. **Zide BM.** The temporomandibular joint. In: McCarthy JG, ed. *Plastic Surgery*. Philadelphia, PA: WB Saunders; 1990:1475–1513.
40. **Taub D, Jacobs JS, Bessette RW.** Treatment of disorders of the temporomandibular joint. In: Guyuron B, Erikkson E, Persing JA, eds. *Plastic Surgery: Indications and Practice*. Philadelphia, PA: Saunders Elsevier; 2009:591–603.
41. **Finn RA.** Treatment of comminuted mandibular fractures by closed reduction. *J Oral Maxillofac Surg* 1996;54:320–327.
42. **Smith BR, Teenier TJ.** Treatment of comminuted mandibular fractures by open reduction and rigid internal fixation. *J Oral Maxillofac Surg* 1996;54:328–331.
43. **Ellis E III.** Lag screw fixation of mandibular fractures. *J Craniomaxillofac Trauma* 1997;3:16–26.
44. **Lee C, Mueller RV, Lee K, Mathes SJ.** Endoscopic subcondylar fracture repair: functional, aesthetic, and radiographic outcomes. *Plast Reconstr Surg* 1998;102:1434–1445.
45. **Buchbinder D.** Treatment of fractures of the edentulous mandible, 1943 to 1993: a review of the literature. *J Oral Maxillofac Surg* 1993;51:1174–1180.
46. **Gruss JS.** Complex craniomaxillofacial trauma: evolving concepts in management. A trauma unit's experience — 1989 Fraser B. Gurd lecture. *J Trauma* 1990;30:377–383.
47. **Clark N, Birely B, Manson PN, *et al.*** High-energy ballistic and avulsive facial injuries: classification, patterns, and an algorithm for primary reconstruction. *Plast Reconstr Surg* 1996;98:583–601.
48. **Markowitz BL, Manson PN.** Panfacial fractures: organization of treatment. *Clin Plast Surg* 1989;16:105–114.
49. **Rodriguez ED, Martin M, Bluebond-Langner R, Khalifeh M, Singh N, Manson PN.** Microsurgical reconstruction of posttraumatic high-energy maxillary defects: establishing the effectiveness of early reconstruction. *Plast Reconstr Surg* 2007;120(7 Suppl 2):103S–117S.
50. **Rodriguez ED, Martin M, Bluebond-Langner R, Manson PN.** Multiplanar distraction osteogenesis of fibula free flaps used for secondary reconstruction of traumatic maxillary defects. *J Craniofac Surg* 2006;17:883–888.

CLEFT LIP 11

Ananth S. Murthy, MD, FACS

11.1 Introduction

The commonly quoted incidence of cleft lip and/or palate of 1 in 1,000 live births[1] does not reveal the complexity of treatment of this congenital anomaly. As a result of a genetic or environmental mishap, the lip, alveolus, and palate may fail to fuse and result in a cleft lip and palate. This cleft may cause problems with breathing, chewing, sucking, speaking, hearing, swallowing, and appearance. It takes a combined effort of teams of health professionals to reverse the effects of this deformity.

Cleft lip represents a failure of the medial nasal process to fuse with the maxillary processes on each side. Several genes are activated and deactivated in the first 3 to 8 weeks of life, which are critical to formation of the lip and nose. Genetic variability of this process of migration results in phenotypic heterogeneity. Consequently, clefts of the lip may be unilateral or bilateral, complete or incomplete. A complete cleft lip may have a skin bridge between the medial edges of the nasal floor, known as a "Simonart's band." A minor form of an incomplete cleft is referred to as a microform cleft lip (Figure 11.1).[2–4]

Types of cleft lip deformities

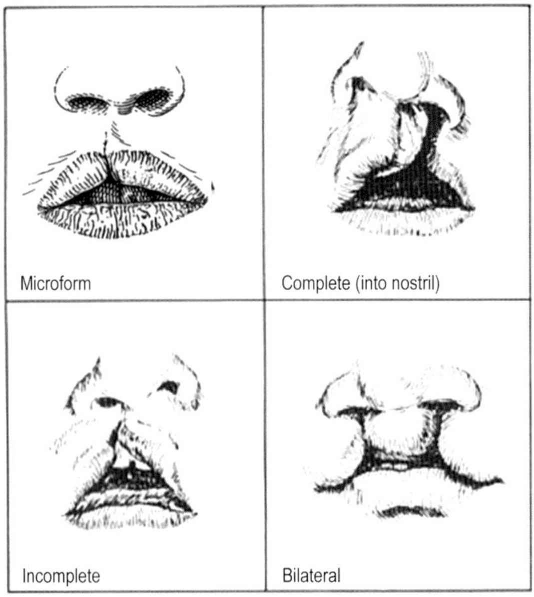

Figure 11.1. Types of cleft lip deformities. Upper left illustration from **Veau V.** *Bec-de-Lièvre: Formes Cliniques — Chirurgie.* Paris: Masson et Cie; 1938.

The same process that produced the cleft can also cause other congenital anomalies. In fact, 35% of all infants with cleft lip and palate have additional associated anomalies. This incidence rises to 54% for infants with a cleft palate alone.[5] Therefore, when evaluating a patient with cleft lip and palate, it is necessary to perform a thorough examination.[6]

Periodically, such anomalies occur together and are named after their descriptor, as there is no apparent singular cause. Presumably, the multiple anomalies that make up the syndrome are related. Numerous syndromes have been delineated that involve orofacial clefting.[6,7] As research in genetics grows, the source of some of these syndromes has been isolated. The most common syndrome to be associated with cleft palate is Stickler syndrome (mutation of collagen genes *COL2A1*, *COL11A1*, or *COL11A2*).[8] Other common syndromes include Shprintzen (velocardiofacial syndrome; 22q11 microdeletion) and van der Woude (*IRF6* mutation) syndromes.[9–11]

With the increasing sophistication of ultrasonography, the anatomy of the lip can now be discerned prenatally. If a complete cleft is present, it may be detected by 16 weeks, and an incomplete cleft can be detected by 27 weeks.[12] A prenatal consultation with the mother can help allay her fears and offer expectations for surgical treatment. Obstetric anxiety can also be reduced with a simple statement of hope, describing accomplishments of other children with cleft lip and palate, ". . . and she plays the trumpet."

Once a child is born with a cleft, the most pressing concern is feeding. Since they are unable to form a seal around the nipple to produce adequate negative pressure required for sucking, these infants are faced with an immediate problem. This can be ameliorated by using a modified nipple (wider aperture and squeeze chamber), such as a Haberman nipple, as well as several others that are commercially available.

After the baby is able to feed and demonstrates growth, surgical correction can be contemplated. Wilhelmsen and Musgrave emphasized the "rule of 10": weight 10 pounds, hemoglobin 10 g, age 10 weeks.[13] In general, however, in a wide cleft of the lip, the option of a lip adhesion may be considered before definitive lip and nasal correction. If the lip adhesion is performed after 10 weeks, a definitive repair can be scheduled 2 to 3 months later.

Before any attempt to correct a deformity, the norm has to be correctly understood. Farkas has documented the normal anthropometry of the face in detail.[14] By using this guide, a lip may be constructed to achieve optimal results. It is crucial to maintain photographic and numeric records, so that an accurate assessment can be done on the results of a surgeon's protocol. Newer three-dimensional anthropometry systems are particularly convenient as they can record accurate measurements in a split second.[15]

11.2 Unilateral Cleft Lip and Nasal Deformity: Surgical Principles

Alexander Limberg first described the concept of extending a rotational flap with the help of a back-cut.[16] Several geometric repairs had been proposed to correct the deficient length of the medial (noncleft) side of the cleft lip. Being dissatisfied with the obvious scars and distortion of key features of the upper lip, Millard proposed using the rotation flap with a back-cut to lengthen the medial portion of the cleft lip.[2,17] This hid the scar along the reconstructed philtral column and was flexible enough to be modified according to the length of the lip. The lateral lip was then advanced across the cleft to complete the closure. This constituted the rotation-advancement correction of the cleft lip, which has withstood the test of time.[18,19] The Millard rotation advancement flap and its variants are the most common methods of cleft lip repair today.

The following principles have been proposed to correct a unilateral cleft lip: (1) symmetry — staged procedures result in better symmetry in the wide unilateral cleft; (2) primary muscular continuity — the abnormal insertion of the orbicularis oris along the cleft edge at the base of the nose is horizontally reoriented across the cleft; (3) proper philtral shape — the rotation flap is hidden along the neophiltrum, and extension of this flap to the opposite philtrum is avoided; (4) augmenting the median tubercle from lateral lip elements — white-roll and vermilion flaps are inserted into the medial, deficient counterparts; (5) primary nasal correction — a C flap is used to augment the hemicolumella, and correct the positioning of the alar cartilage and alar base.[2,20]

11.2.1 *Surgical technique markings*

Important landmarks of the lip and nose should be marked (Figure 11.2). On the lateral side, the subalar point (sbal) on the affected side is marked first. Note that the sbal will be splayed laterally secondary to the under-rotated alar base of the cleft nose. The most important point to mark is the Cupid's bow peak (cphi) on the lateral side. To obtain a desirable result, an equal vertical length of the cutaneous upper lip must be achieved. Landmarks unaffected by the cleft are the sbal and the cphi on the unaffected side. Therefore, this length should serve as a template for the affected side. Calipers are useful to first determine the length of the upper lip on the unaffected side (sbal

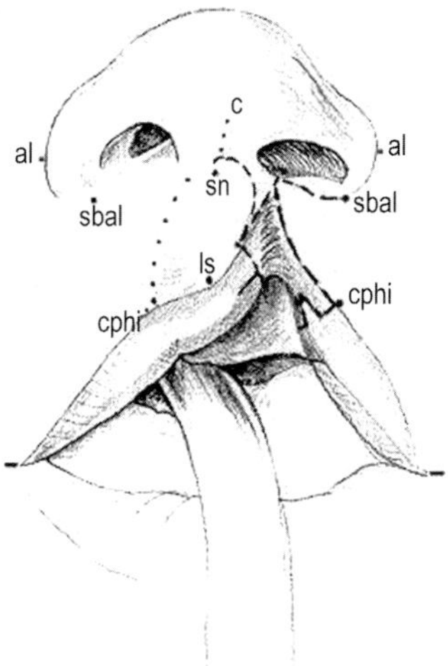

Figure 11.2. Important landmarks and markings for a unilateral cleft lip repair. On the medial element, Cupid's bow peaks (cphi) and low-point (ls), philtral column, subalar point (sbal), subnasal point (sn), lateral alar point (al), and midline of the columella (c). Note that the sbal–cphi distance should be equal on both sides of the cleft. Reprinted with permission from Wolters Kluwer Health in Ref. 20. Copyright © 1999 American Society of Plastic Surgeons.

to cphi), and then to mark the cphi on the affected side by marking the point where the arc of the length of the lip meets the vermilion–cutaneous (white roll) junction. The horizontal length between the cphi and its ipsilateral commissure, or chelion, is recorded. However, it has been shown that a short preoperative horizontal distance lengthens after correction of the complete oral sphincter.[20,21] Once the cphi on the affected side has been determined, the marking can be made for the rotation and advancement flaps.[22]

The rotation flap is marked along the medial margin of the cleft curving toward the columella. The advancement flap is marked on the lateral lip from the proposed cphi to the nasal sill along the cleft margin and is extended to the alar base. The columellar flap (C flap) is marked from the superior edge of the rotation flap to the membranous septum. This flap will be used to augment the hemicolumella and reconstruct the nasal sill. Attention then turns to the vermilion and mucosa of the lip. The vermilion is deficient on the medial edge of the cleft; therefore, a triangular flap of vermilion is designed at the vermilion–mucosal junction ("red line"). The labiobuccal mucosa is also deficient; a triangular flap of mucosa is planned from the lateral lip to elongate it. A gingivobuccal incision is planned from the cleft edge to raise the cheek flap for advancement across the cleft. A third triangular flap carrying the white roll will be designed just before closure of the philtral incision (Figure 11.2).[20,23,24]

11.2.2 *Dissection*

Incisions are made along the markings, and the mucosa lining the cleft is discarded. The buccal sulcus incision is made, although it does not extend to the level of the parotid duct. A supraperiosteal dissection is performed on the maxilla up to the level of the infraorbital foramen. If a lip adhesion has been performed previously, extensive maxillary dissection is not necessary. The alar base is elevated along with this flap off the piriform rim. The orbicularis is first separated from its anomalous attachment to the alar base, then dissected away from skin and mucosa of the lip. A mucosal back-cut in the buccal sulcus assists in advancing the lateral lip elements across the cleft. Scissors are placed between the medial crura (under the columellar flap), and blunt dissection is used to separate it from the opposite medial crura and dome. A sharp back-cut at the top of the rotation flap (on the columella, toward the opposite philtral column) is then created while the affected nostril is held at optimal level with a retractor. The back-cut is performed till the cphi are level.[23] If not addressed during a lip adhesion, the septal mucoperichondrium and the lateral vestibular mucosa are elevated for nasal floor reconstruction.[20,22]

11.2.3 *Closure*

The nasal floor is closed by approximating the septal mucoperichondrium and the lateral vestibular mucosa. While retracting the nostril to a level symmetric to the contralateral side, the columellar flap is retrogressed into the hemicolumella. The alar base flap is rotated endonasally and is approximated (end-to-side) to the columellar flap to form the nasal sill. The buccal sulcus is closed after advancing the back-cut. A triangular mucosal flap at the leading edge of this flap is interdigitated into the labial frenum to augment the mucosa on the cleft side. The buccal side of the lip mucosa is then closed. The orbicularis oris is then apposed from an inferior to a superior accession. The most superior portion of the orbicularis is affixed to the anterior nasal spine to create the appearance of a pout.[20,22]

The alar base is secured to the underlying orbicularis muscle to a point where the interalar distance is symmetric. The cutaneous closure of the lip starts at the vermilion–cutaneous junction. A small triangular flap (the white-roll flap) is inserted into a releasing incision on the medial side to complete the white roll and dictate the balance of the Cupid's bow.[2] The triangular flap of vermilion is inserted into a releasing incision along the vermilion–mucosal line (wet–dry junction or red line) to complete closure of the mucosa of the upper lip.[24] The advancement flap is then trimmed to a convex shape and is closed to the rotation flap in an inferior-to-superior direction. The subnasal portion of the incision is trimmed as needed and closed along the nasal sill. The distal edge of the advancement flap is trimmed and inserted into the superior portion of the philtral incision without any tension.

Through a marginal incision, the lower lateral cartilage is exposed. Using a cotton-tipped applicator, the contralateral dome is delivered through the marginal incision; an interdomal suture is placed between this spot and the proposed dome of the affected cartilage. The lateral portion of the lower lateral cartilage is suspended from the ipsilateral upper lateral cartilage to reconstruct the scroll (which is usually separated due to the stretch across a complete cleft; however, it may be intact in an incomplete cleft and therefore unnecessary). Correction of the alar cartilage usually results in redundancy or webbing of the vestibular mucosa and warrants a lenticular excision to open up the nostril. If necessary, a crescentic excision may be performed just superior to the marginal incision before closure in order to remove some of the stretched, excess skin of the nostril (Figure 11.3).[20,23]

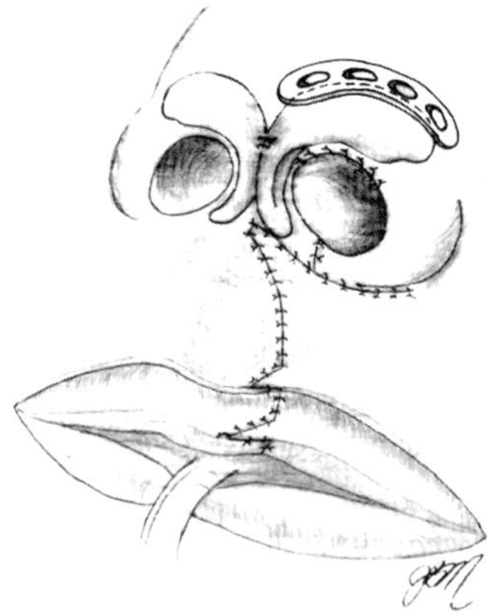

Figure 11.3. Closure of a unilateral cleft lip. Triangular flaps are used to complete the white roll and to augment the vermilion on the medial side. A resorbable splint can be used (after interdomal apposition of the lower lateral cartilages) to maintain the nasal correction.[25] Reprinted with permission from Wolters Kluwer Health in Ref. 25.

11.2.4 *Nasal correction*

Primary correction of the nasal deformity is prescribed in all clefts. Internal resorbable sutures are recommended. The use of percutaneous sutures yields a nonanatomic correction, and the use of bolsters is inadequate since they are usually removed in a week (cartilage healing takes considerably longer).

Owing to incisions along the columella, nasal floor, alar base, and nostril roof (marginal incision), a circumferential contraction of scar can lead to nostril stenosis. To avoid nostril stenosis, a postsurgical silicone conformer can be used during the healing phase.[26] However, an external splint is usually not tolerated by infants and can also cause frictional abrasions and pressure-related ulcerations. To address these challenges, Wong *et al.* recommend the use of an internal resorbable splint.[25] A resorbable plate can be placed over the corrected cartilage to act as an internal splint (Figure 11.3). This splint obviates the need for an external conformer or preoperative nasal molding.[25]

11.2.5 *Dentofacial orthopedics*

There are a variety of options for presurgical treatment of the alveolus. They vary depending on expertise, accessibility, finances, and individual protocols. There are three basic methods of presurgical molding: (1) taping, (2) passive molding, and (3) active orthopedic devices. Taping is the simplest method, with external force placed by gradual approximation of the cleft edges of the lip with adhesive tape. A dental plate may be used in conjunction with taping to prevent collapse of the lesser segment. However, accurate alignment is challenging, and dermatitis and epidermolysis from frequent tape removal can be annoying.[27] Alveolar approximation is also possible by progressive molding of a dental plate. The dental plate is held in place with an adhesive and gradually shaved on the palatal surface. External force by taping assists in moving the arches along this molded surface. Since infant cartilage can be molded nonsurgically, a nasal phalange is added when the interalveolar distance is less than 6 mm. This nasal molding bulb is progressively straightened to achieve an excellent preoperative position of the affected lower lateral cartilage. Usually, this process takes 10 to 12 weeks. A simultaneous correction of the lip, nose, and alveolus (gingivoperiosteoplasty) is possible after nasoalveolar molding.[28]

An active dentomaxillary appliance accomplishes alveolar alignment much more quickly (3–5 weeks). A custom-made prosthesis is secured to the palate with pins (under anesthesia). A screw is turned daily to activate an arm that moves the lesser segment along the radius of the arm. An auxiliary elastic chain can be engaged to assist in decreasing the interalveolar gap. A stronger force is applied on the maxillary segments for proper positioning.[28,29] Presurgical orthopedics effectively narrows the cleft, facilitating primary repair and decreasing the need for secondary repair.[30] No long-term effects have been noted with use of dentofacial orthopedics.[31]

11.2.6 *Lip adhesion*

A lip adhesion can be a useful adjunct in the treatment of a complete cleft lip.[32] An adhesion may be used instead of or in conjunction with dentofacial orthopedics. If access to presurgical orthopedics is unavailable, a lip adhesion can be performed as a staged procedure to narrow the cleft and approximate the dental arches, allowing for staged correction of the nasal deformity. This may decrease the number of secondary procedures necessary.[20,32,33] However, many centers have abandoned a preliminary adhesion as it may increase exposure to anesthesia, complications, scarring, and cost.[34,35]

Markings for a lip adhesion are made beyond any landmarks that are important for the ultimate cleft lip repair. On the medial side, a linear incision is marked 2 mm beyond the vermilion–cutaneous junction that extends along the base of the caudal septum. On the lateral side, a similar, corresponding incision is marked in the lip (beyond the vermilion–cutaneous junction) to the level of the piriform. A perpendicular incision is marked from the vestibular–piriform margin along the lateral buccal sulcus. The lip incisions are made to the level of the submucosa until the underlying muscle is visualized. However, the muscle is not dissected. The cheek is elevated along the supraperiosteal plane so it may be advanced across the cleft for a tension-free closure. A back-cut in the mucosa greatly assists in advancing the flap along the buccal sulcus, and the posterior mucosa of the adhesion is closed. The nasal floor is constructed by apposing the septal mucoperichondrium and the lateral vestibular mucosa. Interrupted sutures are placed in the muscular layer and the anterior mucosa is carefully approximated. Thin adhesive skin-closure strips (Steri-strips) reduce the tension across the adhesion in the immediate postoperative period. Typically, the final correction of the cleft lip is delayed for 2 to 3 months after the adhesion.[20,33]

11.2.7 *Gingivoperiosteoplasty*

Efforts to close the cleft alveolus primarily (with bone grafts) may produce detrimental effects on maxillary growth, especially if dissection is aggressive. Primary bone grafting has been abandoned at most institutions.[36] However, an unrepaired alveolar cleft can result in fluid and air leakage. One option to close the cleft alveolus is a gingivoplasty or gingivoperiosteoplasty.[2,28] After approximation of the arches with dentofacial orthopedics, local gingival tissue can be used with limited undermining to close the alveolar cleft. A gingivoperiosteoplasty effectively closes the alveolar cleft and completes the dental arch to provide a stable platform for nasal correction and tooth eruption.

More commonly, the alveolar cleft is left untreated until secondary bone grafting. Typically, secondary alveolar bone grafting is performed at a stage of mixed dentition, when the canine root has not fully formed (ages 8–10). A bone graft is performed to provide bony support for the teeth adjacent to the cleft and a dental implant (for the missing lateral incisor), or to allow for movement of the permanent canine into the lateral incisor position. Secondary grafting is successful using cancellous bone from the iliac crest.[37]

11.2.8 *Controversy of adjunctive treatment in cleft lip and nasal deformity*

Anecdotally, the incomplete cleft is easiest to correct. The dental arches are well aligned, the alar base is in a good symmetric position, and there is greater orbicularis bulk secondary to tension from partial completion of the oral sphincter.[33] In fact, just the presence of a skin bridge across the cleft (Simonart's band) greatly minimizes the severity of the cleft. Based on these observations, Millard *et al.* introduced a protocol to convert a complete cleft to an incomplete cleft.[38] A dentofacial appliance is first used to approximate the dental arches. Then, a lip adhesion and gingivoperiosteoplasty are performed to set up the foundation for correction of a complete cleft. This protocol has the advantages of arch alignment, preferred alar base position, and increased muscle bulk, as well as a slight lengthening of the medial element of the lip.[33] This can reduce the length of the back-cut necessary for the rotational flap so that it does not encumber the lip or philtrum on the normal side. Staged correction of the nasal deformity also yields better and more consistent results (Figure 11.4).

Alignment of the arches may be performed by either active or passive dentofacial orthopedics.[28,38] Controversy surrounds the use of dentofacial appliances and the effect of gingivoperiosteoplasty. Supporters refer to the advantages of not having an alveolar fistula and obviation of a secondary bone graft without significant effect on maxillary growth.[28,38,39] Detractors point to its effect on restricting maxillary growth and an abnormal bite relationship.[40–42] This is most likely secondary to the closure of the lateral incisor space and

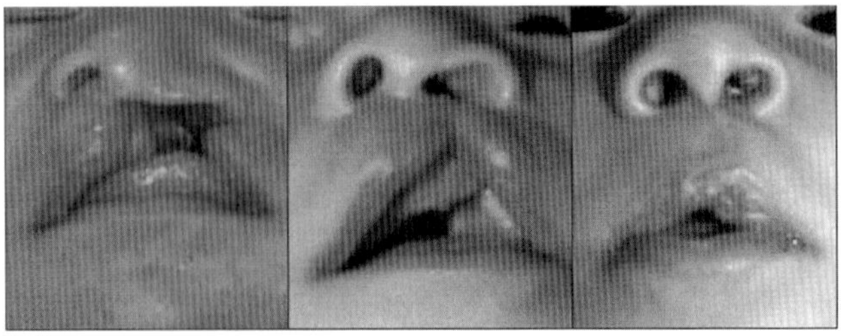
(A) (B) (C)

Figure 11.4. Staged correction of the complete unilateral cleft lip and nasal deformity. (A) Typical uncorrected cleft nasal deformity caused by the stretch of the alae across the cleft and posterior and lateral displacement of the alar base. (B) Stepwise improvement of the cleft nasal deformity after a lip adhesion. (C) Cleft rhinoplasty including tip definition and suspension of the lower lateral cartilage, use of a resorbable internal splint, crescentic excision along the marginal incision, and lenticular excision of the vestibular web. Cleft nasal correction was synchronous with cleft lip correction.

restriction of the sagittal growth of the maxilla.[41] However, recent studies have documented that a cleft of the primary palate rather than operative strategy is the inciting cause of maxillary restriction.[43,44] In the same vein, inherent differences in health care systems, treatment protocols, and ethnic expectations as well as cultural acceptance of concavity of the facial profile have led to inadequate elucidation of treatment outcomes.[43,44]

11.2.9 *Microform cleft lip*

A microform cleft lip, as described by Onizuka *et al.*, includes (1) minimal nasal deformity; (2) philtral groove; (3) thin free-margin of the lip; (4) notch at the vermilion–cutaneous junction (white roll); and rarely, (5) notch in the alveolus.[45] The philtral groove is an indication of an incomplete oral sphincter and should be corrected during the operation. Correction of the microform cleft lip can be done either with a rotation-advancement repair (for severe defects) or by a "double unilimb Z-plasty." Triangular flaps at the vermilion–cutaneous junction and the vermilion–mucosal junction are used to augment the medial element by insetting the flaps into corresponding releasing incisions.[4] The orbicularis is carefully apposed, and the alar base is endonasally rotated in a Y-V advancement. Last, correction of the slumped lower lateral cartilage is performed as previously described.[4,45]

11.3 Bilateral Cleft Lip and Nasal Deformity

A bilateral cleft lip closure is said to be "twice as difficult to repair as a unilateral cleft, and the results are only half as good."[46] Traditional principles concentrated on closure of the lip while postponing nasal correction, and resulted in typical stigmata. Straight-line closure resulted in a widened philtrum with biconvex scars, and retained prolabial vermilion and mucosa. This deformity was further accentuated with the need for an Abbe flap as a secondary operation. Additionally, the orbicularis oris muscle was not apposed, and a whistle deformity resulted.

The splayed lower-lateral cartilages of the nose (due to stretching secondary to the cleft) displayed a short columella, and numerous secondary procedures were devised to lengthen the columella. "Sill" flaps and "forked" flaps resulted in a plexus of scars at the nasolabial junction, resulting in tertiary deformity (Figure 11.5).[47–49]

Unhappy with results that were "half as good" and on the basis of accepted principles of unilateral cleft correction, Mulliken proposed the following principles to guide simultaneous lip and nasal correction in the presence of bilateral cleft lip: (1) symmetry — staged procedures will result in asymmetry; (2) primary muscular continuity — the orbicularis oris is brought across the premaxilla and apposed to form a continuous oral sphincter; (3) proper philtral size and shape — to avoid the previously mentioned stigmata, biconcave incisions are planned and the philtrum is constructed wider inferiorly; (4) formation of median tubercle from lateral labial elements — prolabial white roll, vermilion, and mucosa are discarded; and (5) correct positioning of splayed alar cartilages and construction of nasal tip and columella.[50]

Farkas and colleagues have documented facial anthropometry for Caucasians ages 1 to 18 and noted that certain features are fast

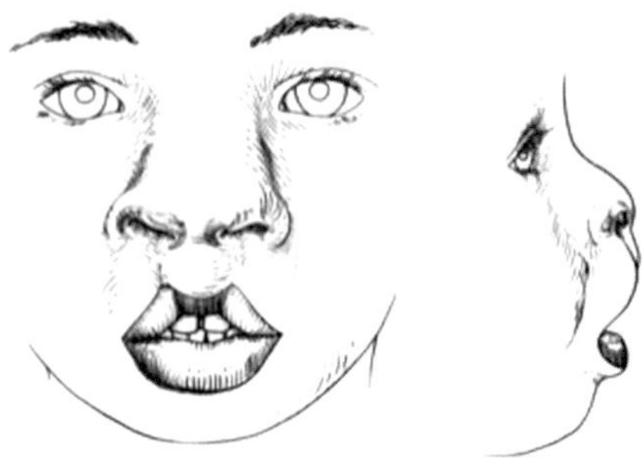

Figure 11.5. Typical stigmata of a traditional repair of a bilateral cleft lip. Straight-line closure resulted in a widened philtrum with biconvex scars. Retained prolabial vermilion and mucosa appears deficient medially. Failure to reorient the muscle by apposing the edges across the cleft may result in bulges under the alar base with animation and an akinetic segment of the upper lip (whistle deformity). The splayed lower-lateral cartilages of the nose (due to stretching secondary to the cleft) may display a short columella. Uncorrected and underrotated alar bases appear wide. Reprinted with permission from Wolters Kluwer Health (**Mulliken JB**. Principles and techniques of bilateral complete cleft lip repair. *Plast Reconstr Surg* 1985;75:477–486). Copyright © 1985 American Society of Plastic Surgeons.

growing (i.e., they reach adult proportions by age 5) and others are slow growing.[51] After analyzing these data, Mulliken *et al.* suggested that fast-growing features are to be constructed on a smaller scale than slow-growing features, which are constructed on a larger scale — "The surgeon . . . must conceive the problems as both third- and fourth-dimensional."[49,52] Accounting for temporal changes prevents the stigmata that are commonly seen with traditional bilateral cleft lip repair.

11.3.1 *Surgical technique markings*

The philtral flap is designed to be biconcave with a V-shaped inferior tip (to simulate the handle of the Cupid's bow). The biconcave incisions straighten from the stretch on the closure and prevent the typical biconvex philtral incisions seen after traditional repair. The prescribed length of the philtrum is 6 to 8 mm for a 4- to 5-month-old infant, and the width is limited to 2 mm superiorly and 3 to 4 mm inferiorly to prevent excessive widening after repair. The proper philtral

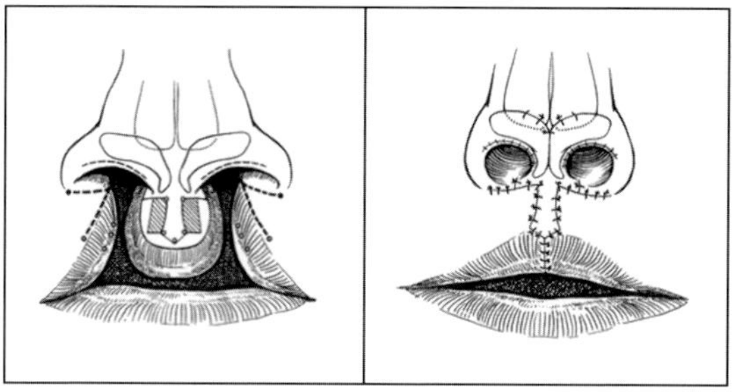

Figure 11.6. Markings and closure of a complete bilateral cleft lip and nasal deformity.[50] (See text for this section.) Reprinted with permission from Wolters Kluwer Health in Ref. 50.

size and shape are paramount for achieving a good result. The actual philtral flap is wider with bilateral flanking de-epithelialized strips. Hypertrophy or widening of the philtral scars is prevented by a tension-free closure across the premaxilla. Premaxillary orthopedics can greatly aid in aligning the protruding premaxilla, alleviating the stretch across the bilateral complete cleft. Corresponding philtral incision length is marked on the lateral lips and continued as a semilunar incision under each alar base. The peak of the Cupid's bow is planned on the lateral labial elements at a symmetric point where there is enough white roll to construct the handle of the bow (Figure 11.6).[50]

11.3.2 *Dissection*

Key landmarks are tattooed, and local anesthesia with epinephrine is injected. After de-epithelializing the flanking strips, the philtral flap is elevated. The remaining prolabial skin and mucosa are discarded. It is important to save a strip of the premaxillary mucosa to augment the gingivolabial sulcus in the midline. Laterally, the white-roll flaps are separated from the philtral incisions. The orbicularis muscle is dissected bilaterally. Bilateral buccal sulcus incisions are made, and lateral lip elements are raised in the supraperiosteal plane. Simultaneous nasal dissection of the alar base flaps as well as lower lateral cartilages (through marginal incisions) is performed.[50]

11.3.3 *Closure*

Closure begins by approximating the septal mucoperichondrium to the lateral vestibular mucosa for nasal floor reconstruction. If presurgical orthopedics were used, gingival flaps are apposed to close the alveolar clefts. The prolabial mucosa is hiked up to the premaxillary periosteum to create a gingivolabial sulcus. The lateral labial elements are advanced across the cleft after a back-cut in the sulcus. Subsequently, the buccal sulcus is closed across the premaxilla and the mucosa is closed in the midline (to form the anterior wall of the gingivolabial sulcus). The orbicularis muscle is then completed across the premaxilla. The superior portion of the orbicularis (pars peripheralis) is attached to the anterior nasal spine. The median tubercle is carefully created from the lateral lip mucosa, and the white roll is completed across the lip. The philtral flap is inset and the philtral incisions are closed. Lastly, the subalar incision is trimmed (for symmetry) and closed around the alar base and nasal floor (Figure 11.6).[50]

For nasal correction, the lower lateral cartilages must be replaced in their normal position. Fibrofatty tissue that has accumulated as a result of splayed alar cartilages must be dissected and pushed superiorly so the domes can be apposed directly. An interdomal suture is performed to secure the middle crura. The lateral crura are suspended from the ipsilateral upper lateral cartilages. The alar bases are cinched to an interalar distance of less than 25 mm. The alar bases are then secured to the underlying muscle to prevent paradoxical elevation with animation.[50]

11.3.4 *"The columella is in the nose"*[49,53]

Once the lower lateral cartilages are secured to their normal position, there is extra skin in the soft triangle of the nose due to the stretch across the bilateral cleft. This skin is carefully excised to sculpt the columella of the nose to the age-appropriate norm of 6 to 7 mm in infants. Redundant mucosa is also seen in the nasal vestibule in the form of a web (Figure 11.7). These vestibular webs are therefore excised to open up the nostril. These steps are performed synchronously with the lip

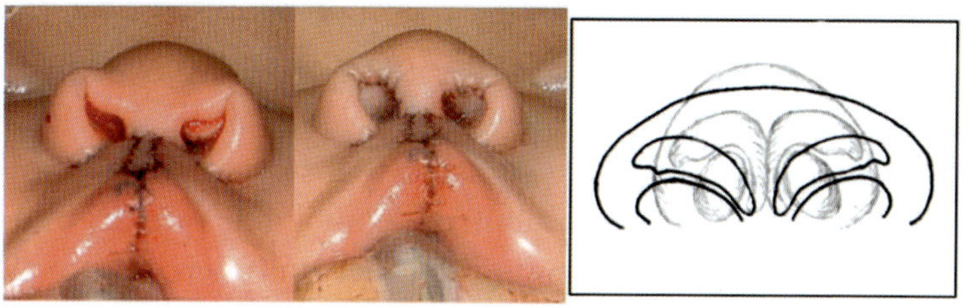

(A) (B) (C)

Figure 11.7. Nasal correction in a complete bilateral cleft lip. (A) The lower lateral cartilages are splayed due to stretching across the cleft. (B) When reoriented and corrected with sutures, there is excess skin along the soft triangle of the nose. (C) After excision of the excess skin, one realizes that "the columella is in the nose."[54] Panel C reprinted with permission from Elsevier in Ref. 54. Copyright © 2004 Elsevier Inc. All rights reserved.

closure so that the cutaneous closure of the lip is not disturbed during nasal correction.[50]

Variation of phenotypic expression will dictate variation in surgical technique. If the cleft is incomplete and the alveolus is intact, the lip and nasal deformity is less severe. However, the median tubercle should still be constructed from the lateral lip elements, and the orbicularis should still be completed across the cleft. Advancement of the buccal sulcus or the alar bases may not be necessary, and limited nasal surgery is prudent. If the cleft is asymmetric (complete/incomplete), then initial lip adhesion will set up a foundation for optimal results. Premaxillary orthopedics and lip adhesion (on the side with the complete cleft) help to centralize the premaxilla and close the alveolar cleft. During planning the definitive correction of the lip, it is important to realize that the side of the complete cleft will cause more stretch. Therefore, the philtrum should be canted slightly toward the side of the incomplete cleft to achieve eventual symmetry.[55] Occasionally, a complete bilateral cleft lip with an intact palate is encountered. This is especially challenging, since premaxillary orthopedics cannot be used with an intact palate. Premaxillary osteotomy and primary positioning can aid in aligning the alveolus. However, this can be costly in the future as it can cause midface retrusion. The only other option is to perform the correction across the protruding premaxilla.[56]

In summary, careful study of the shortcomings of traditional repair as well as anticipation of age-related changes have led to recommendations for simultaneous correction of the bilateral cleft lip and nose. This follows principles of achieving symmetry by using the proper shape and size of the philtrum, obtaining primary muscular continuity across the cleft, creating the median tubercle from the lateral lip mucosa, and simultaneous meticulous correction of the nasal deformity. The results from a careful repair would obviate the need for secondary procedures such as columellar lengthening, forked flaps, and Abbe flaps.

11.3.5 *Postoperative care*

Typically, an infant with a cleft lip operation has an overnight hospital stay. Cardiopulmonary monitoring during narcotic use (for pain control) and intravenous hydration are required. When the infant is feeding well, it may be discharged. Several postoperative adjuncts may assist in reducing anxiety and iatrogenic injury. A semicircular metallic brace (Logan's bow) may be taped to the cheek. This brace not only assists in immediate identification of the patient with a cleft but also protects the repair from direct frontal impact. Feeding is carefully initiated with a Brecht feeder or syringe feeder (with a soft tube attachment). Older children may use cups. The use of instruments (nipples, pacifiers, spoons, forks, straws, and so forth) near the lip should be discouraged. Soft elbow restraints are especially helpful in infants to prevent mischief. Some or all of these adjuncts are used at centers for variable durations (1–3 weeks).[57] If nonabsorbable sutures are used, they should be removed 4 to 5 days after the operation. Scar treatment, such as taping, creams, massage, and sunscreen may be recommended after 3 weeks.

11.4 Secondary Deformity of Cleft Lip and Nose

11.4.1 *Secondary deformities of the lip*

It is rare that final surgical results do not reflect the careful planning and correct technique used to repair a cleft. It is the rule, however, that thoughtless planning and incorrect technique lead to secondary deformity. It is important to evaluate the landmarks of the lip and nose and also to take account of previous procedures, to be able to correct a secondary deformity. Common secondary deformities of the lip can be classified into mucosal, vermilion, Cupid's bow, orbicularis, cutaneous lip scars, philtral, or nasal deformities.[58]

11.4.1.1 *Mucosa*

Mucosal variance (thickness or weakness of the free margin of the upper lip) is very common, as it is difficult to predict the fullness of the lip during the primary repair. A transverse excision along the vermilion–mucosal junction can address fullness. The scar can be hidden along the red line. Thinness of the free margin of the upper lip can be addressed by augmenting with a dermal fat graft, acellular dermis, or fat injection. Dermal fat grafts are reliable and predictable, and are the preferred method; they can be performed in conjunction with other procedures, such as alveolar bone grafts.[59]

It is not uncommon to have prolapse of mucosa from the labiobuccal sulcus after primary bilateral cleft lip repair. It is important to resuspend and recreate the sulcus across the premaxilla.[54]

11.4.1.2 *Vermilion*

Minor stepoffs, mismatch, and notching are commonly encountered. Notching, usually secondary to scar widening, can be corrected by a simple diamond-shaped excision. Stepoffs or mismatch at the vermilion–cutaneous junction (white roll) is typically from incorrect alignment during primary repair. A traditional Z-plasty or a unilimb Z-plasty can be useful to correct these deformities. Vermilion deficiency or stepoff is encountered if there has been no effort to equalize the width during the primary repair. A triangular flap of vermilion from the wider side can be inset into a releasing incision at the vermilion–mucosal junction to achieve symmetry.

Retained prolabial mucosa from primary bilateral cleft lip repair is always deficient, and results in a stepoff with the lateral labial

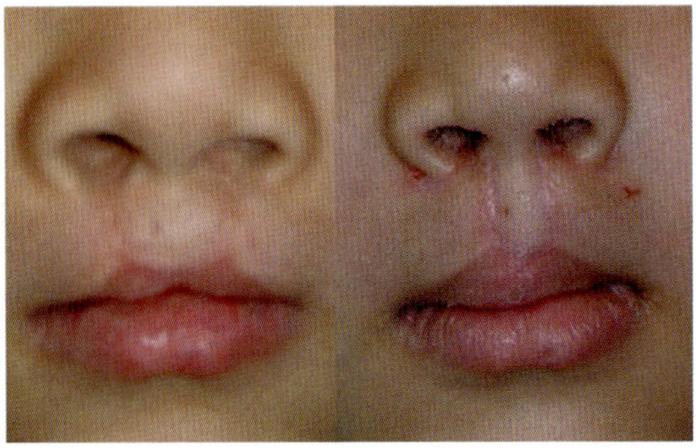

(A) (B)

Figure 11.8. Correction of a secondary bilateral cleft lip and nasal deformity. (A) Typical secondary bilateral cleft lip deformity with widened philtrum with biconvex scars, incomplete orbicularis apposition, retained prolabial mucosa, and no nasal correction. (B) After correction, the philtrum is the correct shape and size. The orbicularis muscle is completed across the cleft (under the philtral flap). The median tubercle is constructed from lateral labial elements (the prolabial mucosa is discarded). Nasal correction includes transdomal suturing and suspension of lower lateral cartilages. The alar bases are rotated and narrowed.

vermilion (whistle deformity). The exposed mucosa usually undergoes parakeratosis ("chapped skin"). This may be prevented by constructing the median tubercle from lateral labial elements and is treated by the same principle (Figure 11.8).[54,57]

11.4.1.3 *Philtrum*

Adult philtral columns narrow under the columella (6 mm) and widen at the Cupid's bow (10 mm). The normal length of the philtrum is 15 to 17 mm. During primary repair (ages 3–5 months), the Cupid's bow is 6 mm wide and 6 mm long. The philtrum and the philtral column scars usually widen after repair. Therefore, it is critical to plan the correct shape and size of the philtrum during primary repair. Abnormal shape and size should be corrected to age-appropriate norms.[14,51]

11.4.1.4 *Cupid's bow*

An upswing of the Cupid's bow, in a corrected unilateral cleft lip, is usually an indication of inadequate rotation of the medial element during primary repair. If the upswing is limited to 1–2 mm, it may be corrected with a traditional Z-plasty or a unilimb Z-plasty (Tennison's triangle). If the discordance is worse (short lip), a takedown and re-rotation will be required.

Traditional bilateral cleft-lip repair can result in secondary deformity. Columellar lengthening, dehiscence, or surgical misadventure can result in circumferential scarring of the philtrum. This results in an abnormal shape and size of the philtrum as well as "pin-cushioning" during animation.[54] One option to reconstruct the philtrum is an Abbe flap. Drawbacks of using an Abbe flap include lack of a Cupid's bow, opposite direction of hair growth (in males), excess bulk, and noticeable scarring of the lower lip. Also, if it is not sandwiched around the orbicularis muscle, it will result in an immobile segment at the philtrum.[60] Therefore, an Abbe flap should be seen as a salvage procedure.

11.4.1.5 *Orbicularis oris*

The continuity of the oral sphincter is paramount in the functional repair of the cleft lip. The orbicularis oris has two parts: (1) the pars peripheralis and the (2) pars marginalis. The pars peripheralis is the functional oral sphincter; the pars marginalis is present in the vermilion–cutaneous junction or Cupid's bow. The most superior portion of the pars peripheralis attaches to the anterior nasal spine. The pathology of the cleft lip results in reorientation of muscle fibers that aberrantly insert into the alar base rather than forming a continuous sphincter. Failure to reorient the muscle by apposing the edges across the cleft may result in a secondary deformity, the contraction of the muscle during animation resulting in bulges under the alar base. Failure to tighten and anchor the superior portion of the pars peripheralis to the anterior nasal spine results in a flat upper lip. Inadequate muscle bulk across the cleft can become thin, allowing the philtral scar to contract. Incorrect approximation of the pars marginalis can result in white-roll abnormalities and notching. In a bilateral cleft, it is imperative to appose the lateral edges of the orbicularis muscle across the premaxilla to prevent an akinetic segment centrally (whistle deformity). If the orbicularis discontinuity is suspected, it is necessary to reopen the previous repair and appropriately repair the muscle.[58]

11.4.1.6 *Lip scars*

The appearance of the philtral scar is dependent on the tension across the cleft repair as well as individual response to injury. It is important to note that philtral scars undergo some contraction immediately after repair. Parents must be counseled to perform scar massage, and, typically, the lip will be balanced after 3 months. Despite best efforts, scars may become hypertrophic, in which case they may have to be revised. A short lip is usually a result of inadequate rotation of the medial elements during the initial correction. A takedown of the original repair and a re-rotation is required. A long lip was traditionally seen after a geometric (triangular or quadrangular) repair of the cleft lip. This is not seen with the advent of the rotation-advancement repair. However, it can be encountered after the correction of an incomplete cleft lip. A complete revision with suspension of the buccal sulcus and crescentic excision along the alar base is required to correct a long lip.[58]

11.4.2. *Secondary deformity of the nose*

Unlike secondary lip deformities, which usually result from inappropriate or inadequate correction, secondary nasal deformities are the rule despite appropriate and adequate correction. The splayed alar cartilage that accompanies a complete cleft lip retains the memory of its fetal position and reverts (to some extent) in spite of correction. Furthermore, the lack of septal retaining ligaments on the side of the cleft allows the deformity to progress throughout childhood and adolescence. Therefore, it is not only important to correct the nasal deformity primarily but it is also important to revise it in childhood and adolescence to maintain the correction. Similarly, it is important to realize that improper secondary correction can lead to tertiary problems. The dogma of waiting until adolescence to correct the cleft nasal deformity is applicable only for osteotomies.

The tripod theory implies progressive nasal tip and septal deviation secondary to asymmetric displacement of the alar base.[2] Septal deformity and abnormal tension of the cartilage due to malalignment of muscles and the skeletal base (maxilla) can lead to the cleft nasal deformity. It is important to remember that the lower lateral cartilage, although misplaced, is inherently normal anatomically and histologically.[61] The unilateral cleft nasal deformity is secondary to an inferolateral displacement of the medial and middle crus of the lower lateral (alar) cartilage as well as a hemicolumellar deficiency. The bilateral cleft nasal deformity consists of splayed lower lateral cartilages with intervening fibrofatty tissue as well as widened alar bases.[19,27,30]

McComb[30] and Potter[62] first recommended primary sutural correction of the lower lateral cartilage to prevent progressive deformity. Later studies showed that primary correction of the nasal cartilage did not affect growth.[30] Mulliken followed McComb's anthem that the "columella is in the nose" and suggested a more aggressive primary nasal correction in an infant with bilateral cleft lip and palate.[49,53] These principles also apply to secondary correction of the bilateral cleft nasal deformity: the replacement of the cartilages in their ideal position and sutural correction (after removal of the intervening fibrofatty tissue); medial advancement and endonasal rotation of the alar bases; and excision of the excess skin in the soft triangle of the nostril to sculpt the columella.[54]

Many adjuncts have been suggested for maintaining the nasal correction. Cartilage can be shaped permanently if molded in the first few months of life. Preoperative nasoalveolar molding has utilized this principle to obtain superior cleft nasal correction and maintenance. Postoperative nasal conformers can be effective but may be cumbersome and cause columellar excoriation. The use of an internal, resorbable splint to maintain the sutural correction of the lower lateral cartilages has been successful in reducing the need for revisions.[25]

In the quest for ideal position and symmetry, primary correction followed by timely revisions can be more effective than delaying nasal correction till adolescence. Gilles and Kilner stated that a "well-mended harelip would go unnoticed at a cocktail party were it not for the nose."[63] However, when judging operative correction of a secondary lip or nasal deformity, it is important to determine the impact on the patient. In other words, substantiating a qualitative improvement rather than a quantitative improvement should be proven to the child, especially *in lieu* of medical, academic, social, familial, and financial obstacles. Marsh stated that the surgeon is often more critical of the result than the child with a cleft. Therefore, it is important to know "when enough is enough" in the search for the ideal.[64]

11.5 Conclusion

In parts of Africa, children with clefts are discarded as cursed souls. A simple operation to correct the appearance of a 2-cm area of the face can change the lifeline of these children. There are so many important functional considerations such as feeding, hearing, speaking, and chewing that are necessary for the child with a cleft lip and palate. However, appearance seems paramount, as explained by William Mayo's oft-quoted canticle: "It is the divine right of man to look human." It is this motivation that forces surgical commandos to descend upon far-off lands in hopes of correcting this disfigurement. Donors pour in money to support such projects so that withdrawn or repressed children can be given a chance to heal not only their appearance but also their psyche. Dr. Joseph Murray, Nobel laureate, perhaps explains it best: "I prefer to think of our work as operating on the soul."[65]

References

1. **Spritz RA.** The genetics and epigenetics of orofacial clefts. *Curr Opin Pediatr* 2001;13:556–560.
2. **Millard DR.** *Cleft Craft: The Evolution of its Surgery. The Unilateral Deformity.* Vol. 1. Boston, MA: Little, Brown; 1976.

3. **Wyszynski DF, Beaty TH, Maestri NE.** Genetics of nonsyndromic oral clefts revisited. *Cleft Palate Craniofac J* 1996;33:406–417.
4. **Mulliken JB.** Double unilimb Z-plastic repair of microform cleft lip. *Plast Reconstr Surg* 2005;116:1623–1632.
5. **Rollnick BR, Pruzansky S.** Genetic services at a center for craniofacial anomalies. *Cleft Palate J* 1981;18:304–313.
6. **Cohen MM Jr.** Syndromes with cleft lip and cleft palate. *Cleft Palate J* 1978;15:306–328.
7. **Cohen MM Jr.** Syndrome delineation. In: Cohen MM Jr., ed. *The Child With Multiple Birth Defects.* 2nd edn. New York, NY: Oxford University Press; 1997:151–163.
8. **Stickler GB, Pugh DG.** Hereditary progressive arthro-ophthalmopathy. II. Additional observations on vertebral abnormalities, a hearing defect and a report of a similar case. *Mayo Clin Proc* 1967;42:495–500.
9. **Shprintzen RJ, Goldberg RB, Young D, Wolford L.** The velo-cardio-facial syndrome: a clinical and genetic analysis. *Pediatrics* 1981;67:167–172.
10. **Nickel RE, Pillers DA, Merkens M, *et al.*** Velo-cardio-facial syndrome and DiGeorge sequence with meningomyelocele and deletions of the 22q11 region. *Am J Med Genet* 1994;52:445–449.
11. **van der Woude A.** Fistula labii inferioris congenita and its association with cleft lip and palate. *Am J Hum Genet* 1954;6:244–256.
12. **Mulliken JB, Benacerraf BR.** Prenatal diagnosis of cleft lip: what the sonologist needs to tell the surgeon. *J Ultrasound Med* 2001;20:1159–1164.
13. **Wilhelmsen HR, Musgrave RH.** Complications of cleft lip surgery. *Cleft Palate J* 1966;3:223–231.
14. **Farkas LG, ed.** *Anthropometry of the Head and Face.* 2nd edn. New York, NY: Raven Press; 1994:344.
15. **Aldridge K, Boyadjiev SA, Capone GT, DeLeon VB, Richtsmeier JT.** Precision and error of three-dimensional phenotypic measures acquired from 3dMD photogrammetric images. *Am J Med Genet A* 2005;138A:247–253.
16. **Fee WE Jr., Gunter JP, Carder HM.** Rhomboid flap principles and common variations. *Laryngoscope* 1976;86:1706–1711.
17. **Millard DR Jr.** A radical rotation in single harelip. *Am J Surg* 1958;95:318–322.
18. **Millard DR Jr.** Complete unilateral clefts of the lip. *Plast Reconstr Surg* 1960;25:595–605.
19. **Millard DR Jr., Morovic CG.** Primary unilateral cleft nose correction: a 10-year follow-up. *Plast Reconstr Surg* 1998;102:1331–1338.

20. **Mulliken JB, Martinez-Pérez D.** The principle of rotation advancement for repair of unilateral complete cleft lip and nasal deformity: technical variations and analysis of results. *Plast Reconstr Surg* 1999;104:1247–1260.
21. **Cutting CB, Dayan JH.** Lip height and lip width after extended Mohler unilateral cleft lip repair. *Plast Reconstr Surg* 2003;111:17–26.
22. **Stal S, Brown RH, Higuera S, *et al.*** Fifty years of the Millard rotation-advancement: looking back and moving forward. *Plast Reconstr Surg* 2009;123:1364–1377.
23. **Mohler LR.** Unilateral cleft lip repair. *Plast Reconstr Surg* 1987;80:511–517.
24. **Noordhoff MS.** Reconstruction of vermilion in unilateral and bilateral cleft lips. *Plast Reconstr Surg* 1984;73:52–61.
25. **Wong GB, Burvin R, Mulliken JB.** Resorbable internal splint: an adjunct to primary correction of unilateral cleft lip-nasal deformity. *Plast Reconstr Surg* 2002;110:385–391.
26. **Nakajima T, Yoshimura Y, Sakakibara A.** Augmentation of the nostril splint for retaining the corrected contour of the cleft lip nose. *Plast Reconstr Surg* 1990;85:182.
27. **Noordhoff MS, Chen PK.** Unilateral cheiloplasty. In: Mathes SJ, ed. *Plastic Surgery.* 2nd edn. Philadelphia, PA: Elsevier; 2006:165–215.
28. **Grayson BH, Santiago PE, Brecht LE, Cutting CB.** Presurgical nasoalveolar molding in infants with cleft lip and palate. *Cleft Palate Craniofac J* 1999;36:486–498.
29. **Latham RA, Kusy RP, Georgiade NG.** An extraorally activated expansion appliance for cleft palate infants. *Cleft Palate J* 1976;13:253–261.
30. **McComb H.** Primary correction of the unilateral cleft lip nasal deformity: a 10-year review. *Plast Reconstr Surg* 1985;75:791–799.
31. **Bongaarts CA, van 't Hof MA, Prahl-Andersen B, Dirks IV, Kuijpers-Jagtman AM.** Infant orthopedics has no effect on maxillary arch dimensions in the deciduous dentition of children with complete unilateral cleft lip and palate (Dutchcleft). *Cleft Palate Craniofac J* 2006;43:665–672.
32. **Randall P.** In defense of lip adhesion. *Ann Plast Surg* 1979;3:290–291.
33. **Vander Woude DL, Mulliken JB.** Effect of lip adhesion on labial height in two-stage repair of unilateral complete cleft lip. *Plast Reconstr Surg* 1997; 100:572–574.
34. **Salyer KE, Genecov ER, Genecov DG.** Unilateral cleft lip-nose repair — long-term outcome. *Clin Plast Surg* 2004;31:191–208.
35. **Hoffman W.** Unilateral cleft lip repair. In: Bentz ML, Bauer BS, Zuker RM, eds. *Principles & Practice of Pediatric Plastic Surgery.* St. Louis, MO: Quality Medical Publishing; 2008:439–453.

36. **Friede H, Johanson B.** A follow-up study of cleft children treated with primary bone grafting. 1. Orthodontic aspects. *Scand J Plast Reconstr Surg* 1974;8:88–103.
37. **Murthy AS, Lehman JA.** Evaluation of alveolar bone grafting: a survey of ACPA teams. *Cleft Palate Craniofac J* 2005;42:99–101.
38. **Millard DR, Latham R, Huifen X, Spiro S, Morovic C.** Cleft lip and palate treated by presurgical orthopedics, gingivoperiosteoplasty, and lip adhesion (POPLA) compared with previous lip adhesion method: a preliminary study of serial dental casts. *Plast Reconstr Surg* 1999;103:1630–1644.
39. **Chan KT, Hayes C, Shusterman S, Mulliken JB, Will LA.** The effects of active infant orthopedics on occlusal relationships in unilateral complete cleft lip and palate. *Cleft Palate Craniofac J* 2003;40:511–517.
40. **Ross RB, MacNamera MC.** Effect of presurgical infant orthopedics on facial esthetics in complete bilateral cleft lip and palate. *Cleft Palate Craniofac J* 1994;31:68–73.
41. **Berkowitz S.** A comparison of treatment results in complete bilateral cleft lip and palate using a conservative approach versus Millard-Latham PSOT procedure. *Semin Orthod* 1996;2:169–184.
42. **Henkel KO, Gundlach KK.** Analysis of primary gingivoperiosteoplasty in alveolar cleft repair. Part I: Facial growth. *J Craniomaxillofac Surg* 1997; 25:266–269.
43. **Daskalogiannakis J, Mehta M.** The need for orthognathic surgery in patients with repaired complete unilateral and complete bilateral cleft lip and palate. *Cleft Palate Craniofac J* 2009;46:498–502.
44. **Good PM, Mulliken JB, Padwa BL.** Frequency of Le Fort I osteotomy after repaired cleft lip and palate or cleft palate. *Cleft Palate Craniofac J* 2007;44:396–401.
45. **Onizuka T, Hosaka Y, Aoyama R, Takahama H, Jinnai T, Usui Y.** Operations for microforms of cleft lip. *Cleft Palate Craniofac J* 1991;28:293–300.
46. **Brown JB, McDowell F, Byars LT.** Double clefts of the lip. *Surg Gynecol Obstet* 1947;85:20–29.
47. **Millard DR Jr.** Columella lengthening by a forked flap. *Plast Reconstr Surg Transplant Bull* 1958;22:454–457.
48. **Cronin TD, Upton J.** Lengthening of the short columella associated with bilateral cleft lip. *Ann Plast Surg* 1978;1:75–95.
49. **Mulliken JB.** Bilateral complete cleft lip and nasal deformity: an anthropometric analysis of staged to synchronous repair. *Plast Reconstr Surg* 1995;96:9–26.

50. **Mulliken JB.** Primary repair of bilateral cleft lip and nasal deformity. *Plast Reconstr Surg* 2001;108:181–194.
51. **Farkas LG, Posnick JC, Hreczko TM, Pron GE.** Growth patterns of the nasolabial region: a morphometric study. *Cleft Palate Craniofac J* 1992;29:318–324.
52. **Mulliken JB, Burvin R, Farkas LG.** Repair of bilateral complete cleft lip: intraoperative nasolabial anthropometry. *Plast Reconstr Surg* 2001;107:307–314.
53. **McComb H.** Primary repair of the bilateral cleft lip nose: a 4-year review. *Plast Reconstr Surg* 1994;94:37–50.
54. **Mulliken JB.** Bilateral cleft lip. *Clin Plast Surg* 2004;31:209–220.
55. **Yuzuriha S, Oh AK, Mulliken JB.** Asymmetrical bilateral cleft lip: complete or incomplete and contralateral lesser defect (minor-form, microform, or mini-microform). *Plast Reconstr Surg* 2008;122:1494–1504.
56. **Friede H, Pruzansky S.** Long-term effects of premaxillary setback on facial skeletal profile in complete bilateral cleft lip and palate. *Cleft Palate J* 1985;22:97–105.
57. **Sommerlad BC, Kangesu T.** Arm restraint in children with cleft lip/palate. *Plast Reconstr Surg* 2003;112:331–332.
58. **Stal S, Hollier LH.** Secondary deformities of the cleft lip, nose and palate. In: Mathes SJ, ed. *Plastic Surgery*. 2nd edn. Philadelphia, PA: Elsevier; 2006: 339–363.
59. **Steinbacher DM, Padwa BL, Mulliken JB.** Simultaneous harvesting of cancellous iliac bone for alveolar cleft closure and dermis for augmentation of median tubercle. *Cleft Palate Craniofac J* 2009;46:295–298.
60. **Jackson IT, Soutar DS.** The sandwich Abbe flap in secondary cleft lip deformity. *Plast Reconstr Surg* 1980;66:38–45.
61. **Park BY, Lew DH, Lee YH.** A comparative study of the lateral crus of alar cartilages in unilateral cleft lip nasal deformity. *Plast Reconstr Surg* 1998;101:915–920.
62. **Potter J.** The nasal tip in bilateral and unilateral harelip. *Ann Plast Surg* 1981;6:85–96.
63. **Gilles HD, Kilner TP.** Operations for correction of secondary deformities. *Lancet* 1932;2:1369.
64. **Marsh JL.** When is enough enough? Secondary surgery for cleft lip and palate patients. *Clin Plast Surg* 1990;17:37–47.
65. **Murray JE.** *Surgery of the Soul: Reflections on a Curious Career*. Canton, MA: Science History Publications; 2001:204.

CLEFT PALATE 12

Joseph E. Losee, MD and Alexander Y. Lin, MD

12.1 Introduction

Plastic surgeons solve problems of form and function that affect the quality of human life, and no unique quality separates humans from animals more than the function of speech. The soft palate, or velum, plays a pivotal role in the production of speech through the orchestrated separation of the nasal and oral cavities during specific phonemes. By closing the velum against the posterior pharyngeal wall (velopharyngeal competence), air can be forced through the mouth without escape through the nose, allowing the normal enunciation of plosives and fricatives. In addition, velopharyngeal competence allows the suckling infant to create negative pressure suction. A baby born with a cleft palate will have problems with velopharyngeal competence, leading to difficulties with feeding and ultimately the development of speech.

Cleft palate can occur alone or in conjunction with cleft lip-nose. Isolated cleft palate, or cleft palate only (CPO), is usually considered a separate entity from cleft lip-nose with or without cleft palate (CL ± P), as the epidemiology of these two diseases appears quite different. CL ± P has male predominance and an incidence that varies by race from about 1:500 in Asians and 1:1,000 in Caucasians to 1:2,000 in Africans. Isolated cleft palate has a female predominance and an incidence that is fairly uniform across races, about 1:1,500 births.[1] There is also a subtype of cleft palate called *submucous cleft palate* (SMCP) in which there is no overt visible clefting of the palate since the overlying mucosa looks normal; however, the submucosal muscles of the velum are sagitally oriented, similar to those of overt cleft palate, and potentially leading to velopharyngeal dysfunction.

CPO has a greater association with syndromic diseases (50%) than CL ± P (about 15–30%).[2] The most common syndromic cleft palate is 22q11.2 deletion syndrome, or the velocardiofacial syndrome spectrum.[3] Other genetic defects that may lead to cleft palates include those in FGFR1, IRF6, and MSX1.[4] A combination of genetic defects and environmental factors interrupts the normal embryogenesis of the palate. As well, CPO may be more influenced by fetal environmental factors than is CL ± P, on the basis of both animal experiments and human observation. Weinzweig *et al.*[5] developed a caprine model in which pregnant goats were gavaged with anabasine, which reduces fetal movement and leads to sustained neck flexion, resulting in a single congenital defect: cleft palate. It is hypothesized that the neck position leaves the tongue interposed between the developing palatal shelves.[6] In humans, neonates with Pierre Robin sequence (micrognathia, glossoptosis, and respiratory distress) often have cleft palates, probably also from the mechanism of the obstructive tongue interrupting palatal development.[7] Additional factors correlated with clefting are smoking, nutritional influences, cholesterol-lowering drugs, anticonvulsants, corticosteroids, and retinoic acid.[4,8]

12.2 Anatomy: Normal and Pathologic

The palate consists of an immobile, bony hard palate anteriorly, and a muscular soft palate (velum) positioned posteriorly such that it can make functional contact with the posterior pharyngeal wall and obtain velopharyngeal competence. The palate can also be divided into the primary palate (anterior to the incisive foramen) and the secondary palate (posterior to the incisive foramen). At 4 weeks of gestational age, facial development begins to develop with five facial prominences or processes: frontonasal, left and right maxillary, and left and right mandibular.[9] The inferior portion of the frontonasal prominence becomes the premaxilla, consisting of the primary palate, four anterior incisors and their alveolar bone, and the labial musculature. The two paired maxillary prominences begin as vertically oriented lateral palatal shelves, which at the 8th week of gestational age rotate into a horizontal position and fuse to form the secondary palate. This rotation is thought to occur due to changes in mouth-opening reflexes, connective tissue swelling, vascularity, or mitotic activity, possibly related to a syndecan cell adhesion molecule.[9] Once the palatal shelves are horizontal, they adhere and fuse, and epithelial apoptosis takes place, possibly caused by differential signaling in TGF-β3, *N*-cadherin, FGF8, and SHH.[9] The junction of the primary and secondary palates is the incisive foramen, which contains the posterior septal branches of the sphenopalatine artery and the nasopalatine nerve (of cranial nerve [CN] V_2).[10] Ossification proceeds from the centers of all three facial processes except for the posterior portion of the secondary palate that instead becomes the velum. The velum comprises the mesenchyme derived from the first and fourth branchial arches. The first branchial arch gives the velum the tensor veli palatini, innervated by the trigeminal nerve (CN V_3), whereas the fourth branchial arch contributes the rest of the velar muscles, including the levator veli palatini, all innervated by the vagus nerve (CN X).

There are five main muscles of the normal velopharyngeal apparatus (Figure 12.1). The levator veli palatini, or motor of the velum, is found transversely oriented in the middle 50% of the velum. Huang *et al.*[11,12] showed in cadaveric dissections that the levator originates from the base of the skull bilaterally at the posteromedial junction of the cartilaginous and bony segments of the eustachian tube. It travels inferiorly, anteriorly, and medially to join its contralateral mate across the midline, spreading its fibers transversely to form a sling across the middle 50% of the velum. Therefore, on contraction, the levator sling readily serves as the main functional muscle of the velum by moving the velum laterally, superiorly, and posteriorly to make contact with the posterior pharyngeal wall.

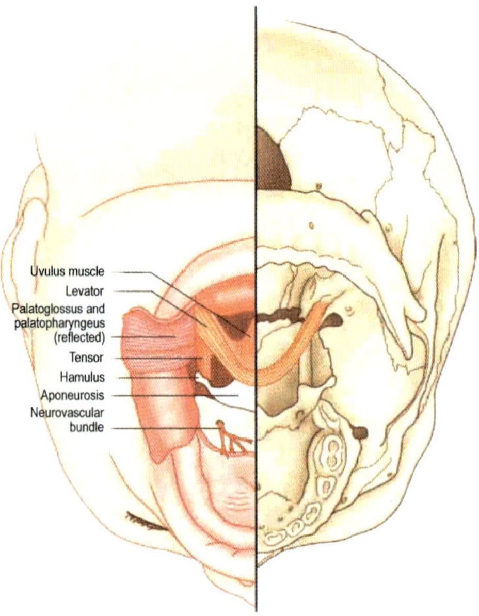

Figure 12.1. Anatomy of the normal palate. Reprinted with permission from Elsevier in Ref. 20, p. 273. Copyright © 2009 Elsevier.

The middle 50% of the velum also contains the insertion of two additional muscles, which extend posteriorly to become the anterior and posterior tonsillar pillars. The anterior tonsillar pillar is the palatoglossus muscle, which originates from the dorsolateral transverse fibers of the tongue and inserts as the most superficial muscle of the base of the soft palate. The posterior tonsillar pillar, the palatopharyngeus muscle, has two origins: an inferior head on the oral surface of the intravelar levator muscle and a superior head on the nasal aspect of the intravelar levator muscle. The palatopharyngeus extends inferiorly toward the larynx, bounded by the posterior pharyngeal walls. It plays a role in elevating the pharynx over the bolus of food when swallowing.

The posterior 25% of the velum contains the remainder of the palatoglossus and palatopharyngeus, as well as the muscularis uvulae. The latter originates from the tensor aponeurosis anteriorly and proceeds as a paired midline structure to the base of the uvula posteriorly.

This muscle controls the shape of the uvula. The anterior 25% of the velum contains the aponeurosis of the tensor veli palatini muscle. The tensor veli palatini muscle takes its origin from the scaphoid fossa of the greater wing of the sphenoid and the length of the superolateral aspect of the eustachian tube. The muscle descends almost vertically to hook around the anterior aspect of the hamulus and continues medially as an aponeurosis, spreading across the midline to join its contralateral mate and forming a fibrous band posterior to the hard palate but anterior to the levator veli palatini sling.

The superior constrictor originates from the posterior pharyngeal raphe and courses inferiorly and anteriorly to insert into the pterygoid hamulus, lateral pterygoid plate, pterygomaxillary ligament, mandible, and floor of the mouth. It may play some role in constricting the posterior pharynx, thus contributing to velopharyngeal function.

The palate is vascularized by two sets of neurovascular bundles, anteriorly the incisive and posteriorly the greater palatine. These vessels do not cross the midline extensively, leaving each half of the palate reliant on its own vasculature. The palate soft tissues extend posteriorly to the soft palate where they cover the functional muscles of the velum.

A cleft of the palate predictably alters the normal functional sling of the paired levator veli palatini (Figure 12.2). The clefted levator veli palatini inserts longitudinally onto the posterior edge of the clefted hard palate, never transversely joining the contralateral muscle. Therefore, a functional levator sling does not exist. Three abnormal attachments or associations of each levator veli palatini muscle have been described and can easily be seen during a cleft palate repair: (1) the posterior medial edge of the hard palate, (2) the aponeurosis of the similarly interrupted tensor veli palatini, and (3) the superior pharyngeal constrictor (Figure 12.3).[13,14] The functional reconstruction of the levator sling therefore requires the complete release of the levator muscles from the three abnormal attachments in order to reposition them anatomically into a transverse position within the middle 50% of the velum.[15]

The tensor and levator veli palatini muscles are both associated with the eustachian tube, and are equally affected in the cleft palate

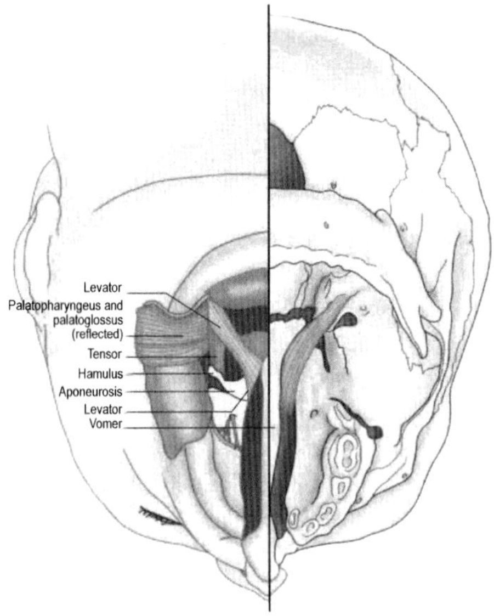

Figure 12.2. Anatomy of the cleft palate. Reprinted with permission from Elsevier in Ref. 20, p. 274. Copyright © 2009 Elsevier.

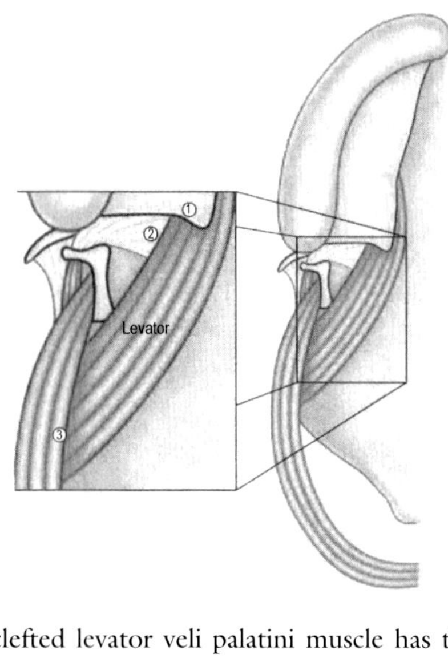

Figure 12.3. The clefted levator veli palatini muscle has three abnormal associations: (1) the hard palate, (2) the tensor aponeurosis of the tensor veli palatini, and (3) the superior pharayngeal constrictor. Reprinted with permission from Elsevier in Ref. 20, p. 275. Copyright © 2009 Elsevier.

anomaly. Classically, the levator elevates the palate, while the tensor tenses, or contracts, to dilate the eustachian tube; however, it is likely that these muscles work synergistically to dilate, or at least modulate, the eustachian tube. The tensor may draw on the lateral aspect to dilate the tubal lumen, and the levator may rotate the lip of the tubal cartilage to maximize the vector of the tensor's contraction.[16] As explained by Huang *et al.*,[11] the paratubal muscles have abnormal insertions in the cleft palate pathology, and therefore their actions as tubal dilators are likely compromised. Patients with cleft palate have eustachian tube dysfunction resulting in chronic effusions and frequent ear infections. Eustachian tube dysfunction secondary to cleft palate can lead to hearing loss, and is regularly treated with ear tube placement.

12.3 Classification

There are many classifications published for CL ± P. The most useful capture the pathologic anatomy concisely to help summarize the diagnosis and the treatment. Two of the simplest and most commonly used are the Veau[17] and the LAHSHAL[18] classifications.

The Veau system specifically classifies cleft palate and is intuitively based on anatomy (Figure 12.4). It classifies the four subtypes of cleft palate as follows: I is a cleft of the soft palate only, II is a cleft of the soft and part of the hard palate, III is a complete unilateral cleft of the palate and alveolus, and IV is a complete bilateral cleft palate and alveolus. Frequently, the Veau III and IV clefts include clefts of the lip as well.

The LAHSHAL system is an acronym, using four initials to describe where the clefts occur, as follows: "L" is lip, "A" is alveolus, "H" is hard palate, and "S" is soft palate.[18] The initials are repeated to denote the right and left sides. A capital letter denotes a complete cleft, a lowercase letter denotes an incomplete cleft, and an "X" denotes a normal structure. Therefore, XXXSHAL would represent a complete left-sided lip and palate, and lXXsXXX would denote an incomplete right-sided cleft lip with a Veau I cleft of the velum.

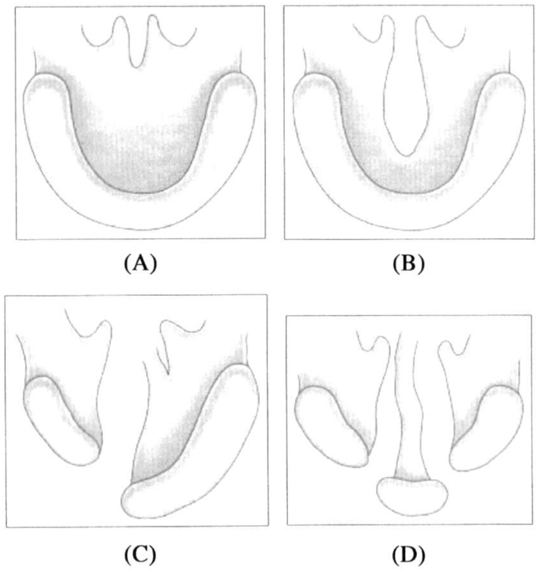

Figure 12.4. Veau classification of palates. (A) Veau I, cleft of the soft palate. (B) Veau II, cleft of the soft and part of the hard palate. (C) Veau III, complete unilateral cleft of the soft and hard palates and alveolus. (D) Veau IV, complete bilateral cleft of the soft and hard palates and alveolus. Reprinted with permission from Elsevier in Ref. 20, p. 276. Copyright © 2009 Elsevier.

An SMCP occurs when the velar muscles are clefted and misoriented, as in the overt cleft palate. However, the overlying mucosa of the soft palate is intact; therefore, the clefting is submucosal and hidden from view. The degree of levator clefting and disorganization is variable, as it is understood that not all SMCPs result in velopharyngeal dysfunction. When complete levator muscle clefting occurs, three cardinal signs may appear: (1) midline notching of the posterior edge of the hard palate, (2) midline translucent blue zona pellucida where the muscles are missing, and (3) a bifid uvula. The three classic signs are actually not commonly present; the Children's Hospital of Pittsburgh series demonstrated that only 29% of patients diagnosed with SMCP possessed all three signs, 34% had any two signs, 17% had only bifid uvula, 14% had only zona pellucida, and 6% had only notched hard palate.[19] Far more clinically practical is the abnormal function of the velum as it can be seen elevating in a "vaulted" V-shaped pattern, indicative of abnormal sagittally oriented levator muscles. Therefore, SMCP is a diagnosis of clinical suspicion on the basis of a physical examination, speech evaluation, and frequently a history of recurrent ear infections. Pure idiopathic velopharyngeal insufficiency, with no signs of SMCP, can be found to have "occult SMCP" on confirmation of the diagnosis intraoperatively.[20]

12.4 Treatment Goals and Preoperative Workup

An infant with orofacial clefting should be seen by a cleft-craniofacial team trained in the unique comprehensive care that will be required. Early evaluation by a qualified feeding specialist (speech language pathologist or occupational therapist) and plastic surgeon will address and assure airway safety and successful feeding. Feeding specialists often assist in optimizing nutrition, with customized bottles that allow easier fluid egress and in positioning the infant in a more upright position to allow for gravity-assisted feeding.[21] We prefer having the infant able to drink from a sippy cup and completely weaned from a bottle before cleft palate repair, as the nipple could potentially injure the repair postoperatively.[20]

Timing of cleft repair depends upon several factors including the size and shape of the mandible, the infant's airway, the nature of the palatal cleft, and the development of speech. There is debate that early cleft palate surgery may impair maxillary growth, whereas late cleft palate surgery may lead to worse speech problems. As normal speech development occurs at about 1 year of age, in general, a cleft palate repair is timed at approximately 12 months of age, although this may be individualized depending on the patient. Children with other medical conditions or syndromes may require additional perioperative evaluation.

An important subset of infants with cleft palate are those with Pierre Robin sequence, characterized by a retrognathic mandible leading to posterior displacement of the tongue (glossoptosis) and airway compromise. These patients often have a wide, U-shaped Veau II cleft. Infants with Pierre Robin sequence may require preparatory airway correction (tongue–lip adhesion or mandibular distraction) before cleft palate repair. Another important subset of patients with cleft palate are those with velocardiofacial syndrome, or 22q11.2 deletion, also known as Shprintzen or DiGeorge syndrome. These patients may have cardiac anomalies, immunoincompetence, hypotonia, or other manifestations that require intervention.[22]

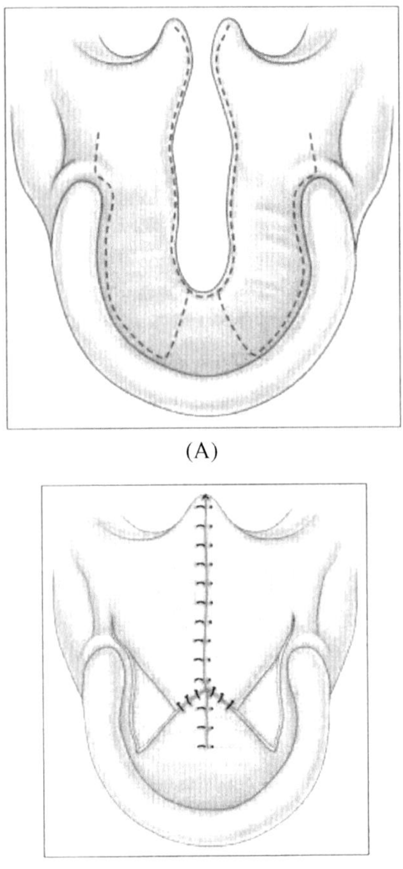

(A)

(B)

Figure 12.5. In a Veau II cleft of the soft and hard palates, unipedicled flaps can be designed to be elevated (A) and set back in a V-Y pushback manner that closes the cleft as well as potentially lengthening the palate (B). Reprinted with permission from Elsevier in Ref. 20, p. 289. Copyright © 2009 Elsevier.

12.5 Primary Repair of the Soft Palate

The earliest soft palate repairs by Von Graefe and Roux in the early 19th century[23] simply reapproximated the separated soft palate, and did not specifically try to reconstruct the muscle. The realization that the length of the palate plays a potential role in velopharyngeal competence did not come until Veau, Wardill, and Kilner designed repairs that "pushed back" the hard palate flaps, potentially adding length to the soft palate[23] (Figure 12.5). It was not until 1969 that Kriens specifically repaired the levator sling to reconstruct the abnormal anatomy of the muscular sling,[23] calling his repair an *intravelar veloplasty* (IVVP). The options for velar repair today include straight-line or Z-plasty closure with or without an IVVP.

12.5.1 *Intravelar veloplasty*

Most modern-day palatoplasties include an attempt at repairing the levator veli palatini muscle sling. However, not all IVVPs are the same, and it is important to distinguish between an "incomplete" IVVP and a "complete" IVVP. An incomplete IVVP occurs when only the most medial ends of the pathologically oriented levator muscles are dissected free and repaired. This unfortunately results in most of the levator muscle remaining in a sagittal orientation and the reapproximated medial ends of the levator muscle positioned anteriorly along the posterior edge of the hard palate. Without completely detaching the levator from its three abnormal attachments (Figure 12.3) and radically repositioning them into an anatomic transverse sling in the middle 50% of the velum, a complete IVVP cannot be performed.[15,24] It is important to identify and release the clefted levator from (1) the medial aspect of the posterior hard palate, (2) the aponeurosis of the tensor veli palatini, and (3) the superior constrictor laterally.

12.5.2 *Z-plasty velar repair*

In the late 1980s, Furlow realized that he could reroute the anomalous sagittal levator veli palatini into its proper transverse orientation.[25] Using double-opposing Z-plasties, two flaps of oral lining and two flaps of nasal lining are created. The posteriorly based oral and nasal flaps each contain their respective levator muscle, which is subsequently transferred with the Z-plasty flap into the middle 50% of the velum. As well, when the muscle is transferred on a Z-plasty flap, it eliminates the need to completely dissect both surfaces of the muscle, thereby potentially reducing scarring. The levator muscles are overlapped, being placed on "functional tension," and the transverse narrowing effect of the Z-plasty produces a secondary pharyngoplasty effect by narrowing the size of the velopharyngeal port. Similarly, the Z-plasty effect sagittally lengthens the velum and prevents longitudinal contracture scarring that can occur with straight-line repairs.

12.5.3 *Preparation*

An oral Ring–Adair–Elwyn endotracheal tube is used to facilitate the placement of the Dingman retractor. A roll is placed beneath the shoulders and the head in a gel doughnut. Loupes and a headlight are donned, and the patient is prepped and draped. Permissive hypotension can be used to potentially decrease blood loss. Simple silk sutures are placed on both sides of the anterior tongue and are used to control positioning. The Dingman mouth gag is positioned, and dental rolls are placed on either side of the endotracheal tube (at the bend) to prevent tube compression (Figure 12.6). The Dingman is "released" for 5 to 10 min every hour, reducing the threat of postoperative tongue-swelling. A 10 French suction catheter passed through the nostril to rest on the posterior pharyngeal wall provides continuous suctioning of irrigation and blood from the operative field, negating the need for a throat pack; as well, leaving this suction catheter in place after completion of the operation gives the anesthesia team a properly positioned tool to suction the hypopharynx. It is removed just before extubation. An appropriately sized nasopharyngeal airway is placed in the other nostril; alternatively, it can be placed under direct vision just before repair of the nasal layer. This nasopharyngeal airway provides postoperative airway maintenance in case there is

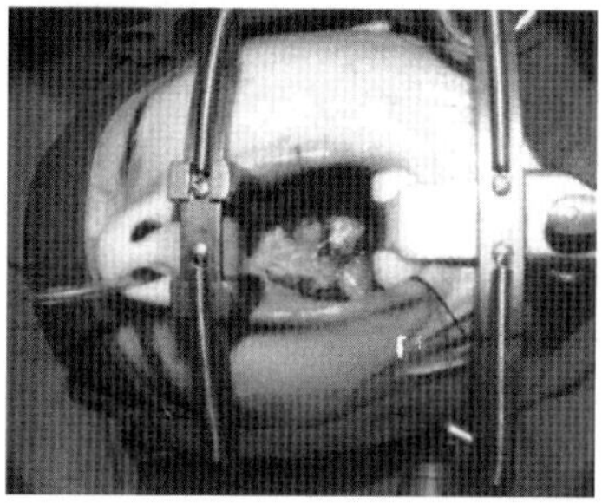

Figure 12.6. At the 90° bend of the oral Ring–Adair–Elwyn endotracheal tube in the Dingman tongue retractor, dental rolls can be placed on either side of the tube to prevent kinking. Reprinted with permission from Elsevier in Ref. 20, p. 278. Copyright © 2009 Elsevier.

undue postoperative tongue-swelling, and is removed on the first postoperative day when it is certain that tongue-swelling and airway compromise are no longer concerns.

12.5.4 *Markings*

The double-opposing Z-plasty refers to two Z-plasties: one on the oral mucosa and one on the nasal mucosa, each containing two flaps. Therefore, there are two oral mucosa flaps (one anteriorly based and one posteriorly based) and two nasal mucosa flaps (one anteriorly based and one posteriorly based). Both posteriorly based flaps include the respective ipsilateral levator muscle.

Furlow's traditional operation did not include "classical" relaxing incisions; however, the operation described herein is the modified procedure made popular by the Children's Hospital of Philadelphia. Relaxing incisions are freely used as necessary to repair the velum without tension. Bilateral velar relaxing incisions, in the crease of the palatal–buccal junction and extending posteriorly from the retromolar trigone of the mandible and anteriorly to the maxillary tuberosity, are marked with a marking pen. They extend anteriorly onto the hard palate between the attached gingiva and the hard palate mucosa (Figure 12.7). The hamulus can be palpated just

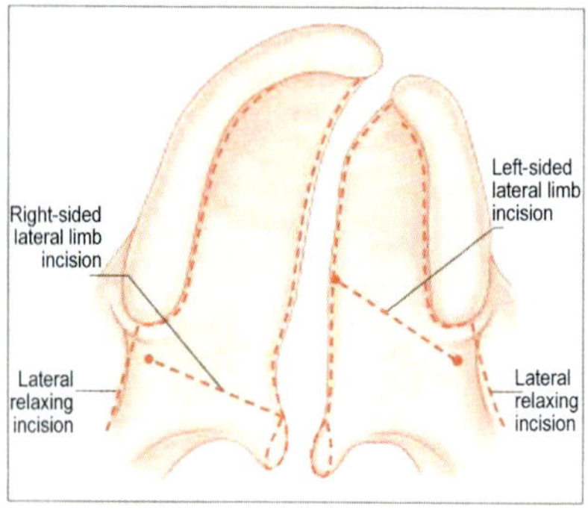

(A)

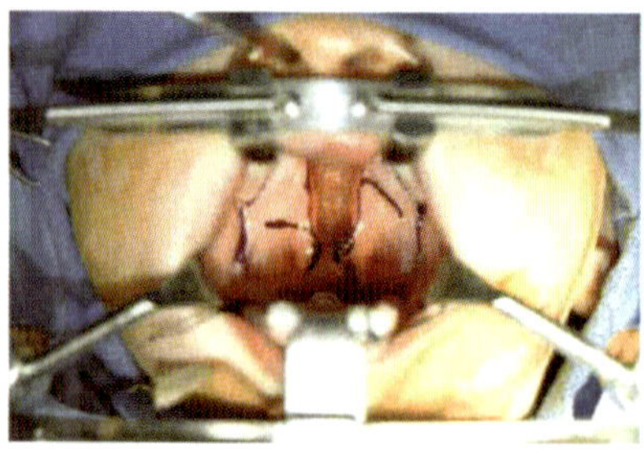

(B)

Figure 12.7. (A) Markings for the double-opposing Z-plasty velar repair. (B) Intraoperative markings. Reprinted with permission from Elsevier in Ref. 20, p. 279. Copyright © 2009 Elsevier.

posterior to the maxillary tuberosity and marked bilaterally, taking care to leave enough tissue between the hamulus mark and the relaxing incision. The posterior edge of the hard palate is identified, and the "normal expected" junction of the hard and soft palates, at the margin of the cleft medially, is marked. Alternatively, this location can be estimated to be on a transverse line connecting the maxillary tuberosities. The bases of the uvulae, at the uvula–velum junction, are marked bilaterally. The medial edge of the entire hard and soft cleft, from uvular base to the anterior extent of the cleft is now outlined, taking care to leave enough additional millimeters of nasal lining to facilitate its repair. The uvular halves are marked to be demucosalized (Figure 12.7).

The limbs of the oral Z-plasty flaps are now marked. The lateral limb of the left-sided posteriorly based oral musculomucosal flap is marked by joining the left hamulus to the junction of the hard and soft palates, creating a 60–90° flap. The lateral limb of the right-sided anteriorly based oral mucosal flap is marked by joining the right hamulus with the right uvular base, creating a 60–90° flap.

The velum and relaxing incisions are infiltrated with epinephrine for hemostasis. We prefer a fresh mixture of epinephrine with a concentration of 10 μg/mL. We consider the maximum dose of epinephrine in the otherwise healthy pediatric patient (not receiving halothane anesthetic) to be 10 μg/kg, so 1 mL/kg can be injected. Every 20 to 30 min, further dosing of the epinephrine may be administered to enhance hemostasis if needed.

12.5.5 *Incisions and elevation of the oral flaps*

Scissors are used to demucosalize the uvular halves, and 4-0 chromic gut suture on a tapered needle is used to mark both uvular tips, making it easier to identify them later (Figure 12.8). A No. 15 blade is used to cut the left lateral limb and cleft-margin incisions (Figure 12.9). Dissecting scissors are used to elevate the left-sided, posteriorly based, oral mucosa and the levator off the nasal mucosa. The levator muscle

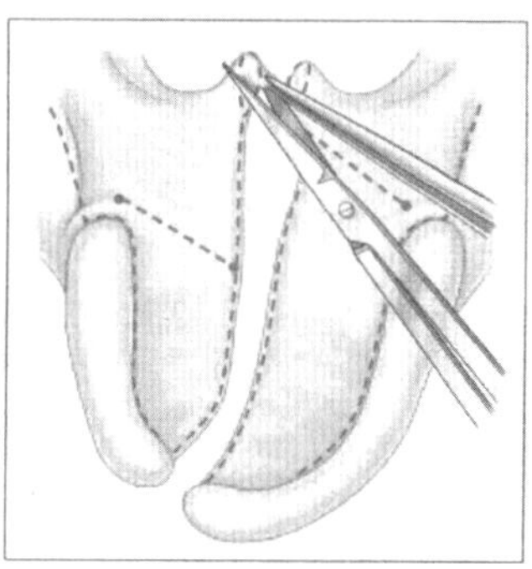

Figure 12.8. Scissors are used to demucosalize the uvular halves, which are then marked with a simple suture for later identification. Reprinted with permission from Elsevier in Ref. 20, p. 280. Copyright © 2009 Elsevier.

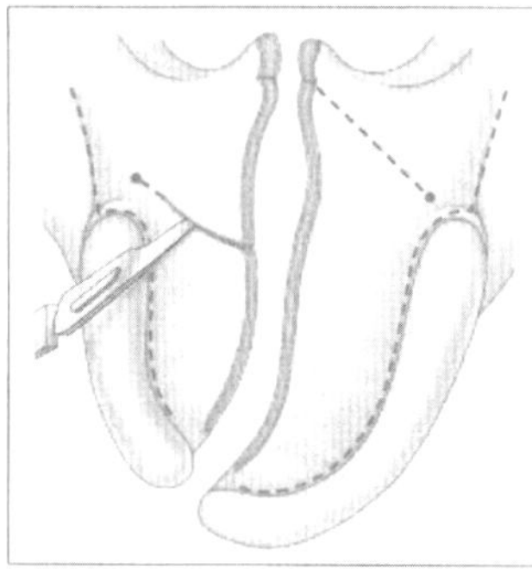

Figure 12.9. Cleft margins are incised. The oral mucosal incisions create a left-sided posteriorly based oral musculomucosal flap and a right-sided anteriorly based oral flap. Reprinted with permission from Elsevier in Ref. 20, p. 280. Copyright © 2009 Elsevier.

can be identified medially where it is attached to the posterior edge of the hard palate and laterally where the tensor aponeurosis is seen tethering the levator. The aponeurosis is cut along the posterior edge of the hard palate, and the dissection continues laterally. Sharp and blunt dissection allows release of the levator from its third and most lateral abnormal attachment — the superior constrictor (Figure 12.10) — and visualization of the levator muscle exiting the skull base. A retraction stitch is placed in the tip of the left-sided posteriorly based oral musculomucosal flap and brought out and draped over the Dingman retractor. Dissection between the muscle and the nasal mucosa continues posteriorly, leaving the submucosa on the nasal mucosa so as to not thin out the nasal lining until the junction of the uvula and velum. With the levator muscle completely released, it can be radically retropositioned in a completely transverse orientation across the middle 50% of the velum. The levator, as it exits the skull base, is now almost 90° to the superior constrictor (Figure 12.11). This complete retropositioning required to reconstruct the levator sling in the native position requires complete release of the levator from its three attachments.

The right-sided anteriorly based oral mucosal flap is similarly incised with a No. 15 blade. Scissors are used to elevate the

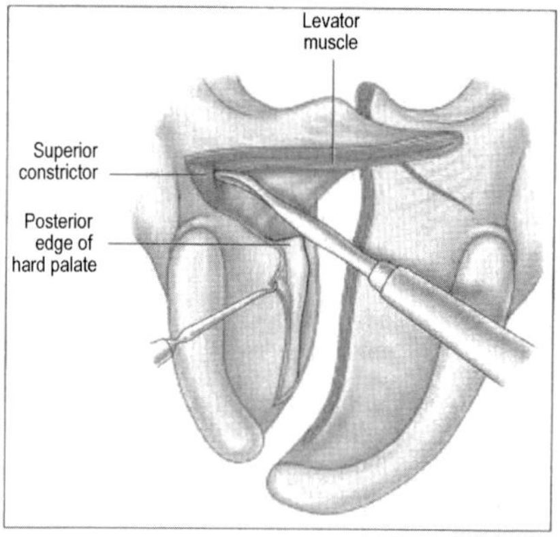

Figure 12.10. After sweeping free from the superior constrictor laterally, the levator muscle is completely released from its three abnormal attachments. The levator can now be radically transposed from its abnormal anterior position to the anatomically correct transverse position. Reprinted with permission from Elsevier in Ref. 20, p. 281. Copyright © 2009 Elsevier.

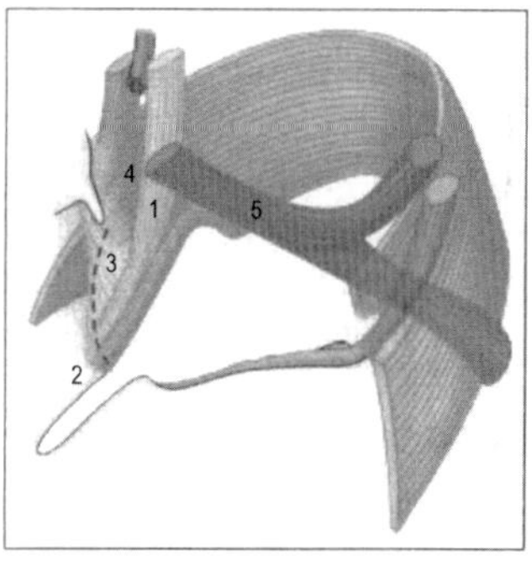

Figure 12.11. Shown is the abnormal longitudinal insertion of the (1) levator muscle into the (2) posterior edge of the hard palate, (3) tensor aponeurosis, and (4) superior constructor. On the right, (5) represents the levator radically retropositioned into a transverse position overlying the middle 50% of the velum. Reprinted with permission from Elsevier in Ref. 20, p. 282. Copyright © 2009 Elsevier.

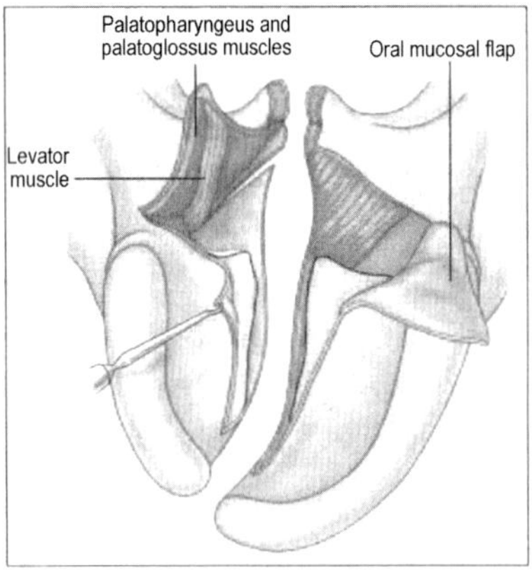

Figure 12.12. Incision and elevation of the right-sided anteriorly based oral mucosal flap. The palatopharyngeus and palatoglossus muscles are left down and uninjured. Reprinted with permission from Elsevier in Ref. 20, p. 282. Copyright © 2009 Elsevier.

submucosa with the flap so that it is not too thin or buttonholed. Beneath the submucosa, the palatopharyngeus and palatoglossus muscles are identified and left down (Figure 12.12). The dissection continues anteriorly until the posterior edge of the hard palate.

12.5.6 *Mobilizing the velar flaps*

The velar relaxing incisions can now be made, from the retromolar trigone posteriorly to the maxillary tuberosity anteriorly. The extent of these incisions is often determined by the width of the cleft. Within the markings along the palate–buccal crease, the knife blade is aimed slightly medial to avoid exposing lateral buccal fat. When the incision continues anteriorly on the hard palate, the knife blade should be aimed perpendicular to the hard palate, to avoid the neurovascular bundle. Through the relaxing incisions, access to completely release the tensor aponeurosis and the posterior edge of the hard palate may be obtained. Scissors are placed in the relaxing incisions with the tips aimed medially. The tips of the scissors palpate the hamulus, and with the blades medial to the hamulus and superior constrictor, they are

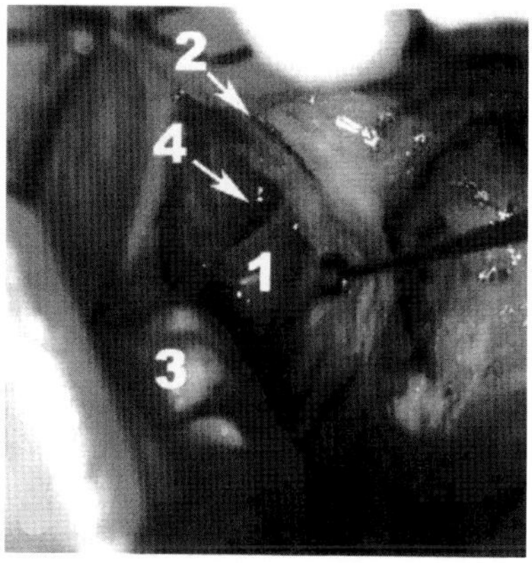

Figure 12.13. Lateral relaxing incisions expose the tensor aponeurosis (1) as it courses medially around the hamulus (2). The maxillary tuberosity is shown (3) and the space of Ernst (4), just medial to the superior constrictor. Reprinted with permission from Elsevier in Ref. 20, p. 283. Copyright © 2009 Elsevier.

gently pushed several millimeters into the space of Ernst (Figure 12.13). The scissors are then gently spread along the course of the relaxing incision. Through the lateral relaxing incision, the tensor tendon is identified as it travels around the hamulus and is sharply divided just medially to the hamulus (Figure 12.13). Some have advocated securing the tensor tendon, with a suture, to the hamulus before its division medial to the hamulus, thereby preventing the theoretical retraction of a freed tendon into the skull base. From the relaxing incision, the posterior edge of the hard palate is palpated with the scissors, and the oral flap released from the posterior edge of the hard palate by blindly cutting along the posterior edge of the hard palate coursing medially.

A hockey-stick-shaped Blair palate elevator is placed in the lateral relaxing incision of the hard palate just anterior to the neurovascular bundles, and subperiosteally dissects the hard-palate mucoperiosteal flaps from the hard palate (Figure 12.14). Gentle rolling of the Blair elevator medially will elevate the oral flaps at the hard–soft junction as well as stretch the tissue in the region of the neurovascular bundle, allowing visualization of the pedicles.

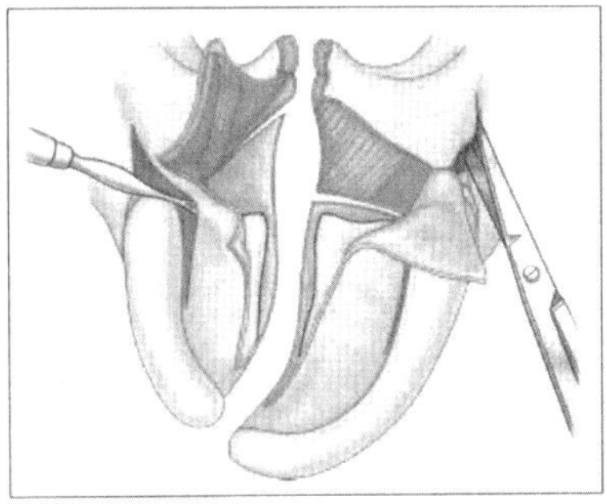

Figure 12.14. Via the lateral relaxing incision extended onto the hard palate, the Blair cleft palate elevator (on the left side of the image) is inserted to elevate the hard palate mucoperiosteal flaps. Reprinted with permission from Elsevier in Ref. 20, p. 284. Copyright © 2009 Elsevier.

The oral flaps can be completely released by placing the tips of the scissors on the medial aspect of the posterior edge of the hard palate and cutting laterally until the scissor tips join the lateral relaxing incision dissection. This maneuver can be blind, so it is important that the scissors are always in contact with the posterior edge of the hard palate, preventing them from migrating anteriorly toward the neurovascular bundle. The nasal mucosa can then also be subperiosteally dissected off the nasal side of the hard palate (Figure 12.15).

12.5.7 *Mobilization of the hard-palate flaps*

If the plan is to create unipedicled hard-palate mucoperiosteal flaps, it is usually easier to create them now to get better exposure. This dissection provides a more direct approach and visualization of the neurovascular bundle. When treating a wider cleft, complete dissection of the greater palatine neurovascular bundles with subperiosteal release at the rim of the bony foramina may be required to free the bundle. Sometimes, the posterior aspect of the bony foramina will require an osteotomy to mobilize the neurovascular bundle posteriorly and medially. The hard-palate repair will be described in greater detail in Sec. 12.6.

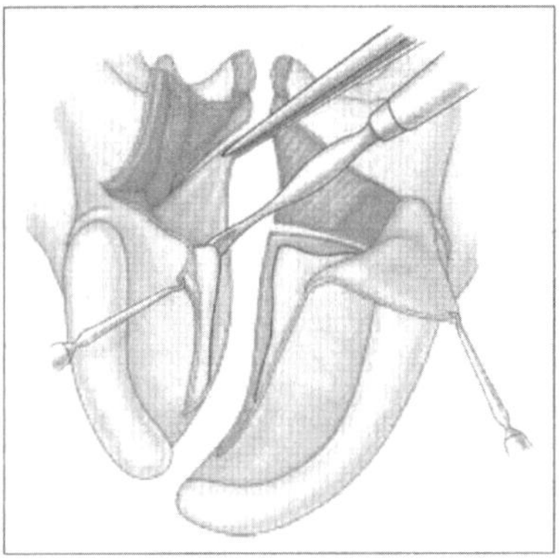

Figure 12.15. The bilateral nasal mucosa can be subperiosteally dissected off the nasal side of the hard palate along the medial cleft edge and posterior edge of the hard palate. Reprinted with permission from Elsevier in Ref. 20, p. 284. Copyright © 2009 Elsevier.

12.5.8 *Creation of the nasal flaps*

The left-sided anteriorly based nasal mucosal flap is made. The incision is started from the base of the uvula medially and moves laterally to where the left levator exits the skull base, near the hamulus. It is helpful to have the left-sided oral flap retracted toward the posterior pharyngeal wall during this maneuver (Figure 12.16).

After the previous elevation of the right-sided anteriorly based oral mucosal flap, the palatal muscles remain on the right-sided posteriorly based nasal musculomucosal flap. The levator is identified and released from its three attachments — the posterior edge of the hard palate, the tensor aponeurosis, and the superior constrictor laterally. The right-sided, posteriorly based nasal musculomucosal flap is now cut from the junction of the hard and soft palate medially to the hamulus laterally in the region where the levator exits the skull base (Figure 12.16). A very important note about making this incision: first, the incision should be made several millimeters away from the posterior edge of the hard palate. Leaving this cuff of nasal mucosa along the posterior edge of the hard palate facilitates the final closure. Second, this incision is carried laterally *only* as far as is needed to transpose it to the other side.

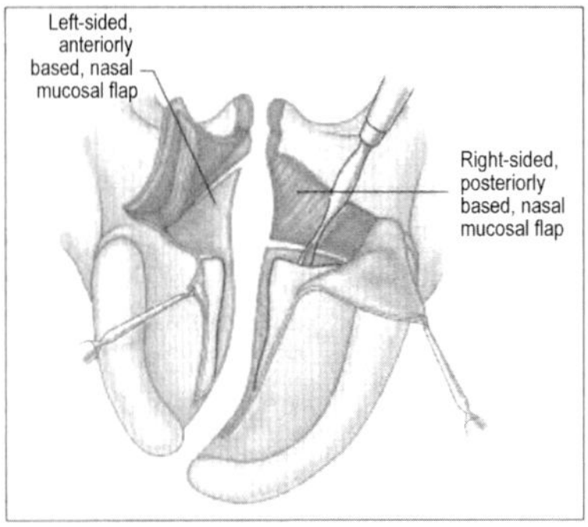

Figure 12.16. The left-sided anteriorly based nasal mucosal flap is created by an incision from the left uvular base toward the left hamulus. For the right-sided posteriorly based nasal musculomucosal flap, the incision from the junction of the hard and soft palate should go laterally only as far as needed to allow the tip of the right-sided posteriorly based nasal musculomucosal flap to be inset into the nasal lining defect on the left side. Reprinted with permission from Elsevier in Ref. 20, p. 285. Copyright © 2009 Elsevier.

Often, this incision is made only partially to the hamulus. Following the creation of the flap, and before inset, the anterior edge of the levator muscle is dissected away from the mucosal edge of the right-sided nasal flap for a few millimeters, allowing a cuff of free mucosal edge to be used for the final inset and preventing the incorporation of muscle into the repair (Figure 12.17).

12.5.9 *Nasal flaps: inset and closure*

Simple sutures with 4-0 chromic gut on a tapered needle are used for the entire repair. Saline irrigation is placed on the surgeon's fingers during tying. The nasopharyngeal tube should be placed at this time if not already done, and placing the nasal flap sutures in the nasopharyngeal tube must be avoided.

The previously placed uvular sutures are identified, and the uvular tips are sutured together. This suture is left long, pulled out of the mouth, and draped with slight traction over the Dingman retractor in the midline for the nasal closure, which helps keep the reconstructed

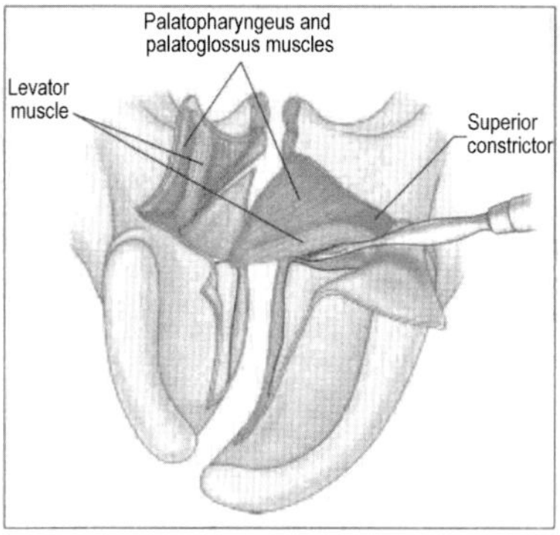

Figure 12.17. The right-sided posteriorly based nasal musculomucosal flap must be similarly released from the posterior edge of the hard palate medially, the tensor aponeurosis anterolaterally, and the superior constrictor laterally to allow complete retroposition of the longitudinal levator into a transverse position over the middle 50% of the velum. Reprinted with permission from Elsevier in Ref. 20, p. 284. Copyright © 2009 Elsevier.

uvula in the midline. The uvular repair is completed with interrupted sutures 1 mm apart on both the oral and nasal sides of the uvula.

The nasal closure begins with a key suture placed through the tip of the right-sided posteriorly based nasal musculomucosal flap. The suture grasps the tip of the flap, capturing the distal free edge of the levator, transposing it across the defect, and insetting it just beneath the contralateral levator as it exits the skull base. This move radically retropositions the levator in a transverse, physiologically functional position across the middle 50% of the new velum. Next, the left-sided anteriorly based nasal mucosal flap is transposed into the corner of the right-sided nasal defect. With the nasal flap tips inset, the three nasal limb incisions can be completely repaired. Given the occasional difference in limb lengths, bisect the limb defects with interrupted sutures until the limb is finished. It is important that only mucosa and not muscle is sewn along these limbs, to reduce scarring or tethering of the muscle (Figure 12.18).

Depending upon the type of cleft, the nasal repair may extend anteriorly into the hard palate, where vomer flaps are sewn to the

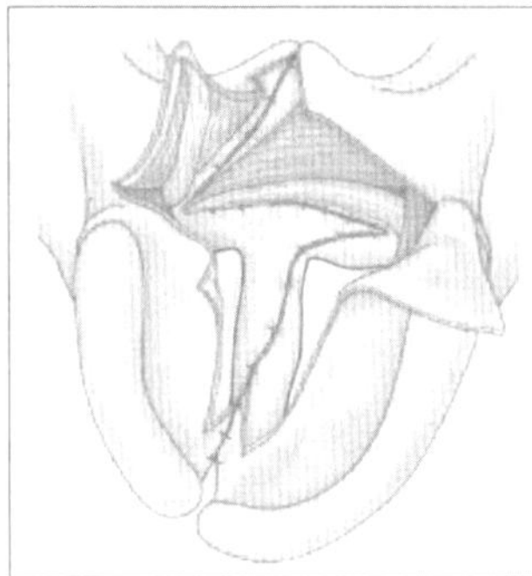

Figure 12.18. Complete closure of the nasal flaps requires insetting of the tips of the right and left nasal flaps, followed by interrupted chromic gut sutures along the limbs and the hard palate mucosa. Reprinted with permission from Elsevier in Ref. 20, p. 285. Copyright © 2009 Elsevier.

nasal lining (Veau III or IV). Unilateral or bilateral vomer flaps (described below) are used for additional nasal lining flaps to complete the hard-palate repair.

Occasionally, there will be challenges in approximating the nasal flaps without tension. Particularly when insetting the left-sided, anteriorly based nasal mucosal flap, there can be a deficiency in nasal lining and a defect results (Figure 12.19A). In these cases, a piece of thin acellular dermal matrix can be sewn into the nasal defect in an onlay manner, patching this defect. Care is taken to place the anchoring points in such a way as not to tether the levator muscle sling. The acellular dermal matrix is then draped over the hard palate nasal lining repair, augmenting this reconstruction and decreasing the risk of fistula formation (Figure 12.19B).

12.5.10 *Oral flaps: inset and closure*

Similarly, the oral flaps are inset and closed. The midline uvular retraction stitch is cut, and the uvula is placed back into the nasal pharynx. When needed, the repaired uvula can be retracted with a forceps into the nasopharynx, facilitating the posterior oral limb repair. The left-sided posteriorly based musculomucosal flap is sutured into its

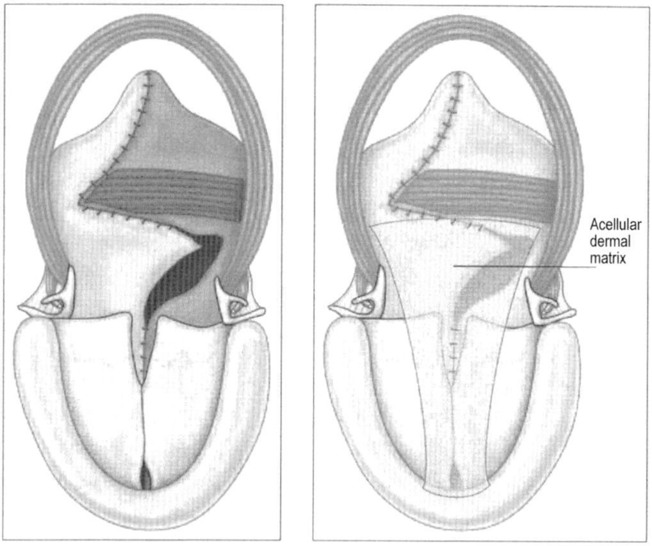

(A) (B)

Figure 12.19. (A) Example of a nasal lining defect that cannot be closed without undue tension. This is most commonly in the right side, where the left-sided anteriorly based nasal mucosal flap has trouble reaching the defect near the right hamulus. This emphasizes the importance of not extending this incision all the way to the right hamulus. (B) Onlay repair of this defect with acellular dermal matrix to cover both the nasal lining defect and to reinforce the nasal lining repair of the hard palate. Reprinted with permission from Elsevier in Ref. 20, p. 286. Copyright © 2009 Elsevier.

receiving corner on the right. This radically retropositions the left levator into an anatomic transverse position. This completes the levator sling reconstruction by overlapping the levator muscles under functional tension (Figure 12.20). The right-sided anteriorly based mucosal flap is similarly inset into the remaining defect on the left. The limbs are then repaired in the same way, with each interrupted suture bisecting each remaining segment of limb. If there is undue tension on the oral repair, the inferior extent of the relaxing incision can be extended to the retromolar trigone of the mandible and even medial to it if necessary. If there still is tension on the oral repair, further dissection and release of the neurovascular bundle may need

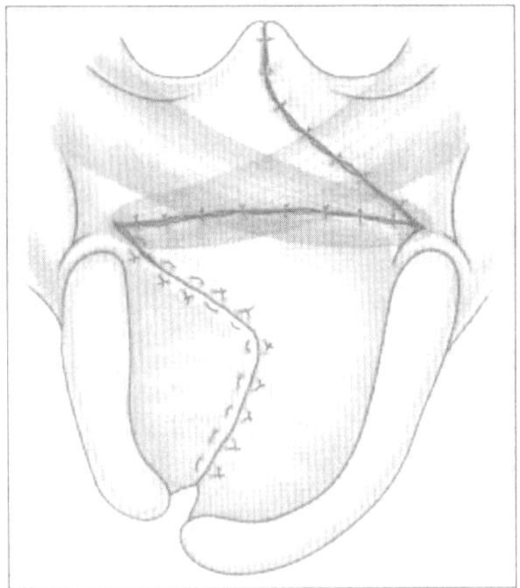

Figure 12.20. Inset of the oral side flaps overlaps the levator muscles under functional tension. Reprinted with permission from Elsevier in Ref. 20, p. 287. Copyright © 2009 Elsevier.

to be performed. If there is a hard-palate repair, then the oral flap closure will become contiguous with the hard-palate closure. Irrigation is performed and hemostasis is checked, especially the raw edges of the lateral relaxing incisions.

12.5.11 *Two-stage velar repair*

The Furlow double-opposing Z-plasty velar repair is our standard for repairing all cleft palates. In rare, very wide cleft defects (greater than 2 cm at the hard–soft palate junction), such as those seen in Veau II clefts in Pierre Robin sequence or in complete bilateral clefts, it can be difficult to do the Furlow palatoplasty without undue tension. In these cases, we choose to perform the velar repair in two stages. The first stage includes a normal repair of the hard palate, and the wide soft palate is approximated in a straight line with an IVVP — essentially, a palatal adhesion. The second stage, at least 3 months later, is a conversion Furlow palatoplasty, where the intact velum is treated as an SMCP and is repaired with a "conversion" double-opposing Z-plasty.

12.6 Primary Repair of the Hard Palate

The hard palate's mucoperiosteum lies directly over bone, and relies primarily on the greater palatine neurovascular bundles and secondarily on the anterior sphenopalatine vessels exiting the incisive foramen. Therefore, hard-palate flaps can be raised either as bipedicled flaps (von Langenbeck) or unipedicled flaps (Bardach and others) relying solely upon the greater palatine vessels. The choice of hard-palate flaps depends on the Veau type, the width of the palatal cleft, and the width of the alveolar cleft. Each side can potentially be raised as either a unipedicle or bipedicle flap. The design may need to be customized further depending on the position of the major and minor segments of the maxillary alveolus and the position of the vomer.

Bipedicled flaps are made with a lateral and medial incision on the hard palate, sparing the anterior connection with the alveolus. The lateral incisions are made by extending the lateral relaxing incisions of the soft-palate repair anteriorly along the junction of the hard palate and the attached gingiva. The medial incisions are made along the medial cleft margin, taking care to leave enough mucosa for turning down to become nasal lining flaps (Figure 12.18). By sparing the anterior tip of the flap, the bipedicle flap has an additional blood supply from both the sphenopalatine vessels via the incisive foramen and the mucosal attachments to the anterior alveolus. The drawback is their relative inability to move, given this anterior attachment; therefore, bipedicle flaps cannot help cover an anterior defect or a wide cleft.

Unipedicled flaps are raised similarly to bipedicled flaps; however, the anterior connection to the alveolus is released. As the sole pedicle is found posteriorly near the junction of the hard and soft palates, the unipedicled flap is elevated in an anterior-to-posterior direction, always keeping in mind the position of the pedicle (Figure 12.21). The advantage of the unipedicled flap is its mobility, as well as the greater access to the neurovascular bundle and its bony foramina. With its free anterior end, the tip of the flap can be placed more medially or laterally to offset the nasal and oral repairs so that they overlap less, and may lessen the chance of an oronasal fistula. In the Veau II cleft, where there is no cleft of the most anterior hard palate, the unipedicled flaps can be pushed back as far as necessary, into a V-Y

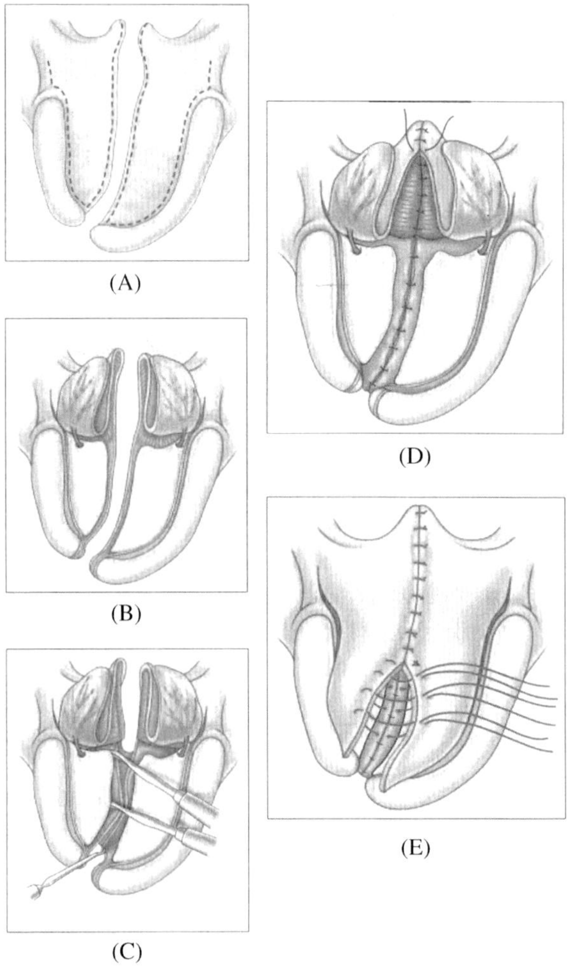

Figure 12.21. (A) Bilateral unipedicled flaps can be designed by extending the lateral relaxing incisions onto the gingival-hard palate line and the medial cleft margin, leaving enough nasal lining tissue to close the nasal side. In this example, the velum has a straight-line repair rather than a double-opposing Z-plasty repair. (B) Elevation of the unipedicled hard-palate mucoperiosteal flaps proceeds in an anterior-to-posterior direction, dissecting around the greater palatine neurovascular bundle to allow more mobility of the flaps. (C) The nasal lining is elevated off the nasal side of the hard palate to allow its closure. (D) Closure of the nasal lining (also shown is a straight-line IVVP repair). (E) Closure of the oral side: for the hard-palate portion, horizontal mattress sutures are utilized to evert and appose the raw surfaces of the thicker mucoperiosteal flaps. Reprinted with permission from Elsevier in Ref. 20, p. 288. Copyright © 2009 Elsevier.

closure (Figure 12.5). The disadvantage of the unipedicled flap is that it is based on a single blood supply, making it an all-or-nothing phenomenon should the pedicle become compromised.

In the Veau IV complete bilateral cleft, bilateral vomer flaps are necessary to repair the nasal lining. The anterior tips of the bilateral unipedicled mucoperiosteal hard-palate flaps are sewn to the tip of the elevated mucoperiosteal raw edge of the posterior premaxilla (Figure 12.22). Acellular dermal matrix in the Veau IV cleft, to

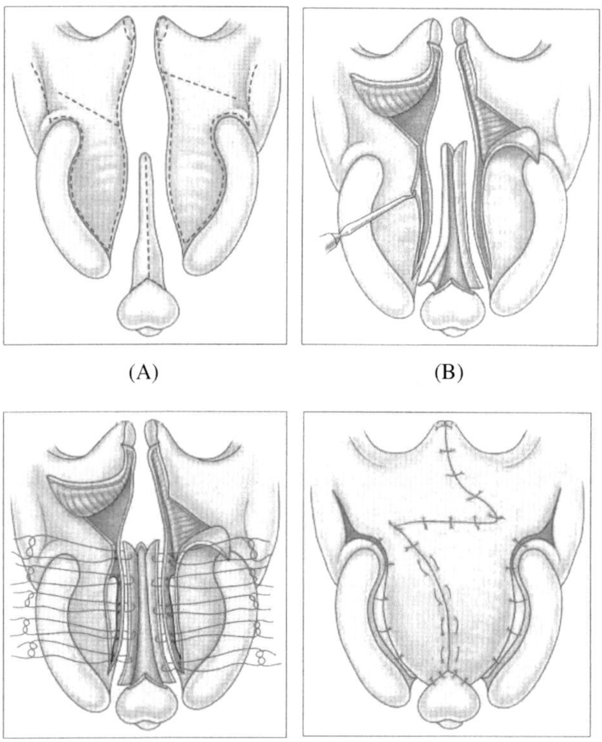

(A) (B) (C) (D)

Figure 12.22. (A) For the bilateral cleft repair, bilateral unipedicled flaps extending from the lateral relaxing incisions and vomer flaps can be designed. Note that in this example, the velum has the markings for a double-opposing Z-plasty velar repair. (B) Elevation of the oral and nasal lining flaps. (C) The vomer nasal lining flaps allow nasal closure. (D) The hard palate mucoperiosteal flaps should be closed in a horizontal mattress manner. Note that the simultaneous double-opposing Z-plasty velar repair is completed. Reprinted with permission from Elsevier in Ref. 20, p. 290. Copyright © 2009 Elsevier.

augment the anterior repair of the palate, is frequently used. Once the nasal lining of the hard palate is closed, usually with a vomer flap, rotated from the major maxillary segment to the nasal lining of the minor maxillary segment, the oral side, or mucoperiosteal flaps are closed. Horizontal mattress sutures are used to assure eversion of the raw edges of the mucoperiosteum.

12.6.1 *Primary repair of the alveolar cleft*

In the Veau III and IV cleft palates, there is a complete cleft of the alveolus. At the primary cleft-lip repair, the alveolar clefts can be repaired via a gingivoperiosteoplasty.[26] To facilitate the gingivoperiosteoplasty, the neonatal alveolar shelves usually must be brought together with a preliminary lip adhesion or presurgical infant orthopedics, such as nasoalveolar molding. If the alveolar clefts are not repaired primarily in infancy, they are repaired during an alveolar bone graft procedure, usually around ages 7 to 9 years, during the age of mixed dentition.

12.6.2 *Bilateral cleft palate repair*

Veau IV clefts are challenging, as they are often wide and the premaxilla may be quite protrusive. Presurgical infant orthopedics is frequently required to bring the premaxilla into the proximity of the posterior segments to allow for a tension-free, complete, hard-palate closure. The hard palate can be repaired with bilateral unipedicled mucoperiosteal flaps and bilateral vomer flaps to close both the nasal lining and oral side, as described above. Finally, acellular dermal matrix can augment the repair, especially over the incisive foramen, where the closure is usually most tenuous.

12.7 Postoperative Care

The primary concerns following palatoplasty are the maintenance of a patent airway and the return of feeding. The tongue can become swollen from pressure caused by the Dingman retractor and can potentially lead to anterior airway obstruction. The placement of a nasopharyngeal airway at the time of the surgery can assure a patent airway should the tongue swell postoperatively. The nasopharyngeal trumpet is removed on the first postoperative day. Pain control is essential, as distress leads to hypertension and bleeding from the fresh relaxing incisions. The patient can be discharged once the airway is deemed safe and the patient is tolerating adequate oral intake. A conservative postoperative diet is often requested, beginning with clear liquids for 48 h, then full liquids for 7 days. If at the first postoperative visit at 1 week the incisions are healing as expected, the diet is slowly advanced to a soft diet for another 1 to 2 weeks before a normal diet is resumed. If children are old enough to understand, they should rinse their mouths after feeding with clear water and chlorhexidine until the normal diet resumes.

12.8 Complications and Secondary Repair

12.8.1 *Oronasal fistulae*

The Pittsburgh Fistula Classification System was originally designed as a consistent system to classify oronasal fistulas that may occur after cleft palate repair, in order to improve outcome analyses[27] (Figure 12.23). Contemporary studies quote a wide range of fistulae

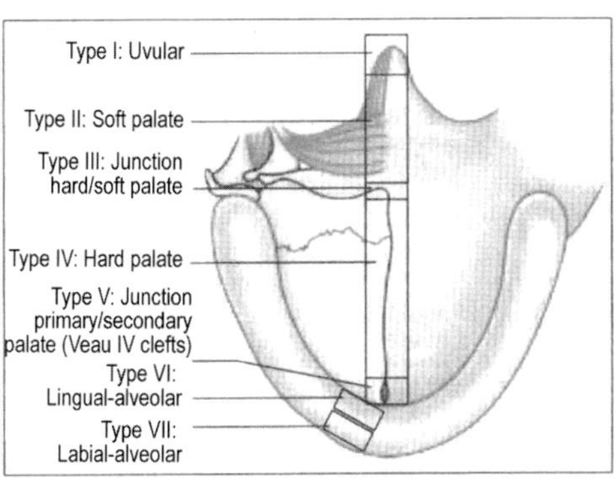

Figure 12.23. Pittsburgh Fistula Classification System. Reprinted with permission from Elsevier in Ref. 20, p. 276. Copyright © 2009 Elsevier.

incidence from less than 1% to 10–15% depending on the type of primary repair. Postoperative fistulae are very difficult to repair since they have a tendency to recur.[14] Prevention is paramount, and the prospective use of acellular dermal matrix may potentially decrease the occurrence of postoperative palatal fistulae.[15]

12.8.2 *Velopharyngeal insufficiency*

Despite the successful repair of a cleft palate, postoperative hypernasality from velopharyngeal insufficiency may occur.[28] The incidence of velopharyngeal insufficiency ranges from less than 10% to significantly higher, depending on the type of palatoplasty and the performance of a complete IVVP.[29] The importance of postoperative speech therapy and evaluation cannot be overemphasized. Standardized speech assessments, such as the Pittsburgh Weighted Speech Score,[30,31] are helpful in assessing and following speech outcomes over time. Once postoperative velopharyngeal insufficiency has been diagnosed by perceptual speech evaluation, objective anatomic evaluation of the velopharyngeal port is obtained (videofluoroscopy, nasendoscopy, or nasometry). When post-palatoplasty perceptual and anatomic velopharyngeal insufficiency is determined, secondary speech surgery is indicated.

12.8.3 *Secondary speech surgery*

Post-palatoplasty surgical treatment of velopharyngeal insufficiency can be performed with three categories of procedures: (i) lengthening the palate, (2) blocking the velopharyngeal port, or (3) narrowing the velopharyngeal port. If the original palatoplasty was performed with a straight-line repair and incomplete IVVP, then a conversion Furlow palatoplasty is the operation of choice, as it both lengthens the palate and narrows the anterior portion of the velopharyngeal port.[24] If the primary palatoplasty consisted of double opposing Z-plasty with a complete IVVP, then the nasendoscopy and videofluoroscopy can help select between posterior pharyngeal flap (PPF) to block the velopharyngeal port, or sphincter pharyngoplasty (SP) to narrow the velopharyngeal port.

If there is adequate lateral wall motion and a sizable velopharyngeal gap, a PPF is the procedure of choice. A PPF is performed by raising a musculomucosal tongue of tissue from the posterior pharyngeal wall and insetting it into the posterior edge of the velum (Figure 12.24).[32] The PPF can be superiorly or inferiorly based. The active lateral pharyngeal wall motion contacts the midline PPF and velopharyngeal competence is obtained. If the nasendoscopy and videofluoroscopy reveal minimal lateral pharyngeal wall motion and a minimal velopharyngeal gap, then an SP is the procedure of choice.

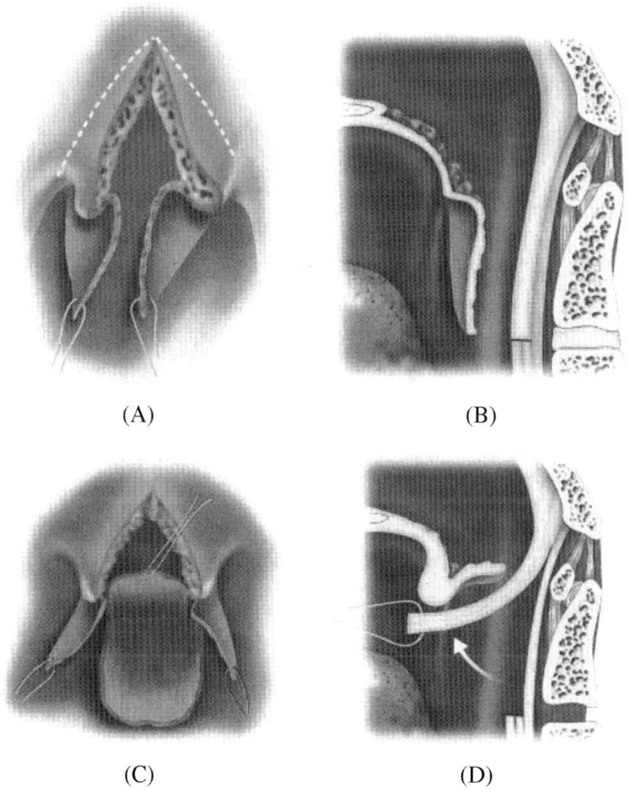

Figure 12.24. Posterior pharyngeal flap. Each pair of illustrations shows both the anterior view and the lateral view. (A and B) The uvula is split down the middle to facilitate in elevating two nasal flaps inferiorly. (C and D) The superiorly based PPF is designed and elevated off the prevertebral fascia.

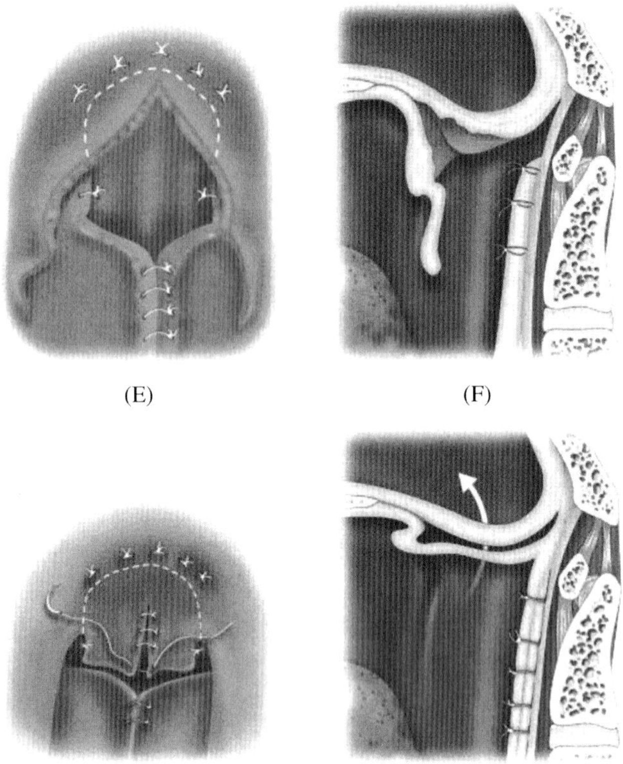

(E) (F)

(G) (H)

Figure 12.24. (*Continued*) (E and F) The PPF is inset above the palate with interrupted horizontal mattress sutures. The posterior pharyngeal donor site may be closed. (G and H) The raw surfaces of the nasal flaps are approximated to the raw edge of the PPF and closed in the midline to reduce contraction of the PPF if it had a raw surface for healing by secondary intention. Reprinted with permission from The McGraw Hill Companies in Ref. 32, Chapter 41, pp. 655, 657 [Figures 41-2 (A-B), 41-3 (A-B), 41-5 (A-B), 41-6 (A-B)].

An SP is performed by raising superiorly based posterior tonsilar pillars containing the palatopharyngeus muscles.[33] The musculomucosal flaps are inset along the posterior pharyngeal wall, thereby narrowing the velopharyngeal port (Figure 12.25).

Overcorrection, hyponasality, and potential obstructive sleep apnea are potential complications of secondary speech surgery. Parents

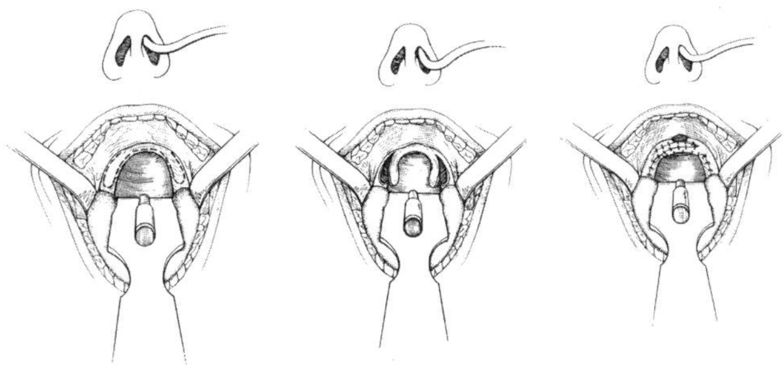

Figure 12.25. Sphincter pharyngoplasty. (A) Superiorly based flaps are designed over the posterior tonsillar pillar. (B) Elevation of the flaps, which incorporate fibers of the palatopharyngeus muscles. (C) Inset of flaps to narrow the central port. Reprinted with permission from The McGraw Hill Companies in Ref. 33, Chapter 42, pp. 668–669 [Figures 42-2, 42-3, 42-4].

should preoperatively be counseled regarding this potential complication, and frequent evaluation of obstructive sleep apnea is important over time.

12.9 Conclusions

The palate plays an important role in one of the most fundamental of human functions — speech. Whether a child is born with CL ± P, an isolated CPO, or SMCP, surgical repair can make a significant difference in the child's development and life. Soft- and hard-palate flaps can be elevated safely with knowledge of the anatomy; however, closure without tension is the key to avoiding wound healing problems and postoperative oronasal fistulae. Likely, the most important factor in successful palatoplasty is the reconstruction of the levator veli palatini sling to its transverse anatomic location in the middle 50% of the velum. This requires the complete release of the abnormally positioned levator muscle and its radical retroposition during sling reconstruction. Despite these maneuvers, velopharyngeal insufficiency may result, requiring secondary speech surgery. The diagnosis and treatment of speech problems requires both the plastic surgeon and the speech pathologist working together in the setting of a multidisciplinary cleft-craniofacial team.

References

1. **Fraser FC.** The genetics of cleft lip and cleft palate. *Am J Hum Genet* 1970;22:336–352.
2. **Mitchell LE.** Epidemiology of cleft lip and palate. In: Losee JE, Kirschner RE, eds. *Comprehensive Cleft Care.* New York, NY: McGraw-Hill Medical; 2009: 35–42.
3. **Goldberg R, Motzkin B, Marion R, Scambler PJ, Shprintzen RJ.** Velo-cardio-facial syndrome: a review of 120 patients. *Am J Med Genet* 1993; 45:313–319.
4. **Jugessur A, Murray JC.** Orofacial clefting: recent insights into a complex trait. *Curr Opin Genet Dev* 2005;15:270–278.
5. **Weinzweig J, Panter KE, Pantaloni M, *et al.*** The fetal cleft palate: I. Characterization of a congenital model. *Plast Reconstr Surg* 1999;103: 419–428.
6. **Panter KE, Bunch TD, Keeler RF, Sisson DV, Callan RJ.** Multiple congenital contractures (MCC) and cleft palate induced in goats by ingestion of piperidine alkaloid-containing plants: reduction in fetal movement as the probable cause. *J Toxicol Clin Toxicol* 1990;28:69–83.
7. **Randall P, Hamilton R.** The Pierre Robin syndrome. In: Grabb WC, Rosenstein SW, Bzoch KR, eds. *Cleft Lip and Palate: Surgical, Dental, and Speech Aspects.* Boston, MA: Little, Brown and Company; 1971:559–570.
8. **Eppley BL, van Aalst JA, Robey A, Havlik RJ, Sadove AM.** The spectrum of orofacial clefting. *Plast Reconstr Surg* 2005;115:101e–114e.
9. **Marazita ML, Mooney MP.** Current concepts in the embryology and genetics of cleft lip and cleft palate. *Clin Plast Surg* 2004;31:125–140.
10. **Kahn DM, Schendel SA.** Anatomy and classification of alveolar and palatal clefts. In: Mathes SJ, ed. *Pediatric Plastic Surgery.* Vol. 4. 2nd edn. Philadelphia, PA: Saunders Elsevier; 2006:69–89.
11. **Huang MH, Lee ST, Rajendran K.** A fresh cadaveric study of the paratubal muscles: implications for eustachian tube function in cleft palate. *Plast Reconstr Surg* 1997;100:833–842.
12. **Huang MH, Lee ST, Rajendran K.** Anatomic basis of cleft palate and velopharyngeal surgery: implications from a fresh cadaveric study. *Plast Reconstr Surg* 1998;101:613–629.
13. **Furlow LT.** Double-opposing Z-plasty palate repair. In: Losee JE, Kirschner RE, eds. *Comprehensive Cleft Care.* New York, NY: McGraw-Hill Medical; 2009:371–389.

14. **Losee JE, Smith DM, Vecchione L, *et al.*** Post-palatoplasty fistulae: diagnosis, treatment, and prevention. In: Losee JE, Kirschner RE, eds. *Comprehensive Cleft Care.* New York, NY: McGraw-Hill Medical; 2009:525–554.
15. **Losee JE, Smith DM, Afifi AM, *et al.*** A successful algorithm for limiting postoperative fistulae following palatal procedures in the patient with orofacial clefting. *Plast Reconstr Surg* 2008;122:544–554.
16. **Dayan JH, Smith D, Oliker A, Haring J, Cutting CB.** A virtual reality model of eustachian tube dilation and clinical implications for cleft palate repair. *Plast Reconstr Surg* 2005;116:236–241.
17. **Veau V.** *Division Palatine.* Paris, France: Masson et Cie; 1931.
18. **Kriens O.** LAHSHAL: a concise documentation system for cleft lip, alveolus and palate diagnosis. In: Kriens O, ed. *What Is a Cleft Lip and Palate?* New York, NY: Thieme; 1989:32–33.
19. **Worrall CI, Smith DM, Vecchione L, *et al.*** Detection and treatment options for submucous cleft palate: the Pittsburgh experience. Presented at the 64th Annual Meeting of the American Cleft Palate-Craniofacial Association; April 23–28, 2007; Broomfield, CO.
20. **Losee JE, Smith D.** Cleft palate repair. In: Butler CE, ed. *Head and Neck Reconstruction.* Philadelphia, PA: Saunders Elsevier Ltd; 2009.
21. **Musgrave RH.** General aspects of the unilateral cleft lip repair. In: Grabb WC, Rosenstein SW, Bzoch KR, eds. *Cleft Lip and Palate: Surgical, Dental, and Speech Aspects.* Boston, MA: Little, Brown and Company; 1971:175–194.
22. **Kirschner RE, Kaye AE.** Pierre Robin sequence. In: Losee JE, Kirschner RE, eds. *Comprehensive Cleft Care*: New York, NY: McGraw-Hill Medical; 2009:791–802.
23. **LaRossa D.** The state of the art in cleft palate surgery. *Cleft Palate Craniofac J* 2000;37:225–228.
24. **Noorchashm N, Dudas JR, Ford M, *et al.*** Conversion Furlow palatoplasty: salvage of speech after straight-line palatoplasty and "incomplete intravelar veloplasty." *Ann Plast Surg* 2006;56:505–510.
25. **Furlow LT Jr.** Cleft palate repair by double opposing Z-plasty. *Plast Reconstr Surg* 1986;78:724–738.
26. **Hopper RA, Birgfeld CB.** Gingivoperiosteoplasty. In: Losee JE, Kirschner RE, eds. *Comprehensive Cleft Care.* New York, NY: McGraw-Hill Medical; 2009:829–836.
27. **Smith DM, Vecchione L, Jiang S, *et al.*** The Pittsburgh Fistula Classification System: a standardized scheme for the description of palatal fistulas. *Cleft Palate Craniofac J* 2007;44:590–594.

28. **Witt PD.** Velopharyngeal dysfunction. In: Losee JE, Kirschner RE, eds. *Comprehensive Cleft Care.* New York, NY: McGraw-Hill Medical; 2009:627–640.
29. **LaRossa D, Jackson OH, Kirschner RE, *et al.*** The Children's Hospital of Philadelphia modification of the Furlow double-opposing z-palatoplasty: long-term speech and growth results. *Clin Plast Surg* 2004;31:243–249.
30. **Dudas JR, Deleyiannis FWB, Ford MD, Jiang S, Losee JE.** Diagnosis and treatment of velopharyngeal insufficiency. *Ann Plast Surg* 2006;56:511–517.
31. **McWilliams BJ, Phillips BJ.** *Velopharyngeal Incompetence: Audio Seminars in Speech Pathology.* Philadelphia, PA: WB Saunders; 1979.
32. **Forrest CR, Klaiman PM, Mason AC.** Posterior pharyngeal flaps. In: Losee JE, Kirschner RE, eds. *Comprehensive Cleft Care*: New York, NY: McGraw-Hill Medical; 2009:649–664.
33. **Marsh JL.** Sphincter pharyngoplasty. In: Losee JE, Kirschner RE, eds. *Comprehensive Cleft Care.* New York, NY: McGraw-Hill Medical; 2009: 665–671.

CRANIOSYNOSTOSIS 13

Steven R. Cohen, MD; Ryan C. Frank, MD; Hal S. Meltzer, MD and Michael L. Levy, MD, PhD

13.1 Introduction

Craniosynostosis can be defined as the premature fusion of one or more sutures of the skull.[1] When skull sutures fuse prematurely as an isolated event, the process is referred to as *nonsyndromic craniosynostosis*.[2] When skull sutures fuse in conjunction with other anomalies in a clinically recognizable pattern, the process is referred to as *syndromic craniosynostosis*.[1] There have been as many as 90 reported syndromes that are associated with craniosynostosis. The most common of these syndromes are Apert's, Crouzon's, Pfeiffer's, Saethre–Chotzen, and Carpenter's.[1] These syndromes are usually genetic and can be inherited via autosomal dominant, autosomal recessive, or X-linked patterns. Although there are some key distinguishing features for each syndrome, there are many more common traits. These include multiple-suture craniosynostosis, midface retrusion, exorbitism, and limb anomalies.[1]

The etiology of craniosynostosis remains unclear. However, molecular genetic analysis has helped to identify a relationship between the above syndromes and an abnormal gene encoding for fibroblast growth factor.[1,2] There is still debate about the exact relationship between the cranial base synchondroses and the cranial vault sutures. Some argue that the primary issue lies within the cranial base, thus resulting in abnormal fusion in the cranial vault. Others believe that the cranial vault is at fault, which translates into abnormal cranial base and subsequent abnormal facial development.[1–3]

13.2 Functional Issues in Craniosynostosis

Normal craniofacial growth depends on patent sutures between the cranial vault and base bones as well as the presence of a rapidly expanding brain.[1,2] The brain typically triples in size during the first year of life and continues to grow at a high rate until approximately 6 years of age. As the brain grows, it displaces the overlying cranial vault bones which, in turn, grow and remodel. If the cranial vault sutures are fused during this rapid growth phase of the brain, growth and development are unable to occur, and functional issues may develop.[1,2] One of the more significant of these issues is an increased intracranial pressure (ICP). This problem develops as a result of a discrepancy between brain size and cranial vault volume. Clinical symptoms suggesting raised ICP include headaches, irritability, and difficulty sleeping. Clinical signs include papilledema on funduscopy, and *luckenschadel* (beaten metal) appearance of the inner table of the vault as seen in plain radiography and computed tomography (CT).[1,2,4] This abnormal appearance of the inner table of the vault is, however, a late finding. Marchac *et al.* report that up to 42% of children with multiple-suture craniosynostosis will have intracranial hypertension. This is markedly higher than their reported incidence of 13% in those children with single-suture synostosis.[5] The diagnosis of raised ICP is often made clinically, since the signs on CT are often unreliable.[1,2]

Disturbance of vision can accompany multiple-suture synostosis and can manifest by three main mechanisms. The first is a result of exorbitism, which is defined as the displacement of the globe from its normal position due to underdeveloped or abnormally shaped orbits. This is a result of the severe midface and orbital hypoplasia that often occurs within the syndromes. This exorbitism can result in corneal exposure and keratitis, which can in turn lead to infection, pain, ulceration, or even blindness. The second mechanism of visual disturbance is a result of ocular dysmotility secondary to the abnormal shape and size of the orbits and extraocular muscles. This form of disturbance will often present as strabismus or exotropia. The third mechanism relates to the aforementioned raised ICP. Intracranial hypertension can lead to optic atrophy and blindness as a result of diminished vascular perfusion to the retina.[1,2,6]

Another issue that can arise in this patient population is hydrocephalus. The most popular theory explaining it is, that increased venous pressure within the sagittal sinus as a result of craniosynostosis prevents outflow from the sinus. The diminished outflow can result in communicating hydrocephalus or, less commonly, the noncommunicating form. Hydrocephalus can be identified either clinically, with findings similar to those of raised ICP, or radiographically, as enlarged ventricles.[4]

The final functional issue that can develop is neuropsychiatric disturbance.[7] This can present on a spectrum, from mild behavioral abnormality to overt mental retardation. Several studies have demonstrated differing results when it comes to mental retardation associated with craniosynostosis and the role of surgery in preventing this issue. It is generally accepted that the rate of mental dysfunction in children with both syndromic and nonsyndromic craniosynostosis is higher than in the normal population. However, it remains disputed whether the primary cause of this issue is a result of a poorly developed brain or of a calvaria restricting the growth of an otherwise normal brain.[4,7] The former is thought to be more likely in the setting of a single-suture craniosynostosis.[4] It is also important to consider the psychological disturbance that can be involved with having a severely misshapen calvaria.[7]

13.3 Nonsyndromic Craniosynostosis

The major sutures of the cranial vault include the metopic, sagittal, coronal, and lambdoid.[2] "Nonsyndromic craniosynostosis" encompasses fusion of one of these sutures in a sporadic occurrence without any other systemic abnormalities. Assessment of the patient with an abnormal head shape should focus on obtaining a focused history, performing an appropriate physical examination, and acquiring any necessary diagnostic imaging studies. Finally, it should involve consultation with a geneticist, neurosurgeon, and/or ophthalmologist.[2]

Important points to elicit on history include family history of craniosynostosis, as well as signs and symptoms of raised ICP (nausea, headache, irritability). Genetic testing and counseling can help to both establish a diagnosis and inform the parents of current and future issues. Physical examination should involve palpating the cranial vault sutures for ridging and the fontanelles for patency and bulging. Close attention should be paid to the facial and calvarial morphology. The eye and periorbital structures should be evaluated. Jaw size and position, including occlusion, should be noted. Acquiring diagnostic images, including 3-dimensional CTs, continues to be controversial for patients with isolated, single-suture craniosynostosis.[2] It is common practice at our center to obtain a CT with 3-dimensional reconstructions because we feel it is important not only for assessing the underlying brain, but also for aiding in perioperative reconstruction (Figure 13.1).

The plagiocephaly associated with craniosynostosis must be distinguished from the plagiocephaly associated with external, positional factors (positional plagiocephaly).[2,7] That deformity is the result of external pressure on the developing skull, either in utero or in early

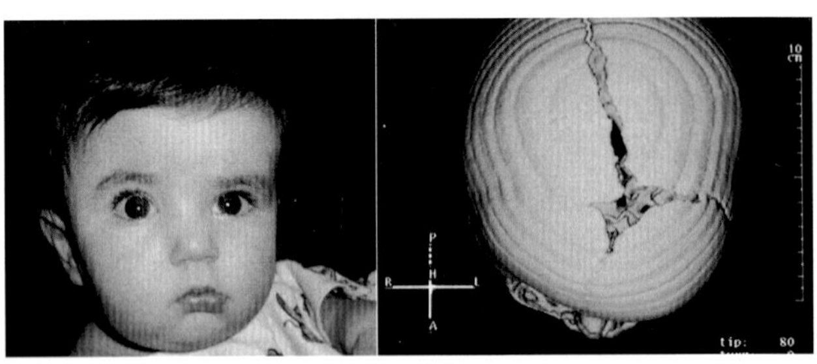

(A) (B)

Figure 13.1. (A) Photograph of a child with right unicoronal craniosynostosis. (B) 3-dimensional CT image of the same child. Notice the patent anterior fontanelle and left unicoronal suture, along with the fused right unicoronal suture.

infancy, leading to an abnormal head shape that often mimics craniosynostosis. This distinction is important because, although operative intervention is the standard of care for most moderate to severe craniosynostotic deformities, nonoperative helmet-molding therapy is typically used for most positional deformities. The distinction between these two entities can usually be made during the physical examination. Signs of positional plagiocephaly include absent cranial suture ridging, patent fontanelles, and the parallelogram head deformity, which is characterized by ipsilateral occipital flattening and frontal bossing with an anteriorly displaced ear.[2,7]

13.3.1 *Types of synostosis*

Listed below are the major types of cranial vault synostoses and their associated characteristics.

13.3.1.1 *Sagittal synostosis*

Affected suture: Sagittal

Resulting deformity: Scaphocephaly

Incidence: 1 in 2,000 (40% of all nonsyndromic craniosynostosis)

Epidemiology: Sporadic, male:female of 4:1

Physical examination: Palpable midline ridge with narrowing of the skull in a biparietal and bitemporal dimension. Frontal and occipital bossing are also present.[2,7]

13.3.1.2 *Metopic synostosis*

Affected suture: Metopic

Resulting deformity: Trigonocephaly

Incidence: 1 in 2,500 to 15,000 (10–20%; recent studies have shown an increase of metopic synostosis up to 40% of all nonsyndromic craniosynostosis)

Epidemiology: Sporadic, male:female of 3:1

Physical examination: Can present on a spectrum of deformities ranging from a palpable mid-forehead ridge to a severely pointed forehead associated with bitemporal narrowing, biparietal flaring, and hypotelorism.[2,7]

13.3.1.3 *Unicoronal synostosis*

Affected suture: Coronal

Resulting deformity: Anterior plagiocephaly

Incidence: 1 in 10,000 (20% of all nonsyndromic craniosynostosis)

Epidemiology: Sporadic, female:male of 3:2

Physical examination: Ipsilaterally, there is widening of the palpebral fissure, elevation and anterior displacement of the ear, nasal root deviation to the affected side, a prominent malar eminence, and an elevated and recessed supraorbital bar. Contralaterally, there is frontal bossing and the chin is usually deviated to the unaffected side.

Imaging: The harlequin orbit is present due to a lack of descent of the greater wing of the sphenoid. This deformity consists of loss of lateral orbital height with an elevated and recessed supraorbital bar.[2,7]

13.3.1.4 *Bicoronal synostosis*

Affected suture: Coronal
Resulting deformity: Turribrachycephaly

Incidence: 1 in 10,000 (20% of all nonsyndromic craniosynostosis)

Epidemiology: Sporadic, male:female of 1:1

Physical examination: The skull is typically shortened in an anterior/posterior dimension. There tends to be a widened forehead with hypoplastic supraorbital rims.[1,2,7]

13.3.1.5 *Lambdoid synostosis*

Affected suture: Lambdoid

Resulting deformity: Posterior plagiocephaly

Incidence: Rare, less than 3% of all nonsyndromic craniosynostosis

Epidemiology: Sporadic, male:female of 2:1

Physical examination: Ipsilaterally, there is occipital flattening and an occipitomastoid boss, and the ear is displaced inferiorly and posteriorly. Contralaterally, there is a parietal and occipital boss as well as an occipitofrontal boss.[2,7]

13.3.2 *Surgical treatment strategies*

Many variables go into the decision-making process regarding the type of surgical intervention for nonsyndromic craniosynostosis. They include the age of the patient, the location and degree of the deformity, the overall health of the patient, and the potential need for repeat surgery.[7–9] Generally speaking, limited (endoscopic, linear craniectomy) approaches are typically reserved for properly selected younger patients (less than 6 months old) with mild deformities affecting only one suture.[10] These procedures rely on the growth of the underlying brain to aid in vault reshaping and often employ postoperative helmet-molding therapy to facilitate appropriate changes.[10] The larger, more invasive approaches (open cranial vault remodeling with fronto-orbital advancement) are usually used for older children (older than 6 months) who have more severe deformities affecting one or more sutures.[11] The open procedures often involve removal of the affected bones, with osteotomies and adjustments of those bones performed on a side table in the operating room. These remodeled bones are then placed back onto the exposed dura in a more anatomic position and stabilized in place using a number of different methods (suture, wire, plates, screws).[11] The modern trend of fixation involves resorbable plating systems that are beneficial in that they (1) do not need to be removed since they are resorbed over time and (2) are less likely than titanium plates to interfere with facial growth. The main features of any operation for craniosynostosis include (1) releasing of the fused sutures, and (2) remodeling the hypoplastic and compensatory abnormalities of the craniofacial skeleton.[11]

It is generally agreed that in cases where functional issues are present (raised ICP, globe exposure), early intervention is the standard of care.[5,8,12–15] In the absence of these functional issues, advocates of early surgery believe that a better, more naturally shaped skull can be obtained by reshaping the vault during early infancy, when the brain is in its most rapid-growth phase.[8,15] Advocates of delayed surgery believe that the risk of blood loss and other complications is greater in early infancy, and that the deformity is more likely to recur if dealt with too early.[6,14] Another consideration regarding the timing of operative intervention has to do with bone formation and development. Early in infancy, bone is very malleable and easier to remodel than it is beyond 1 year of age. The surrounding soft tissue of the infant cranium is also very osteogenic and permits the surgeon the flexibility of not having to fill in all bony gaps. These factors can lead to a technically easier surgery and perhaps a better result.[12–14]

The most important preoperative consideration for most skull-altering procedures involves dealing with blood loss. All patients must have blood products prepared preoperatively in case of significant loss during surgery.[16–18] Optimization of medical comorbid conditions is critical, with appropriate consultations made well before the planned surgery.[1,2]

Choice of patient positioning intraoperatively involves providing the most complete access to the involved portions of the skull. The most common incision is the bicoronal incision. It is typically created in a zigzag fashion to help hide its appearance within the hair, especially in the temporal regions.[19,20]

Air embolism is a concern whenever the head is in a position above the heart. Cardiac Doppler monitoring as well as end-tidal carbon dioxide measurement are useful tools for detecting air entering the blood stream during large craniofacial operations.[2,20]

There are several different approaches to the various deformities in craniosynostosis. Outlined below is our center's approach to each form of nonsyndromic craniosynostosis.

13.3.2.1 *Sagittal synostosis*

Endoscopic linear craniectomy of the fused sagittal suture is performed in those children presenting early (less than 3 months of age) with a mild to moderate deformity.[11,21,22] Our goal is to release the fused suture at around 3 months of age, followed by placement of the child into helmet-molding therapy by 1 week postoperatively (Figures 13.2–13.8).

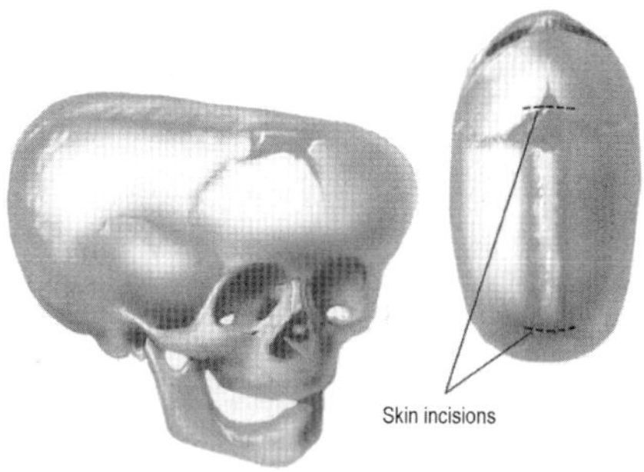

Figure 13.2. Planned endoscopic cranial vault remodeling for sagittal craniosynostosis. Skin incisions are made anterior and posterior to the fused suture. Reprinted with permission from Wolters Kluwer Health (Ref. 10). Copyright © 2002 by Mutaz B. Habal, MD.

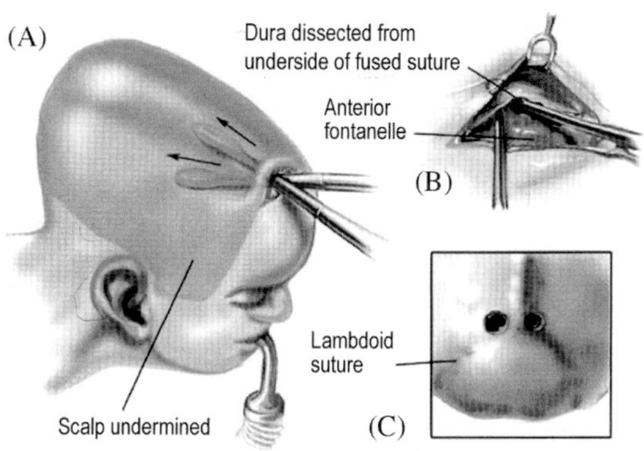

Figure 13.3. (A) Dissection is first performed in the subgaleal plane superficially. (B) The dura is then carefully dissected from the overlying calvarial bone, using the anterior fontanelle as the port of access. (C) Bur holes are drilled posterior to the fused suture. Dissection of the dura posteriorly is then performed through these access ports. Reprinted with permission from Wolters Kluwer Health (Ref. 10). Copyright © 2002 by Mutaz B. Habal, MD.

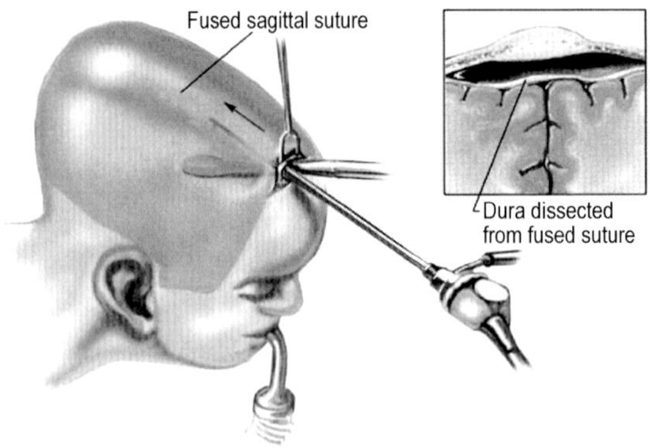

Figure 13.4. The endoscope is introduced to assist in careful dissection of the dura from the overlying fused suture. Reprinted with permission from Wolters Kluwer Health (Ref. 10). Copyright © 2002 by Mutaz B. Habal, MD.

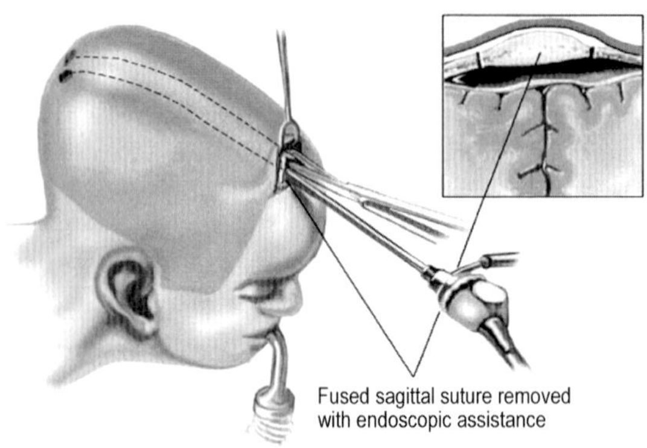

Figure 13.5. The endoscope is then used to assist in careful osteotomy of the calvaria on either side of the fused suture. Reprinted with permission from Wolters Kluwer Health (Ref. 10). Copyright © 2002 by Mutaz B. Habal, MD.

For those children with severe deformities or those who present late (beyond 4–6 months of age), either a one-stage or a two-stage open cranial vault remodeling is performed. Two-stage procedures are reserved for those patients with severe deformities affecting the posterior skull and in whom the risk of blood loss is greater. Major attention intraoperatively is paid to addressing the diminished width of the skull in the biparietal region as well as the bossed frontal and occipital regions[23] (Figure 13.9).

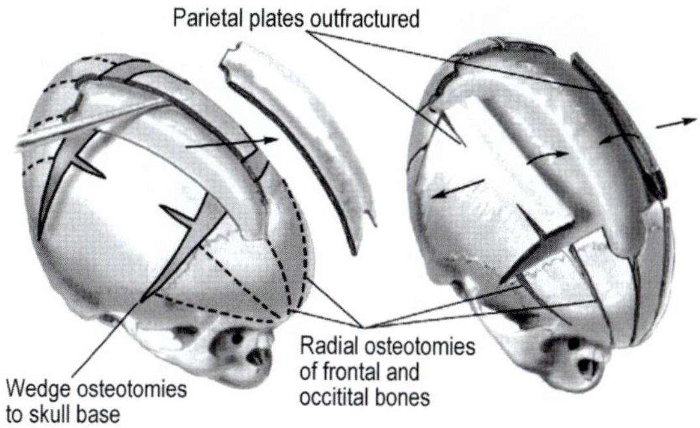

Figure 13.6. For more severe deformities, radial and wedge osteotomies can be performed to further reduce the scaphocephalic head shape. Reprinted with permission from Wolters Kluwer Health (Ref. 10). Copyright © 2002 by Mutaz B. Habal, MD.

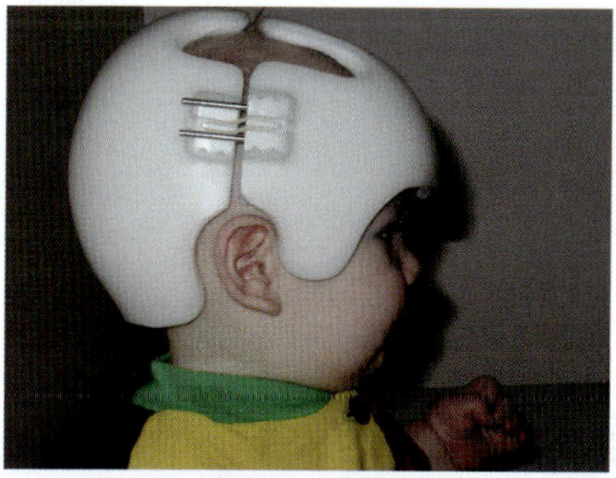

Figure 13.7. Lateral view of a molding helmet used in the postoperative phase after endoscopic sagittal cranial vault reshaping.

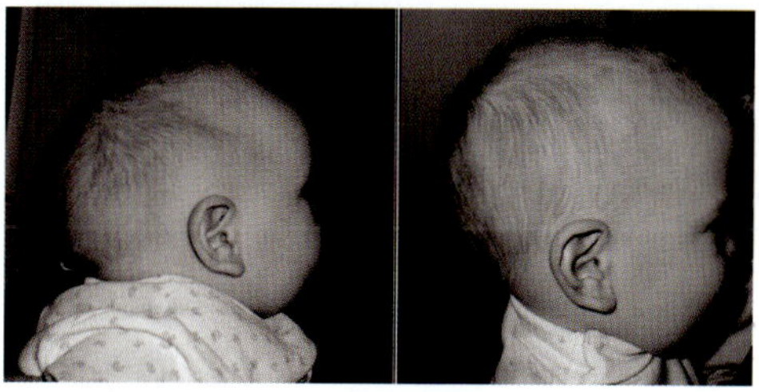

(A) (B)

Figure 13.8. (A) Preoperative view of a 3-month-old child with sagittal craniosynostosis. (B) Three-month postoperative view of the same child (6 months old) after endoscopic cranial vault reshaping, followed by helmet-molding therapy. Panel A reprinted with permission from Wolters Kluwer Health (Ref. 10). Copyright © 2002 by Mutaz B. Habal, MD.

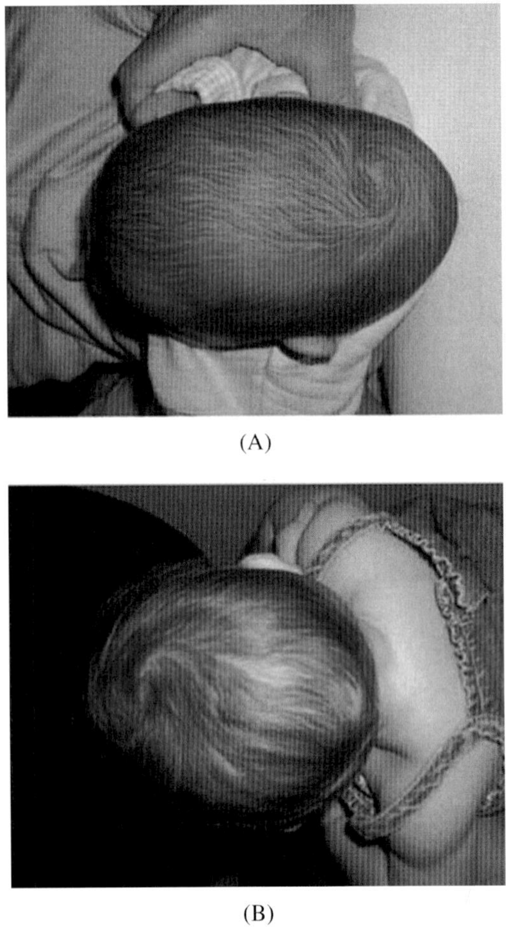

Figure 13.9. (A) Preoperative photograph of a 4-month-old child with sagittal synostosis and severe scaphocephaly. (B) Six months after endoscopic cranial reconstruction and 4 months of helmet therapy.

13.3.2.2 *Metopic synostosis*

Open cranial vault remodeling with fronto-orbital advancement is performed for those patients with moderate to severe deformities (Figure 13.10).[24–26] The fronto-orbital advancement component of the procedure is usually deferred in those children with mild deformities (those with an unaffected supraorbital bar). The preferred age to

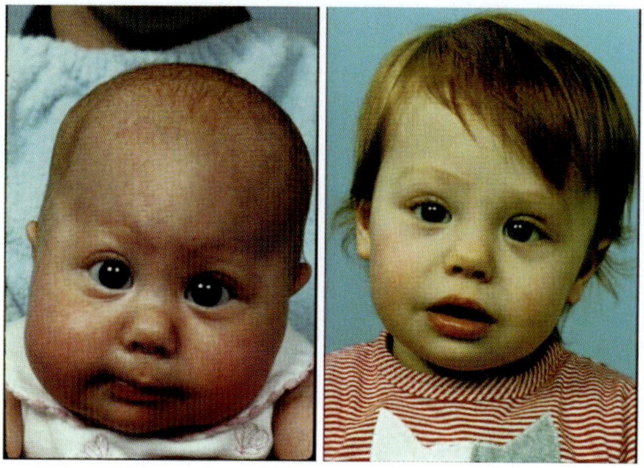

(A) (B)

Figure 13.10. (A) Six-month-old female infant with metopic synostosis. Preoperative photograph. Note the trigonocephalic shape of the skull. (B) Two years after fronto-orbital remodeling and cranial reshaping of 1-month-old female with metopic synostosis.

treat these patients is from 6 to 9 months because it is thought that this age represents the optimal balance between bone malleability and the diminished operative risk involved with major cranial vault surgery. The aim is to expand the pinched bitemporal region and to advance the supraorbital bar that often accompanies this deformity. The supraorbital bar is also widened in cases of hypotelorism.[24,25]

13.3.2.3 *Unicoronal synostosis*

Open cranial vault remodeling with fronto-orbital advancement is performed for those patients with moderate to severe deformities (Figure 13.11). This procedure is typically performed at around 6 to 9 months of age. The goals of operative intervention include advancement of the retruded supraorbital bar with remodeling of the contralateral bossed forehead.[27,28]

13.3.2.4 *Bicoronal synostosis*

Open cranial vault remodeling with fronto-orbital advancement from 6 to 9 months of age is the procedure of choice for this population.

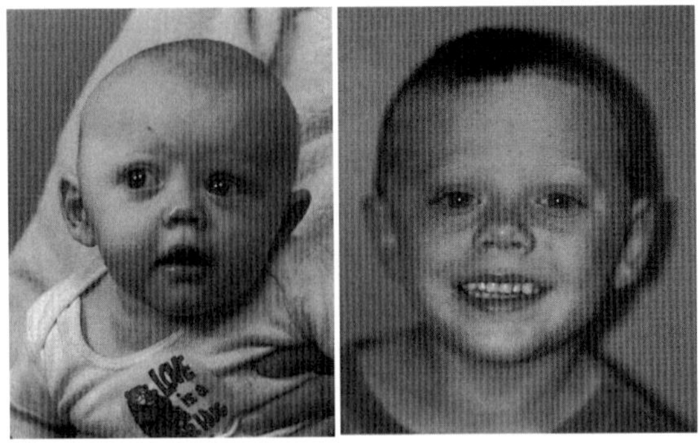

Figure 13.11. (A) Six-month-old male infant with right unicoronal synostosis. (B) Five years after fronto-orbital advancement for right unicoronal synostosis.

Supraorbital bar advancement with forehead vertical reduction is key in addressing this deformity.[27–29]

13.3.2.5 *Lambdoid synostosis*

Open cranial vault remodeling at 6 to 9 months of age is the preferred treatment. The affected bone posteriorly is removed and expanded before being replaced and secured.[30]

Postoperatively, it is important to ensure that the patient remains hemodynamically stable, with adequate hemoglobin. Monitoring is often done in either an ICU setting or a unit specialized in critical care.[18]

13.4 Syndromic Craniosynostosis

When skull suture(s) fuse in conjunction with other anomalies in a clinically recognizable pattern, the process is referred to as *syndromic craniosynostosis.* There have been as many as 90 reported syndromes that are associated with craniosynostosis. The most common are Crouzon's, Apert's, Pfeiffer's, Saethre–Chotzen, and Carpenter's.[1]

13.4.1 *Description of syndromes*

13.4.1.1 *Crouzon's syndrome*

This syndrome was initially described in 1912 by a French neurosurgeon, Octave Crouzon. At that time, he characterized four essential elements of the syndrome: exorbitism, retromaxillism, inframaxillism, and paradoxical retrogenia. Today, it is recognized that there are many variations of the syndrome, and that not all key elements are present in every case.[1]

Crouzon's syndrome is inherited in an autosomal dominant fashion and is present in approximately 1 in 25,000 births.[1]

The typical craniofacial deformities in this syndrome include frontal bone recession, midface retrusion, exorbitism, and craniosynostosis usually involving multiple sutures. The most common form of craniosynostosis associated with this syndrome is bicoronal suture fusion; however, sagittal, metopic, and pansutural synostosis patterns have all been observed. These patients often have normal intelligence, and limb anomalies are typically absent.[1]

13.4.1.2 *Apert's syndrome*

This syndrome was first described in 1906 by Apert as a collection of deformities that included craniosynostosis, exorbitism, midface retrusion, and symmetric syndactyly involving hands and feet.[1]

Apert's syndrome is typically sporadic, although it has occasionally been found in an autosomal dominant inheritance pattern. The incidence of this syndrome is estimated to be approximately 1 in 160,000.[1]

Turribrachycephaly (elongation of the skull in the transverse and foreshortened anterior–posterior dimensions) resulting from fused bicoronal sutures is the most common form of synostosis in this syndrome. In addition to frontal and midface hypoplasia with associated exorbitism, hypertelorism and downslanting palpebral fissures are usually present. Symmetric hand syndactyly typically involves a middigital hand mass fusion of the second, third, and fourth fingers. A similar pattern is usually seen involving the toes bilaterally. Mental

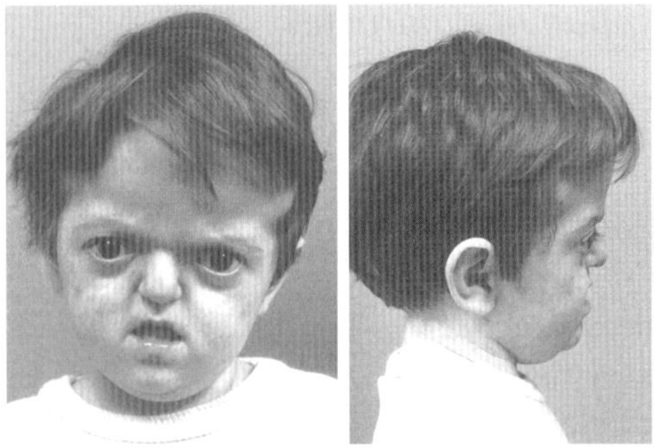

(A) (B)

Figure 13.12. Photograph of a 3-year-old boy with Apert's syndrome. Notice the significant midface retrusion. Reprinted from *Seminars in Orthodontics* (Cohen SR. Midface distraction. Semin Orthod 1999;5:52–58). Copyright © 1999 with permission from Elsevier.

retardation is commonly associated with Apert's syndrome; however, many patients still develop normal intelligence[1] (Figure 13.12).

13.4.1.3 *Pfeiffer's syndrome*

This syndrome was originally described by Pfeiffer in 1964 as a collection of deformities that included craniosynostosis, midface hypoplasia, broad thumbs, and broad great toes.[1]

Pfeiffer's syndrome is inherited in an autosomal dominant pattern.[1]

The midface deformities in Pfeiffer's syndrome are very similar to those in Apert's syndrome; however, the craniosynostosis is usually not as severe. The key distinguishing features of this syndrome are the broad thumbs and broad great toes. Partial syndactyly of both hand and foot digits 2 and 3 may be present.[1]

13.4.1.4 *Saethre–Chotzen syndrome*

This syndrome was first described by Saethre and Chotzen in 1931 and 1932, respectively.[1] Common craniofacial features include turribrachycephaly, low-set frontal hairline, and eyelid ptosis.[1]

Saethre–Chotzen syndrome is inherited in an autosomal dominant fashion, but has wide variability in expression.[1]

This syndrome was referred to by Tessier as "upper Apert" because the midface is often normally developed while the cranial vault is turribrachycephalic and the supraorbital rim is recessed. The low-set hairline is a constant feature. Intelligence is often normal. Short stature and partial finger and toe syndactyly of digits 2 and 3 is commonly observed.[1]

13.4.1.5 *Carpenter's syndrome*

This syndrome was first described by Carpenter in 1901 as a collection of deformities that included variable craniosynostosis, partial syndactyly of the digits, preaxial polydactyly, congenital heart disease, hypogenitalism, and obesity.[1]

Carpenter's syndrome is inherited in an autosomal recessive pattern and is very rare.[1]

The craniosynostosis pattern in this syndrome is often variable, resulting in asymmetric head shape. Midface retrusion tends to be minimal. Low-set ears and lateral displacement of the medial canthi are typical features. Up to 75% of patients will have some degree of mental retardation.[1]

13.4.2 *Surgical treatment approaches*

13.4.2.1 *General approach*

There has been a significant evolution in the treatment of syndromic craniosynostosis since the early 1900s. Initially, treatment was aimed at minimizing functional compromise of the premature skull fusion. This was accomplished by performing linear craniectomies and fragmentation of components of the cranial vault. Although successful brain decompression was obtained with these procedures, it was temporary, and the remaining deformity was still significant, often requiring further reconstructive surgery.[31–34] Dr. Paul Tessier, in 1967, described the first intracranial cranial vault and midface reconstruction that completely altered the method of craniosynostosis treatment.[33] Today, his treatment principles are widely accepted as the standard of care for these patients.

Surgical care of the patient with syndromic craniosynostosis can begin shortly after birth. Airway patency must be assessed immediately, as some patients will have severe midface retrusion resulting in an unstable airway. Failing the ability to secure a stable airway with nonsurgical methods (prone positioning, nasal pharyngeal airway, supplemental oxygen), tracheostomy must be considered. Globe protection must be ensured. Severe exorbitism may result in corneal exposure and keratitis, and this must be prevented at all costs. Simple methods including lubrication and/or taping may be considered in cases with mild deformity, but surgical tarsorrhaphy must be performed early if the cornea is unprotected. Rarely, early fronto-orbital advancement or monobloc osteotomies with distraction osteogenesis may be required. If the child cannot obtain enough calories through oral feeding, placement of a gastrostomy tube should be considered. Consultation with a nutritionist and general surgeon should be done if this issue is present. Finally, the newborn should be worked up for any other associated congenital defects. Heart, lung, renal, and other vital organ deficiencies need to be detected early, and appropriate management undertaken.[1,31–34]

The next phase of potential surgical intervention typically occurs in early infancy. The main issues to monitor for in the first few months of life include increased ICP and hydrocephalus. Clinical and radiologic suspicion of raised ICP will warrant early cranial vault expansion. Radiologic evidence of hydrocephalus may require ventriculoperitoneal shunting. Early neurosurgical consultation should be performed in all patients to ensure that these issues are dealt with early and appropriately.[1,31,32,34]

If the cranial vault deformity is severe, reconstruction can be staged. The posterior cranial vault is often dealt with first in these severe cases at around 6 months of age. At this time, a posterior cranial vault expansion with a posterior skull reduction is performed. At 9 to 15 months of age, the anterior cranial vault is reshaped and fronto-orbital advancement is performed. The more advanced age within this window is preferred for two main reasons. First, by 9 months and beyond, the bone has ossified enough such that manipulation is significantly easier. Second, delaying the anterior reconstruction potentially and theoretically will lead to diminished relapse of deformity. In the setting of raised ICP or other functional issues, earlier remodeling must be considered.[1,31,33,34]

Repeat cranial vault expansion may need to be considered around 2 to 3 years of age if the deformity has significantly recurred. In the 4- to 7-year-old, this may be performed as a monobloc-type procedure if significant midface retrusion is present in association with supraorbital deficiency. Large full-thickness cranial defects should be filled in with autogenous bone and, rarely, alloplastic material at this time, to ensure sufficient brain protection.[35,36]

Early Le Fort III and monobloc should be considered for those patients around 3 years of age who have severe obstructive sleep apnea or significant lack of globe protection. This procedure is preferably delayed till 5 to 9 years of age in the absence of these issues because recurrence of the deformity is likely to recur. The Le Fort III procedure addresses the midface retrusion by advancing the entire midface, including maxillae, zygomas, and nasal bones. The monobloc procedure advances the supraorbital rims as well as the entire Le Fort III segment. Monobloc procedures combined with distraction osteogenesis have significantly reduced the previously high morbidity seen with monobloc advancement alone. When the monobloc is combined with distraction, extradural dead space in continuity with the paranasal sinuses is avoided, reducing the infection rate.[1,19,20]

Further surgical intervention can then often be delayed until skeletal maturity. Orthognathic surgery, rhinoplasty, and mild calvarial contour irregularities can be dealt with at this time.[1,19,20]

13.4.2.2 *Surgical procedures*

Many different types of surgical procedures have been described for the treatment of a child with syndromic craniosynostosis.

13.4.2.2.1 *Posterior cranial vault expansion*

Indication: Posterior cranial flatness or turribrachycephaly with or without lamdoidal synostosis; early (nonshuntable) raised ICP.[19]

Timing: Age from 2 to 6 months

Goal: (1) To increase cranial vault capacity. (2) To delay need for definitive anterior cranial vault remodeling.[19]

Limitations: The bone is typically very poorly ossified at this age, rendering the chance of bony healing to be minimal and the ability to achieve a stable reconstruction to be very difficult.

Perioperative considerations: Type and crossmatch for potential blood loss is extremely important. 3-dimensional CT is often very helpful for operative planning.[19]

13.4.2.2.2 *Fronto-orbital advancement, with cranial vault reshaping*

Indication: Turribrachycephaly

Timing: Age from 9 to 18 months

Goal: (1) To decompress the anterior cranial vault. (2) To reshape the cranial vault and properly advance the frontal bone into a more anatomic position. (3) To provide the globe with improved superior protection.

Limitations: If the deformity is extremely severe, it may be very difficult to sufficiently advance the fronto-orbital bar without compromising the ability to close the bicoronal incision.

Perioperative considerations: Ensure type and crossmatch have been performed. 3-dimensional CT is helpful for intraoperative planning. Perform an eye examination, clearly documenting eye movements. This is important for postoperative comparison.[19]

13.4.2.2.3 *Monobloc and facial bipartition*

Indication: Supra- and infraorbital retrusion with or without midfacial flatness and hypertelorbitism

Timing: Age from 5 to 9 years

Goal: (1) To advance the recessed supraorbital bone into a more protective, anatomic position. (2) To advance the retruded midface to improve occlusion and to provide increased globe protection. (3) To improve the aesthetics of the upper and middle third of the face.[19]

Limitations: Within the last 15 years, distraction osteogenesis has been applied to the advancement of craniofacial bones. Applied specifically to the monobloc, distraction osteogenesis enables surgeons to advance the upper and midface structures gradually, while stretching out the enveloping soft tissue without producing a large retrofrontal dead space. Benefits of performing the monobloc procedure in this fashion include increased advancement distances, shorter operative times, less blood loss, and decreased risk of infection. The facial bipartition component of this procedure involves medializing the orbits by resecting excess midline bone, followed by mobilization of the orbits in a midline direction (Figure 13.13).

Perioperative considerations: Ensure type and crossmatch have been performed. 3-dimensionsal CT is used for intraoperative planning. Perform an eye examination, clearly documenting eye movements. This is important for postoperative comparison.[19]

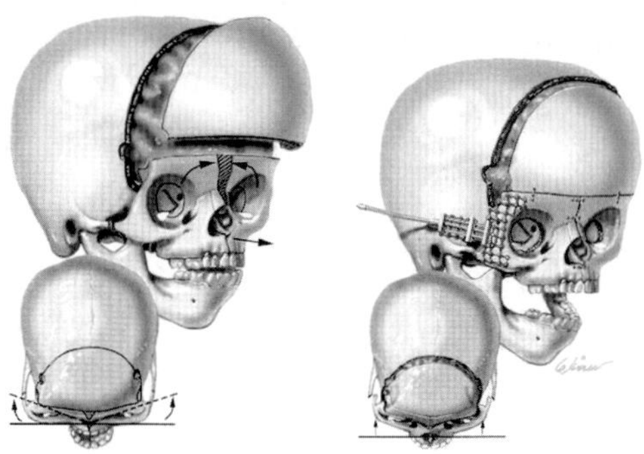

(A) (B)

Figure 13.13. Monobloc with facial bipartition. (A) The middle and upper thirds of the face are advanced simultaneously once the orbits have been osteotomized and medialized. (B) Internal distractors, used to advance the monobloc segment gradually, are illustrated. Reprinted from *Seminars in Orthodontics* (Cohen SR. Midface distraction. *Semin Orthod* 1999;5:52–58). Copyright © 1999 with permission from Elsevier.

13.4.2.2.4 *Le Fort III*

Indication: Midface retrusion

Timing: Early (2–3 years of age); delayed (5–9 years of age); may be done in adolescence

Goal: (1) To advance the retruded midface to improve occlusion and provide increased globe protection. (2) To improve the aesthetics of the midface.

Limitations: There are currently two schools of thought regarding the timing of this procedure. Advocates of early (2–3 years of age) advancement believe improved self-esteem can be gained, although accepting the likely need for repeat advancement once the child has reached skeletal maturity. In situations where severe apnea or globe exposures are present, early advancement is the accepted standard of care. Advocates of delayed advancement (beyond skeletal maturity) believe the risk of recurrent deformity is too great in those treated early and would prefer to wait until cessation of growth has occurred before undertaking this large operation. Distraction osteogenesis has been applied to this operation as well, with great success. This topic is discussed in detail in Chapters 7 and 8 of this handbook.

Perioperative considerations: Ensure type and crossmatch have been performed. 3-dimensional CT is helpful for intraoperative planning. Perform an eye examination, clearly documenting eye movements. This is important for postoperative comparison.[19]

13.4.2.2.5 *Orthognathic surgery*

Indication: Severe Angle class III malocclusion that cannot be corrected with orthodontics alone

Timing: Skeletal maturity

Goal: To improve maloccusion

Limitations: Operative intervention to improve occlusion is best performed beyond skeletal maturity. This is to prevent disruption of both maxillary and mandibular growth, as well as to avoid relapse of the deformity, requiring further operative intervention. Several orthognathic procedures have been developed to address the various occlusal deformities, and these are described in Chapter 5 of this book.

Perioperative considerations: Cephalometric analysis and dental model construction are essential to obtain normal occlusion.[19]

13.4.2.2.6 *Final facial contouring*

Indication: Residual deformities that are present once all osteotomies have been performed and the child has ceased to grow.

Timing: Beyond skeletal maturity

Goal: To improve craniofacial aesthetics

Limitations: Despite the fact that most patients with syndromic craniosynostosis will never look "normal," many procedures, including rhinoplasty, scar revision, and contour revision can be performed once the child has completed growth, to improve the overall aesthetics.

Perioperative considerations: It is important to ensure that both patient and parents have realistic and obtainable goals before opting to pursue further "touch-up" procedures.[19]

13.5 Complications

Early complications include blood loss, infection, seroma, dural tears, air embolus, and respiratory complications. It has been stressed throughout this chapter that proper planning for blood loss is performed and strategies are employed to deal with this issue. Infants undergoing large procedures are at a significant risk for detrimental blood loss, and strategies to counter this loss include intraoperative procoagulant materials and methods, and donor blood infusion. Infection is rare, owing to the extremely well-vascularized scalp. Perioperative antibiotics are given at some centers to help prevent this complication. Dural tears can occur and need to be dealt with promptly. Intraoperatively, the tear should be treated with suture and/or patch. If discovered postoperatively, observation or insertion of a lumbar drain may be most appropriate, depending on the severity and the rate of recovery. Air embolus may occur in any intraoperative position and can result in severe hemodynamic instability. Monitoring is best performed with precordial Doppler and end-tidal carbon dioxide measurement. Management of a patient with an air embolus involves fluid resuscitation and air evacuation with the help of a central venous line. Airway compromise may occur secondary to soft-tissue swelling or tube disruption during advancement procedures. It is crucial to ensure airway patency before extubation, either in the operating room, or in an ICU setting.[19,32,35]

Late complications include bony defects, contour irregularities, and recurrence of deformity. Children older than 1 year will typically be unable to fill in bony defects, as their surrounding soft tissue is less osteogenic than that of younger children. Defects of greater than 2 cm will typically require some form of filling material (autogenous calvarial bone graft, which is preferred to alloplastic). Contour irregularities can be dealt with by using a mechanical bur and/or a calcium phosphate cement material once the child's skull shape has stabilized. This is usually performed around age 4 to 5 years. Deformity recurrence is often unpredictable but is more commonly seen in those children with severe deformities. Repeat advancements or reshapings are sometimes required to deal with these deformities, depending on their severity.[19,32,35]

References

1. **Bartlett S.** Craniosynostosis syndromes. In: Thorne CH, Beasley RW, Aston SJ, Bartlett SP, Gurtner GC, Spear SL, eds. *Grabb and Smith's Plastic Surgery.* 6th edn. Philadelphia, PA: Lippincott Williams & Wilkins; 2007:237–247.
2. **Shin J, Persing JA.** Nonsyndromic craniosynostosis and deformational plagiocephaly. In: Thorne CH, Beasley RW, Aston SJ, Bartlett SP, Gurtner GC, Spear SL, eds. *Grabb and Smith's Plastic Surgery.* 6th edn. Philadelphia, PA: Lippincott Williams & Wilkins; 2007:226–236.
3. **Virchow R.** Uber den cretinismus, namentlich in Franken, und uber pathologiside Schadeelformen. *Verh Phys Med Gesamle Wurzburg* 1851;2:230–256.
4. **Noetzel MJ, Marsh JL, Palkes H, Gado M.** Hydrocephalus and mental retardation in craniosynostosis. *J Pediatr* 1985;107:885–892.
5. **Marchac D, Renier D, Broumand S.** Timing of treatment for craniosynostosis and facio-craniosynostosis: a 20-year experience. *Br J Plast Surg* 1994;47:211–222.

6. **Harrop CW, Avery BS, Marks SM, Putnam GD.** Craniosynostosis in babies: complications and management of 40 cases. *Br J Oral Maxillofac Surg* 1996;34: 158–161.
7. **Pertschuk MJ, Whitaker LA.** Psychosocial considerations in craniofacial deformity. *Clin Plast Surg* 1987;14:163–168.
8. **Whitaker LA, Bartlett SP, Schut L, Bruce D.** Craniosynostosis: an analysis of the timing, treatment, and complications in 164 consecutive patients. *Plast Reconstr Surg* 1987;80:195–212.
9. **Williams JK, Cohen SR, Burstein FD, Hudgins R, Boydston W, Simms C.** A longitudinal, statistical study of reoperation rates in craniosynostosis. *Plast Reconstr Surg* 1997;100:305–310.
10. **Cohen SR, Holmes RE, Meltzer HS, Nakaji P.** Immediate cranial vault reconstruction with bioresorbable plates after endoscopically assisted sagittal synostectomy. *J Craniofac Surg* 2002;13:578–584.
11. **Persing JA.** MOC-PS(SM) CME article: Management considerations in the treatment of craniosynostosis. *Plast Reconstr Surg* 2008;121(Suppl):1–11.
12. **Jimenez DF, Barone CM, Cartwright CC, Baker L.** Early management of craniosynostosis using endoscopic-assisted strip craniectomies and cranial orthotic molding therapy. *Pediatrics* 2002;110:97–104.
13. **Jane JA, Edgerton MT, Futrell JW, Park TS.** Immediate correction of sagittal synostosis. *J Neurosurgery* 1978;49:705–710.
14. **di Rocco C, Marchese E, Velardi F.** Craniosynostosis: surgical treatment during the first year of life. *J Neurosurg Sci* 1992;36:129–137.
15. **Barone CM, Jimenez DF.** Endoscopic craniectomy for early correction of craniosynostosis. *Plast Reconstr Surg* 1999;104:1965–1975.
16. **Meyer P, Renier D, Arnaud E, *et al.*** Blood loss during repair of craniosynostosis. *Br J Anaesth* 1993;71:854–857.
17. **Hentschel S, Steinbok P, Cochrane DD, Kestle J.** Reduction of transfusion rates in the surgical correction of sagittal synostosis. *J Neurosurgery* 2002;97: 503–509.
18. **Eaton AC, Marsh JL, Pilgram TK.** Transfusion requirements for craniosynostosis surgery in infants. *Plast Reconstr Surg* 1995;95:277–283.
19. **Hopper R.** MOC advanced craniofacial surgery lecture. Presented at the meeting of the American Society of Plastic Surgeons; October 2009; Seattle, WA.
20. **Hunt J, Flood J.** Craniofacial anomalies II: syndromes and surgery. *Selected Readings in Plastic Surgery* 2002;9:1–67.
21. **Greene CS Jr, Winston KR.** Treatment of scaphocephaly with sagittal craniectomy and biparietal morcellation. *Neurosurgery* 1988;23:196–202.

22. **Vicari F.** Endoscopic correction of sagittal craniosynostosis. Presented at the American Society of Plastic and Reconstructive Surgeons Presymposium; 1994; San Diego, CA.
23. **Albright AL.** Operative normalization of skull shape in sagittal synostosis. *Neurosurgery* 1985;17:329–331.
24. **Anderson FM.** Treatment of coronal and metopic synostosis: 107 cases. *Neurosurgery* 1981;8:143–149.
25. **Shaffrey ME, Persing JA, Delashaw JB, Shaffrey CI, Jane JA.** Surgical treatment of metopic synostosis. *Neurosurg Clin N Am* 1991;2:621–627.
26. **Cohen SR, Maher H, Wagner JD, Dauser RC, Newman MH, Muraszko KM.** Metopic synostosis: evaluation of aesthetic results. *Plast Reconstr Surg* 1994;94:759–767.
27. **Mohr G, Hoffman HJ, Munro IR, Hendrick EB, Humphreys RP.** Surgical management of unilateral and bilateral coronal craniosynostosis: 21 years of experience. *Neurosurgery* 1978;2:83–92.
28. **Jane JA, Park TS, Zide BM, Lambruschi P, Persing JA, Edgerton MT.** Alternative techniques in the treatment of unilateral coronal synostosis. *J Neurosurg* 1984;61:550–556.
29. **Persing JA, Jane JA, Delashaw JB.** Treatment of bilateral coronal synostosis in infancy: a holistic approach. *J Neurosurg* 1990;72:171–175.
30. **Jimenez DF, Barone CM.** The Sunrise Technique: the correction of occipital plagiocephaly using bandeau occipital plate and radial osteotomies. *Pediatr Neurosurg* 1995;22:162–166.
31. **Whitaker LA, Bartlett SP.** The craniofacial dysostoses: guidelines for management of the symmetric and asymmetric deformities. *Clin Plast Surg* 1987;14:73–81.
32. **Posnick JC.** The craniofacial dysostosis syndromes: current reconstructive strategies. *Clin Plast Surg* 1994;21:585–598.
33. **McCarthy JG, Glasberg SB, Cutting CB, *et al.*** Twenty-year experience with early surgery for craniosynostosis. II. The craniofacial synostosis syndromes and pansynostosis — results and unsolved problems. *Plast Reconstr Surg* 1995;96:284–298.
34. **Cohen SR, Kawamoto HK Jr, Burstein F, Peacock WJ.** Advancement-onlay: an improved technique of fronto-orbital remodeling in craniosynostosis. *Childs Nerv Syst* 1991;7:264–271.
35. **Wall SA, Goldin JH, Hockley AD, Wake MJ, Poole MD, Briggs M.** Fronto-orbital re-operation in craniosynostosis. *Br J Plast Surg* 1994;47:180–184.
36. **Prevot M, Renier D, Marchac D.** Lack of ossification after cranioplasty for craniosynostosis: a review of relevant factors in 592 consecutive patients. *J Craniofac Surg* 1993;4:247–256.

MICROTIA 14

James A. Lehman, Jr., MD

14.1 Definition

Microtia is defined as a severe hypoplasia of the external ear with a constricted, blind, or absent auditory canal and varying vestigial remnants (Figure 14.1). The incidence varies, with Asians and American Indians having a high incidence (1:2,000) and Caucasians having a low incidence (1:12,000). About 90% of cases are unilateral, and there is a 2:1 male-to-female ratio. About 50% have some form of mandibular deformity in association with hemifacial microsomia (Figure 14.2).

14.2 Embryology

Embryologically, the auricle develops from six auricular hillocks around the margins of the first pharyngeal groove. As the auricle grows, the contribution by the first arch is reduced. The lobule is the last part to develop. The auricles begin to develop in the base of the neck, which can account for their displaced position in some patients[1] (Figure 14.3). As the mandible develops, the auricles move to their normal position at the side of the head. The parts of the ear derived from the first branchial arch (tragus, crus helix, and helix) are supplied by its nerve, the mandibular branch of the trigeminal nerve. The parts derived from the second branchial arch (concha, antehelix, scapha,

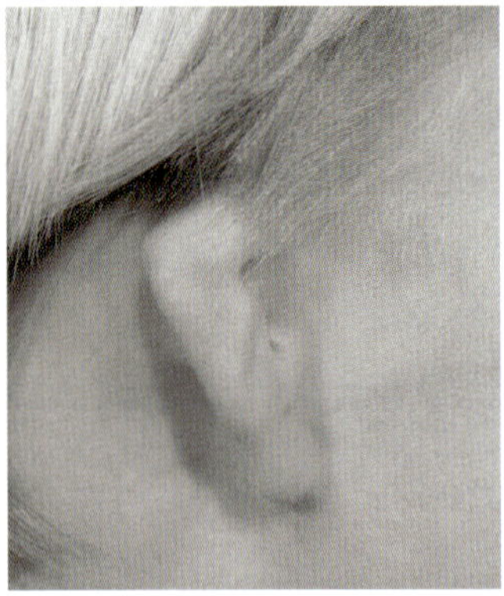

Figure 14.1. A typical case of lobular microtia.

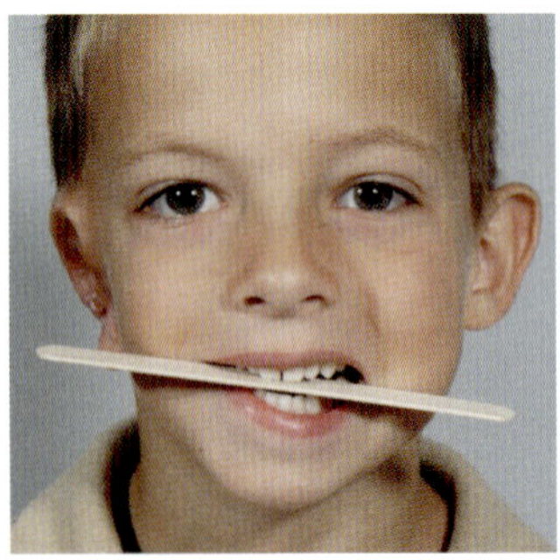

Figure 14.2. Approximately 50% of patients with microtia have some mandible deformity. This patient has conchal-type microtia and a significant cant to his occlusal plane.

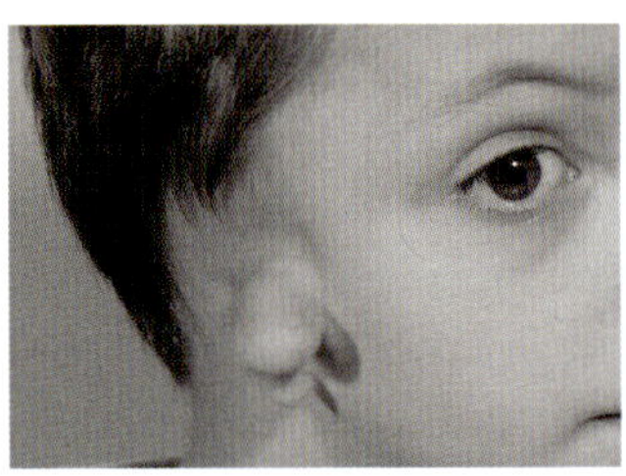

Figure 14.3. The low-set position of the conchal microtia can be accounted for by the early position of the auricles in the base of the neck.

antetragus, and lobule) are supplied by cutaneous branches of the cervical plexus.

Poswillo[2] postulated a hematoma in the area of the first and second branchial arches as the major cause of microtia and first and second branchial arch syndrome. The varying size of the hematoma can account for the variations in the clinical presentation.

14.3 Anatomy

There is wide variation in the size and shape of the auricle. Auricular appendages are common and result from accessory hillocks. The normal ear length varies from 5.5 to 7.5 cm in the adult, and its width is approximately 50% of its length. The long axis of the ear is parallel to the nasal bridge and approximately one ear's length lateral to the lateral orbital rim.[3] The delicate skin draped over the complex framework, consisting of a conchal complex, a helix lobule complex, and an antehelix fossa triangularis complex, make reconstruction a challenge for any surgeon.

14.4 Classification

A simplified classification divides defects into lobular-type microtia, conchal-type microtia, and anotia (Figure 14.4). Anotia is very rare, and will not be discussed in this chapter.

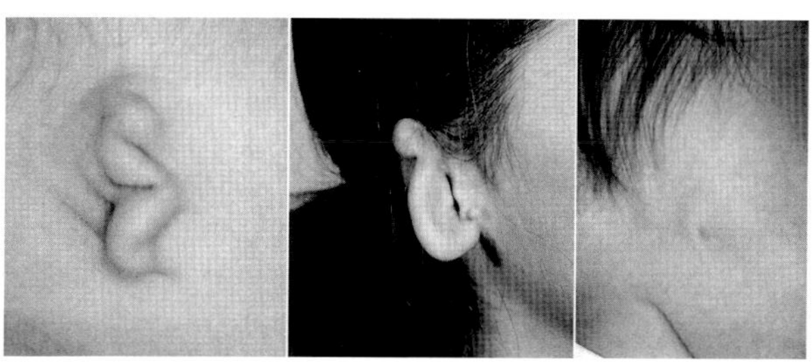

(A) (B) (C)

Figure 14.4. (A) Lobular microtia, (B) conchal microtia, (C) anotia.

14.5 Ear Reconstruction

The goal for the plastic surgeon is to reconstruct an auricle that appears normal and closely matches the opposite side. The 3-dimensional feature makes it a complex reconstruction and one that requires practice in carving the framework before working on a patient. The modern era of autogenous costal cartilage reconstruction began with principles presented by Tanzer,[4] was refined by Brent,[5,6] and has been augmented by Nagata.[7–11] The best material for reconstruction is autogenous costal cartilage because of the low number of complications and its long-term durability. Alloplastic materials have no place in pediatric reconstruction because the risk of exposure and extrusion of these materials is great, and the primary flap available for salvage of problems is expended in reconstruction with alloplastic materials.[12]

Reconstruction is generally performed around age 7 to 8 years. At that point the ear is close to an adult size, and the chest is large enough for an adequate cartilage graft.[13] Nagata[7] waits until age 10 years, but his Asian patients are probably of smaller stature than Westerners, and therefore the cartilage available for the graft would be less at age 7 years.

The method of auricular reconstruction that has evolved for my understanding is a combination of the principles outlined by Brent[5,6] and the recent refinements described by Nagata.[8–11] Nagata's technique has reduced the steps from four to three for lobular microtia and to two stages for conchal microtia.

14.5.1 *Lobular microtia*

The first stage of reconstruction consists of lobule rotation, excision of the auricular remnant, fabrication of the cartilage framework, and insertion of the framework. Stage 2 consists of elevation of the reconstructed auricle, support with a cartilage wedge, and split-thickness grafting of the posterior ear. Stage 3 consists of tragus reconstruction and setback of the opposite ear.

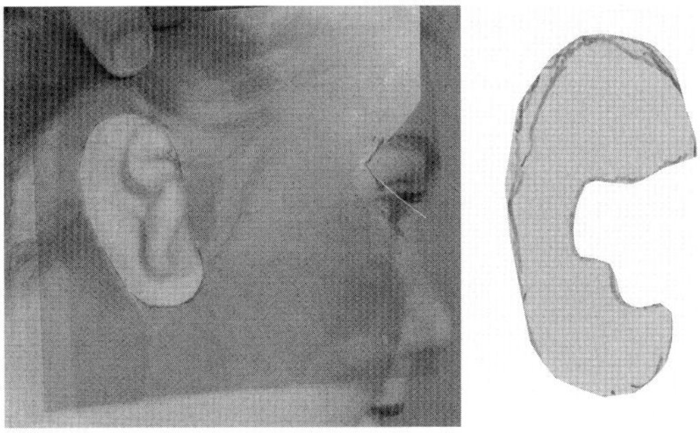

(A) (B)

Figure 14.5. Radiographic film template.

14.5.1.1 *Stage 1 surgical procedure*

Placement of the auricle and the size of the auricle are the two most important preoperative steps. Before surgery, the opposite normal ear is traced on radiographic films. This pattern is cut and then reversed to design the framework from the rib cartilage (Figure 14.5). At the same time, the radiographic film is marked using the lateral canthus as a landmark. The pattern is placed on the affected side, and the placement for the reconstructed ear is marked. The film is then autoclaved for use during surgery.

The rib graft is harvested from the opposite chest, using an incision parallel to the costal margin. This scar usually heals quite well (Figure 14.6). After exposing the sixth, seventh, and eighth ribs, the template is used to mark the sixth and seventh ribs and the synchondrosis. The template often does not match the rib anatomy exactly, and the surgeon must do some creative planning. I have found that if you leave a gap where the fossa triangularis will be, the helix will bridge the area and you will be carving out the fossa triangularis anyway (Figure 14.7). The rib graft is removed along with the entire cartilaginous eighth rib. The perichondrium of the donor site is maintained *in situ* as much as possible, and then the perichondrium is closed as a separate layer. Before muscle closure is started, a pain pump is inserted, and the remainder of the incision is closed. The pain pump has resulted in greatly reduced need for narcotics in the postsurgical period.

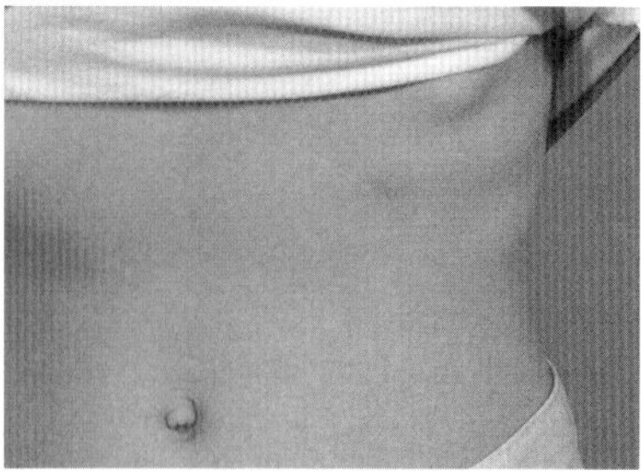

Figure 14.6. Healed scar on chest.

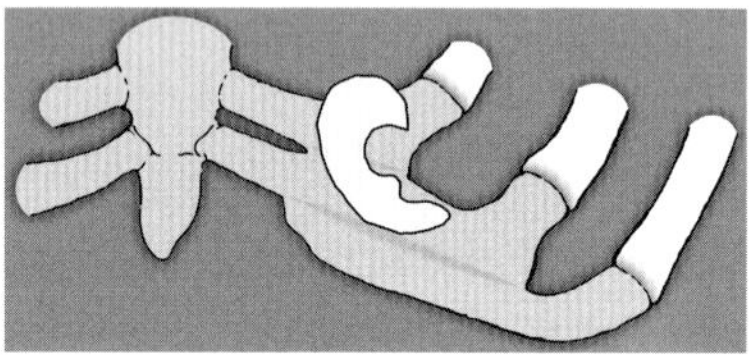

Figure 14.7. Diagram of template on rib showing how to compensate for rib anatomy that does not fit the template exactly.

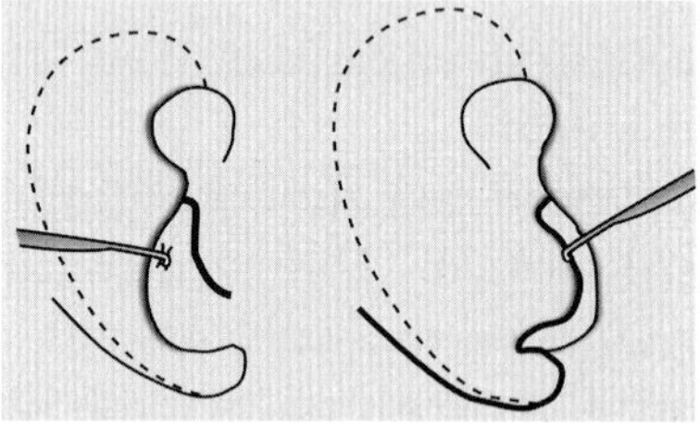

Figure 14.8. Incision in lobule (left) and area of undermining (right).

While the one team is harvesting the cartilage, the second team makes a W-shaped incision on the posterior aspect of the lobule and extends that into the mastoid area for the inset of the lobule (Figure 14.8). The incision extends anteriorly on the lobule, and this allows excision of the cartilage remnant as well as rotation of the lobule. Often there are deep sinus tracks in this skin, and perforations can be made in dissecting the skin off the cartilage remnant. It is important to recognize those, and to excise the margins and close the opening. A large subcutaneous pocket is then dissected for the framework (Figure 14.8). Inferiorly, a subcutaneous pedicle is left attached in the area of the lobule to maintain circulation to the skin. At this point, gauze is placed in the pocket and the framework is constructed.

The base framework is made from the sixth and seventh ribs, and frequently part of the fossa triangularis will be constructed through a gap in the framework. The helix and crus helix are constructed from the eighth rib, carving it on one side to create the necessary curvature. Using an X-Acto blade, the helical rim can be hollowed to create a natural look. The helical rim is sutured to the base to create the crus helix and rim. Creating the crus helix is an important improvement in the appearance of the final result. We use 4-0 clear nylon to suture the helical rim to the base. After this, the fossa triangularis and scapha are carved using a 15C blade and an X-Acto blade (Figure 14.9). The superior and inferior crus antehelix unit can be augmented if necessary with an onlay cartilage graft fixed with sutures, as described by Nagata.[8] With the framework completed (Figure 14.9), the pocket is inspected for bleeding, and the framework is then inserted and positioned. A suction tube is inserted, and the incisions are closed

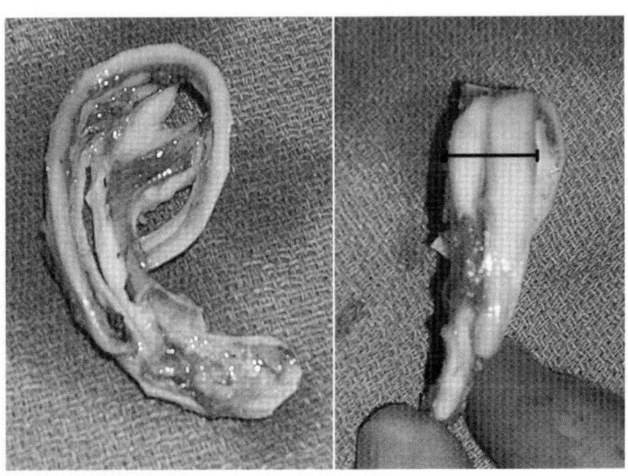

(A) (B)

Figure 14.9. (A) Cartilage framework. The framework on the left has the carved-out fossa triangularis and the scapha, along with the crus helix, which gives a better appearance to the reconstructed ear than previous techniques. (B) The side view is important because the height of the framework should be at least 1 cm to get the detail in the reconstructed ear.

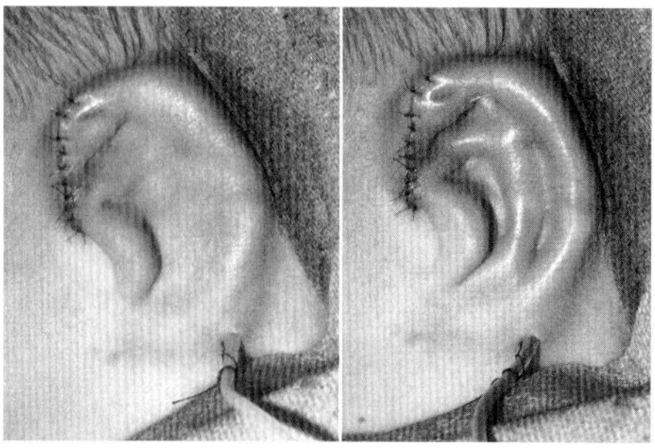
(A) (B)

Figure 14.10. (A) Framework in place. (B) After suction applied.

(Figure 14.10). Petroleum gauze dressing rolled into small cylinders is then packed to the contours, and suction is obtained with the vacuum tube. A large dressing is applied. The dressing is removed after 5 to 7 days, along with the suction tube.

14.5.1.2 *Stage 2 surgical procedure*

We usually wait 2 to 3 months for the second stage, but it can be performed as early as 6 weeks.

The skin incision around the periphery is made and carried down through the fascia. This allows elevation of the ear without exposure of the cartilage. The ear must be elevated to the midpoint of the conchal bowl. If cartilage is exposed, it is important to cover the area with fascia so the skin graft will heal. The skin on the margins of the ear is sutured back to the fascia so that the contour looks uniform and the skin graft does not show.

The scalp flap is undermined so it can be advanced downward; thus, when one sees the patient on a side view, only the ear and hair can be seen. No skin graft is visible. If cartilage has been saved it can be wedged with the junction of the framework and skull and covered with mastoid fascia (Figure 14.11). This maintains the ear position away from the skull. The scalp flap is advanced and the remaining raw surface is covered with a skin graft. It is wise to take a piece of skin

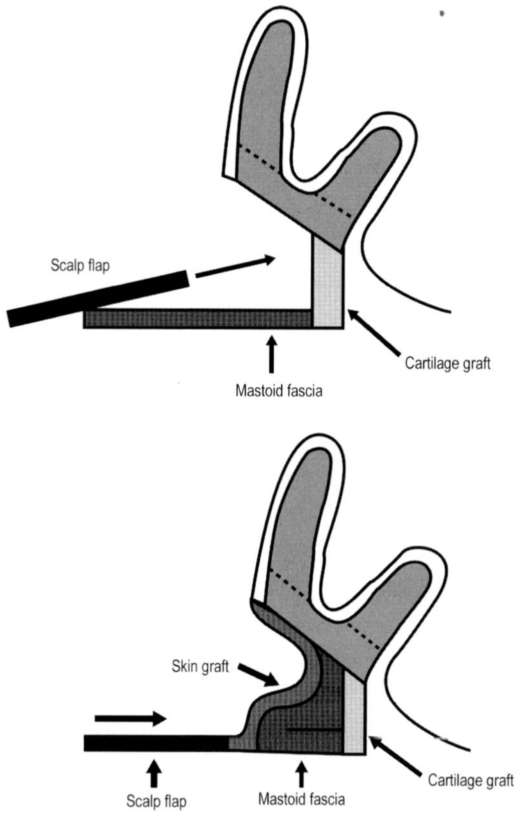

Figure 14.11. Diagram of cartilage wedge for Stage 2.

10 ➡ 10 cm to allow for adequate resurfacing, because the curvature of the posterior ear requires a large piece of skin for coverage.

14.5.1.3 *Stage 3: Construction of tragus*

We usually wait 6 to 8 weeks for this stage. Reconstruction of the tragus is performed using a chondrocutaneous graft from the opposite ear concha along with a full-thickness graft from the opposite postauricular area.[5] Use of the opposite ear allows the surgeon to set back the normal ear, which is usually necessary to get frontal symmetry. Nagata[10] carves the tragus into his framework at the first stage.

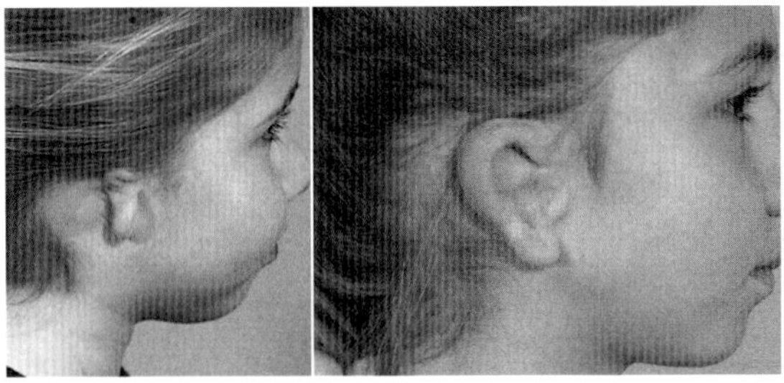

Figure 14.12. Pre- and postoperative photos of lobular microtia.

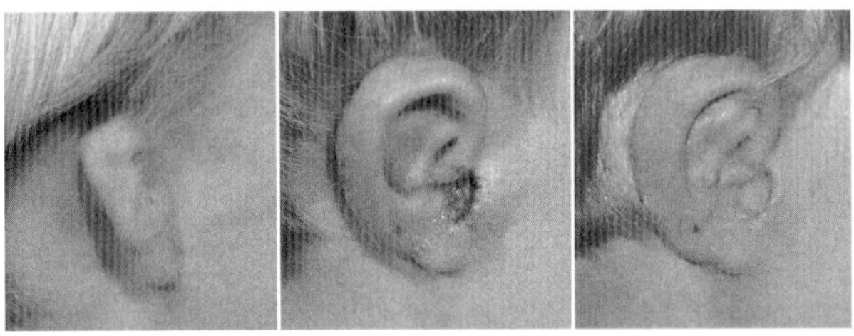

Figure 14.13. Pre- and postoperative photos of lobular microtia.

A J-shaped flap is elevated at the site of the proposed tragus as described by Brent.[5] The composite graft is sutured to the undersurface of the flap, and the open area is covered with the skin from the opposite ear. A dressing is applied, which usually heals without a problem. Figures 14.12 and 14.13 show results of reconstruction of lobular microtia at 5 years post-reconstruction.

14.5.2 *Conchal microtia*

Conchal microtia presents with a more normal-appearing inferior portion, but it is smaller and rotated anteriorly. For conchal microtia, the lobule, conchal bowl, tragus, meatus, and canal are all present in various forms. Conchal microtia requires repositioning of the lobule with a higher position to the lobular incision. The auricular cartilage remnant is excised. A pocket is then created similar to that in the lobular type, and the tail of the helix is inserted into a pocket made in the lobule. The remainder of the procedure is similar to the

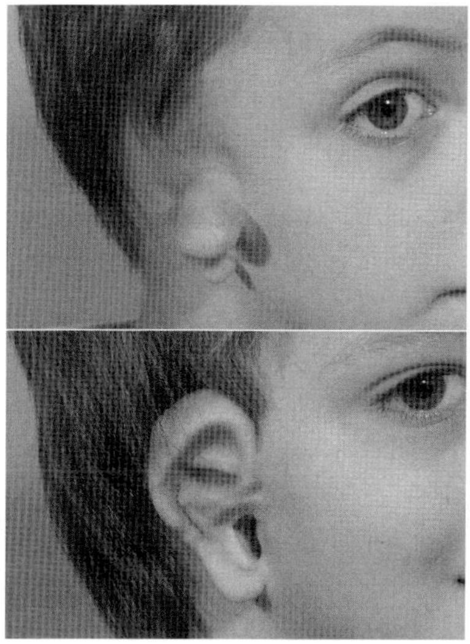

Figure 14.14. Pre- and postoperative photos of conchal microtia.

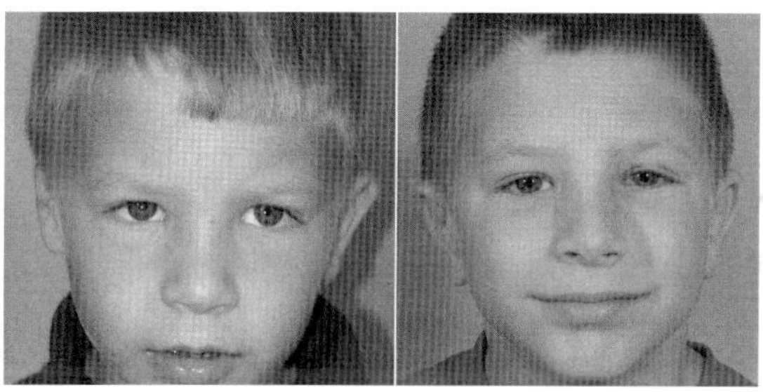

(A) (B)

Figure 14.15. (A) Result after tragus construction and setback of normal ear in lobular microtia. (B) Same child in 2004, 4 years older.

lobule-type procedure. The second stage, with ear elevation, is less involved than in lobule microtia. No tragus reconstruction is necessary (Figure 14.14). Setback of the normal ear may be required to get balance in auricular position between the two ears (Figure 14.15).

In patients with a low-set hairline, one can reconstruct the ear and then replace the hair-bearing area with a skin graft or use the temporoparietal fascial flap with a skin graft. I prefer the temporoparietal

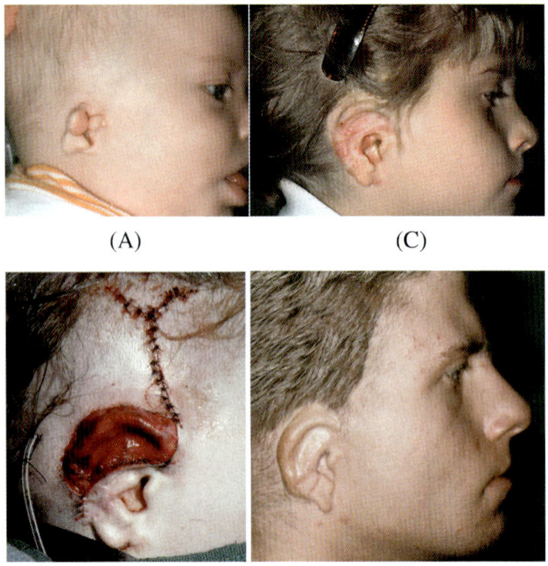

(A) (C)

(B) (D)

Figure 14.16. Result of reconstruction of low-set ear with temporoparietal fascial flap and skin graft with a 15-year follow-up. (A) Preoperative. (B) Intraoperative. (C) 3 months postoperative. (D) 15-year follow-up.

fascial flap (Figure 14.16). When possible, it is better to avoid the temporoparietal flap in boys unless there is no other choice, because the scar is very visible with short hair.

14.5.2.1 *Secondary auricular reconstruction*

Secondary auricular reconstruction after failed primary reconstruction presents a number of difficult issues. The skin at the site is usually scarred and not usable and the primary graft-donor site has been used, so the cartilage from the ipsilateral side must be used. The patient should be made aware of the reduced expectations. The temporoparietal flap should be used to cover the framework, followed by a skin graft (Figure 14.17). Elevation and tragus reconstruction are similar to that for lobular microtia.

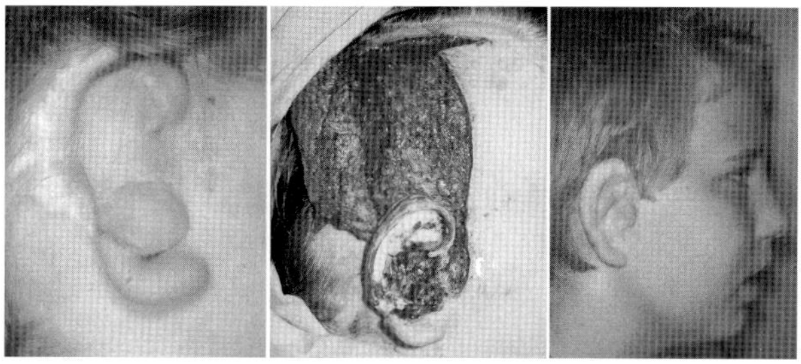

Figure 14.17. Result of reconstruction of a failed primary reconstruction using the ipsilateral rib and temporoparietal fascial flap. (A) Appearance of ear at presentation for secondary reconstruction. (B) Intraoperative view before temporoparietal flap. (C) Final result, 2 years later.

14.6 Acquired Deformities

Acquired deformities present their own unique problems depending on the mechanism of injury. The missing or deformed ear can result from an accident, a burn, or a gunshot wound.

Traumatic injuries can be partial or complete, but the tragus and ear canal are usually present. If it is a clean amputation and the auricular skin is undamaged, it can be used for covering the framework (Figure 14.18). If there is a burn injury, the skin is usually damaged and the temporoparietal fascial flap will need to be used for framework coverage (Figure 14.19). The steps are similar to those in lobular microtia. In some burn injuries, only the helix and antehelix are lost, and the retroauricular skin may be satisfactory for skin coverage (Figure 14.20).

If the temporoparietal flap is not available on the ipsilateral side, a free tissue transfer from the contralateral side can be used to solve the problem, as in this shotgun injury (Figure 14.21). The first phase was a scalp flap, using expansion to resurface the temporal bone defect, and then the ear reconstruction was performed (Figure 14.21).

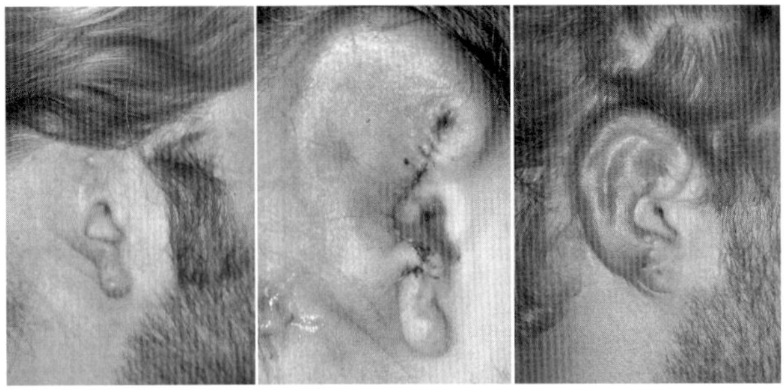

Figure 14.18. Result of reconstruction of a subtotal ear amputation using the postauricular skin and rib cartilage graft in a 25-year-old.

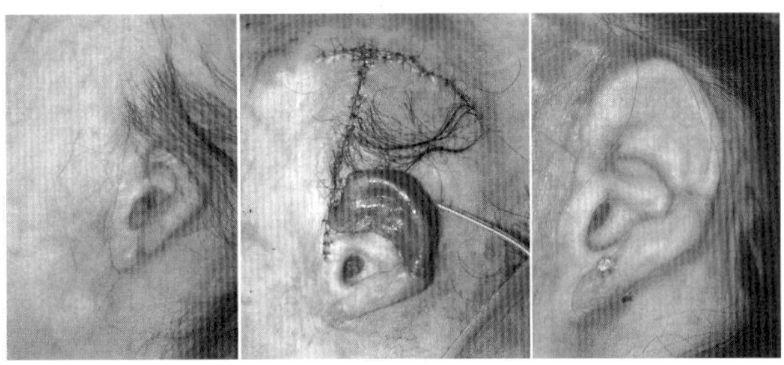

Figure 14.19. Result after reconstruction of a burn ear deformity using a temporoparietal fascial flap. The hair was reconstructed using a tissue expander.

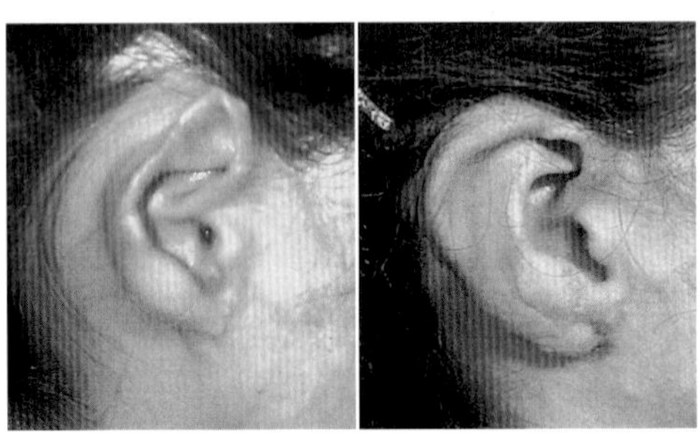

Figure 14.20. Reconstruction of a burnt ear deformity involving only the helix and scapha. The cartilage framework was placed under the postauricular skin.

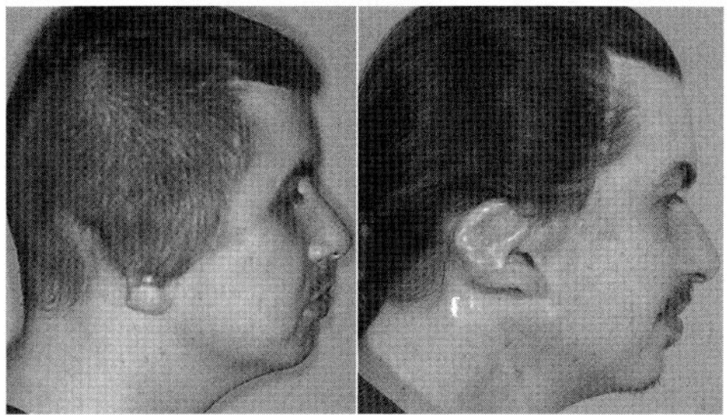

Figure 14.21. Patient who lost scalp, temporal bone and ear from a shotgun injury. Result using free microvascular temporoparietal fascial flap and cartilaginous framework.

14.7 Summary

The techniques described in this chapter to reconstruct congenital and acquired defects of the ear have been developed by modifying the contributions made by previous authors. My approach has been to present a technique that can be easily learned by any pediatric plastic surgeon who wants to practice carving a framework and that will give reproducible results. The future looks bright as research with chondrocytes leads us toward "growing" an ear in the desired shape and then transferring it onto a microvascular pedicle.

References

1. **Moore KL, Persand TV.** *The Developing Human.* Philadelphia, PA: Saunders; 2003:478–483.
2. **Poswillo D.** The pathogenesis of the first and second branchial arch syndrome. *Oral Surg Oral Med Oral Pathol* 1973;35:302–328.
3. **Tolleth H.** Artistic anatomy, dimensions, and proportions of the external ear. *Clin Plast Surg* 1978;5:337–345.
4. **Tanzer RC.** Total reconstruction of the external ear. *Plast Reconstr Surg* 1959;23:1–15.
5. **Brent B.** The correction of microtia with autogenous cartilage grafts. I. The classic deformity. *Plast Reconstr Surg* 1980;66:1–12.
6. **Brent B.** The correction of microtia with autogenous cartilage grafts. II. Atypical and complex deformities. *Plast Reconstr Surg* 1980;66:13–21.

7. **Nagata S.** A new method of total reconstruction of the auricle for microtia. *Plast Reconstr Surg* 1993;92:187–201.
8. **Nagata S.** Modification of the stages in total reconstruction of the auricle. Part I. Grafting the three-dimensional costal cartilage framework for lobule-type microtia. *Plast Reconstr Surg* 1994;93:221–230.
9. **Nagata S.** Modification of the stages in total reconstruction of the auricle. Part II. Grafting the three-dimensional costal cartilage framework for concha-type microtia. *Plast Reconstr Surg* 1994;93:231–242.
10. **Nagata S.** Modification of the stages in total reconstruction of the auricle. Part III. Grafting the three-dimensional costal cartilage framework for small concha-type microtia. *Plast Reconstr Surg* 1994;93:243–253.
11. **Nagata S.** Modification of the stages in total reconstruction of the auricle. Part IV. Ear elevation for the constructed auricle. *Plast Reconstr Surg* 1994;93:254–266.
12. **Jones CE, Wellisz T.** External ear reconstruction: use of a pivoting helix, porous polyethylene implant. *AORN J* 1994;59:411–415, 418–422.
13. **Bauer BS.** Reconstruction of the microtic ear. *J Pediatr Surg* 1984;19:440–445.

MAXILLOFACIAL AND SALIVARY PATHOLOGY TREATED BY SURGERY

15

Julien Ghannoum, DMD

This chapter offers a brief overview of the immense complexity of maxillofacial and salivary gland pathology. Discussion will be restricted to common or distinctive lesions treated by surgery.

15.1 Soft Tissue and Bone Lesions

The head and neck can give rise to a plethora of different mesenchymal tumors and non-neoplastic conditions. Whether benign or malignant, many of these tumors are classified according to the mature tissue counterpart they resemble. Further subclassification is an exercise in intricacy and depends on numerous factors such as phenotype, clinical behavior, and genotype.

In the past 2 decades, soft tissue pathology has evolved greatly in our understanding of tumor biology and in developing new diagnostic tools. Indeed, molecular genetics plays an increasingly important role, and specific genotypes may even dictate treatment and prognosis in some tumors. Conversely, strict reliance on immunohistochemical stains and electron microscopy may lead to diagnostic pitfalls, since many different soft tissue tumors share similar antigen expression and ultrastructural features.

The pathologist must be able to correlate clinical and radiographic features with histology, especially for matrix-producing lesions. Such features may be imperative in differentiating benign from malignant mesenchymal tumors.

15.1.1 *Aneurysmal bone cyst*

An aneurysmal bone cyst (ABC) is a benign, expansive, pseudocystic lesion that can affect any bone. The exact pathogenesis is unknown, although one of the prevailing hypotheses is that ABCs are the result of vascular events. ABCs can present in combination with a wide variety of bone lesions. Primary ABCs (i.e., those not associated with other bone lesions) are now viewed as tumors because they show consistent gene rearrangements. Symptoms vary according to location and degree of expansion. ABCs are characterized as blood-filled spaces surrounded by fibrous tissue containing multinucleated giant cells, osteoid, and woven bone. Different treatment modalities can be applied, including curettage with or without cryotherapy, selective embolization, and resection.

15.1.2 *Benign fibrous histiocytoma*

Benign fibrous histiocytomas are benign tumors composed of spindle cells exhibiting fibroblastic and histiocytic differentiation. They occur in the submucosa and, less likely, within bone. The cutaneous counterpart of a benign fibrous histiocytoma is called a *dermatofibroma*. Histologic features are those of a storiform proliferation of spindle cells. Scattered lymphocytes, multinucleated giant cells, and foamy histiocytes may be seen and represent an important diagnostic clue. Complete conservative excision is usually curative.

15.1.3 *Benign peripheral nerve sheath tumors*

Benign peripheral nerve sheath tumors (BPNST) represent a range of disease that includes neurofibromas, true neuromas (i.e., nontraumatic),

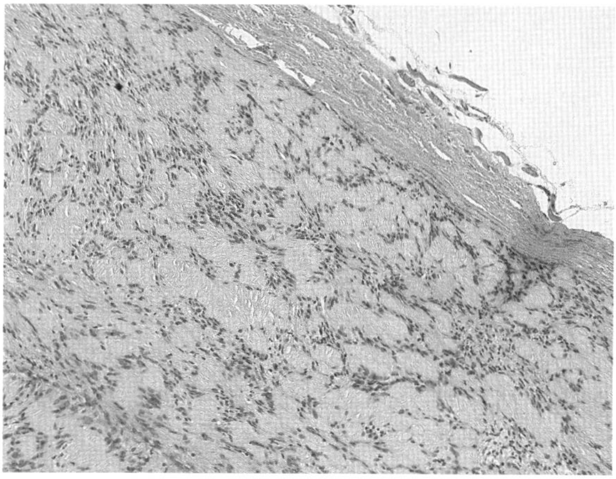

Figure 15.1. Schwannoma (hematoxylin-eosin, 203). This tumor is encapsulated and shows typical palisaded nuclei surrounding acellular areas (Verocay bodies).

schwannomas (neurilemomas), neurothekeomas, and perineuriomas. These last two entities are rare and are treated by complete excision.

Schwannomas are fairly common in the head and neck and can elicit pain and other symptoms. They are typically well circumscribed and often encapsulated. The histologic hallmark of schwannomas is the presence of a cellular "Antoni A" pattern (Figure 15.1) with palisading nuclei (Verocay bodies) and an "Antoni B" pattern with a hypocellular loose stroma. Marked cellular atypia may be present in degenerated or "ancient" schwannomas, although mitoses are virtually absent.

Neurofibromas present as solitary (circumscribed), diffuse, or plexiform lesions. They are composed of spindle cells with wavy nuclei arranged either haphazardly, in short fascicles, or in a storiform pattern. The stroma contains varying amounts of wire-like wavy collagen and myxoid areas. Solitary neurofibromas are cured by conservative excision.

Syndromic association with multiple BPNST can occur as follows: neurofibromas in neurofibromatosis (NF) type 1, schwannomas in NF type 2, mucosal neuromas in multiple endocrine neoplasia syndrome type 2B (Figure 15.2), and perineuriomas in NF type 2, although these are exceedingly rare.

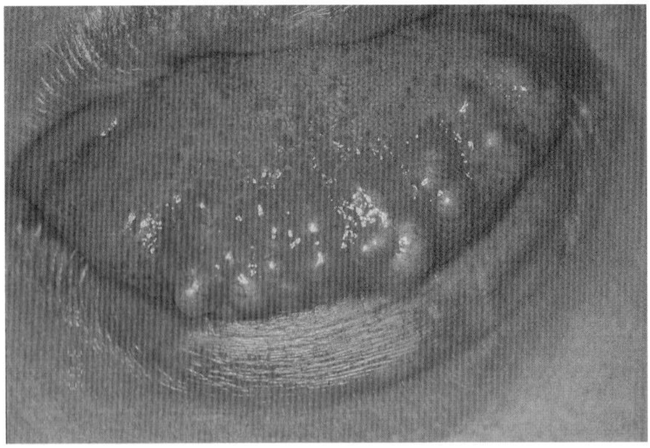

Figure 15.2. Multiple neuromas in multiple endocrine neoplasia 2B syndrome presenting as multiple submucosal nodules.

15.1.4 *Bisphosphonate-associated osteonecrosis of the jaws*

Bisphosphonate-associated osteonecrosis is defined as bone necrosis in patients with a history of previous or current bisphosphonate therapy who have not received radiotherapy in the involved area. It is much more common in *i.v* forms of therapy, due to which osteoclastic activity is severely compromised. Clinically, bisphosphonate-associated osteonecrosis may arise *de novo* or secondary to odontogenic infections or invasive dental procedures. Patients present with exposed necrotic bone and may develop pain, abscess formation, and pathologic fracture (Figure 15.3). There is no proven cure thus far. Treatment can include cessation of bisphosphonate therapy followed by debridement (depending on the patient's medical condition and overall prognosis), vascularized grafts, prevention of acute infections, and palliative care. Patients under other forms of bone-targeted therapy, such as receptor activator of nuclear factor-κB ligand inhibitors, may also develop osteonecrosis of the jaws, clinically indistinguishable from bisphosphonate-associated osteonecrosis.

15.1.5 *Cemento-osseous dysplasia*

Also known as osseous dysplasia, cemento-osseous dysplasia (COD) is a common benign fibro-osseous disease of the alveolar processes of

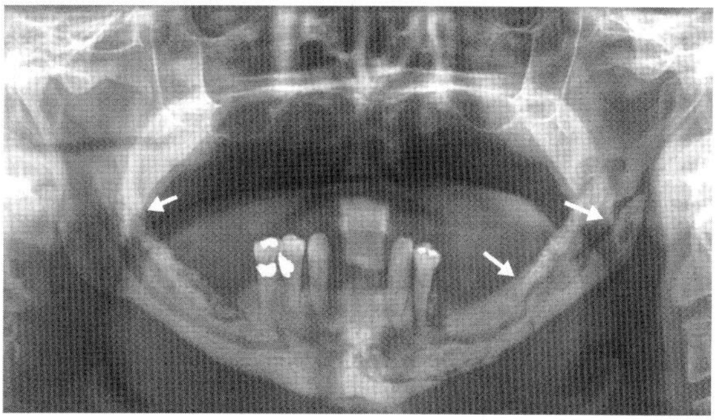

Figure 15.3. Bisphosphonate-associated osteonecrosis of the mandible. Panoramic radiograph showing a complex and open pathologic fracture involving the entire mandible (arrows).

the jaws. COD is classified into three distinct clinicoradiologic entities: periapical, focal, and florid. Periapical COD by definition involves the periapex of anterior mandibular teeth. It has a marked predilection for women, and is more common in black patients. Focal COD is confined to a single site of involvement, typically in the posterior mandible. Florid COD involves multiple foci and may cause slight expansion of the cortices. In early stages of disease, all three forms of COD present as asymptomatic radiolucencies on conventional radiographs and computed tomography, gradually becoming more calcified. Eventually, lesions may become completely sclerotic and hypovascular, and hence prone to necrosis after trauma or odontogenic infections. CODs may be associated with the formation of simple bone cysts (SBCs). Histologically, CODs are composed of cementum-like calcifications and irregular islands of trabecular and woven bone set in a moderately cellular fibrovascular stroma (Figure 15.4). In cases where lamellar bone is prominent, CODs can be mistaken for chronic osteomyelitis. Unlike other calcifying bone lesions, CODs normally do not require any treatment, unless in the presence of secondary osteomyelitis.

Familial gigantiform cementoma is a very rare autosomal dominant disorder characterized by multifocal fibro-osseous lesions of the jaws, leading to dramatic expansion of the cortices and disfigurement.

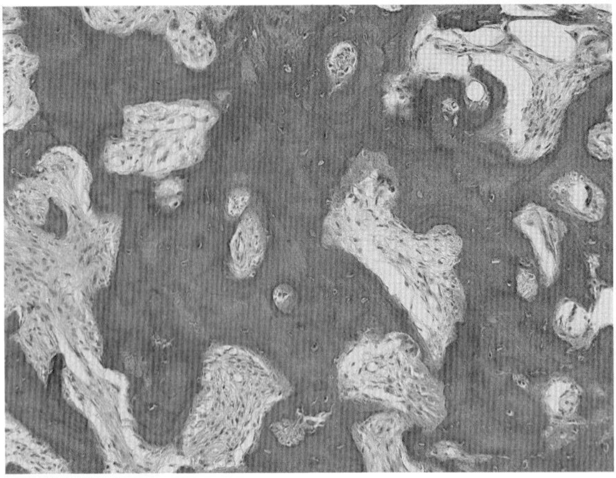

Figure 15.4. COD (hematoxylin-eosin, 203). Interconnecting trabeculae of woven bone in a moderately cellular and fibrovascular stroma. This case was diagnosed clinically as periapical cemental dysplasia.

It is regarded by some as a part of the COD disease spectrum because of similar histopathologic features and occurrence in the tooth-bearing area of the jaws. Partial excision leads to recurrence or secondary osteomyelitis. Therefore, extensive resection and reconstruction may be required.

15.1.6 *Central giant cell granuloma*

Central giant cell reparative granulomas (CGCGs) are benign osteolytic lesions composed of osteoclastic giant cells, fibrous tissue, extravasated red blood cells, and reactive bone formation (Figure 15.5). They have a predilection for the mandible and may be associated with significant expansion and osteolysis. Histologic features are not predictive of clinical behavior. Furthermore, because CGCGs are histologically identical to brown tumors of hyperparathyroidism, the latter must be excluded clinically. The histologic differential diagnosis also includes cherubism, ABC, and giant cell-rich variants of osteosarcoma. Again, clinicopathologic correlation is required. Treatment of small lesions consists of conservative curettage, whereas large lesions

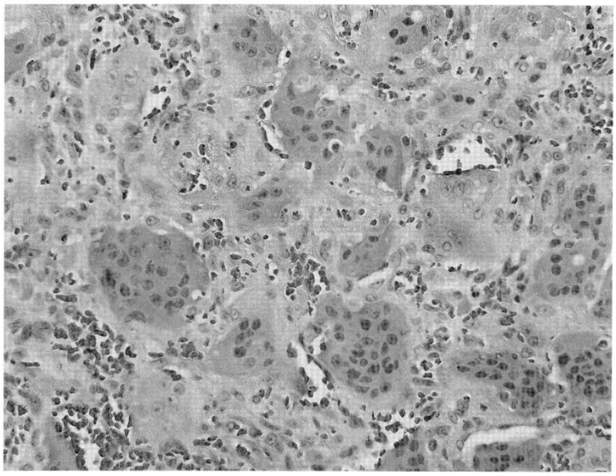

Figure 15.5. CGCG (hematoxylin-eosin, 403). Densely packed multinucleated giant cells obscuring the fibrovascular background stroma.

may respond to intralesional injections of corticosteroids or alpha-interferon in combination with intranasal calcitonin therapy.

Giant cell tumors are common tumors of the long bones, but their occurrence in the jawbones is a controversial topic. They are histologically comparable to CGCG, to a point where they may be impossible to differentiate from aggressive types of CGCG. In general, giant cell tumors are benign but behave more aggressively than CGCGs.

15.1.7 *Central ossifying fibroma*

Central ossifying fibroma (COF), also known as cemento-ossifying fibroma, is a rare neoplasia of the jawbones with a predilection for the posterior mandible of female patients. Eventually, if left untreated, COFs may cause significant expansion of the cortices and dental displacement. In early stages of disease, radiographic features may be indistinguishable from those of focal COD or osteoblastoma. Histologic features can resemble those of other benign fibro-osseous lesions, although COFs tend to show osteoblastic rimming and varying levels of mineralization. An important distinguishing feature is that the lesions are easily separated from surrounding bone, as opposed to focal COD or fibrous dysplasia, both of which merge with adjacent bone. Complete enucleation is the treatment of choice.

Juvenile active ossifying fibroma is an aggressive variant of COF that is seen in young patients, typically in the maxilla or paranasal sinuses. Histologic features include a cellular stroma containing spindle cells and giant cells, strands of immature osteoid with numerous osteoblasts, and variable amounts of psammomatoid calcifications. Recurrences are much more common than in conventional COF, thereby justifying complete resection.

Hyperparathyroidism-jaw tumor syndrome is a very rare autosomal dominant disease characterized by parathyroid tumors, renal lesions, uterine polyps, and occasional multicentric fibro-osseous lesions of the jaws that resemble COFs.

15.1.8 *Cherubism*

A rare autosomal dominant inherited disease, cherubism is characterized by osteolytic fibrous lesions resulting in bilateral enlargement of the jaws (Figure 15.6). It occurs in the first decade of life and tends to stabilize at puberty, at which point lesions may evolve into mature

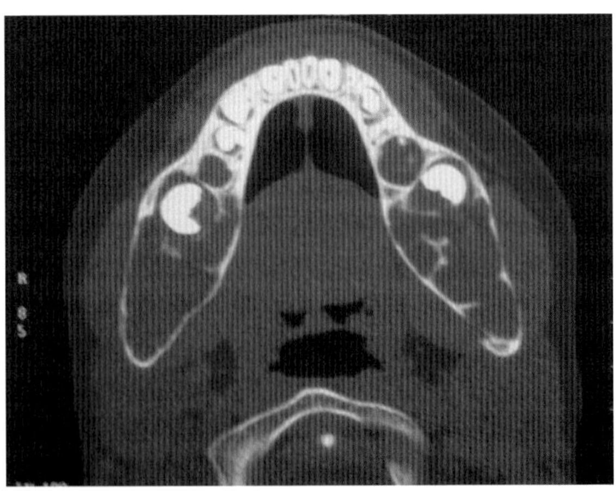

Figure 15.6. Cherubism. Axial computed tomogram showing bilateral and symmetric expansion of the mandibular cortices.

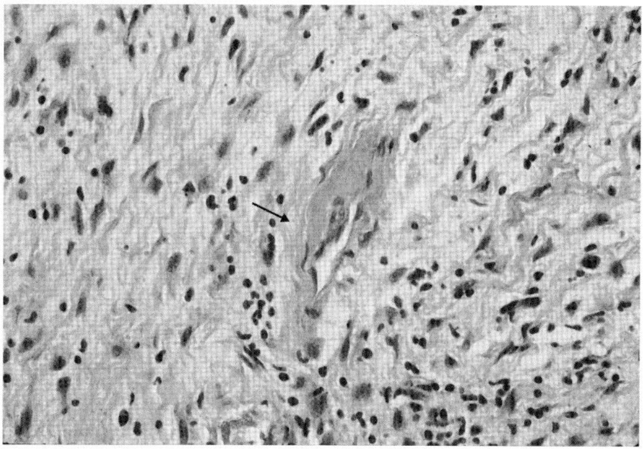

Figure 15.7. Cherubism. Perivascular hyalinization (arrow) and fibrous stroma (hematoxylin-eosin, 403). Other areas (not shown here) contained numerous multinucleated giant cells.

bone. Histologic features include cellular fibrous stroma in which are scattered varying amounts of multinucleated giant cells, extravasated red blood cells, and hemosiderin. Perivascular hyalinization is a distinguishing feature (Figure 15.7). Treatment is the topic of ongoing debate and varies according to the extent of cosmetic or functional involvement.

15.1.9 *Chondrosarcoma*

Chondrosarcoma is one of the most common malignancies of bone. In the head and neck area, the most frequent site of occurrence is the larynx, followed by the jaws, the maxillary sinus walls, the nasal cavity, and the base of the skull. Most cases arise centrally within bone, but they may also occur in periosteal locations from preexisting benign cartilaginous tumors. Incidentally, any intraosseous lesion of the jaws that produces cartilage should be viewed with extreme suspicion; such lesions are malignant until proven otherwise. Well-differentiated chondrosarcomas (grade 1) are composed of rather uniform cells whereas poorly differentiated tumors (grade 3) are characterized by pleomorphic tumor cells, necrosis, and a lesser amount of chondroid matrix. Clear cell and dedifferentiated variants have been described.

Prognosis and treatment depend on histologic grade. Treatment ideally consists of complete resection with uninvolved margins. The efficacy of conventional radiotherapy is not clearly established, although proton therapy is showing promise.

A *mesenchymal chondrosarcoma* is a related malignancy composed of a dense population of small, round cells with a hemangiopericytoma-like vasculature. Cartilaginous differentiation can be bland and minimal. Mesenchymal chondrosarcomas of the jaws seem to have a better prognosis than nongnathic tumors. However, overall prognosis is worse than for conventional chondrosarcomas.

15.1.10 *Chordoma*

Chordomas are relatively rare malignant neoplasms that recapitulate embryonic remnants of the notochord. In the head and neck area, they have a tendency to occur in the base of the skull and may present with various symptoms depending on their exact location. The periphery of these tumors is often well demarcated by a pseudocapsule. Histologic examination of chordomas typically reveals "bubbly" or vacuolated epithelioid cells (physaliphorous cells) arranged in chords and pseudoglandular structures. The stroma is markedly mucoid, which confers a gelatinous consistency to the tumor. The treatment of choice may include complete resection and combined proton radiotherapy. The 5-year survival rate is distinctly poorer after age 40.

15.1.11 *Craniopharyngioma*

Craniopharyngiomas are benign, slow-growing but aggressive epithelial tumors thought to be derived from remnants of Rathke's pouch. Although most of these tumors occur in the suprasellar or intrasellar region, they may also occur in ectopic locations such as the nasopharynx and sphenoid bone. There are two histologic types: adamantinomatous (by far the most common) and papillary squamous. Adamantinomatous craniopharyngiomas are composed of ameloblastoma-like epithelium with peripheral palisading and central

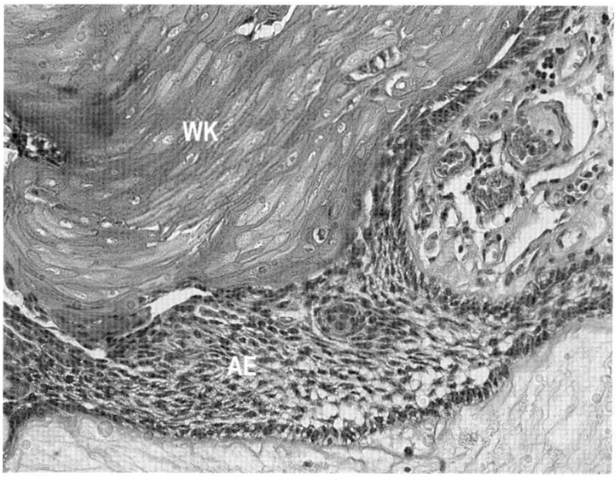

Figure 15.8. Craniopharyngioma (hematoxylin-eosin, 403). Ameloblastic epithelium (AE) with "wet" keratin (WK).

stellate reticulum, as well as nests of keratotic and calcifying cells ("wet" keratin) (Figure 15.8). These combined features can also be seen in odontogenic ghost cell tumors and, to a lesser extent, in calcifying odontogenic cysts (Gorlin's cysts). Whenever feasible, complete conservative resection is the treatment of choice; adjuvant radiotherapy may be required in cases of partial excision. Prognosis worsens with age.

15.1.12 *Ewing's sarcoma/primitive neuroectodermal tumor*

Ewing's sarcoma/primitive neuroectodermal tumor (ES/PNET) are high-grade primitive malignancies generally occurring in bone but occasionally arising in extraskeletal sites such as the sinonasal tract. The typical onset is usually in the first 2 decades of life. Histologically, they are composed of a diffuse population of small round blue cells often containing intracytoplasmic glycogen. PNET shows neuroepithelial differentiation in the form of rosettes and pseudorosettes, and reacts to neural/neuroendocrine markers. In opposition, ES lacks neuroepithelial differentiation and neural/neuroendocrine immunoreactivity. Treatment of ES/PNET generally consists of chemotherapy and radiotherapy, although surgical management is indicated in localized disease.

15.1.13 *Fibrous dysplasia*

Fibrous dysplasia is considered a benign genetic fibro-osseous condition resulting in bone alteration and expansion. This rare disease can be localized to one bone ("monostotic") or may involve multiple bones ("polyostotic"), in which case endocrine and cutaneous abnormalities may be present (McCune–Albright syndrome) as well as marked facial deformity. Fibrous dysplasia can be a component of Mazabraud syndrome, which includes intramuscular myxomas and fibrous dysplasia. The typical radiographic feature is replacement of medullary bone by an ill-defined, expansive, "ground-glass" radiopacity. SBC may be also present. Microscopic features include irregular trabeculae of woven bone lacking osteoblastic rimming and set in a cellular fibrous stroma (Figure 15.9). Treatment usually consists of bone recontouring for cosmetic purposes or to prevent compression of vital structures, although this inevitably leads to recurrence since the bulk of the lesion is not removed. Smaller lesions can be resected. Malignant transformation occurs only rarely.

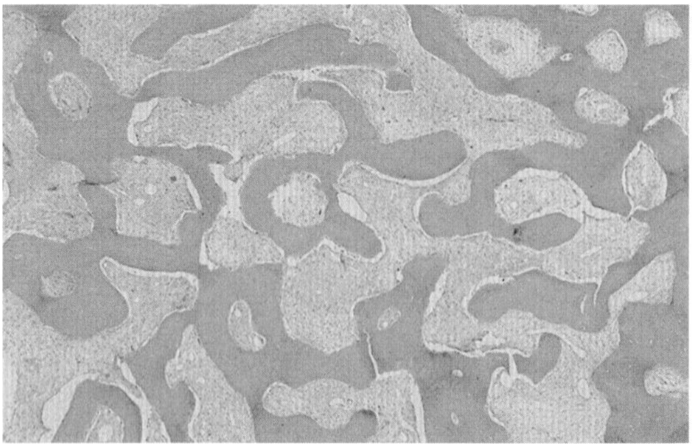

Figure 15.9. Fibrous dysplasia (hematoxylin-eosin, 103). Smooth-contoured islands of woven bone lacking osteoblastic rimming and set in a fibrous stroma.

15.1.14 *Glomangiopericytoma*

Glomangiopericytoma, also known as sinonasal-type hemangiopericytoma, is a rare neoplasm occurring mostly in the sinonasal tract and paranasal sinuses. Even though the very existence of hemangiopericytoma as a distinct entity is debatable, glomangiopericytoma deserves to be classified separately. It is characterized by a dense proliferation of spindled or ovoid cells arranged in a fascicular, storiform, or whorled pattern. The stroma contains abundant vascular channels, often exhibiting characteristic perivascular hyalinization. Treatment consists of complete excision. Recurrences are relatively common, even decades after surgery, and tumors may occasionally behave as low-grade malignancies.

15.1.15 *Gorham's disease*

Gorham's disease, also known as massive osteolysis or vanishing bone disease, is a very rare disease of unknown origin characterized by vascular proliferation leading to dramatic osteolysis. Patients present with spontaneous and progressive bone resorption. There is no proven cure, although successful disease stabilization through radiation therapy or *i.v.* bisphosphonates has been reported. Surgery alone has had unpredictable results.

15.1.16 *Granular cell tumor*

Granular cell tumors are relatively common benign tumors with a predilection for the tongue and larynx. They often present as asymptomatic, slow-growing, submucosal masses exhibiting a faint yellow-pink color. Laryngeal dysfunction may occur. The exact pathogenesis of this entity is unknown, although the tumor cells share some similarities with Schwann cells. Histologically, granular cell tumors are composed of sheets of large cells with abundant cytoplasm containing eosinophilic granules. A significant proportion of these tumors demonstrate marked pseudoepitheliomatous hyperplasia of the surface epithelium, which may be mistaken for an invasive squamous cell carcinoma by the untrained eye (Figure 15.10). Conservative excision is the treatment of choice.

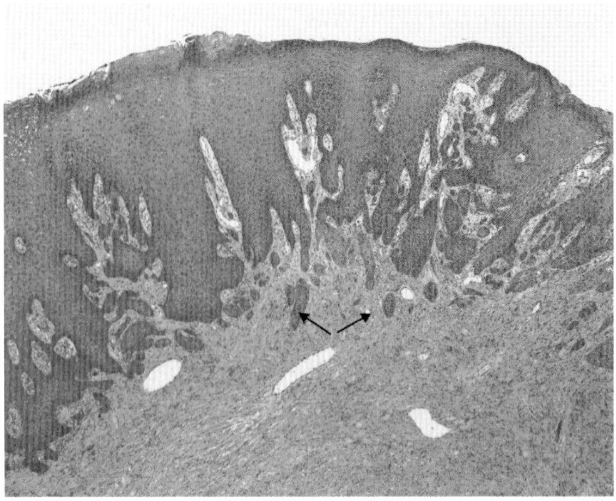

Figure 15.10. Granular cell tumor. The surface epithelium displays prominent pseudoepitheliomatous hyperplasia (arrows), mimicking superficially invasive squamous cell carcinoma (hematoxylin-eosin, 103).

15.1.17 *Langerhans cell histiocytosis*

Langerhans cell histiocytosis is characterized by a proliferation of Langerhans cells that can either be localized (eosinophilic granuloma) or multifocal with possible multiorgan involvement. In the head and neck area, it typically presents as an intraosseous lesion. Langerhans cells are large antigen-presenting cells with grooved or convoluted nuclei. Numerous eosinophils are typically seen admixed with the tumor cells (Figure 15.11). The ultrastructural hallmark of Langerhans cells is the Birbeck granule, a disk- or tennis racquet-shaped cytoplasmic organelle. Eosinophilic granulomas respond well to conservative surgery, whereas multifocal forms require chemotherapy. Malignant versions of Langerhans cell histiocytosis have been described.

15.1.18 *Leiomyoma*

Leiomyomas are benign tumors of smooth muscle that typically present as well-defined, occasionally painful, submucosal masses. Noncutaneous leiomyomas can arise in the walls of vascular channels (vascular leiomyomas or angioleiomyomas). Histologically, they are composed of fascicles of mature spindle cells with blunt-ended nuclei

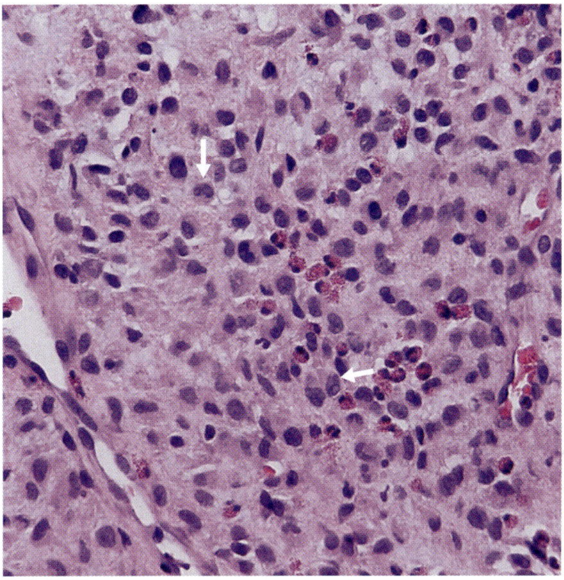

Figure 15.11. Langerhans cell histiocytosis. Scattered Langerhans cells with pale cytoplasm and grooved or convoluted nuclei (arrows). Eosinophils are also present (hematoxylin-eosin).

and perinuclear vacuolization. Different histologic variants have been described, such as the solid, granular cell and epithelioid types. Conservative excision is usually curative.

15.1.19 *Lipoma*

Lipomas are benign tumors of adipose tissue and represent the most common benign mesenchymal tumors. Distinct histologic variants have been described, such as pleomorphic, myxoid, chondroid, spindle-cell, intramuscular (infiltrating), and so forth. Complete surgical excision is the treatment of choice in many, if not all, types of lipomas. Recurrence is rare.

15.1.20 *Liposarcoma*

Liposarcomas are among the most common soft tissue sarcomas. In the head and neck, they occur most commonly in the larynx, hypopharynx, and neck. Much like their benign counterparts, liposarcomas are classified into numerous subtypes. The histologic hallmark of liposarcomas is the presence of vacuolated lipoblasts, which can be frustratingly lacking in well-differentiated tumors. Treatment and prognosis depend on histologic variants. Well-differentiated and myxoid variants have the best 5-year survival rate.

15.1.21 *Lymphangioma*

Lymphangiomas are benign lesions of lymphatic channels. They have a predilection for the head and neck and can be seen in the setting of genetic or congenital anomalies. Lymphangiomas are sometimes classified into three histologic types: cystic (cystic hygroma), capillary, and cavernous. Cystic hygromas are most often present at birth and may undergo spontaneous involution during childhood. They typically spread along tissue planes and may extend downward into the thoracic cavity. Cystic hygromas are characterized by dilated lymphatic spaces containing proteinaceous fluid. The treatment of choice is complete surgical excision, although sclerotherapy and laser therapy have been useful in selected cases. Even though lymphangiomas remain benign, death may occur as a result of pulmonary complications or impingement on vital structures.

15.1.22 *Malignant peripheral nerve sheath tumors*

In the head and neck, malignant peripheral nerve sheath tumors (MPNST) are rare and have a predilection for the neck. Although they may arise *de novo* in peripheral nerves, they usually develop in the setting of NF type 1 or from a preexisting BPNST. Histologically, MPNST are often composed of spindle cells arranged in long intersecting fascicles. Heterologous elements, such as metaplastic bone and cartilage, can be seen. MPNST can also exhibit divergent differentiation (muscular or glandular), in which case synovial sarcoma and melanoma should be ruled out. Low-grade tumors contain very few atypical mitotic figures and no necrosis, resembling atypical BPNST; therefore, demonstration of infiltrative growth is essential. Treatment includes wide resection with postoperative radiotherapy and chemotherapy. Prognosis is poorer in NF-1-related tumors.

15.1.23 *Meningioma*

Meningiomas are common benign intracranial neoplasms of meningothelial cells, although extracranial tumors are possible. Meningiomas are usually slow-growing, and may cause bone erosion and extension into the central nervous system. Different histologic subtypes have been described. Among these, the meningothelial subtype is the most common in extracranial sites of the head and neck. It is characterized by the presence of whorls and confluent islands of epithelioid cells with occasional nuclear inclusions (Figure 15.12). Concentric calcifications (psammoma bodies) can be seen but are not required for the diagnosis. Complete resection is the treatment of choice; recurrences are common in cases where surgical access is limited.

15.1.24 *Nodular fasciitis*

Nodular fasciitis is a benign, fast-growing, tumor-like proliferation of myofibroblasts that is part of the same spectrum of disease as cranial

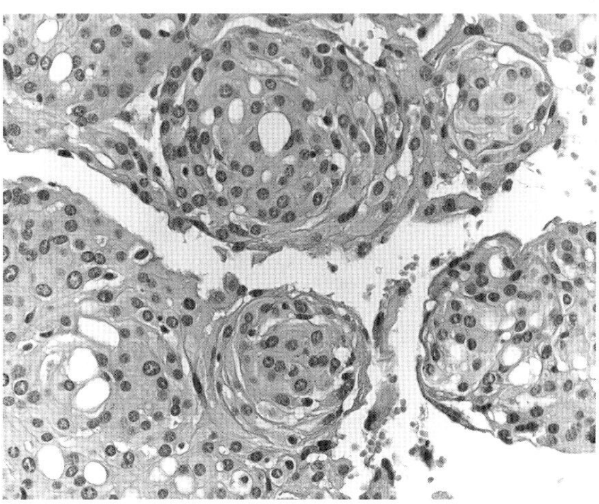

Figure 15.12. Meningioma. Whorls of epithelioid tumor cells (hematoxylin-eosin).

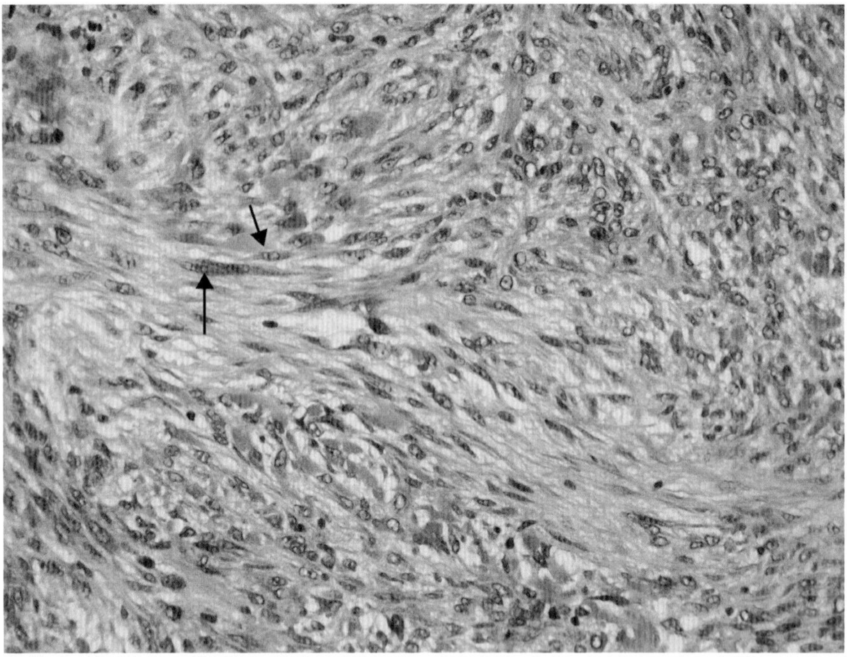

Figure 15.13. Nodular fasciitis. Fascicles of bipolar spindle cells (arrows) (hematoxylin-eosin).

fasciitis and intravascular fasciitis. It may affect any age, although young patients are more often affected. Trauma is thought to be a possible etiologic factor. Histologically, nodular fasciitis is vaguely infiltrative and composed of fascicles of immature bipolar spindle cells that can display a fair amount of pleomorphism and typical mitotic figures (Figure 15.13). The stroma contains inflammatory cells and extravasated red blood cells, and also exhibits keloidal collagen deposition as the lesions age. Misdiagnosis as a sarcoma is a common diagnostic pitfall. Conservative surgical excision is generally considered curative.

15.1.25 *Osteoblastoma*

Osteoblastomas are benign bone-forming tumors. By definition, the term "osteoid osteoma" is used instead when the lesion is less than 2 cm in its greatest dimension. Osteoblastomas can occur in any bone but have a predilection for the mandible. The male-to-female ratio is roughly 2:1, and patients in the second decade are most often affected. Nocturnal pain is a characteristic symptom. Histologic features include anastomotic trabeculae of woven bone and osteoid with prominent osteoblastic rimming set in a markedly vascularized intertrabecular stroma. Osteoblastomas are analogous to cementoblastomas (not discussed in this chapter) except that the latter are attached to dental roots. Complete excision is the treatment of choice.

15.1.26 *Osteoma*

Osteomas are benign slow-growing tumors of the craniofacial bones (Figure 15.14). Multiple osteomas of the maxillofacial complex are pathognomonic of Gardner's syndrome (gastrointestinal adenomatous polyps, osteomas, skin cysts, and numerous types of tumors). Osteomas are to be differentiated from exostoses and tori, which are hamartomatous by nature and lack significant growth potential. The histologic appearance of osteomas is one of mature and

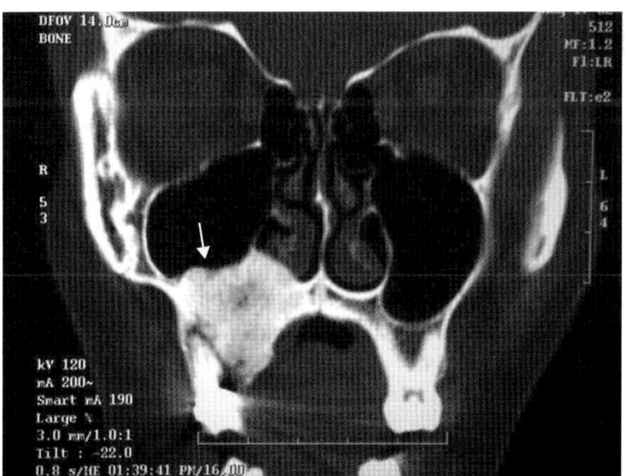

Figure 15.14. Osteoma. Coronal computed tomogram showing a dense mass of the right maxillary sinus (arrow).

predominantly lamellar bone. Nonsyndromic osteomas are cured by local excision, although surgery is recommended only in the presence of symptoms or functional disturbance.

15.1.27 *Osteoradionecrosis*

Osteoradionecrosis (ORN) is a relatively common complication of radiation treatment with a predilection for the mandible. Irradiated bone becomes less vascularized, hypoxic, and hypocellular, thus less able to regenerate or respond to infections. ORN is rare in patients who received radiation doses less than 5000 cGy. Acute and chronic infections often complicate ORN. Early cases may not be visible through imaging studies. Chronic ORN may present just like chronic osteomyelitis, i.e., as ill-defined, mixed radiolucent-radiopaque lesions with periosteal duplication, formation of sequestra, and possible pathologic fracture (Figure 15.15). Histologic examination reveals bone trabeculae deprived of osteocytic lacunae set in inflamed fibrous tissue. Epithelialized fistulous tracts with reactive cytologic atypia may be seen. Biopsy specimens of ORN must be thoroughly inspected to rule out radiation-induced sarcomas or recurrent disease. Treatment ranges from conservative curettage to resection of diseased bone, with cessation of smoking. Most studies indicate that hyperbaric oxygen therapy is a useful therapeutic adjunct.

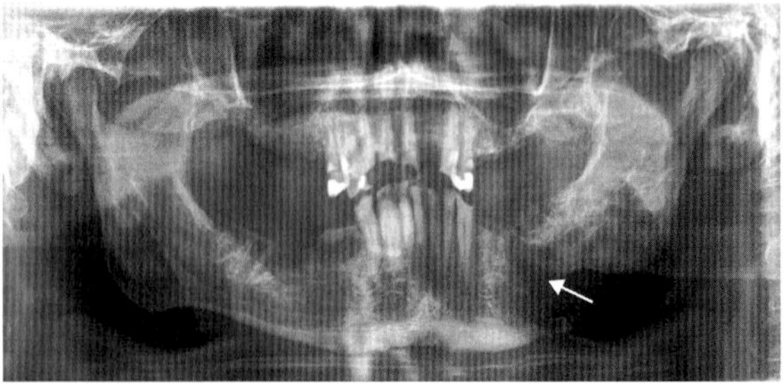

Figure 15.15. ORN. Panoramic radiograph showing an irregular pathologic fracture of the left mandibular body (arrow).

15.1.28 *Osteosarcoma*

Osteosarcoma is the most common primary malignancy of bone. It can be classified according to its localization, whether intraosseous (conventional), juxtacortical, orextraosseous, and according to the histologic grade. Regardless of the histologic variant, all osteosarcomas demonstrate production of either malignant bone or osteoid (Figure 15.16). Differentiating low-grade osteosarcomas from osteoblastomas or even fibrous dysplasia can be an arduous task on small biopsies; therefore, clinicopathologic correlation is paramount. Distinguishing osteosarcomas from giant cell tumors can also prove to be challenging in lesions with little osteoid and numerous giant cells. Treatment consists of wide resection with tumor-free margins, possibly with neoadjuvant or postoperative chemotherapy.

Osteosarcomas of the jaw have a distinctly better prognosis than extragnathic tumors. Nevertheless, tumors arising in irradiated bone or in preexisting bone lesions, such as Paget's disease of bone, tend to have a poorer prognosis.

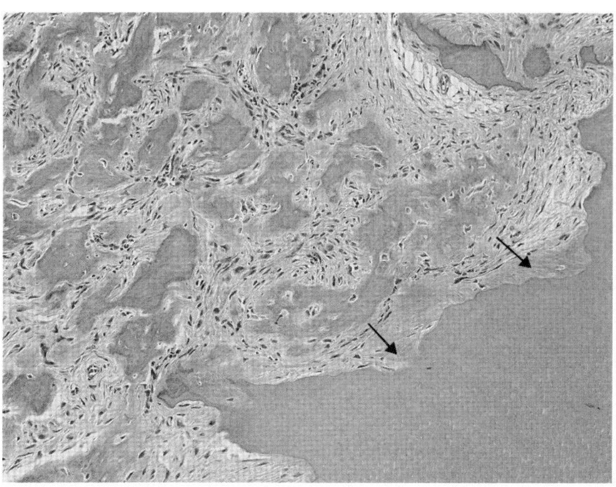

Figure 15.16. Well-differentiated osteosarcoma (hematoxylin-eosin). Somewhat atypical stromal cells associated with the formation of osteoid and bone. Adjacent dentin is showing irregular resorption (arrows).

15.1.29 *Paraganglioma*

Paragangliomas are slow-growing neuroendocrine neoplasms arising from paraganglia, some of which are distributed in the jugular bulb (glomus jugulare), the medial cochlea promontory (glomus tympanicum), the carotid, and the vagal body. They are morphologically similar to pheochromocytomas but are not to be confused with glomus tumors or glomangiomas, which are entirely different entities and are exceedingly rare in the head and neck. A significant proportion of paragangliomas is linked to inherited mutations (hereditary paragangliomatosis) and must be ruled out in multicentric tumors. Histologically, these tumors are composed of nests ("Zellballen") of granular tumor cells surrounded by spindled sustentacular cells (Figure 15.17). The stroma of paragangliomas is extremely vascularized, which may cause extensive bleeding and may justify preoperative embolization. Since there are no well-recognized histopathologic criteria for the diagnosis of malignant paragangliomas, such a diagnosis can almost be rendered only in the presence of metastases in sites that do not usually contain

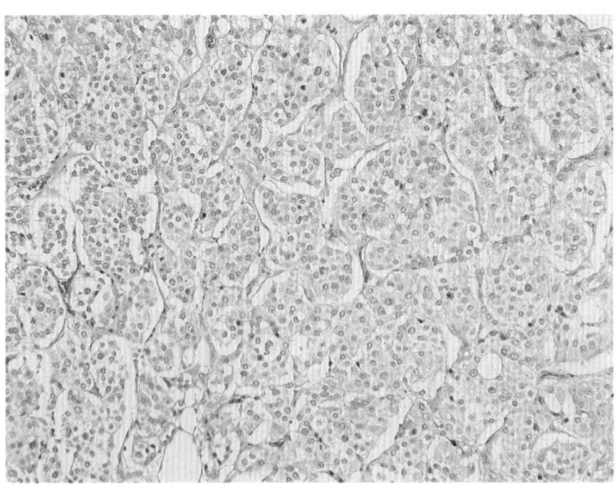

Figure 15.17. Paraganglioma (hematoxylin-eosin). Nests of tumor cells ("Zellballen") surrounded by spindled sustentacular cells. This tumor was later found to be metastatic.

normal paraganglia. Nonetheless, MIB-1 immunostaining, extensive invasion, atypical mitotic features, and confluent *de novo* necrosis can be harbingers of malignancy.

15.1.30 *Rhabdomyoma*

Rhabdomyomas are be.nign lesions of striated muscle. Although quite rare, adult and fetal subtypes have a strong predilection for the head and neck area and can be multifocal. Fetal rhabdomyomas may be a component of basal cell nevus syndrome (Gorlin's syndrome) and are composed of spindled rhabdomyoblasts with centrally placed nuclei. Adult subtypes are composed of eosinophilic polygonal cells with granular cytoplasm, peripherally placed nuclei, and frequent cross-striations (Figure 15.18). Surgical excision tends to be curative, and recurrence is rare.

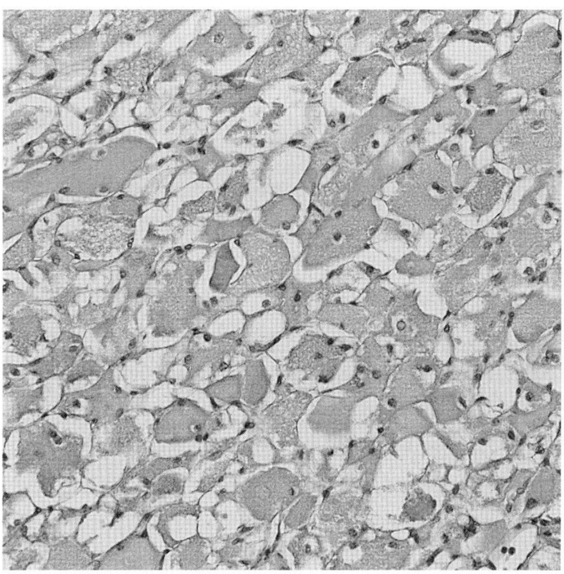

Figure 15.18. Adult rhabdomyoma. Polygonal tumor cells with granular cytoplasm (hematoxylin-eosin).

15.1.31 *Rhabdomyosarcoma*

Rhabdomyosarcoma (RMS) is a malignancy of striated muscle and is the most common sarcoma of the head and neck. It occurs predominantly in the first decade of life and has a predilection for the nasopharynx and sinonasal tract. Even though several subtypes have been described, RMS can be classified into three broad categories: embryonal, alveolar, and pleomorphic. Embryonal RMS occasionally displays a distinct polypoid appearance, which defines the "botryoid" variant. The embryonal type displays cellular zoning and is composed of an admixture of elongated cells and smaller tadpole-shaped cells. Alveolar RMS is characterized by discohesive small cells grouped in alveolar spaces. The pleomorphic type is a high-grade variant of RMS and is rare in the head and neck. It is composed of large bizarre cells of varying shape with deeply eosinophilic cytoplasm. Treatment consists of combined surgery, chemotherapy, and radiotherapy. Prognosis worsens in adults, in non-orbital cases, in nonembryonal RMS, in tumors larger than 5 cm and, of course, in the presence of positive lymph nodes or metastatic disease.

15.1.32 *Simple bone cyst*

SBC, also known as traumatic bone cyst, is a benign, intraosseous pseudocyst of unknown etiology with a predilection for the mandible. Most cases are asymptomatic and are detected as incidental findings, and may even be associated with fibro-osseous lesions. Well-delineated "scalloping" around dental roots, with little or no cortical expansion, are typical features of gnathic SBCs. Upon surgical exploration, the cavity of SBCs is either empty or fluid-filled, and may be lined by a thin fibrous capsule lacking epithelium. SBCs occurring in the jaws are usually cured by simple trepanation or conservative curettage.

15.1.33 *Solitary fibrous tumor*

Solitary fibrous tumors (SFTs) are benign mesenchymal tumors occurring in a wide variety of soft tissue locations. Some tumors formerly diagnosed as hemangiopericytomas have been reclassified as SFTs. In fact, some authorities believe that they essentially represent the same entity. Histologically, SFT is usually composed of spindle cells arranged in growth patterns varying within the same tumor. Vascularity is often prominent, and large "staghorn-shaped" vessels are noted. Malignant variants have been described. Complete conservative excision is curative, and the prognosis is good.

15.1.34 *Synovial sarcoma*

Synovial sarcomas are among the most common soft tissue sarcomas. They are histologically separated into two main patterns, biphasic and monophasic. The biphasic type is composed of gland-like epithelial elements surrounded by fascicles of spindle cells. The monophasic type is composed strictly of either mesenchymal or epithelial elements, in which case differentiation from other tumors may be challenging. The search for a specific gene translocation, namely t(x;18)(p11;q11), can be of great use in cases of diagnostic doubt. Complete surgical excision with possible chemotherapy and radiotherapy is the treatment of choice.

15.1.35 *Teratoma*

Teratomas are tumors derived from each of the three germinal layers (endoderm, mesoderm, and ectoderm). In the head and neck area, teratomas have a predilection for the neck. They are seen mostly in neonates and are benign. In contrast, teratomas in adults are more often malignant. Clinically, functional or developmental anomalies are often present, especially in cervical teratomas, thus warranting prompt treatment. Polyhydramnios is another well-known, albeit uncommon, complication of neonatal teratomas. All tumors typically contain cystic areas; in fact, a "dermoid cyst" is considered a type of benign teratomatous cyst. Teratomas may contain a wide range of tissues of variable maturity, including adnexal structures, adipose tissue, glial tissue, thyroid parenchyma, cartilage, and so forth. Treatment of benign teratomas consists of complete conservative removal. Malignant teratomas have a poor prognosis and are treated primarily by surgery, sometimes with chemotherapy and radiotherapy.

15.1.36 *Traumatic fibroma*

Traumatic fibromas ("irritation fibromas") of the oral cavity are extremely common reactive proliferations of dense fibrous connective tissue caused by chronic mechanical irritation. If the causative irritant is removed, conservative excision is curative. These tumors are histologically different from "giant cell fibromas," which are thought to be true benign fibrous neoplasms of the oral cavity. The latter are also composed of dense collagenous tissue, although with a multitude of giant stellate-shaped fibroblasts and a papillary surface on occasion.

15.1.37 *Vascular tumors and hamartomas*

Hemangiomas are among the most common soft tissue tumors/ hamartomas of the head and neck area. They may occur in any site and as multifocal lesions. Histologic features vary according to the subtype of hemangioma and the patient's age. For instance, cellularity decreases as the lesions mature. Most congenital tumors involute at least partially before puberty; hence, treatment can be delayed in cases where function or aesthetics is not impinged upon.

Arteriovenous malformations are persistent communications between arterial and venous channels. They may occur in any location, even within bone, and can elicit pain. A bruit may be detected upon auscultation. Histopathologic features are those of mature blood vessels lacking endothelial proliferation. *Sturge-Weber angiomatosis* is a related nonhereditary, developmental condition characterized by angiomas of the leptomeninges and facial skin ("port-wine stains").

Nasopharyngeal angiofibromas are benign, unencapsulated, aggressive vascular tumors that occur almost exclusively in young males. They typically involve the posterior nasal wall and can cause significant expansion and destruction of underlying bone. Histopathologic features include dense fibrous tissue containing numerous thin-walled vascular channels, some of which are dilated

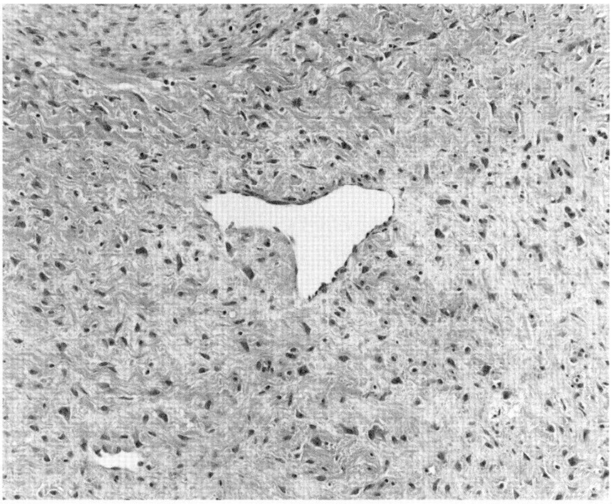

Figure 15.19. Nasopharyngeal angiofibroma (hematoxylin-eosin). Cellular fibrous stroma with a single angular and dilated blood vessel.

and angular (Figure 15.19). Complete endoscopic or external surgical removal, with possible preoperative embolization, is the treatment of choice. Inaccessible or aggressive lesions could benefit from postoperative radiotherapy. Because some tumors may express androgen receptor, patients may respond favorably to hormonal therapy; however, this has not been thoroughly established.

15.2 Odontogenic Lesions

The tooth is composed of four types of tissue found nowhere else in the human body: enamel, dentin, pulp, and cementum. These unique tissues are the result of complex embryologic interactions carried into an extensive range of dental pathology. Unsurprisingly, many odontogenic lesions recapitulate sequences of dental formation to a certain extent.

15.2.1 *Adenomatoid odontogenic tumor*

Adenomatoid odontogenic tumors are benign epithelial odontogenic tumors with a predilection for the anterior maxilla of young patients.

The tumor is typically well circumscribed and can be associated with the crown of unerupted permanent teeth. Microscopically, adenomatoid odontogenic tumors exhibit characteristic whorls of spindled epithelial cells and formation of duct-like cystic structures surrounded by ameloblastic cells. An important diagnostic pitfall is to misinterpret these areas as ameloblastomas, especially on a small biopsy specimen. Conservative curettage is curative and prognosis is excellent.

15.2.2 *Ameloblastoma*

Ameloblastoma is one of the most common benign odontogenic neoplasms. It can affect any age group. It has a predilection for the posterior mandible, which it eventually expands significantly (Figure 15.20), but it can arise in any portion of the jaws and may even occur in extragnathic sites such as the sinonasal tract. There are numerous histologic variants, such as acanthomatous (follicular), desmoplastic, granular cell, and the rare papillary subtypes. Histologic subtyping of these tumors has failed to reveal a consistent prognostic significance. Therefore, ameloblastomas are classified into three broad clinical forms: cystic (which includes unicystic and mural types), solid (or "multicystic"), and peripheral, i.e., limited to the soft tissue.

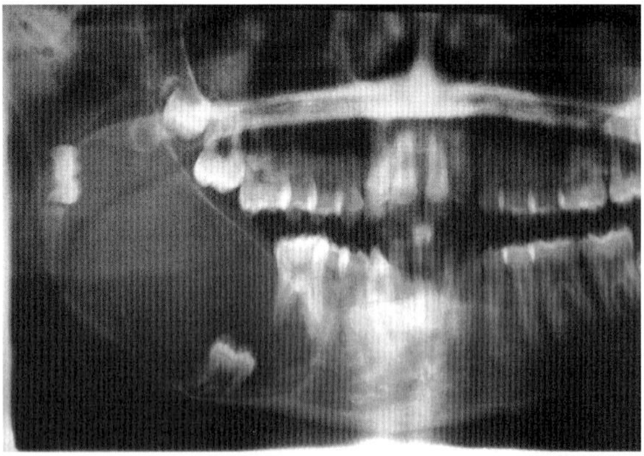

Figure 15.20. Ameloblastoma. Panoramic radiograph showing a well-defined radiolucency causing significant cortical expansion and displacement of developing teeth.

Common histologic features include interconnecting islands of basophilic epithelial cells exhibiting peripheral palisading with reverse nuclear polarization and vacuolization. The central portion of these islands is looser and edematous, thus mimicking the stellate reticulum of the enamel organ (Figure 15.21). These characteristic features might be less obvious in desmoplastic ameloblastomas, wherein epithelial islands are compressed by densely fibrous connective tissue. Otherwise, the presence of hypercellularity, pleomorphism, and increased mitotic figures in any ameloblastoma is atypical and can suggest malignant degeneration. The existence of pure unicystic ameloblastomas is debatable, as thorough sampling of the cystic wall often shows discrete islands of tumor cells, which can be interpreted as a sign of mural ameloblastoma. Nevertheless, unicystic and mural ameloblastomas can be dealt with more conservatively than solid ameloblastomas. The latter are locally aggressive and are associated with a high recurrence rate; therefore, wide excision with uninvolved

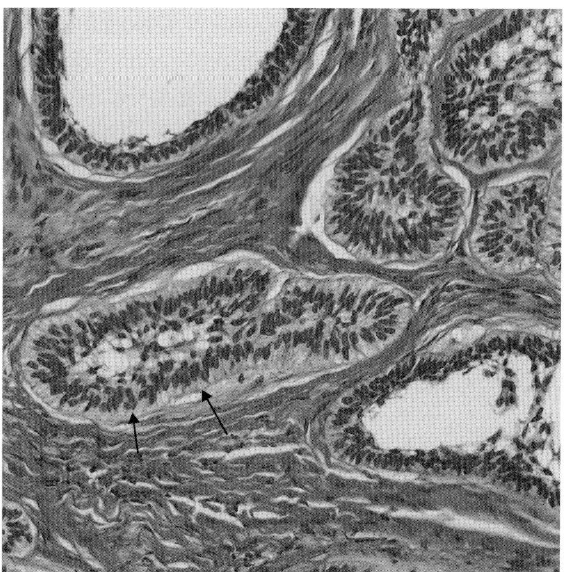

Figure 15.21. Ameloblastoma. Islands of AE (arrows), showing typical palisading of peripheral cells and reverse polarization of the nuclei (hematoxylin-eosin).

margins is the treatment of choice. Conversely, peripheral ameloblastomas are cured with simple excision.

Ameloblastomas may on rare occasions give rise to distant but cytologically benign metastatic foci ("malignant ameloblastoma"). An ameloblastic carcinoma is described as an ameloblastoma with malignant cytolopathologic features. It occurs most often in the posterior mandible and is locally aggressive, with a potential for regional and distant metastases. Prognosis is poor.

15.2.3 *Ameloblastic fibroma*

An ameloblastic fibroma (AF) is a rare, benign, mixed neoplasm of odontogenic epithelium and mesenchyme. It has a predilection for young patients and may be associated with an odontoma ("ameloblastic fibro-odontoma"). If left untreated, it can grow very large and present radiographically as a multilocular expansive radiolucency. Treatment is complete excision, the aggressiveness of which is debatable because of the relatively high recurrence rate.

Malignant degeneration of the mesenchymal component may occur and is termed "ameloblastic fibrosarcoma." Histologically, the stroma appears more cellular and composed of atypical and hyperchromatic cells. The epithelial component is much less conspicuous than in AF. Consequently, the pathologist may require thorough sampling in order to identify it and confirm the diagnosis. Wide surgical resection with tumor-free margins appears to be the treatment of choice.

15.2.4 *Calcifying epithelial odontogenic tumor*

Calcifying epithelial odontogenic tumor (CEOT), also termed "Pindborg tumor," is a rare, benign, and aggressive epithelial tumor. It is composed of islands of polyhedral cells that display nuclear pleomorphism. Amyloid production is a pathognomonic feature. Concentric psammomatoid calcifications can be seen but are not required for the diagnosis. A clear cell variant of CEOT has also been described, and must be distinguished from a clear cell odontogenic carcinoma. Conservative resection is the treatment of choice, since management by curettage is associated with a high recurrence rate.

15.2.5 *Central odontogenic fibroma*

Central odontogenic fibroma is a rare benign tumor composed of fibrous tissue of varying density and obligatory islands of odontogenic epithelium. This tumor is usually well defined and can arise in association with crowns of erupting teeth. Conservative enucleation is usually curative.

15.2.6 *Clear cell odontogenic carcinoma*

Clear cell odontogenic carcinomas are very rare malignancies of odontogenic epithelium that tend to affect the jaws of adult patients. They are characterized histologically by nests and strands of glycogen-rich epithelial cells, showing at least focal peripheral palisading with reverse nuclear polarization. They do not contain amyloid or mucous cells, thus ruling out clear-cell rich CEOT and central mucoepidermoid carcinoma (MECa), respectively. Clear cell odontogenic carcinoma must also be differentiated from metastatic clear cell tumors, such as renal cell carcinoma. Treatment may involve complete resection with wide margins, neck dissection, and postoperative radiotherapy.

15.2.7 *Inflammatory odontogenic cysts*

Inflammatory odontogenic cysts encompass a broad gamut of benign cysts derived from odontogenic rests in the jawbones or from the epithelial lining of dental follicles. They are finally diagnosed by correlating their histologic findings with clinical location and relation to teeth. For instance, an inflammatory odontogenic cyst associated with the crown of an erupting tooth is designated a "follicular" or "dentigerous" cyst. An inflammatory odontogenic cyst associated with the periapex of a nonvital tooth is a "periapical" cyst. Conservative enucleation is curative, provided that sources of infection have been removed. Untreated cysts can give rise to odontogenic tumors and carcinomas, although this is rare.

15.2.8 *Melanotic neuroectodermal tumor of infancy*

Melanotic neuroectodermal tumor of infancy is a very rare, pigmented, congenital or perinatal tumor derived from the neural crest. It occurs most commonly in the anterior maxillary bone and often displays radiographic signs of aggressiveness. Patients may demonstrate high levels of urinary vanillylmandelic acid, although this feature is nonspecific. Histopathologic features include a biphasic proliferation of large pigmented epithelioid cells and smaller, hyperchromatic round cells set in a fibrous stroma. Tumor behavior varies unpredictably from benign to malignant, therefore warranting complete surgical removal with close follow-up.

15.2.9 *Odontogenic keratocyst*

Odontogenic keratocysts (OKCs) are benign aggressive cysts with biologic features of neoplasia, which is why they have been recently reclassified as "keratocystic odontogenic tumors." They are fairly common and have a predilection for the mandible. Two histologic variants have been described: parakeratinized and orthokeratinized. Parakeratinized OKC may occur at any age and can be the first presenting sign of basal cell nevus syndrome (Gorlin's syndrome). They are lined by a uniform and narrow epithelial membrane exhibiting palisading of the basal cell layer (Figure 15.22). The epithelial-connective tissue interface is flat, which facilitates epithelial cleavage and often leads to piecemeal enucleation. The fibrous capsule is thin and friable, and may harbor small cysts ("daughter" or "satellite" cysts). Because of these features, parakeratinized OKCs tend to recur. Effective treatment options include enucleation with or without peripheral osteoectomy, cryotherapy, marsupialization, and chemical fixation.

Orthokeratinized cysts are much rarer and are not a feature of Gorlin's syndrome. In essence, the only feature they share with

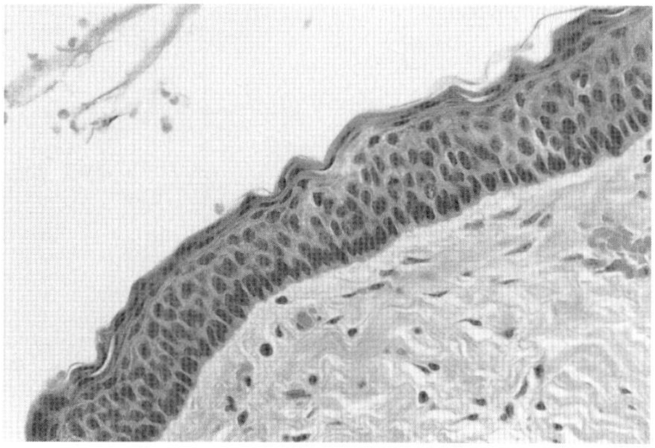

Figure 15.22. Parakeratinized OKC. A thin epithelial membrane with palisaded basal cells and a flat epithelial-connective tissue interface (hematoxylin-eosin).

parakeratinized OKCs is the production of keratin. They behave much less aggressively and are treated by conservative curettage.

15.2.10 *Odontogenic myxoma*

Odontogenic myxomas are benign aggressive mesenchymal tumors composed of loose hypocellular tissue (Figure 15.23). They occur more often in young adults, and typically expand cortices and displace teeth. Macroscopically, myxomas display a somewhat gelatinous texture and are well circumscribed but never encapsulated. Unlike soft tissue myxomas, they are not part of Carney's syndrome (pigmented skin lesions, endocrine abnormalities, and various tumors), nor are they related to Mazabraud's syndrome (fibrous dysplasia and intramuscular myxomas). Treatment involves complete resection with uninvolved surgical margins; simple curettage is insufficient.

15.3 Salivary Gland Tumors

Salivary gland neoplasms represent a vast group of tumors with seemingly endless histologic variations and architectural patterns. Treatment and outcome are usually dictated by the tumor type and clinical stage. However, in some types of salivary gland tumors, other clinical and

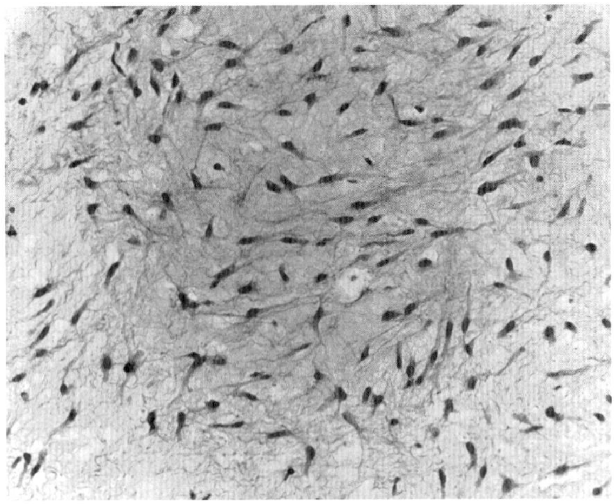

Figure 15.23. Odontogenic myxoma. Immature spindle cells in a loose hypocellular stroma (hematoxylin-eosin).

histologic parameters are as crucial. Most tumors initially present as asymptomatic masses.

Many salivary gland malignancies are cytologically benign and show rare mitoses. Therefore, malignancy is often diagnosed according to tumor behavior (e.g., perineural invasion, infiltration, lack of demarcation, and so forth). Even so, acinic cell carcinomas and other rare tumors do not obey that rule as they can be very well defined and cytologically benign. Because of the aforementioned reasons and because of the great histologic variability of salivary gland tumors, interpreting fine-needle aspirations can be both challenging and misleading. Necrosis should not be expected in low- or medium-grade malignancies. Nonetheless, *de novo* necrosis should be regarded as highly suspicious in any salivary gland tumor that has not been previously traumatized or aspirated.

15.3.1 *Benign salivary gland tumors*

15.3.1.1 *Cystadenoma*

Cystadenomas are benign cystic tumors of minor and major salivary glands. They can affect a wide age range and may present clinically as mucoceles. Histologic features include a single or multiple cystic space often lined by papillary projections. The differential diagnosis includes intraductal or inverted papillomas and other cystic salivary gland tumors. Conservative surgery is curative. Malignant versions (cystadenocarcinoma) can occur and are characterized by papillary cystic growth lacking any defining feature of other salivary gland tumors. Necrosis and mitotic figures are scarce. Therefore, malignant behavior is diagnosed by the presence of infiltrative growth.

15.3.1.2 *Monomorphic adenomas*

Monomorphic adenomas form a subgroup of benign epithelial neoplasms that include basal cell adenomas and canalicular adenomas. Basal cell adenomas have a marked predilection for the parotid gland whereas canalicular adenomas tend to arise in the upper lip. Monomorphic adenomas tend to be well circumscribed and have a good prognosis after complete surgical removal. It is worth mentioning that the membranous subtype of basal adenoma and canalicular adenomas may initially present as multifocal disease, not to be confused with a malignant feature. Furthermore, membranous basal cell adenomas can occur synchronously with dermal eccrine tumors. Basal cell adenomas are composed of basaloid cells, frequently arranged in nests or anastomosing bands. In contrast, canalicular adenomas are composed of interconnecting tubules in a rather loose connective tissue. Malignant transformation has been reported, especially in basal cell adenomas.

15.3.1.3 *Myoepithelioma*

Myoepitheliomas are viewed by some to be biologically similar to pleomorphic adenomas (PAs), but lack ductal and myxochondroid differentiation. They occur more commonly in the parotid gland and in the palate. Histologically, they can easily be mistaken for a wide variety of benign and malignant tumors, given the broad array of growth patterns they may display. Treatment consists of complete intact removal.

15.3.1.4 *Oncocytoma*

Oncocytomas are benign tumors composed entirely of oncocytes, which are polygonal epithelial cells with eosinophilic and granular cytoplasm. They tend to be well delineated but may lack a well-formed fibrous capsule. Mitotic figures are rare, and constitute an important feature in ruling out malignancy. Multifocal foci or infiltrative nests of benign oncocytes raise the possibility of oncocytosis or oncocytic hyperplasia, which are benign non-neoplastic conditions.

15.3.1.5 *Pleomorphic adenoma*

PA, also termed benign mixed tumor of salivary glands, represents the most common tumor of salivary gland origin. It can affect any age group and may occur synchronously with other salivary gland tumors. PA arising in the major glands tends to be encapsulated, whereas in the minor salivary gland, it often lacks a well-formed capsule. Histologically, PA demonstrates both epithelial/myoepithelial and mesenchymal differentiation. The former is typically characterized by bilayered ducts in association with nonductal cells exhibiting several cell types. Squamous metaplasia can be prominent and must not be misinterpreted as a sign of malignancy. Mesenchymal areas are characterized by myxoid, chondroid, hyalinized, or osseous differentiation (Figure 15.24). Complete integral excision is the treatment of choice, and great care should be taken to ensure that the tumor margins are uncompromised. Tumors ruptured or damaged during surgery have a much higher recurrence rate; in those cases, patients may benefit from postoperative radiation therapy. Malignant transformation can occur (see Section 15.3.2.5 of this chapter).

15.3.1.6 *Sebaceous lymphadenoma and sebaceous adenoma*

Sebaceous lymphadenoma and sebaceous adenoma are rare, benign, epithelial, salivary gland tumors thought to be derived from sebaceous lobules normally found in salivary glands, in the oral mucosa, or in

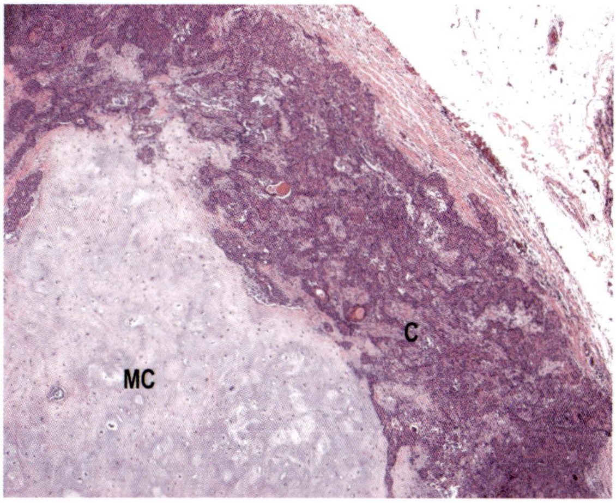

Figure 15.24. PA. Encapsulated tumor showing hypocellular (myxoid-chondroid) (MC) areas and cellular (C) areas (hematoxylin-eosin).

parotid lymph nodes. Both tumors are well delineated and often encapsulated. Histologic features include solid and cystic areas displaying mature sebaceous differentiation. In sebaceous lymphadenoma, epithelial elements are surrounded by benign lymphoid tissue. Sebaceous adenoma and sebaceous lymphadenoma are cured by complete conservative excision. Malignant counterparts are extremely rare.

15.3.1.7 *Sialoblastoma*

Sialoblastomas are rare congenital or perinatal tumors that have a strong predilection for the parotid gland and the submandibular gland. They are regarded as low-grade malignancies because of their high recurrence rate and possible regional node metastasis. Histopathologic features include a proliferation of basaloid islands of primitive cells with focal ductal differentiation. Mitotic features can be numerous, but are scarcely atypical.

15.3.1.8 *Warthin's tumor*

Warthin's tumor is the second most common benign salivary gland tumor. It has a strong predilection for the parotid gland and for smokers.

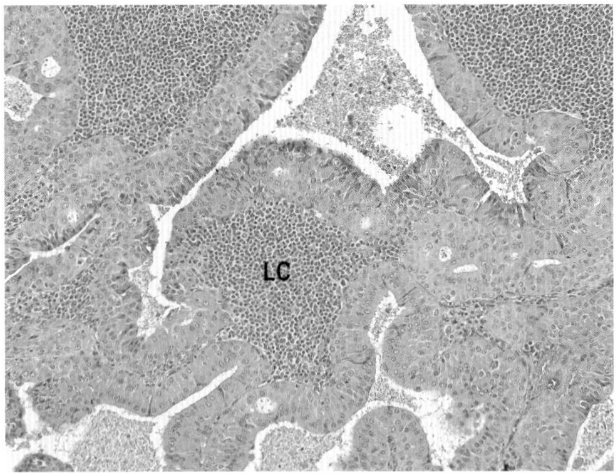

Figure 15.25. Warthin's tumor. Cystic spaces surrounded by double-layered papillary projections of tumor cells, admixed with lymphoid cells (LC) (hematoxylin-eosin).

It can be bilateral or multicentric within the same gland. Warthin's tumors are well delineated and encapsulated. They are composed of cystic spaces lined by papillary growth of a double layer of columnar oncocytes, admixed with benign lymphoid tissue (Figure 15.25). Recurrence rate is low in cases of unifocal Warthin's tumor.

15.3.2 *Malignant salivary gland tumors*

15.3.2.1 *Acinic cell adenocarcinoma*

Acinic cell adenocarcinoma (ACA) is a relatively common low-grade salivary gland malignancy that has a predilection for the parotid gland. Synchronous bilateral involvement is possible, although very rare. As its name implies, an ACA is composed of acinic cells that display a basophilic cytoplasm containing diastase-resistant, periodic acid-Schiff–positive, zymogen-like granules. Additional cell types are present, such as vacuolated cells, which can also be encountered in other salivary gland tumors. ACA is typically classified according to four growth patterns: solid, microcystic, papillary-cystic, and follicular. The latter resembles follicular tumors of the thyroid. ACA are typically well circumscribed and can even be encapsulated. In a manner comparable with MECa, ACA often harbors a mature lymphoid reaction. Complete surgical resection is the treatment of choice, with adjuvant radiotherapy in cervical metastases or incompletely excised tumors.

15.3.2.2 *Adenocarcinoma*

Adenocarcinomas NOS (ANOS) are defined as salivary adenocarcinomas that do not fit any specific diagnosis. Basically, ANOS is a diagnosis of exclusion. By definition, all tumors show ductal differentiation, although they display a dazzling array of growth patterns and cell types. Necrosis, hemorrhage, abnormal mitoses, and cellular atypia are features seen in high-grade ANOS. However, perineural invasion can be seen in all grades of ANOS and should not be used as a discriminatory criterion. Tumors arising in the minor salivary glands have a better overall prognosis. High-grade ANOS are among the deadliest salivary gland tumors and should be dealt with aggressively.

15.3.2.3 *Adenoid cystic carcinoma*

Adenoid cystic carcinoma (ACC), formerly known as cylindroma, is one of the most common malignancies of salivary or seromucous gland origin. It may arise in any location containing salivary glands. It is rare in children. Clinically, patients with ACC can present with pain and paralysis, likely due to a typically high incidence of sweeping neurotropism. Three growth patterns have been described: cribriform (the most common), tubular, and solid. The cribriform type is characterized by the formation of circular cyst-like areas referred to as a Swiss cheese pattern (Figure 15.26). The tubular type exhibits obvious ductal differentiation and often extensive hyalinized material. Lastly, solid ACCs are composed of dense nests and sheets of tumor cells with minimal ductal or pseudocystic areas. All three types of ACC contain myoepithelial cells with archetypical dark and angular nuclei. ACCs are indolent but relentless tumors with a poor

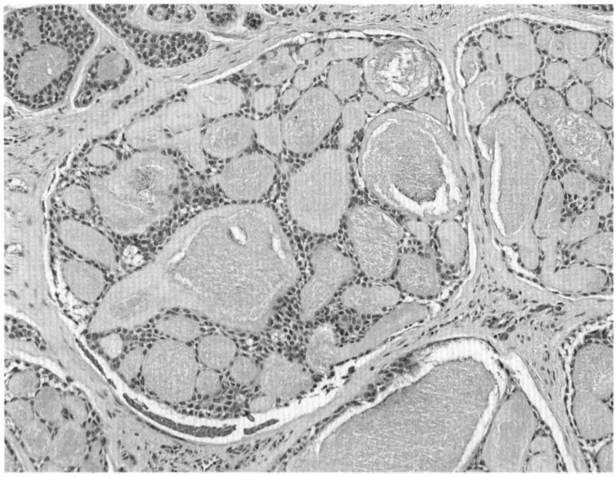

Figure 15.26. ACC. Cribriform ("Swiss cheese") pattern (hematoxylin-eosin).

long-term outcome. Prognosis is poorer in tumors larger than 4 cm, in seromucous gland ACC, and in predominantly solid tumors. The primary treatment of ACC is wide surgical excision, including assessment of tumor spread along peripheral nerves through intraoperative frozen sections. Radiotherapy may be useful in controlling microscopic residual disease.

15.3.2.4 *Basal cell adenocarcinoma*

Basal cell adenocarcinoma is a rare low-grade malignancy, with a propensity for the parotid gland and for adults. Since it is cytologically benign and rarely shows necrosis, its malignant nature is often confirmed solely by the presence of infiltrative growth. Assessing malignancy on small biopsy samples is a perilous endeavor, which can also be said of many salivary gland tumors. Complete excision is the treatment of choice.

15.3.2.5 *Carcinoma ex PA*

Carcinoma ex PA is defined as a malignant epithelial neoplasm arising in a PA. It is associated with a poor prognosis, especially with

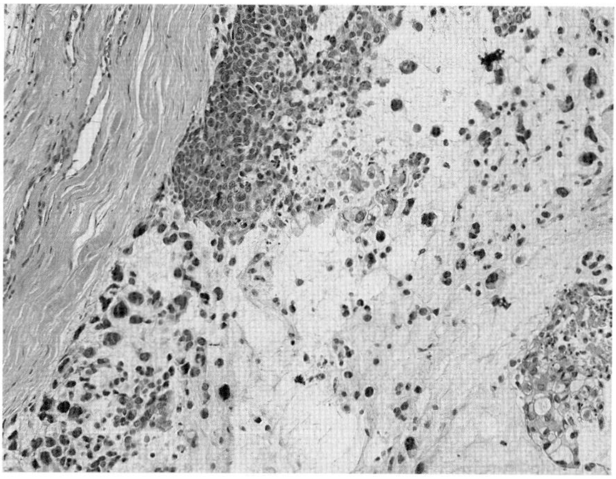

Figure 15.27. Malignant mixed tumor/carcinosarcoma. Malignant epithelial and mesenchymal cells. This tumor arose in a preexisting encapsulated PA (hematoxylin-eosin).

high-grade carcinomas and extensively invasive tumors. However, further subclassification of the malignant portion is not clinically relevant. When both epithelial and mesenchymal components of a PA are synchronously malignant, the term "carcinosarcoma" (or malignant mixed tumor) is applied (Figure 15.27).

Metastasizing PA is an unusual condition characterized by metastatic foci of histologically benign PA. Metastatic deposits have been reported in numerous sites, but are more common in bone and lungs. There is no established form of therapy, although metastatectomy has been used with success.

15.3.2.6 *Clear cell carcinoma*

Clear cell carcinoma is a very rare low-grade malignancy of the salivary gland, composed of a uniform population of clear cells. Since these can be seen in other salivary gland tumors, clear cell carcinoma can be regarded as a diagnosis of exclusion. The background stroma can vary from delicate to densely fibrous, to hyalinized and sclerotic. Mitotic figures are scarce and necrosis is absent. Differential diagnosis includes mainly odontogenic clear cell carcinomas, clear cell-rich MECa, and metastatic renal cell carcinomas. Surgery with or without radiotherapy is the treatment of choice.

15.3.2.7 *Epithelial-myoepithelial carcinoma*

Epithelial-myoepithelial carcinoma is a rare, low-grade salivary gland tumor that has a predilection for the parotid gland and older patients. It is composed of a biphasic cell population arranged in double-layered ductal structures. Sometimes a prominent deposition of hyalinized material is seen, which, in combination with ductal differentiation, may suggest a diagnosis of tubular ACC or PA. Epithelial-myoepithelial carcinoma is associated with a relatively high recurrence rate and a tendency to metastasize to regional lymph nodes.

15.3.2.8 *Mucoepidermoid carcinoma*

MECa is one of the most common malignancies of salivary gland origin. As its designation implies, a MECa is composed of both epidermoid (squamous) and mucous cells (Figure 15.28). However,

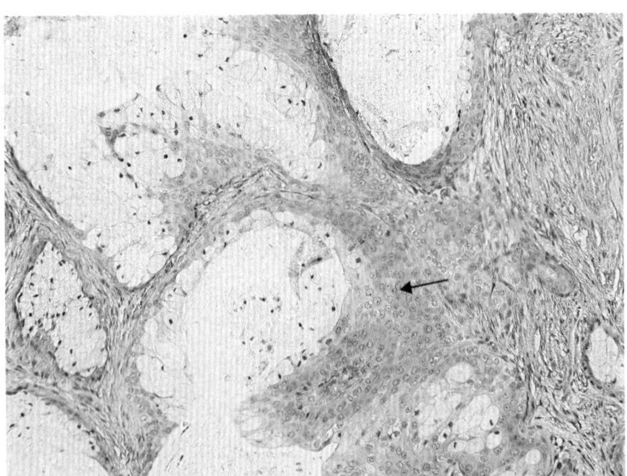

Figure 15.28. Low-grade MECa (hematoxylin-eosin). Cystic areas lined by mucous, epidermoid (arrow), and clear cells.

other cell types are also present, such as the so-called intermediate cell and clear cells. A common diagnostic pitfall would be to mistake MECa and necrotizing sialometaplasia (a reactive and self-limiting process), or vice versa, as these entities share comparable histologic features. MECa can occur within the jawbones and must be differentiated from benign glandular odontogenic cysts, which lack complex architecture and invasion into adjacent bone.

Cystic areas are common in MECa, especially in low-grade tumors, although true ductal differentiation is seldom present. High-grade tumors tend to display cytologic atypia and a higher mitotic rate as well as necrosis and frank anaplasia (Figure 15.29). High-grade tumors may be composed almost exclusively of squamous cells with very few other cell types, thus emulating poorly differentiated squamous cell carcinomas. MECa tends to be infiltrated by lymphocytes, and may also elicit an intense inflammatory response. The most widely accepted classification of MECa is the Armed Forces Institute of Pathology grading proposed by Auclair *et al.* (Table 15.1). Treatment of MECa depends on tumor location, clinical stage, and tumor grade. Tumors of the submandibular gland, floor of mouth, tongue, and maxillary sinus behave more aggressively.

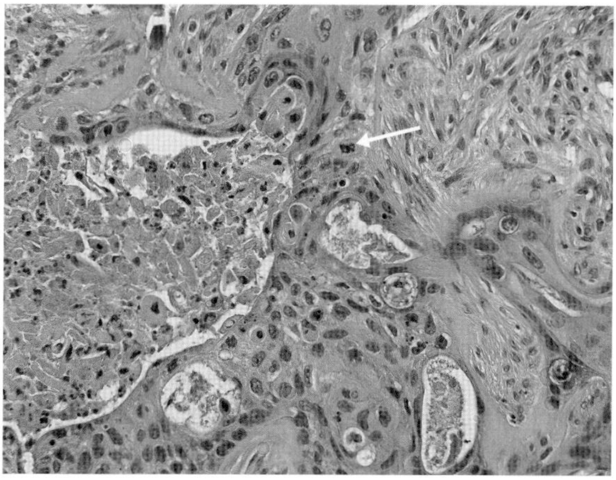

Figure 15.29. High-grade MECa. Microcystic areas filled with necrotic debris and lined by epidermoid tumor cells. Nuclear pleomorphism and mitoses (arrow) are present (hematoxylin-eosin).

Table 15.1. Armed Forces Institute of Pathology Grading of MECa.

Histologic parameter	Parameter point value
Intracystic component less than 20%	+2
Neural invasion present	+2
Necrosis present	+3
Mitotic figures (4 or more per 10 high-power fields)	+3
Anaplasia	+4
Grade	**Total score**
Low grade	0–4
Intermediate grade	5–6
High grade	7 or more

15.3.2.9 *Polymorphous low-grade adenocarcinomas*

Polymorphous low-grade adenocarcinomas (PLGAs) are slow-growing tumors, the overwhelming majority of which involve intraoral minor salivary glands. As their name implies, PLGAs exhibit a wide variety of growth patterns. They are cytologically very bland and can even be partially well delineated. PLGAs may contain myxoid or mucoid areas which, combined with their unremarkable cytomorphic features, can be reminiscent of PAs. However, infiltration into the adjacent tissue and perineural involvement are extremely common features that are not seen in PAs (Figure 15.30). Complete surgical excision is often the only treatment required. Nodal metastasis is very rare.

15.3.2.10 *Salivary duct carcinoma*

Arguably the most aggressive malignancy of salivary gland origin, salivary duct carcinoma arises mostly in the major glands and has a predilection for male patients. Histologic findings include large duct-like structures with comedonecrosis and the formation of characteristic "Roman arches" and cribriform areas (Figure 15.31). Cytologic atypia is marked, and mitotic figures are readily identifiable. Since all these features may also be seen in ductal carcinoma of the breast, metastatic disease must be ruled out. Prognosis decreases with large primary tumor size, HER2/neu overexpression, and micropapillary areas.

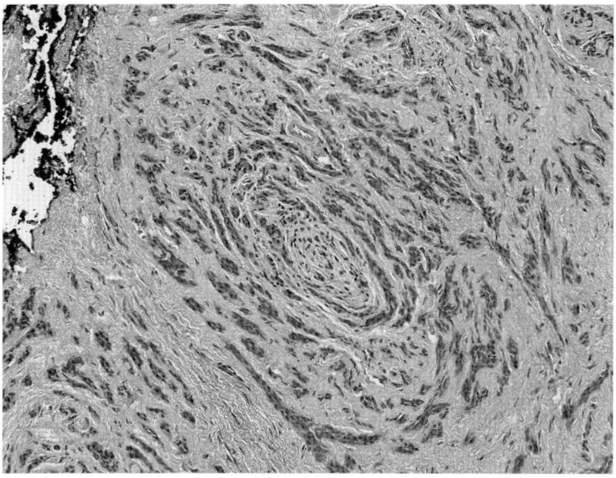

Figure 15.30. PLGA. Typical "targetoid" perineural infiltration, resembling lobular carcinoma of the breast (hematoxylin-eosin).

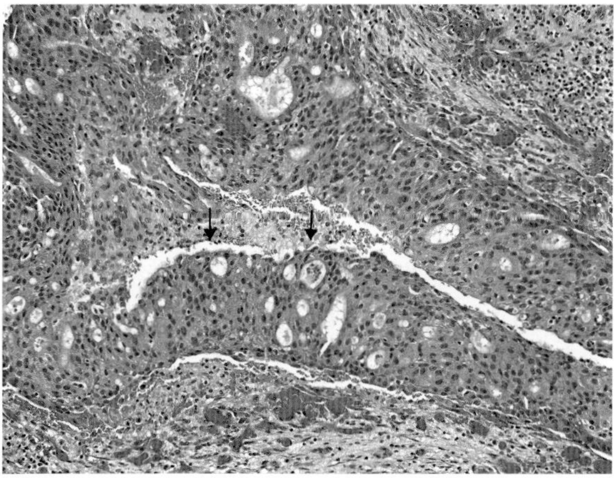

Figure 15.31. Salivary duct carcinoma. Cystic area with central necrosis. The epithelium exhibits typical "Roman arches" (arrows) and cribriform areas (hematoxylin-eosin).

15.4 Mucosal Neoplasia

15.4.1 *Melanoma*

Mucosal melanomas are less common than their cutaneous counterpart. They may arise from any mucosa of the head and neck area, the most common locations being the sinonasal tract, gingiva, and hard palate (Figure 15.32). Melanomas are known among pathologists as "the great mimickers" since they can easily be confused with carcinomas, sarcomas, and all the "round blue cell tumors" (Table 15.2). Indeed, they display an astonishing array of different growth patterns and cell types, often requiring immunohistochemical stains to confirm

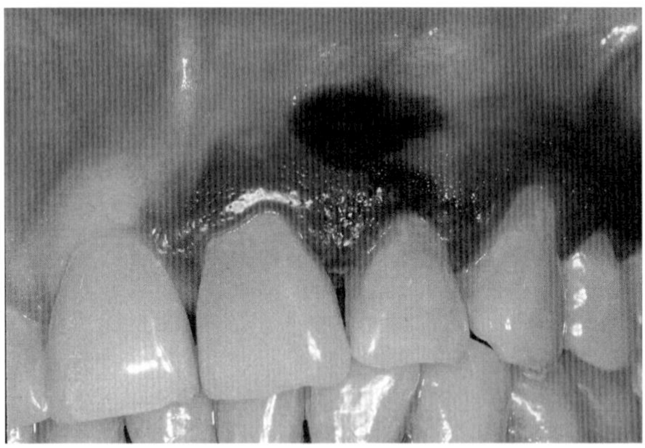

Figure 15.32. Melanoma. Diffuse and heterogeneous pigmentation of the left maxillary gingiva.

Table 15.2. Differential Diagnosis of Round Blue Cell Tumors of the Head and Neck.

Melanoma
Rhabdomyosarcoma
Sinonasal undifferentiated carcinoma
Lymphoma
Extramedullary plasmacytoma
Olfactory neuroblastoma
Ewing's sarcoma/primitive neuroectodermal tumor
Neuroendocrine carcinoma/small cell carcinoma
Ectopic pituitary adenoma
Melanotic neuroectodermal tumor of infancy
Mesenchymal chondrosarcoma
Small cell variant of osteosarcoma
Occult metastasis

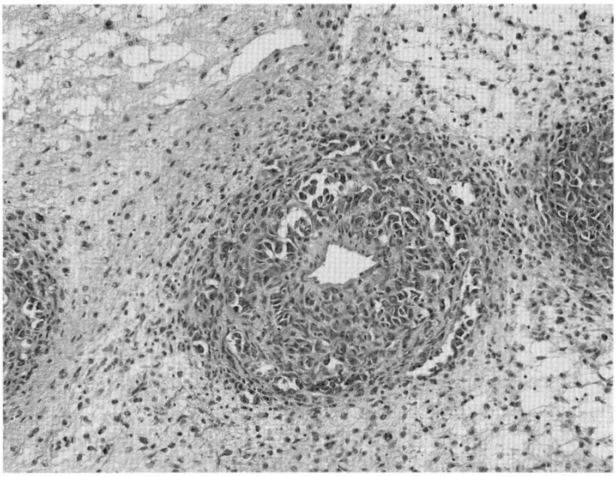

Figure 15.33. Melanoma (hematoxylin-eosin). Pathognomonic peritheliomatous distribution of pigmented and atypical cells.

the diagnosis. Desmoplastic melanomas are especially challenging to diagnose on routine histologic sections. In all melanomas, the presence of melanin pigment and junctional activity is certainly helpful for the diagnosis but is often lacking. A perivascular (peritheliomatous) distribution is pathognomonic (Figure 15.33). Treatment consists of wide excision with radiotherapy. Prognosis is very poor, and decreases with advanced stage, multifocal tumors, and the presence of angioinvasion.

15.4.2 *Nasopharyngeal carcinoma*

Nasopharyngeal carcinoma, formerly known as lymphoepithelial carcinoma, is a group of malignancies arising in the nasopharyngeal mucosa. They are separated into three categories: nonkeratinizing (the most common), keratinizing, and basaloid squamous. The tumor is epidemic in East Asian countries, and affects males more often than females. It initially presents with cervical lymphadenopathy followed by nasal symptoms.

The nonkeratinizing type is characterized by variably shaped epithelial cells with ill-defined borders, admixed with lymphocytes and occasional eosinophils. It is strongly associated with Epstein-Barr virus.

The keratinizing type resembles typical squamous cell carcinoma. It is radio resistant, is rarely associated with Epstein-Barr virus, and has a poor prognosis.

The basaloid squamous type is identical to basaloid squamous carcinoma of other anatomic sites. It is extremely rare in the nasopharynx and is associated with a very poor prognosis.

The primary treatment is radiotherapy with or without chemotherapy. Surgery is reserved for tumors that do not respond to radiotherapy or for recurrences.

15.4.3 *Olfactory neuroblastoma*

Olfactory neuroblastoma, also known as esthesioneuroblastoma, is a neuroectodermal malignancy thought to be derived from the olfactory membrane. It occurs in all age groups. By far the most common site of occurrence is the upper nasal cavity, with frequent involvement of the ethmoid sinus. Rare ectopic cases in the nasopharynx and paranasal sinuses have been reported. Olfactory neuroblastomas are often divided into four grades according to the Hyams grading system, which depends on several factors such as lobular architecture, pleomorphism, neurofibrillary matrix, rosette and pseudorosette formation, mitoses, necrosis, and calcifications. In essence, low-grade tumors contain abundant neurofibrillary matrix, lack mitoses and necrosis, and contain pseudorosettes (Homer Wright type). High-grade tumors have larger tumor cells and display marked pleomorphism and mitotic activity, as well as true rosette formation (Flexner–Wintersteiner); neurofibrillary matrix is scant or absent. Olfactory neuroblastoma is treated by endoscopic or open surgery and postoperative radiotherapy, sometimes with chemotherapy and bone marrow transplantation. Patients with tumors confined to the nasal cavity (stage A) fare much better than those whose tumors extend beyond the sinonasal cavities (stage C) (Figure 15.34). Prognosis is also dependent on histologic grading and proliferation rate.

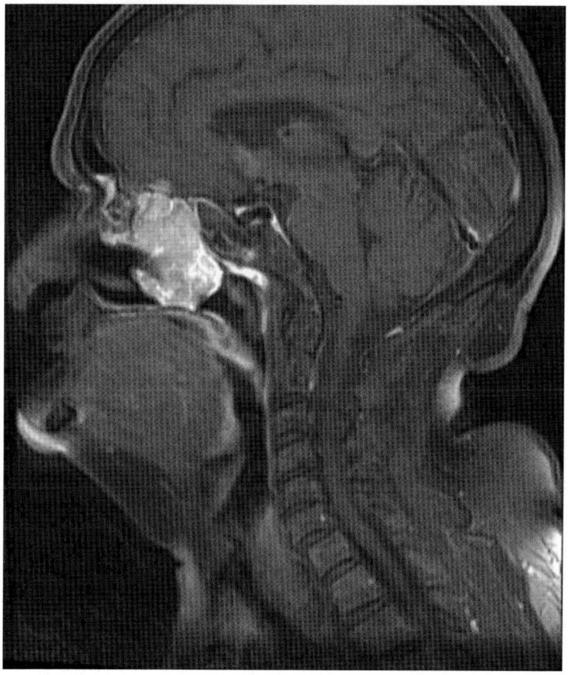

Figure 15.34. Olfactory neuroblastoma. Sagittal view of a T1-weighted, fat-saturated magnetic resonance image showing involvement of the superior aspect of the nasal cavity with slight intracranial extension.

15.4.4 *Sinonasal undifferentiated carcinoma*

Sinonasal undifferentiated carcinoma (SNUC) is a rare high-grade epithelial malignancy of the paranasal sinuses and nasal cavity lacking glandular differentiation. At the time of diagnosis, patients present with advanced disease along with multiple nasal symptoms, pain, and cranial nerve disturbances. Histologic features include the formation of lobules or sheets of poorly differentiated round blue cells (Table 15.2). These tumors are usually Epstein-Barr virus–negative. Cytologic atypia, mitoses, and necrosis are prominent features. SNUCs are treated by combined surgery, radiotherapy, and chemotherapy. Prognosis is very poor.

15.4.5 *Squamous cell carcinoma*

Squamous cell carcinoma is by far the most common malignancy of the head and neck area, excluding cutaneous neoplasms. Known risk factors include tobacco, alcohol, some human papillomavirus (HPV) subtypes, carcinogen exposure, genomic instability, immunosuppression (acquired immunodeficiency syndrome), and a diet poor in fresh vegetables and fruits. Most squamous cell carcinomas arise from preexisting dysplastic mucosal alterations presenting as erythroplakia, leukoplakia, or nonhealing ulcers. Advanced stages of involvement may appear as indurated ulcers, irregular osteolytic lesions, and exophytic masses with well-defined raised edges and coarse surfaces (Figures 15.35 and 15.36). Tumor, node, metastasis staging depends on the exact anatomic site, partly because of different lymphatic drainage.

Squamous cell carcinomas are histologically classified according to their level of differentiation and whether they produce keratin. Well-differentiated tumors are reminiscent of normal squamous mucosa, albeit with several atypical features such as invasion, disorganized growth, nuclear pleomorphism, increased mitotic figures, keratin "pearl" formation, single-cell keratinization, and acantholysis. The term *adenoid squamous carcinoma* is used when epithelial islands demonstrate pseudoglandular spaces due to extensive acantholysis; this is not to be confused with adenosquamous carcinoma (see below).

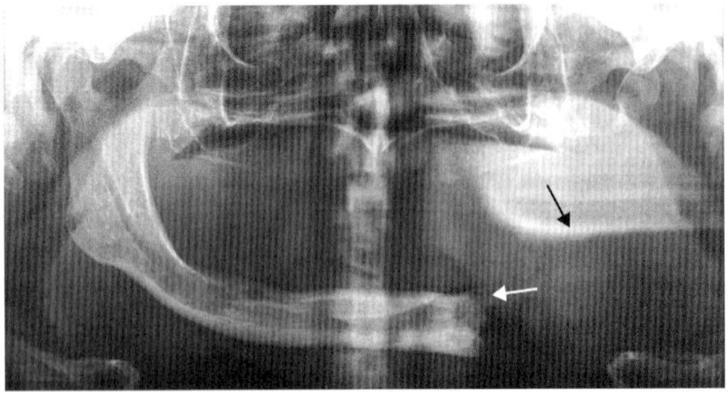

Figure 15.35. Squamous cell carcinoma. Panoramic radiograph showing massive and irregular resorption of the left mandible (arrows).

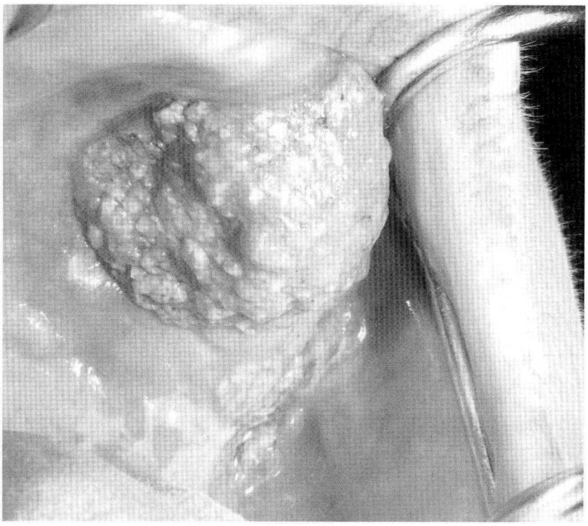

Figure 15.36. Squamous cell carcinoma of the left maxilla.

15.4.5.1 *Squamous cell carcinoma variants*

15.4.5.1.1 *Verrucous carcinoma (VC).* VC is an extremely well-differentiated squamous cell carcinoma variant, presenting clinically as a locally destructive lesion with limited metastatic capabilities. The oral cavity and the larynx are the most common sites of occurrence. The exact pathogenesis is unknown, although a strong association with HPV has been demonstrated. Histologically, VC is characterized by warty and hyperkeratotic epithelium exhibiting an exophytic and endophytic growth pattern. Epithelial dysplasia is either absent or minimal. Invasion occurs as a broad pushing border; therefore, it may sometimes be difficult to distinguish VC from benign verrucous hyperplasia, especially on small or mangled biopsy specimens. VC is treated by complete surgical excision and has a better prognosis than squamous cell carcinoma. It is important to thoroughly sample the surgical bed to rule out foci of concurrent conventional squamous cell carcinoma.

15.4.5.1.2 *Spindle cell carcinoma (sarcomatoid).* This variant of squamous cell carcinoma is widely underdiagnosed and often mistaken for a sarcoma. It usually presents clinically as polypoid and ulcerated lesions,

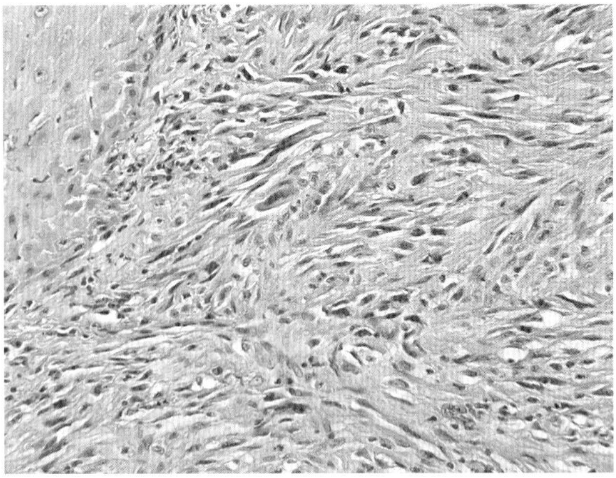

Figure 15.37. Spindle cell carcinoma. Atypical spindle cells merging with the surface epithelium (upper left) (hematoxylin-eosin).

and has a propensity for older men. These tumors are composed of atypical spindle cells arranged in a fascicular or storiform pattern. When visible, merging of squamous cell carcinoma in situ with the spindle cell population is pathognomonic of spindle cell carcinoma (Figure 15.37). Diffuse cytokeratin expression or lack of expression of other markers helps in confirming the diagnosis. However, focal cytokeratin staining should not be used as the sole diagnostic criterion because sarcomas and melanomas may exhibit partial keratin expression. Spindle cell carcinoma should be treated as a carcinoma and not as a sarcoma. Surgery is the primary treatment modality, and patients may benefit from radiotherapy and chemotherapy, depending on clinical stage.

15.4.5.1.3 *Papillary squamous cell carcinoma.* This variant typically occurs in the larynx of older patients and presents as exophytic finger-like projections. HPV may be involved in its pathogenesis. The treatment of choice is surgery with possible radiotherapy. Prognosis is comparable to that of conventional squamous cell carcinoma.

15.4.5.1.4 *Basaloid squamous carcinoma.* The most aggressive variant of squamous cell carcinoma. It has a strong predilection for the base of the tongue, and typically presents with cervical lymphadenopathy. Histologic findings consist of islands of dark, basaloid cells with peripheral palisading and central necrosis. Squamous differentiation can be minimal, and cytologic features of malignancy are conspicuous. Basaloid squamous carcinoma is treated by complete resection, with neck dissection, radiotherapy, and chemotherapy.

15.4.5.1.5 *Adenosquamous carcinoma.* This is a rare and highly aggressive variant of squamous cell carcinoma, characterized by combined squamous and true glandular differentiation. *In situ* carcinoma is often present and is helpful in differentiating this tumor from an adenocarcinoma displaying squamous differentiation. There is an enduring controversy as to whether this is a true, distinct entity or a high-grade variant of MECa.

Acknowledgments

I would like to thank Dr. Faizan Alawi, assistant professor of pathology at University of Pennsylvania School of Dental Medicine, for his help in preparing this chapter.

I am also grateful to the following mentors for their invaluable teachings and sheer talent: Drs. Paul D. Freedman, Stanley Kerpel, Renée Reich, Ronald A. DeLellis, Amy Chadburn, Mark Edgar, Syed A. Hoda, Glauco Frizzera, Sandra J. Shin, Paul P. Rosen, Gilles Lavigne, Satish K. Tickoo, Douglas Flieder, and others.

Further Reading

Head and neck pathology

1. **Thompson LDR.** *Head and Neck Pathology: A Volume in Foundations in Diagnostic Pathology Series.* Philadelphia, PA: Elsevier; 2006.
2. **Wenig BM.** *Atlas of Head and Neck Pathology.* 2nd edn. Philadelphia, PA: Elsevier; 2008.
3. **Gnepp DR.** *Diagnostic Surgical Pathology of the Head and Neck.* 2nd edn. Philadelphia, PA: Saunders; 2009.

Salivary gland pathology

1. **Ellis GL, Auclair PL.** *Tumors of the Salivary Glands. AFIP Atlas of the Tumor Pathology.* Series 4. Silver Spring, MD: American Registry of Pathology; 2008.

Soft tissue pathology

1. **Weiss SW, Goldblum JR.** *Enzinger and Weiss's Soft Tissue Tumors.* 5th edn. St. Louis, MO: Mosby; 2007.

Oral and maxillofacial pathology

1. **Neville B, Damm DD, Allen CM, Bouquot J.** *Oral and Maxillofacial Pathology.* 3rd edn. Philadelphia, PA: Saunders; 2008.

Selected Bibliography

1. **Alawi F.** Benign fibro-osseous diseases of the maxillofacial bones: a review and differential diagnosis. *Am J Clin Pathol* 2002;118 (Suppl):S50–S70.
2. **Alawi F, Stratton D, Freedman PD.** Solitary fibrous tumor of the oral soft tissues: a clinicopathologic and immunohistochemical study of 16 cases. *Am J Surg Pathol* 2001;25:900–910.
3. **Al-Daraji W, Lasota J, Foss R, Miettinen M.** Synovial sarcoma involving the head: analysis of 36 cases with predilection to the parotid and temporal regions. *Am J Surg Pathol* 2009;33:1494–1503.
4. **Auclair PL, Goode RK, Ellis GL.** Mucoepidermoid carcinoma of intraoral salivary glands: evaluation and application of grading criteria in 143 cases. *Cancer* 1992;69:2021–2030.
5. **Brandwein M, Said-Al-Naief N, Gordon R, Urken M.** Clear cell odontogenic carcinoma: report of a case and analysis of the literature. *Arch Otolaryngol Head Neck Surg* 2002;128:1089–1095.
6. **Chen JD, Morrison C, Zhang C, Kahnoski K, Carpten JD, Teh BT.** Hyperparathyroidism-jaw tumour syndrome. *J Intern Med* 2003;253:634–642.
7. **Crowley TE, Kaugars GE, Gunsolley JC.** Odontogenic keratocysts: a clinical and histologic comparison of the parakeratin and orthokeratin variants. *J Oral Maxillofac Surg* 1992;50:22–26.
8. **Czader M, Eberhart CG, Bhatti N, Cummings C, Westra WH.** Metastasizing mixed tumor of the parotid: initial presentation as a solitary kidney tumor and

ultimate carcinomatous transformation at the primary site. *Am J Surg Pathol* 2000;24:1159–1164.

9. **David LA, Sàndor GK, Evans AW, Brown DH.** Hyperbaric oxygen therapy and mandibular osteoradionecrosis: a retrospective study and analysis of treatment outcomes. *J Can Dent Assoc* 2001;67:384.
10. **Davis SE, Rice DH.** Langerhans' cell histiocytosis: current trends and the role of the head and neck surgeon. *Ear Nose Throat J* 2004;83:340, 342, 344.
11. **Dunbar SF, Rosenberg A, Mankin H, Rosenthal D, Suit HD.** Gorham's massive osteolysis: the role of radiation therapy and a review of the literature. *Int J Radiat Oncol Biol Phys* 1993;26:491–497.
12. **Ellis GL, Corio RL.** Acinic cell adenocarcinoma: a clinicopathologic analysis of 294 cases. *Cancer* 1983;52:542–549.
13. **Ellis GL, Wiscovitch JG.** Basal cell adenocarcinoma of the major salivary glands. *Oral Surg Oral Med Oral Pathol* 1990;69:461–469.
14. **Frierson HF Jr, Mills SE, Fechner RE, Taxy JB, Levine PA.** Sinonasal undifferentiated carcinoma: an aggressive neoplasm derived from schneiderian epithelium and distinct from olfactory neuroblastoma. *Am J Surg Pathol* 1986;10: 771–779.
15. **Hicks J, Flaitz C.** Rhabdomyosarcoma of the head and neck in children. *Oral Oncol* 2002;38:450–459.
16. **Koch BB, Trask DK, Hoffman HT, *et al.*** National survey of head and neck verrucous carcinoma: patterns of presentation, care, and outcome. *Cancer* 2001; 92:110–120.
17. **Kruse-Lösler B, Gaertner C, Bürger H, Seper L, Joos U, Kleinheinz J.** Melanotic neuroectodermal tumor of infancy: systematic review of the literature and presentation of a case [published online ahead of print June 8, 2006]. *Oral Surg Oral Med Oral Pathol Oral Radiol Endod* 2006;102:204–216. doi:10.1016/j.tripleo.2005.08.010.
18. **Kumaki N, Kajiwara H, Kameyama K, *et al.*** Prediction of malignant behavior of pheochromocytomas and paragangliomas using immunohistochemical techniques. *Endocr Pathol* 2002;13:149–156.
19. **Lewis JE, Olsen KD, Sebo TJ.** Carcinoma ex pleomorphic adenoma: pathologic analysis of 73 cases. *Hum Pathol* 2001;32:596–604.
20. **Li TJ, Sun LS, Luo HY.** Odontogenic myxoma: a clinicopathologic study of 25 cases. *Arch Pathol Lab Med* 2006;130:1799–1806.
21. **Marx RE, Cillo JE Jr., Ulloa JJ.** Oral bisphosphonate-induced osteonecrosis: risk factors, prediction of risk using serum CTX testing, prevention, and treatment. *J Oral Maxillofac Surg* 2007;65:2397–2410.

22. **Mills SE, Frierson HF Jr.** Olfactory neuroblastoma: a clinicopathologic study of 21 cases. *Am J Surg Pathol* 1985;9:317–327.
23. **Nagao T, Gaffey TA, Visscher DW,** *et al.* Invasive micropapillary salivary duct carcinoma: a distinct histologic variant with biologic significance. *Am J Surg Pathol* 2004;28:319–326.
24. **Oliveira AM, Perez-Atayde AR, Inwards CY,** *et al.* USP6 and CDH11 oncogenes identify the neoplastic cell in primary aneurysmal bone cysts and are absent in so-called secondary aneurysmal bone cysts. *Am J Pathol* 2004;165: 1773–1780.
25. **Ordóñez NG.** Granular cell tumor: a review and update. *Adv Anat Pathol* 1999;6:186–203.
26. **Philipsen HP, Reichart PA.** Calcifying epithelial odontogenic tumour: biological profile based on 181 cases from the literature. *Oral Oncol* 2000;36:17–26.
27. **Philipsen HP, Reichart PA, Zhang KH, Nikai H, Yu QX.** Adenomatoid odontogenic tumor: biologic profile based on 499 cases. *J Oral Pathol Med* 1991;20:149–158.
28. **Pryor SG, Moore EJ, Kasperbauer JL.** Endoscopic versus traditional approaches for excision of juvenile nasopharyngeal angiofibroma. *Laryngoscope* 2005;115:1201–1207.
29. **Reichart PA, Philipsen HP, Sonner S.** Ameloblastoma: biological profile of 3,677 cases. *Eur J Cancer B Oral Oncol* 1995;31B:86–99.
30. **Rushing EJ, Bouffard JP, McCall S,** ***et al.*** Primary extracranial meningiomas: an analysis of 146 cases [published online ahead of print May 20, 2009]. *Head Neck Pathol* 2009;3:116–130. doi:10.1007/s121050-0901181-1.
31. **Sheahan P, Byrne M, Hafidh M, Toner M, Simon C.** Neck dissection findings in primary head and neck high-grade adenocarcinoma. *J Laryngol Otol* 2004;118:532–536.
32. **Simpson RH, Clarke TJ, Sarsfield PT, Gluckman PG.** Epithelial-myoepithelial carcinoma of salivary glands. *J Clin Pathol* 1991;44:419–423.
33. **Su L, Weathers DR, Waldron CA.** Distinguishing features of focal cemento-osseous dysplasia and cemento-ossifying fibromas. II. A clinical and radiologic spectrum of 316 cases. *Oral Surg Oral Med Oral Pathol Oral Radiol Endod* 1997;84:540–549.
34. **Thompson LD, Miettinen M, Wenig BM.** Sinonasal-type hemangiopericytoma: a clinicopathologic and immunophenotypic analysis of 104 cases showing perivascular myoid differentiation. *Am J Surg Pathol* 2003;27:737–749.
35. **Thompson LD, Wieneke JA, Miettinen M.** Sinonasal tract nasopharyngeal melanomas: a clinicopathologic study of 115 cases with a proposed staging system. *Am J Surg Pathol* 2003;27:594–611.

36. **Thompson LD, Wieneke JA, Miettinen M, Heffner DK.** Spindle cell (sarcomatoid) carcinomas of the larynx: a clinicopathologic study of 187 cases. *Am J Surg Pathol* 2002;26:153–170.
37. **Trodahl JN.** Ameloblastic fibroma: a survey of cases from the Armed Forces Institute of Pathology. *Oral Surg Oral Med Oral Pathol* 1972;33:547–558.
38. **Vincent SD, Hammond HL, Finkelstein MW.** Clinical and therapeutic features of polymorphous low-grade adenocarcinoma. *Oral Surg Oral Med Oral Pathol* 1994;77:41–47.
39. **Young SK, Markowitz NR, Sullivan S, Seale TW, Hirschi R.** Familial gigantiform cementoma: classification and presentation of a large pedigree. *Oral Surg Oral Med Oral Pathol* 1989;68:740–747.

FACIAL NERVE PARALYSIS AND ITS MANAGEMENT 16

Richard Y. Ha, MD
and Claude-Jean Langevin, MD, DMD

16.1 Introduction

Facial nerve paralysis is a devastating condition with functional, cosmetic, and psychosocial consequences. Since the paralysis can affect multiple facial anatomic units, the surgeon needs to choose a surgical plan tailored to the specific functional deficit and having the most optimal aesthetic outcome. Numerous techniques have been developed in recent years, with various levels of successes. The advent of free tissue transfer has revolutionized the surgical management of the paralyzed face, and continued research in the field of nerve regeneration will no doubt contribute to further advancement in the treatment of this condition. To provide the best outcome for the patient afflicted with facial paralysis, a multidisciplinary team approach should be used, consisting of neurology, ophthalmology, otolaryngology, neurosurgery, physical medicine and rehabilitation, speech therapy, and plastic surgery.

16.2 Facial Nerve Anatomy and Function

Cranial nerve (CN) VII is a mixed nerve consisting of motor and sensory nerves containing approximately 10,000 fibers, of which 7,000 are motor fibers. The facial nerve is divided into three portions, and knowledge of this anatomy is essential for understanding the signs and symptoms associated with CN VII dysfunction.

16.2.1 *Intracranial portion*

This portion of CN VII originates in the lower segment of the precentral gyrus and crosses the caudal pontine region to form the facial nucleus in the contralateral pons between the olive and the inferior cerebellar peduncle. The nerve passes medial to the abducens nerve (CN VI) as it leaves the nucleus and exits the brainstem at the pontomedullary junction before entering the internal auditory canal (porus acusticus). This portion is approximately 24 mm long from the brainstem to the internal auditory canal of the temporal bone, and no epineurium covers this section.

A central CN VII palsy from a lesion affecting the supranuclear corticobulbar pathway results in a contralateral lower-face paralysis with preservation of upper facial musculature function, such as forehead and periorbital animation, and including the blink reflex. The lower muscles of facial expression receive contralateral cortical input exclusively. In comparison, a peripheral CN VII palsy will affect both the ipsilateral upper and lower facial musculature.

16.2.2 *Intratemporal portion*

The intratemporal portion travels within the fallopian canal and measures approximately 30 mm from the internal auditory canal to the stylomastoid foramen.[1] It is divided into three segments: the labyrinthine, tympanic, and mastoid. Epineurium surrounds the facial nerve in the tympanic and mastoid segments, while proximally, the nerve is covered with pia mater and bathed in cerebrospinal fluid.

1. The labyrinthine segment (3–4 mm) travels from the internal auditory canal to the geniculate ganglion and represents the narrowest portion (0.68 mm) of the fallopian canal.[2] The facial nerve occupies 83% of the available space in this segment compared with 23% in

the mastoid portion.[3] This is the most likely area of compression when there is edema of the facial nerve trunk, as in Bell's palsy.

   a. The greater superficial petrosal nerve carries parasympathetic secretory fibers to the nose, mouth, and lacrimal gland and sensory taste fibers from the palate.
   b. The lesser superficial petrosal nerve carries parasympathetic secretory fibers to the parotid gland.

2. The tympanic or horizontal segment (8–11 mm) runs from the geniculate ganglion to the bend at the lateral semicircular canal.
3. The mastoid or vertical segment (10–14 mm) continues up to the stylomastoid foramen.
   a. The stapedial branch provides motor function to the stapedial muscle, which dampens loud sounds.
   b. The chorda tympani joins the lingual nerve (CN V_3) and carries parasympathetic secretory fibers to the submandibular and sublingual glands as well as afferent sensory taste fibers from the anterior two-thirds of the tongue.

Physical examination may help determine the level of injury within the temporal bony canal. For example, if the injury affects the geniculate ganglion, a loss of secretory function of nose, mouth, and lacrimal gland can be expected, whereas a lesion affecting the stapedial branch may cause hyperacusis.

16.2.3 *Extratemporal portion*

As it exits the stylomastoid foramen, this purely motor facial nerve is protected by the mastoid process and gives off the posterior auricular nerve, which innervates the posterior auricular and occipitalis muscles. In infants, the facial nerve is located more superficially as it exits the lateral aspect of the temporal bone, and is vulnerable to injury either by compression (intrauterine) or iatrogenically (forceps delivery). The nerve will eventually assume a less superficial position as the mastoid process and tympanic ring develop.

The facial nerve travels approximately 15 mm to 20 mm between the posterior belly of the digastric and the stylohyoid muscles, sending out branches to both these muscles before entering the parotid gland, where it gives rise to two trunks at the pes anserinus: the temporofacial and cervicofacial divisions. Within the parotid gland, the nerve is located between the superficial and deep portions of the gland and further divides into five branches: frontal (temporal), zygomatic, buccal, mandibular, and cervical.

The facial nerve travels under the superficial musculoaponeurotic system (SMAS). The SMAS invests the facial musculature and is continuous with the platysma inferiorly and the temporoparietal fascia (also known as the superficial temporalis fascia) superiorly. Branching patterns of the five divisions have variable distributions and numbers of branches. Davis *et al.* described six patterns (Figure 16.1), with type III being the most common (28%). This specific pattern has a single connection between the frontozygomatic and cervicofacial

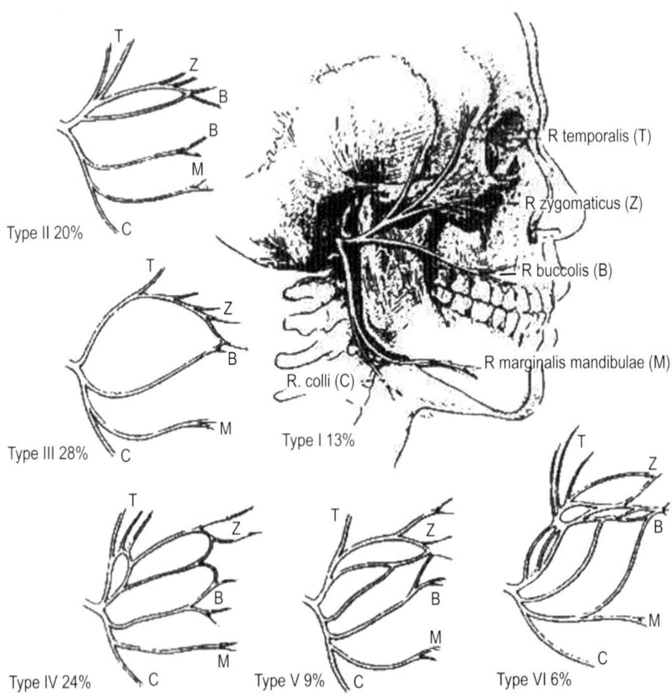

Figure 16.1. Common patterns (and incidences) of facial nerve branching, illustrated. Reprinted with permission from the *Journal of the American College of Surgeons*, formerly *Surgery Gynecology & Obstetrics* (Ref. 4).

divisions, with a connecting loop between the zygomatic and buccal branches.[4] This is relevant when the nerve is dissected for oncologic or reconstructive reasons. Significant overlap and arborization occur as the nerve branches course distally, especially between the zygomatic and buccal branches, which are often referred to as the "zygomaticobuccal" branches. Tzafetta and Terzis reported significant interconnections between the buccal and marginal mandibular branches.[5]

The frontal and marginal mandibular branches usually are minimally interconnected with the other facial nerve branches, resulting in major sequelae when injured. The frontal nerve is composed of an average of 2.8 branches that become more superficial as they enter the temporal region superior to the zygomatic arch, traveling under the temporoparietal fascia.[5] The course of the frontal nerve can be approximated by tracing a line from 5 mm below the tragus to 15 mm above the lateral aspect of the eyebrow.[6] The marginal mandibular nerve consists of an average of 2.3 branches and is located within the superficial layer of the deep cervical fascia under the platysma. The marginal mandibular nerve lies superficial to the facial artery and vein. Posterior to the facial vessels, it travels below the inferior border of the mandible in 19% of the population. Anterior to the facial vessels, it is located above the inferior border of the mandible.[7]

The facial nerve innervates the facial musculature used for facial movement and expression (emotion, psychosocial functioning, and social interaction), eye function and protection (blinking, tear production and distribution, and lacrimal pumping action), nasal airway patency, and oral competence (speaking, eating, and drinking) (Figure 16.2).

16.3 Facial Musculature

The muscles of facial expression innervated by the different branches of the facial nerve consist of multiple paired muscles and the single orbicularis oris muscle (Figure 16.3). The mentalis, levator anguli oris, and buccinator are the deepest of the facial muscles and receive innervation superficially. The remaining facial muscles receive their innervation along their deep surfaces. The frontalis, orbicularis oculi, zygomaticus major, orbicularis oris, and depressor labii inferioris have

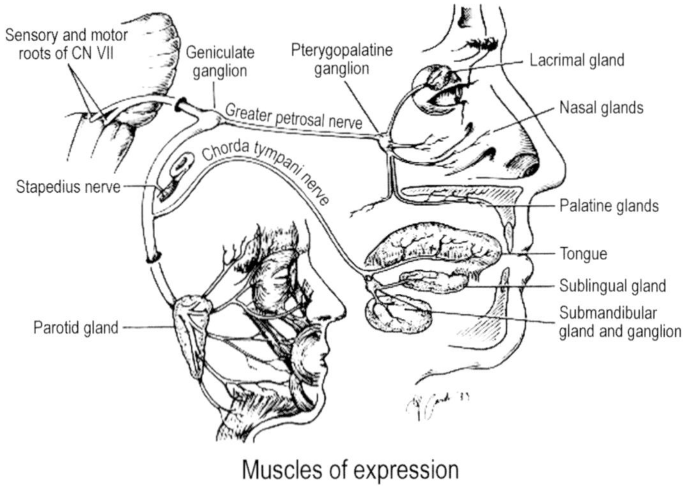

Figure 16.2. Facial nerve innervation and functions, illustrated. Reprinted with permission from Elsevier (Jackson CG, *et al.* The facial nerve: current trends in diagnosis, treatment, and rehabilitation. *Med Clin North Am* 1999;83:179–195). Copyright © 1999 Elsevier.

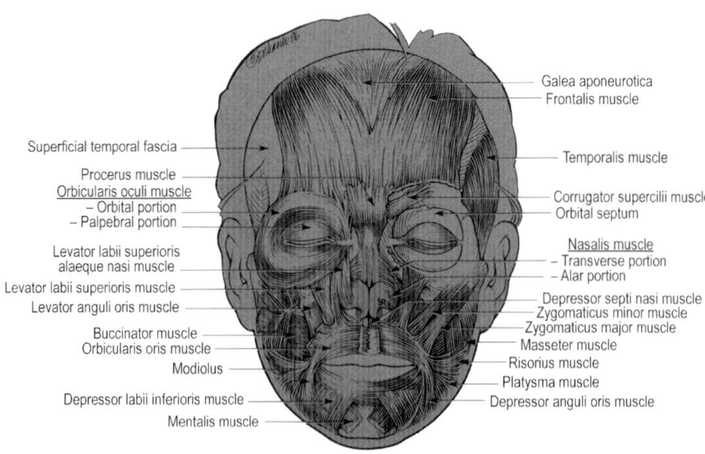

Figure 16.3. Muscles of facial expression. Reprinted with permission from The McGraw-Hill Companies (**Salasche SJ, Bernstein C, Senkarik M**. Surgical Anatomy of the Skin. Chapter 7. Norwalk, CT: Appleton & Lange; 1988:69).

key roles in facial animation. Knowledge of their function and their respective neural innervation helps determine the affected facial nerve branch (Table 16.1). The modiolus represents the point of common

Table 16.1. Innervation and Actions of Facial Mimetic Muscles.

Branch of CN VII	Facial muscle	Actions
Temporal	Frontalis	Elevates eyebrow
	Corrugator supercilii	Pulls eyebrow medially and downward
	Procerus	Pulls medial eyebrow downward
Temporal and zygomatic	Orbicularis oculi	Closes eyelids and contracts skin around eye
Zygomatic and buccal	Zygomaticus major	Elevates corner of mouth
Buccal	Zygomaticus minor	Elevates upper lip
	Levator labii superioris	Elevates upper lip and mid-portion nasolabial fold
	Levator labii superioris alaeque nasi	Elevates medial nasolabial fold and nasal ala
	Risorius	Aids smile with lateral pull
	Buccinator	Pulls corner of mouth backward and compresses cheek
	Levator anguli oris	Pulls angles of mouth upward and toward midline
	Orbicularis oris	Closes and compresses lips
	Nasalis, dilator naris	Flares nostrils
	Nasalis, compressor naris	Compresses nostrils
Buccal and marginal mandibular	Depressor anguli oris	Pulls corners of mouth downward
	Depressor labii inferioris	Pulls lower lip downward
Marginal mandibular	Mentalis	Pulls skin of chin upward
Cervical	Platysma	Pulls down corners of mouth

attachment for the zygomaticus major and minor, orbicularis oris, buccinator, risorius, levator anguli oris, and depressor anguli oris. It is often considered an anchor point when performing reanimation or static elevation procedures.

The action and specific vector orientation created by the facial musculature must be analyzed in the non-symptomatic face before attempting reconstruction on the affected side.

- Lip elevator vector:
  a. Zygomaticus major and minor muscles: 45° superior lateral
  b. Levator anguli oris: superior and medial
  c. Levator labii superioris: superior and lateral
  d. Levator labii superioris nasi alaeque: superior
- Lip depressor vector:
  a. Depressor labii inferioris: inferior and lateral with eversion of the vermilion
  b. Depressor anguli oris: depresses the angle of the mouth

The mentalis muscle is not a lip depressor; it elevates the lip indirectly since it arises from the anterior mandible and inserts into the skin of the chin in a downward direction.

16.4 Causes of Facial Paralysis

Approximately 127,000 cases of permanent facial paralysis occur annually.[8] The differential diagnosis of facial paralysis constitutes a myriad of medical conditions. Etiologies may be classified in the following categories: idiopathic, traumatic, neoplastic, infectious, congenital/genetic/metabolic, neurologic, and toxic (Table 16.2).

16.4.1 *Idiopathic (Bell's palsy)*

The most common cause of facial paralysis is Bell's palsy with an annual incidence of 11 to 40/100,000.[9,10] It is usually unilateral, can be complete or partial, and accounts for 85% of all cases of facial paralysis. Bell's palsy is primarily a diagnosis of exclusion with a proposed viral

Table 16.2. Causes of Facial Paralysis.

Causes	Conditions
Idiopathic	Bell's palsy, **sarcoidosis**, Melkersson–Rosenthal syndrome, **systemic lupus erythematosus**, multiple sclerosis, temporal arteritis, eosinophilic granuloma, amyloidosis, immunization
Infection	Otitis media, herpes simplex, varicella-zoster, **syphilis**, poliomyelitis, botulism, mastoiditis, coxsackievirus, **encephalitis**, tetanus, diphtheria, **HIV/AIDS**, **tuberculosis, meningitis, Lyme disease**, **cryptococcal meningitis, mononucleosis, leprosy**, **pregnancy**
Neoplastic	Schwannoma, teratoma, parotid tumor, cholesteatoma, glomus jugular tumors, neurofibromas (von Recklinghausen's disease), germ cell tumors, meningioma, hemangioma, sarcoma and carcinoma (metastasis)
Congenital/genetic/ metabolic	**Möbius syndrome**, craniofacial (hemifacial) microsomia, **diabetes mellitus**, **pregnancy**, hyperthyroidism, hypothyroidism
Neurologic	**Guillain-Barré syndrome**, **pontine glioma**, opercular syndrome, Wernicke–Korsakoff syndrome, pseudotumor cerebri, cerebrovascular accident (lacunar infarct), **myasthenia gravis**
Trauma	Traumatic delivery, forceps delivery, head injury, facial skeleton and soft-tissue injuries, barotrauma (scuba diving), surgery complication, anesthetic nerve block, postembolization
Toxins	Thalidomide, interferon, **linezolid**, ethylene glycol, ethanol

HIV/AIDS = human immunodeficiency virus/acquired immune deficiency syndrome. Conditions shown in bold are frequently associated with bilateral facial nerve palsy.[22,23]

and inflammatory etiology.[11] The resulting edema of the nerve within the fallopian canal (labyrinthine segment), the canal with the smallest diameter, causes nerve compression and disruption of the neural microcirculation. The incidence is increased during pregnancy (last trimester) and in patients suffering from diabetes mellitus.[12] It manifests as a unilateral palsy and may be associated with other CN neuropathies.

The following signs and symptoms exclude a diagnosis of Bell's palsy[13]:

- simultaneous bilateral facial palsy
- slowly progressive unilateral facial weakness beyond 3 weeks
- slowly progressive unilateral facial weakness associated with facial hyperkinesis
- no improvement in facial nerve function within 6 months after an abrupt onset of palsy
- ipsilateral lateral rectus palsy (CN VI — abducens nerves)

The prognosis is usually good, with 86% of patients recovering within 3 weeks. Therefore, diagnostic testing is deferred until that time.[10] The recurrence risk of Bell's palsy has been reported to be as high as 10%, with women carrying a higher risk.[14]

16.4.2 *Traumatic*

The second most common cause of facial paralysis is trauma, which can be further divided into accidental and surgical causes. Accidental trauma includes temporal bone fracture, sharp injuries, avulsion, and burns. Head injury may result in a temporal bone fracture that usually affects the facial nerve within the labyrinthine segment. The junction of the labyrinthine and tympanic segments forms an acute angle and is therefore at risk for shearing injury. Computed tomography (CT) is helpful in localizing the injury, and immediate exploration is recommended in the setting of acute onset of paralysis.

Penetrating sharp injuries have a more favorable prognosis than crush injury. Injuries located anterior to an imaginary vertical line at the lateral canthus do not require surgical repair because of the extensive arborization between the different facial nerve branches, especially the zygomaticobuccal branches. The most distal nerve ends are also very difficult to identify. If the injury is located posterior to this imaginary vertical line at the lateral canthus, immediate repair should be done within 72 h. In cases of infection or inadequate soft-tissue coverage, identification of the nerve ends should be attempted for delayed repair. Facial nerve stimulation resulting in movement of the facial muscles is possible only within 72 h post injury. Repair of the frontal and mandibular branches should be attempted regardless of the location of the injury because of the morbidity associated with injury to these branches.

Trauma during delivery occurs at an incidence of 1.8 per 1,000 births annually; 91% are associated with forceps delivery, and 89% have complete recovery.[15] Surgical causes of CN VII paralysis may be secondary to resection of a tumor at the cerebellopontine angle, such as a schwannoma (acoustic neuroma). Parotid gland manipulation secondary to a superficial parotidectomy often results in a transient neuropraxia that improves over several months.

16.4.3 *Neoplastic*

Presentation may be quite variable depending on the tumor; however, a prolonged, relapsing, or slowly progressive onset of facial paralysis suggests a neoplasm.[16] Hearing loss, either conductive or sensorineural, is often an associated symptom. A schwannoma is the most common neoplasm of the facial nerve. The index of suspicion for a neoplastic process should be high in cases of slowly progressive facial paralysis lasting more than 3 weeks, abrupt onset with no return of function within 6 months, or facial weakness associated with hyperkinesis (twitching).[13] Imaging studies such as CT or magnetic resonance imaging (MRI) are mandatory if suggestive signs or symptoms are present.

16.4.4 *Infectious*

Varicella-zoster presenting as Ramsay Hunt syndrome (herpes zoster oticus) is one of the more common causes in this category. It is generally severe. Signs and symptoms include peripheral facial paralysis, ear pain, vesicular rash in the external auditory canal, and possible tinnitus and hearing loss. Treatment consists of steroid and antiviral therapy.

Lyme disease (caused by *Borrelia burgdorferi*) presents with cutaneous (erythema chronicum migrans), musculoskeletal, cardiovascular, and neurologic symptoms after a tick bite. Bilateral facial paralysis is common and often resolves within 2 months with antibiotic therapy consisting of doxycycline or erythromycin.

16.4.5 *Congenital/genetic/metabolic*

Craniofacial (hemifacial) microsomia, which is a first and second branchial arch disorder, is the most common congenital cause of unilateral paralysis. It may also be present in Goldenhar's syndrome, which is a variant of craniofacial microsomia associated with epibulbar dermoids and vertebral anomalies.

Congenital unilateral lower lip palsy (also known as asymmetric crying facies) is found in 1 in 160 births and involves the depressor angularis oris.[17,18] There is isolated paralysis of the marginal mandibular branch of the facial nerve (Figure 16.4). These patients may be associated with a 22q11.2 deletion and have cardiac anomalies.[19] Genetic/chromosomal workup should be considered in patients with this disorder.

Möbius syndrome is a rare congenital disorder with a multifactorial pathogenesis that includes genetic, vascular, and toxic causes. It occurs in 0.002% of births.[20] It is characterized by unilateral or bilateral developmental impairment of CN VI and VII. It may also involve CN V, IX, and XII and, less frequently, CN III, IV, and VIII. Other abnormalities associated with this syndrome include orofacial malformations (epicanthal folds, micrognathia, ear anomalies), limb malformations (brachydactyly, syndactyly, talipes equinovarus), musculoskeletal defects (absence of pectoralis and trapezius muscles), and mental retardation (Figure 16.5). Feeding and respiratory problems are frequent in the newborns due to lack of respiratory drive, insufficient sucking, uncoordinated swallowing, and regurgitation.

Treatment of Möbius syndrome is very challenging in these mask-like faces. It usually consists of a dynamic reconstruction with free tissue transfer, such as a bilateral gracilis muscle with masseteric branch innervation. Speech may be improved with direct tongue neurotization with CN VII or CN XI used in combination with a sural nerve graft.[21]

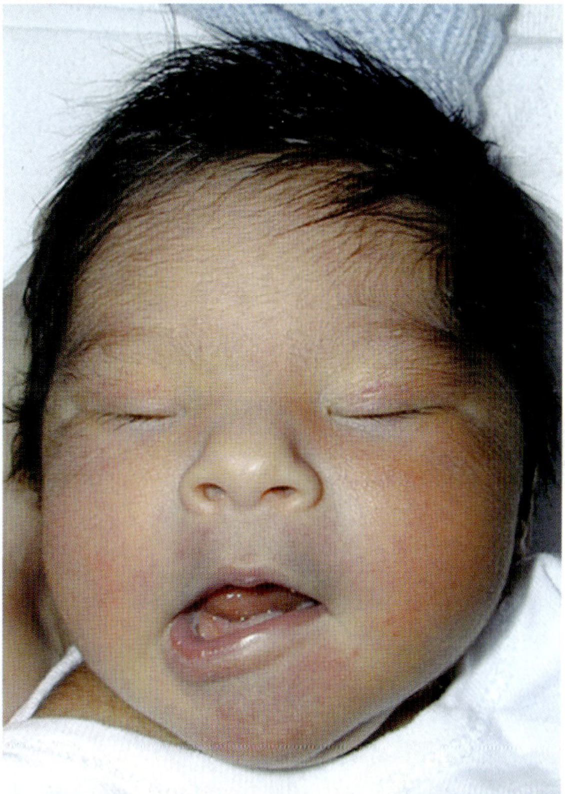

Figure 16.4. Photograph of an infant who has congenital unilateral lower lip palsy, exhibiting paralysis of the left marginal mandibular branch of the facial nerve.

16.5 Evaluation and Treatment of Acute Facial Paralysis

The goal in evaluating a patient afflicted with acute facial paralysis is to identify the site of the lesion, the degree of dysfunction and, ideally, the cause. The history and physical examination are of paramount importance and should include a detailed history of the onset, progress, and associated signs and symptoms of the CN VII dysfunction as well as a careful head and neck examination. The House–Brackmann classification provides an overall facial-function grading scale with measurements of range of motion of the eyebrows and a quantification

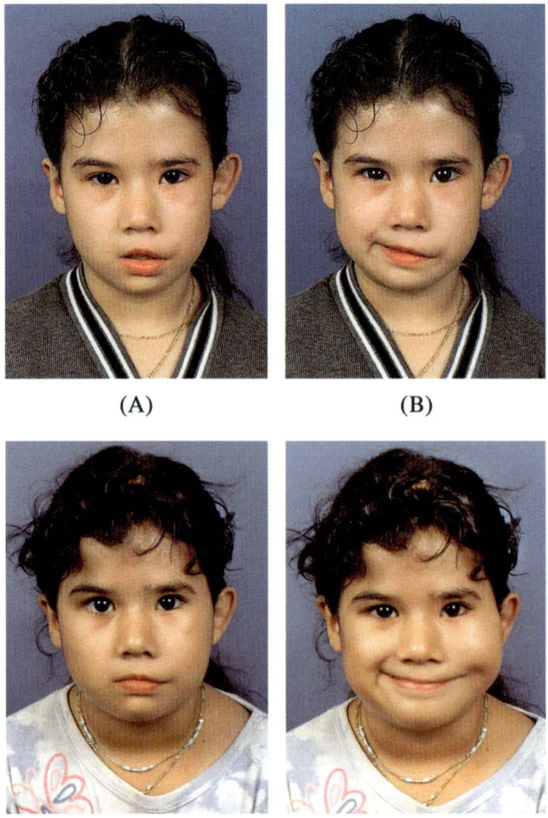

(A) (B)

(C) (D)

Figure 16.5. Photographs of a 6-year-old girl with Möbius syndrome associated with congenital bilateral abducens and a left facial paralysis in repose (A), and in an attempted smile (B). Photographs taken 1 year after she underwent free gracilis muscle transfer to the motor nerve of the masseter at rest (C), and smiling (D).

of the ability to close the eye and to lateralize the oral commissure (Table 16.3).[24] Several new scales such as the Sunnybrook, Yangihara, and Sydney have been introduced with various degrees of objectivity. However, the House–Brackmann grading scale remains to be the gold standard.

Radiologic imaging consisting of MRI and CT may be helpful in determining the location of a disease process affecting the facial

Table 16.3. The House–Brackmann Classification.

Grade	Description	Characteristics
I	Normal	Normal functioning in all branches of the facial nerves
II	Slight	*Gross:* Slight weakness on close inspection, slight synkinesis *At rest:* Normal tone and symmetry ***Motion*** Forehead: Moderate to good function Eye: Complete closure with minimal effort Mouth: Slight asymmetry
III	Moderate	*Gross:* Clear facial asymmetry but not complete or disfiguring, synkinesis or mild hemifacial muscular spasms noticeable in the area of the facial nerve *At rest:* Normal tone and symmetry ***Motion*** Forehead: Slight to moderate movement Eye: Complete closure with moderate effort Mouth: Slight weakness with maximal effort
IV	Moderately severe	*Gross:* Total facial asymmetry that is disfiguring with obvious facial weakness *At rest*: Normal tone and symmetry ***Motion*** Forehead: No movement Eye: Incomplete closure Mouth: Asymmetric weakness with maximal effort
V	Severe	*Gross*: Minimal, barely perceptible movement *At rest:* Asymmetric facial appearance ***Motion*** Forehead: No movement Eye: Incomplete closure Mouth: Slight, barely perceptible movement
VI	Total	No facial function

Modified with permission from Sage (Ref. 24).

nerve. Gadolinium-enhanced MRI is ideal for detecting soft-tissue inflammation and tumors. CT provides detailed anatomy of the temporal bone including the course of the facial nerve, which can be particularly useful after trauma.

Numerous electrodiagnostic tools measuring the neurophysiologic status of the facial nerve itself are available to help in the diagnosis, treatment, and prognosis of facial paralysis.[25] The most commonly used tests include the following:

- Nerve excitability test (NET) is a subjective minimal stimulation test measuring the current threshold required to elicit minimal muscle contraction on the normal side compared with that of the affected side. An abnormal test result is defined as a difference of 3.0 to 3.5 milliamperes between the two sides of the face.
- Maximal stimulation test (MST) is similar to NET but uses maximal stimulation and is therefore painful and subjective. An abnormal test result consists of any difference in facial movement between the two sides of the face. Both NET and MST rely on percutaneous stimulation of the facial nerve, are subjective, and do not show abnormalities until 72 h after nerve degeneration.
- Electroneuronography (ENOG) records the compound action potential after a supramaximal electrical stimulation of the facial nerve. The percentage of nerve fiber degeneration (amplitude of the compound action potential) compared with the non-paralyzed face is helpful in predicting the prognosis of the facial paralysis and selecting an appropriate treatment plan.[26] ENOG is an objective test, and is the most accurate reproducible test to determine the prognosis for return of facial nerve function, although it is expensive and at times impractical.[27] A current is delivered percutaneously to the stylomastoid foramen, and the amplitude of evoked compound muscle action potentials (CMAPs) is measured from electrodes on the nasolabial fold. Maximal muscle response is elicited on each side regardless of the electrical current required. Results are analyzed, and in most cases of Bell's palsy, there is no further decline in CMAP by the 10th day. A 95% decrease in CMAP on the affected side, compared with the

normal side, showed 50% of patients had an unsatisfactory return of facial nerve function.[28] As such, the threshold for recommending surgical decompression has been a 90% decrease in CMAP within the first 2 weeks postparalysis.

- Electromyography (EMG) evaluates muscle activity and provides an approximate measure of the intensity of denervation when performed early in the paralysis. Fibrillation potentials are observed in the denervated muscle, polyphasic potentials are found in muscle undergoing reinnervation, and complete electrical silence is noted in denervated muscle with significant fibrosis. This test should be performed at least 3 weeks from the onset of paralysis to be reliable.[29]

16.6 Management of Acute Facial Paralysis

Most patients with Bell's palsy recover to House–Brackmann I or II function grade without intervention. However, treatment with prednisolone for 10 days within 72 h of symptom onset significantly improves recovery compared with placebo.[30] Patients with Bell's palsy are commonly treated with corticosteroids in the acute setting despite controversy regarding their effectiveness. Another recommended protocol suggests high-dose prednisone, starting with 60 mg/day for the first 5 days and tapered over 10 days.[31] Should the paralysis become progressive and complete or if otalgia occurs, recurs, or worsens, a second 10-day course is recommended. Risk factors for incomplete recovery are complete facial weakness, non-ear pain, and hypertension.[10] Some patients develop disabling sequelae such as synkinesis or severe facial spasm despite targeted medical treatment.

Surgical decompression for Bell's palsy is still highly controversial. Facial nerve decompression from the middle cranial fossa through the tympanic segment performed within 12 days of onset has demonstrated modest but statistically significant improvement in severe cases with unfavorable electrodiagnostic profiles.[32] The procedure involves removal of the bony covering of the fallopian canal with or without incision of the periosteum/epineurium. The decision for decompression usually depends on data derived from ENOG. This is a time-consuming test, requiring daily evaluation for the first 10 days postparalysis. If the patient cannot comply with daily testing or if a surgeon is unwilling to decompress should the test become positive, ENOG may be of little value.

Patients with acute facial paralysis often experience problems with dry eyes, speech, and oral competence. Medical management of ocular symptoms in facial paralysis includes frequent use of artificial tears and lubricating ophthalmic ointment to prevent and treat exposure keratopathy. Other options include eyelid taping (especially at bedtime), moisture chamber goggles, and patches. Speech therapy can help patients cope with drooling and speech difficulties.

16.6.1 *Repair of facial nerve injuries*

A severed facial nerve must be diagnosed early and repaired expeditiously. Delayed repair should be considered in cases of contaminated wounds or inadequate soft-tissue coverage after careful identification of the nerve stumps with permanent sutures. In either case, repair or identification (and "tagging") should be performed within 72 h of the injury. Facial nerve stimulation can result in end muscular movement up to 72 h after the injury. Thereafter, identifying terminal nerve targets becomes extremely difficult.

At the time of repair, both nerve ends are first evaluated to determine the condition of the nerve and its potential for regeneration. For example, a nerve that has sustained a sharp laceration will have a better prognosis once coapted than a crushed or avulsed nerve. An epineural neurorrhaphy consisting of a tensionless coaptation of the nerve ends is the preferred method of repair since epineural neurorrhaphy was proven to be equivalent to intrafascicular repair.[33] If tension is present at the repair site, it encourages disoriented axonal sprouting and the development of painful neuromas.[34] Mobilization of both nerve ends may help to reduce the tension at the repair site and may be able to close gaps up to 1 cm wide. However, mobilization of nerve ends should be done carefully, as it may lead to neural devascularization and further neural injury. Nerve conduits or autologous vein grafts are useful when bridging a gap of less than 3 cm;

however, an interpositional nerve graft is recommended for a larger gap.[35] The graft serves as a conduit through which sprouting axons travel from the proximal nerve end to the distal nerve end and then all the way to the motor end-plate. A nerve graft should ideally be placed in a well-vascularized bed. In the presence of a significant mismatch between the proximal and distal nerve ends, a cable graft may be needed.

The greater auricular nerve and the sural nerve are the most common donor nerves for facial nerve grafting. The greater auricular nerve is located one-half the distance between the mastoid tip and the angle of the mandible and perpendicular to the line adjoining the two. It innervates the lower half of the pinna and posterior auricular region. This nerve provides only 5 cm to 10 cm of nerve and contains two or three fascicles. It is easily harvested since it is located within the surgical field, and it usually provides a good match size. The sural nerve is located 1 cm posterior to the lateral malleolus and innervates the side and back of the distal one-third of the leg, ankle, and heel. It has a larger axonal volume than the greater auricular nerve and provides up to 35 cm of nerve graft.

The reoccurrence of facial nerve function is usually anticipated in the following 4–6 months after nerve grafting since axonal growth occurs at a rate of 1 mm/day.[36] The success of a graft depends on the number of axons in the damaged nerve, the potential for regeneration of these axons through the graft, and the duration of the facial musculature denervation. Radiation does not seem to influence facial nerve regeneration.[37] Primary neurorrhaphy is expected to have a better result than a nerve repair with interpositional grafting.

With regard to facial muscle viability, reinnervation may be attempted up to 3 years after the onset of paralysis in young patients when the affected nerve is not severely atrophic.[38] However, the practical window of surgical intervention is about 18 months to 2 years, before muscle motor end plates degenerate and become incapable of creating an action potential. Also, secondary changes occurring within the muscle itself lead to disuse atrophy, characterized by replacement of muscle fibers by lipofibrous tissue. Other studies indicate that the longer the period of denervation, the smaller the degree of recovery after reinnervation.[39,40] Other factors acting against a successful outcome include advanced age (>40 years old) and disuse.

16.7 Management of Chronic Facial Paralysis

It is often a struggle to juggle multiple reconstructive options and develop a logical treatment plan for a patient with chronic or subacute facial paralysis. The difficulty in determining the appropriate course of action lies in the ambiguity of a patient's prognosis from a facial nerve injury against the backdrop of temporal factors — essentially a race against time.

Facial paralysis should be considered chronic if it has duration longer than 6 months, or what would be expected for complete recovery from Bell's palsy. There are several important considerations for management of chronic acquired facial paralysis:

- timing
- mechanism of injury
- potential for spontaneous recovery
- surgical procedures

Patients may have sustained paralysis for a number of reasons — blunt vs. sharp trauma, incomplete recovery from viral/Bell's palsy, tumor resection, and so forth. Each of these may have a differing prognosis for spontaneous recovery.

First, regarding a facial paralysis, what is the status of the facial nerve itself — was there a traumatic injury with contusion or transection? Or was there a viral or congenital cause of the facial paralysis? If it is thought that a facial palsy may resolve or improve with observation, how long should one wait before proceeding with reconstruction or reinnervation? When does the denervation of the facial musculature reach a point of such degeneration of the motor end plates that effective reinnervation is not possible, leading to suboptimal functional recovery?

Surgical options for improvement include nerve grafting, nerve transfers, and delayed dynamic vs. static reconstruction. Nerve grafting and nerve transfers may be acutely appropriate if indicated, such as for a nerve transected from sharp trauma or a known facial nerve resection due to tumor involvement. The more controversial decisions occur with those injuries that may have a potential for spontaneous recovery but exhibit marginal or no improvement — is there a benefit to intervening with a nerve graft or transfer?

Although it is accepted that target muscles irreversibly degenerate by 18 to 24 months, outcomes for nerve repair or nerve grafting are better when attempted earlier. The length of a nerve graft must be considered when making the decision about surgery. A cross-face nerve graft to the trunk of the paralyzed facial nerve should be attempted within 1 year of the injury for optimal outcomes. With an average length of 200 mm (20 cm) and a regeneration rate of 1 mm/day, 200 days, or 7 months, is required. If this procedure is attempted 18 months postinjury, the time to regeneration will have surpassed any reasonable potential for return of muscular function.

There is little consensus in answers to these questions, and surgeons develop treatment algorithms based on temporal factors or on diagnostic evaluation of facial muscle viability (EMG, for example). We suggest a maximal observation period of 1 year for spontaneous recovery of a nerve palsy — provided that there is not a known transection or discontinuity to the facial nerve. Should there be no improvement, reinnervation procedures (such as cross-facial nerve grafting) are recommended. Nerve regeneration across a graft at 1 mm/day will require 6 to 10 months for reinnervation, still within the motor end-plate degeneration threshold of 2 to 3 years from the time of injury. While it is possible to allow further observation before starting reinnervation procedures, successful functioning of the facial musculature diminishes with increasing time from injury. We recommend EMG evaluation for motor potentials if there is no clinical improvement noted at all during the first 6 months of the observation period. If no activity can be elicited, further spontaneous recovery is unlikely, and reinnervation procedures can be considered at this earlier time. Patients with complete transections of the facial nerve, through trauma or tumor resection, can be treated with ipsilateral nerve grafting, cross-face nerve grafting, or nerve transfers without the obligatory observation period.

Often, incomplete recovery can occur, with asymmetric muscle function. In these cases, the degree of recovery (or lack thereof) will determine whether to:

- accept the recovered function
- transect the underperforming nerve and reinnervate with a donor nerve (cross-face nerve graft or ipsilateral hypoglossal transfer, for example)
- perform free muscle transfer to regional nerve or cross-face nerve graft
- perform static reconstruction for asymmetries

By virtue of the reinnervation procedures, facial nerve transection is required for neurorrhaphy, eliminating any recovered function up to this point. As a result of dissection during procedures for static reconstruction or for reanimation with free muscle transfers, the recovering facial nerve may become further injured. Treatment decisions become difficult in these cases of suboptimal or incomplete recovery, or when the prognosis for recovery is uncertain.

For patients with long-standing facial paralysis (>18–24 months from injury), delayed static or dynamic reconstructive options (i.e., fascial slings or free functional muscle transfer in one or two stages) would be appropriate. Nerve transfers or grafting at this point would no longer be useful.

Before reconstruction, an evaluation of the facial symmetry and function in static and dynamic conditions is performed. As expected, the level of asymmetry is amplified on animation. Key measurements to record are the dynamic vector at the upper lip and commissure, strength of movement, and position of nasolabial and labiomental folds.[41] Older patients will have a greater degree of asymmetry in the lower face secondary to descent and deflation of the soft tissue. Photography and videography at rest and during motion are essential tools to document and monitor improvement of the severity of impairment as well as postoperative progress.

16.8 Management of Congenital Facial Paralysis

Whether congenital facial paralysis stems from birth trauma or from genetic causes such as craniofacial microsomia or Möbius syndrome, surgical options for dynamic facial reanimation are preferred. Free muscle transfers (e.g., gracilis) innervated to either a cross-face nerve graft or to the motor nerve of the masseter are typical procedures. Recreation of smiling is of great psychosocial importance, and timing of surgery is generally recommended between ages 4 and 6 when peer interactions increase. We advocate delaying free muscle transfers for congenital cases until this age, when there has been sufficient growth of the donor muscle, and for improved technical ease of the microsurgery.

Electrical stimulation therapy has been advocated by some to help improve facial muscle contraction and functionality. There have been limited data to indicate any real short-term or long-term benefit.

Static procedures are generally avoided and often unnecessary. Children with facial paralysis often do not exhibit symptomatic lagophthalmos or drooling secondary to oral incompetence. Should these conditions develop, eyelid weight insertion or canthopexy, or both, can be performed for improved eyelid closure. A fascial sling may be indicated for excessive oral incompetence.

16.9 Reconstructive Options

A patient with facial palsy may be treated with numerous reconstructive options. An accurate diagnosis of facial muscle viability is essential to determine the best course of treatment.[42] Ideal reconstructive goals include restoration of symmetry at rest and with animation in addition to eyelid closure, oral competence, and improvement of the nasal airway.

16.9.1 *Static reconstruction*

Static reconstruction techniques aim to suspend the soft-tissue structures of the face to improve function or aesthetics. For example, a static suspension sling of the oral commissure can greatly improve oral competence as well as facial symmetry at rest. Correcting lagophthalmos and lower eyelid laxity by means of static reconstructive procedures protect the cornea. No animation function is achieved with these techniques, although they can be used in conjunction with dynamic procedures. The principal indication for this type of reconstruction alone includes multiple comorbidities, previously failed reanimation procedures, and the patient's (or family's) unwillingness to undergo extensive procedures.

The materials used for a sling include fascia (tensor fascia lata), tendons (palmaris longus, extensor digitorum longus, plantaris), allograft, and alloplastic materials (polytetrafluoroethylene). When performing a static reconstruction, a slight overcorrection is preferable to undercorrection to account for stretching of the sling over time.

16.9.1.1 *Static procedures by zones*

16.9.1.1.1 *Forehead.* Brow ptosis occurs secondary to the loss of the frontalis muscle tone, which may constrict the superior visual field by causing a mechanical eyelid ptosis. Compensatory contralateral eyebrow elevation is usually noted. Various brow-lift procedures such as open (coronal), endoscopic, and supraciliary direct excision with or without a fascial graft suspension are some examples of static reconstructive options.

In addition to a brow lift, a blepharoplasty may be needed to improve the visual field if excess skin is present in the upper eyelid. Other available options to correct the forehead asymmetry if no impairment of the visual field is present include paralyzing the contralateral frontalis muscle with botulinum toxin injections, transection of the contralateral frontal nerve, and resection of the contralateral frontalis muscle.

16.9.1.1.2 *Eyelids.* The periorbital area is one of the most difficult to treat. The orbicularis oculi is a concentric muscle innervated by the frontal and zygomatic branches of the facial nerve that provides tone to the upper and lower eyelids, promoting normal lid position and eyelid closure. Paresis of the orbicularis oculi muscle results in lagophthalmos, which is defined as a partial or complete inability to close the eyelids due to unopposed action of levator palpebrae (CN III innervation) and Müller's muscle (sympathetic innervation) (Figure 16.6). A patient with lagophthalmos is at risk for inadequate corneal protection, causing dryness, irritation, and even corneal ulceration and infection. An intact Bell's phenomenon (an upward movement of the eye when attempting to close eyelids) can partially protect the cornea and help prevent exposure keratopathy. In addition to lagophthalmos, paresis of the orbicularis oculi muscle results in ectropion and retraction of the lower eyelid with a scleral show that can exacerbate epiphora. Ectropion of the lower eyelid results in inadequate apposition of the inferior punctum against the globe and an ineffective nasolacrimal pumping mechanism, which leads to epiphora. Exposure keratopathy triggers reflex tearing due to perceived ocular dryness, which also contributes to excessive tearing. Ocular dryness experienced in central facial paralysis is secondary to diminished tear production caused by a lesion at the geniculate ganglion, which gives rise to the first branch of the facial nerve, the greater superficial petrosal nerve. This in turn yields parasympathetic innervation to the lacrimal gland. A concomitant CN V palsy resulting in decreased corneal sensation is especially concerning because of corneal exposure and ulceration.

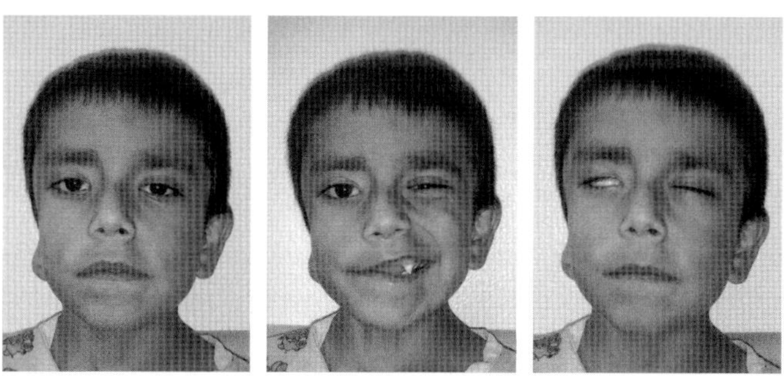

(A) (B) (C)

Figure 16.6. (A) Photograph of a 6-year-old boy with craniofacial microsomia associated with right facial paralysis and right microtia. (B) Characteristic right facial flaccidity when smiling. (C) Evidence of lagophthalmos on the right side when closing eyelids.

Medical management of ocular symptoms in facial paralysis includes frequent use of artificial tears and lubricating ophthalmic ointment to prevent and treat exposure keratopathy; eyelid taping, especially at bedtime; moisture chamber goggles; and patches.

Multiple surgical options with variable success are available to correct lagophthalmos. Static procedures are usually needed to address the eye in facial paralysis since most dynamic procedures do not provide adequate reanimation and protection of the eye.

Tarsorrhaphy can be an effective measure to protect the cornea. It is a simple procedure, and multiple surgical techniques have been described with a primary goal of temporarily or permanently closing the eyelids. The disadvantage of tarsorrhaphy includes loss of field of vision and poor cosmetic appearance. It should not be considered as a first line of treatment because of its considerable functional and aesthetic drawbacks.

Gold weight implantation is a highly effective option in the management of lagophthalmos and corneal protection.[43,44] The prosthesis is fabricated from 24-carat gold and ranges in weight between 0.6 g and 1.8 g in 0.2 g increments. The lightest weight that will bring the eyelid within 2–4 mm of the lower lid should be chosen, with 1.2 g and 1.4 g being the most commonly used weights. An incision is made at the upper eyelid crease, and dissection proceeds through the orbicularis muscle down to the tarsal plate, where a pocket is created to accommodate the implant (Figure 16.7). The gold weight is placed such that the top border of the weight is aligned with the superior edge of the tarsus and centered at the pupil. Sutures are placed to secure it onto the inferior aspect of the tarsal plate, medially and laterally. An additional suture is placed superiorly on the tarsus. Inferior positioning of the gold weight on the tarsus may result in lash ptosis and visibility. Complications associated with the placement of a gold weight include pseudoptosis, migration, extrusion, infection, astigmatism, lash ptosis, and entropion with trichiasis.[45] Fewer complication rates have been reported when the gold weight is substituted for a flexible platinum-chain implant.[46] Placement of the gold weight can be performed more superiorly on the tarsus/septum with less visibility; however, lagophthalmos correction may be lessened.

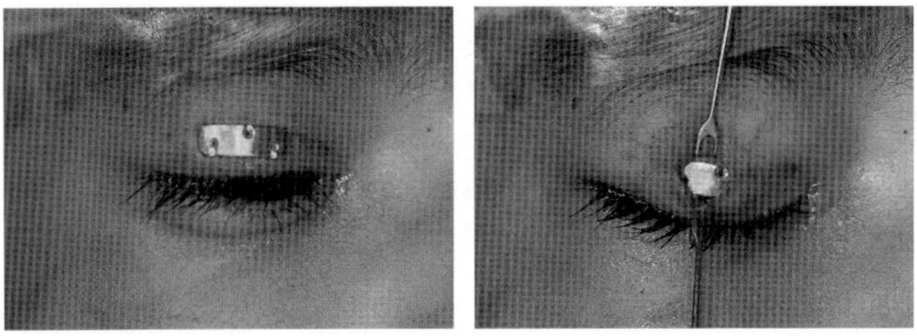

(A) (B)

Figure 16.7. (A) Clinical photograph demonstrating the ideal placement of a gold weight implant. (B) A superior eyelid crease incision is performed, allowing the suturing of a gold weight onto the superior edge of the upper eyelid tarsus.

Paralyzing the levator palpabrae muscle with botulinum toxin is another option in attempting to protect the cornea. It will result in temporary blepharoptosis, thereby preventing corneal exposure.

Lower eyelid ectropion and retraction correction can be addressed with lateral canthoplasty with lid shortening and lid suspension. Lateral canthoplasty consists of resuspending the lateral lower-lid tarsal strip from the inner aspect of the lateral orbital rim through the periosteum or drill hole with appropriate shortening of the tarsal strip as needed. Lid-shortening procedures should be used with caution in patients with prominent eyes or negative vectors. A mid-face lift in conjunction with lateral canthoplasty is a good way to achieve additional support and correct lower eyelid ectropion and retraction.

16.9.1.1.3 Nose. Nasal airway difficulties are secondary to the collapse of nostrils caused by the loss of muscle tone of the dilator naris and levator labii superioris alaeque nasi, resulting in a reduction in airflow. The external and the internal nasal valves together account for about 70% of nasal inspiratory resistance. The internal valve alone can be responsible for up to 50% of the total airway resistance. Nasal lateralization procedures in which a sling is secured intraorally to the deep tissue of the lateral alar base and suspended from the periosteum or a fixation device at the zygoma will help open the external valve. The internal valve can be addressed with the use of a spreader graft, septoplasty, and inferior turbinectomy.

16.9.1.1.4 *Oral commissure and upper lip.* Descent of the oral commissure and upper lip leads to oral incompetence (drooling and difficulty with chewing), facial asymmetry (loss of nasolabial fold, philtral deviation, and incisor show), inability to smile, cheek-biting, and speech difficulty (especially with labial sounds such as *b*, *p*, and *m*). Static reconstruction with slings, wedge resections, or orbicularis muscle transposition will improve the oral sphincter tone and symmetry without providing any animation. When creating a static sling, the suspension vector is determined by analyzing the position of the mouth on the unaffected side. The sling is sutured to the modiolus or split into two tongues and fixed to the orbicular muscle of the upper and lower lip. The other end is secured onto the zygomatic arch or infraorbital rim, depending on the vector desired. Multiple strips of sling material can be utilized to create different vectors of suspension.

Advancement procedures with soft-tissue excision, such as a rhytidectomy with or without SMAS modification, are good adjuncts to static and dynamic techniques. Nasolabial fold excision should be avoided since it has a poor aesthetic result.

16.9.1.1.5 *Lower lip.* Loss of function of the marginal mandibular branch of the facial nerve results in paralysis of the depressors on the lower lip with debilitating cosmetic and functional deficits. On animation, the affected side remains elevated while the non-paralyzed side moves inferiorly and away from the teeth; this is mainly due to the loss of function of the depressor labii inferioris muscle. Temporary correction can be obtained by injecting botulinum toxin on the unaffected contralateral depressor labii inferioris muscle. Permanent measures addressing the contralateral side include the resection of the depressor labii inferioris muscle or transection of the marginal mandibular branch on the unaffected side. Oral continence is minimally affected with these procedures.

16.9.2 *Dynamic reconstruction*

The main objective of dynamic reconstruction is to restore facial symmetry at rest and ultimately provide spontaneous animation. Corneal protection remains a paramount goal when performing reanimation procedures in a patient with facial paralysis.

16.9.2.1 *Reinnervation by nerve transfer*

An adjacent motor nerve may be transferred and coapted to a distal facial nerve stump in a patient with viable facial musculature who lacks the proximal facial nerve segment. The sooner the coaptation is performed, the higher the likelihood that the facial musculature will be reinnervated and hence facial function will return. If the viability status of the distal neuromuscular unit is uncertain, an EMG or muscle biopsy, or both, should be performed before the reinnervation procedure.

Potential donor nerves include the ipsilateral facial nerve, the trigeminal mandibular nerve (CN V_3), the spinal accessory nerve (CN XI), and the hypoglossal nerve (CN XII). Significant morbidities are involved in sacrificing a nerve for transfer. For example, full transfer of CN XII will cause paralysis and atrophy of the ipsilateral tongue, causing significant problems with speech, mastication, and swallowing. Furthermore, it is contraindicated in ipsilateral CN dysfunction of CN IX, X, and XI as it can impair the patient's ability to swallow.[47] A preferable option is to perform a jump graft, which is a partial transfer of hypoglossal nerve fascicles that allows preservation of the ipsilateral hypoglossal nerve function. In general, facial motor function achieved is not as strong after a jump graft as in a full transfer; however, the morbidity is reduced and patients tend to experience less synkinesis.[48] Other alternatives include the use of the ipsilateral masseteric branch (CN V_3) with an interpositional nerve graft to reach the distal nerve stump or a cross-facial nerve graft from the contralateral facial nerve.

16.9.2.2 *Regional muscle transfer*

Regional muscle transfer may be an option when non-viable ipsilateral facial muscles are present. It consists of rotating adjacent innervated muscles and inserting them at key areas such as the oral commissure and eyelids. The masseter and temporalis muscle, both innervated by

CN V, are the most commonly used donor options.[49] This type of reconstruction needs a voluntary action to activate the transferred muscle in order to secondarily achieve a smile or eyelid closure. In the case of the masseter and temporalis muscle transfer, clenching of the teeth, thereby activating the transferred muscle, must be initiated by the patient.

It is important to determine the main vector needed when choosing a muscle transfer graft. The masseter muscle provides a horizontal-lateral vector when used in oral reconstruction, simulating the action of the buccinator-risorius complex (Figure 16.8). It may be used in its entirety or limited to the anterior portion just anterior to the masseteric nerve. The smile generated with this vector often appears unnatural, since there is no elevation generated at the commissure.

The temporalis muscle provides a superolateral vector, simulating the action of the zygomaticus major muscle when attached to the commissure while providing a horizontal-lateral vector when used in reconstruction of the eyelids (Figures 16.9 and 16.10). The central temporalis muscle flap is inferiorly based, and the temporalis fascia is preserved to serve as anchorage. An extension fascial graft may be required in order to reach the eyelid or the commissure. The main disadvantages with this type of transfer are the resulting temporal hollow defect after transfer; the bulge of muscle over the lateral orbit or zygomatic arch, depending on the targeted area; and the slitlike palpebral aperture caused by the horizontal vector pull when used in eyelid reconstruction. Both the temporalis and masseter muscles can be used in conjunction to reanimate the eyelid and the oral commissure.

Another muscle-transfer option is the anterior belly of the digastric muscle, which can be used to correct lower lip asymmetry after the loss of function of the marginal mandibular branch of the facial nerve. The anterior digastric muscle is innervated by the mylohyoid branch of CN V, and once transferred to the lower lip, it helps recreate the vector pull of the depressor muscles.[50]

Regional muscle transfers are often suboptimal for treatment of facial paralysis since accurate vector orientation may be difficult to achieve with limited spontaneous function, and donor site morbidity

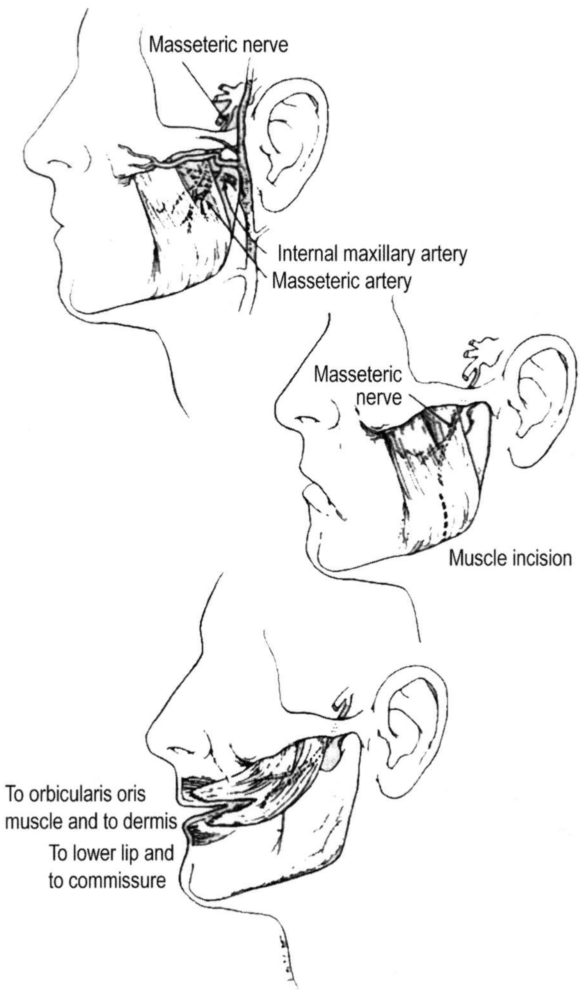

Figure 16.8. Illustration of masseter muscle transfer for reanimation of the lower face. (Modified from Baker DC, Conley J. Regional muscle transposition for rehabilitation of the paralyzed face. *Clin Plast Surg* 1979;6:317–331.)

can be significant. Increasingly, free muscle transfers for facial reanimation are preferred, and regional muscle transfers are reserved for patients who are poor candidates for free muscle transfer or have significant comorbidities.

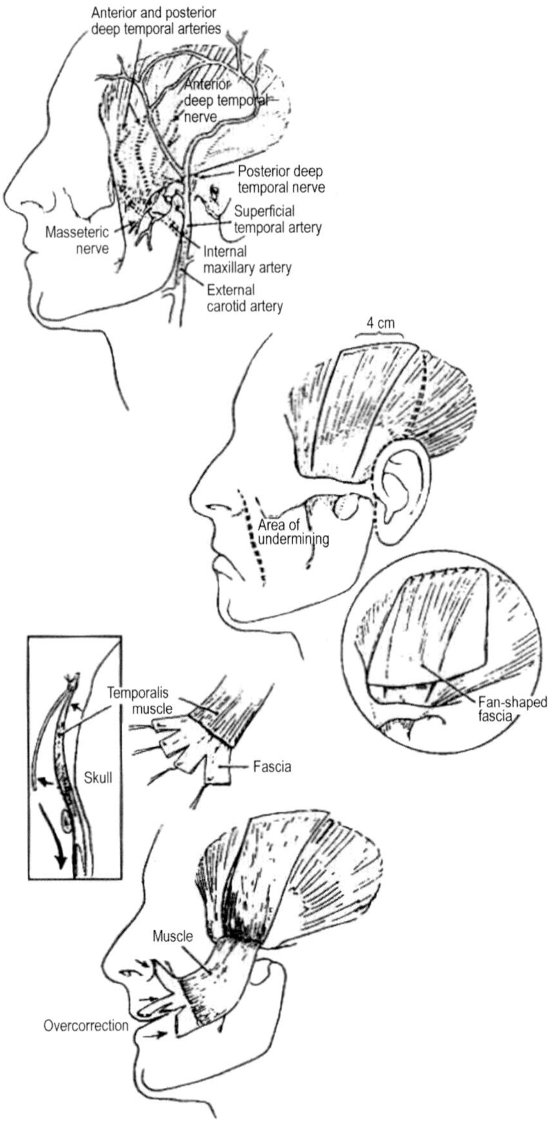

Figure 16.9. Temporalis muscle transfer for reanimation of the lower face including nasal lateralization. (Modified from Baker DC, Conley J. Regional muscle transposition for rehabilitation of the paralyzed face. *Clin Plast Surg* 1979;6:317–331.)

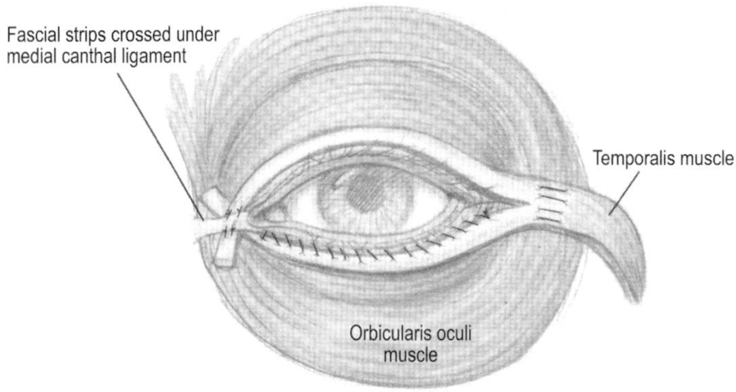

Figure 16.10. Illustration of temporalis muscle transfer with fascial sling to reanimate the upper and lower eyelids. Reprinted with permission from Elsevier (Salimbeni G. Eyelid reanimation in facial paralysis by temporalis muscle transfer. *Oper Tech Plast Reconstr Surg* 1999;6:159–162).

16.9.2.3 *Free neuromuscular tissue transfer*

Free-tissue transfer is a very good reconstructive option when there is no potential for muscle reinnervation or for patients with suboptimal facial nerve recovery.[51–54] There are several proposed advantages over regional muscle transfers. It allows for greater flexibility and precision in vector orientation and the capability of restoring spontaneous mimetic facial expression. This approach works best in younger populations but is now considered an excellent treatment option for older individuals as well.[55,56] Several potential donor muscles are available for free tissue transfer; however, the gracilis muscle has become the workhorse in facial reanimation for the following reasons: relative ease of harvest, expendability, inconspicuous donor scar, adequate muscle length and caliber, reliable neurovascular pedicle, and potential for a two-team approach[57] (Table 16.4). Other candidate muscles, like the latissimus dorsi, do not allow for simultaneous harvest and recipient vessel/nerve dissection because of the close proximity and difficult positioning requirements.

Facial reanimation with free neuromuscular transfer may be performed in a one-stage or two-stage fashion, depending on the recipient nerve neurotizing the flap.

Table 16.4. Potential Donor Muscles in Free Tissue Transfer for Facial Reanimation.

Donor muscle	Blood supply (pedicle length)	Nerve supply (length)	Advantages	Disadvantages
Gracilis	Ascending branch of medial circumflex femoral from profunda femoris (6 cm)	Anterior branch of the obturator nerve (10–12 cm)	Two-team approach, independent neuromuscular units	Bulky
Rectus abdominis	Deep inferior epigastric (5 cm)	Segmental 7th to 12th thoracic intercostal nerve (3–15 cm)	Two-team approach, segmental innervation, tendinous inscriptions	Bulky
Serratus anterior	Lateral thoracic (6–8 cm)	C5–7 roots of long thoracic nerve	Two-team approach, segmental innervation	Bulky
Latissimus dorsi	Thoracodorsal (8 cm)	Thoracodorsal nerve (13–14 cm)	Segmental innervation	Bulky, one-team approach
Pectoralis major	Pectoral branch of thoracoacromial (4 cm)	Lateral pectoral nerve (4–5 cm)	Two-team approach	Bulky, short pedicle
Pectoralis minor	Pectoral branch of thoracoacromial and branch of lateral thoracic (5–6 cm)	Medial and lateral pectoral nerve (4–5 cm)	Two-team approach, dual nerve supply, ideal shape/weight	Short, complex and variable neurovascular pedicle anatomy
Extensor digitorum brevis	Dorsalis pedis (3–4 cm)	Anterior tibial nerve (3–4 cm)	Two-team approach	Short pedicle, insufficient bulk and strength
Rectus femoris	Descending branch of lateral circumflex femoral (5 cm)	Muscular branch of femoral nerve	Two-team approach	Bulky, short pedicle

16.9.2.3.1 *Two-stage operation.* The first stage consists of performing a cross-facial nerve graft. Approximately 20–25 cm of sural nerve is harvested. This donor nerve is coapted to the normal contralateral facial nerve. It is preferable to select a recipient nerve branch that innervates cheek muscle function (zygomaticus major). Branches contributing to the orbicularis oculi or oris function should not be sacrificed. Facial nerve mapping with a nerve stimulator is performed to help determine candidate nerve branches during surgical dissection. The sural nerve graft is tunneled subcutaneously to the contralateral preauricular area. A central sublabial incision is performed to assist with nerve tunneling across the face. The terminal end of the graft is marked with a permanent suture for later identification at the second stage. Nerve regeneration occurs across the graft over 9 to 12 months, and progress can be followed clinically with a Tinel's sign. In some cases, the Tinel's sign may not be appreciated during the regeneration period. We advocate waiting an appropriate time before the second-stage muscle transfer; this corresponds to a length based on regeneration of 1 mm/day, and typically is 9 months for a cross-face nerve graft.

During the second stage, donor muscle with its motor nerve is coapted to the distal end of the cross-facial nerve graft. The distal end of the sural nerve graft stump can be identified and harvested for frozen sections to confirm the presence of myelinated motor fibers within the graft and to select the fascicles with the largest concentration of viable axons. Selection of the donor muscle depends on the surgeon's preference and experience. A patient with a larger face or more robust facial muscle activity on the non-paralyzed side can accommodate bulkier donor muscles. Before full harvest of the muscle from its donor site, the motor nerve to the muscle is dissected adequately for optimal length. It is stimulated, and the muscle is inspected to determine functional vs. non-functional components. The maximally contracting portion of the muscle is preserved along with the neurovascular bundle, and the remainder is excluded. This allows for optimal muscle harvest without adding unnecessary bulk to the face.

The dimensions of the donor muscle harvest are based upon the length required at the recipient site with the oral commissure in slight lateral excursion. The donor muscle is harvested while it is under resting tension length.

A limited rhytidectomy approach is performed to expose the recipient vessels (facial or superficial temporal artery/vein) and nerve, and to create adequate space for muscle inset. We prefer a sub-SMAS dissection for muscle inset. Attaching the muscle to the oral commissure is a critical portion of the procedure. Preoperative assessment of the contralateral muscle function and vector helps determine the appropriate suture placement. In general, the muscle is anchored to the anteromedial aspect of the modiolus and along the upper lip medially. The zygomatic body, temporal fascia, and preauricular fascia serve as the opposite points of attachment of the muscle being transferred. Microvascular anastomosis is performed to the facial or superficial temporal vessels. The vascular anastomosis and the nerve coaptation are placed on the undersurface of the muscle to allow for debulking of the muscle at a later stage if needed. Muscle function can typically be expected 5 to 8 months postoperatively (Figure 16.11).

Another donor muscle for facial reanimation is the serratus anterior muscle. This particular muscle can be divided along its fascial planes, generating up to 10 separate force vectors and thereby allowing restoration of multiple independent functions such as the smile and eyelid closure.[58]

Disadvantages of the two-stage approach include the additional donor site, violation of the contralateral normal facial nerve anatomy, regeneration across two neurorrhaphy junctions, and a long time interval before function is regained. Reduced muscle excursion and strength can sometimes be associated with an inadequate number of axons from the motor donor nerve[59,60] and from an increased nerve-graft length.[61] Nerve-graft failure can lead to secondary cross-face nerve grafting, with the associated delay in achieving reanimation and additional donor facial nerve-branch sacrifice or denervation.

16.9.2.3.2 *One-stage operation.* The one-stage operation consists of performing the free muscle transfer and nerve coaptation to a donor CN in the primary setting (Figure 16.12). Primary neural anastomosis

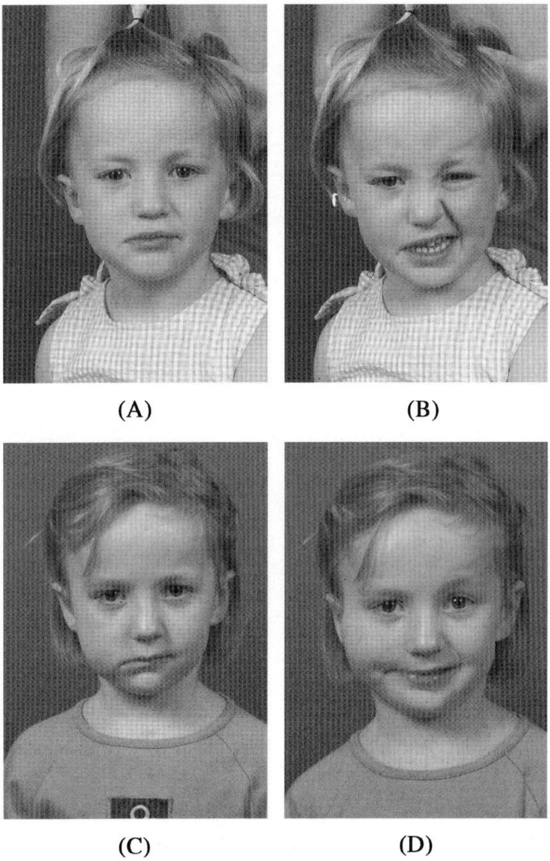

Figure 16.11. A 4-year-old girl with right congenital facial paralysis in repose (A), and in attempted smile (B). Twenty-four months postoperatively after a two-stage free gracilis muscle flap coapted to a cross-facial nerve graft at rest (C) and smiling (D).

may be at the contralateral facial nerve as long as the free tissue transfer has a long nerve segment (such as the latissimus dorsi or gracilis muscles) in order to reach the contralateral facial donor nerve. Another option is to innervate the free tissue transfer with the ipsilateral masseteric nerve branch, which was previously considered only in patients with Möbius syndrome. The motor nerve of the masseter is located on the undersurface of the deep head of the masseter muscle approximately 2 cm below the zygomatic arch. The masseteric branch

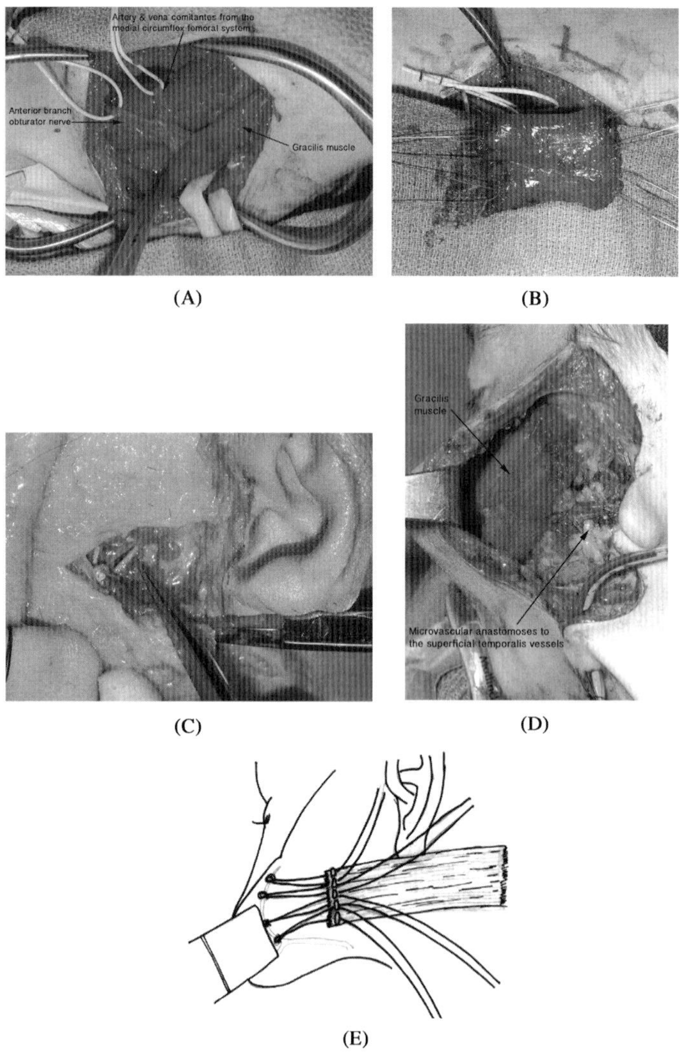

Figure 16.12. (A) Gracilis muscle in situ with its blood and nerve supply. (B) Harvested gracilis muscle with suture plication at proximal and distal ends. Note the significant contraction of the muscle after myotomies. (C) Cadaveric dissection using a limited rhytidectomy approach to expose the superficial temporal vessels and masseteric nerve branch (shown) and to create adequate space for muscle inset. (D) Gracilis muscle is inset with sutures to the oral commissure at four points. The proximal end of the gracilis muscle is secured under appropriate tension at the zygomatic body, temporal fascia, and preauricular fascia. Microscopic neurorrhaphy and microvascular anastomoses are completed. (E) Schematic indicating four suture placements to the oral commissure and "parachuting" of muscle into sub-SMAS pocket.

is a good option for a patient with bilateral facial paralysis but can also be considered for unilateral cases. In addition, when a masseteric branch is used, the onset of movement tends to occur sooner and often with greater strength than with a cross-facial nerve graft.[62] The motor branch of the masseter can be transferred in an end-to-side fashion to preserve muscle function. Muscle activation is often noted as early as 8 to 12 weeks postoperatively, and initially requires a volitional act of biting down. Rapidly, the muscle activation occurs without mouth/biting movements and can be integrated into social situations.

In general, onset of facial movement can be expected 3 to 5 months after one-stage tissue transfer with improvement in function over the following 1 to 2 years. The only donor nerve that will produce a naturally spontaneous smile is the branch of the contralateral facial nerve (CN VII). However, facial reanimation utilizing the motor nerve of the masseter has been shown to exhibit near spontaneity in several cases.[53,63] A smile "training" protocol is beneficial in improving muscle strength and functionality in social settings. Advantages of a one-stage operation include fewer operations, one neurorrhaphy, less time from paralysis to function, stronger power of the innervated muscle, and independent facial motion. Complications include flap failure, poor cortical integration/training resulting in suboptimal muscle function, contour asymmetry, and lack of spontaneity. Revisional surgeries may be beneficial, such as readjustment of insertion and tension of the transferred muscle, addition of a static suspension sling, and procedures for improved symmetry including muscle debulking or fat injections to the contralateral face.[64]

16.9.2.4 *Muscle neurotization*

Muscle neurotization can potentially provide functionality to denervated muscle. It consists of directly implanting a distal nerve or a nerve graft such as a cross-facial or, in cases of bilateral palsy, an ipsilateral motor nerve (masseteric nerve, CN XI, CN XII, or cervical plexus) into the substance of the targeted muscle. The nerve should be divided into a few fascicles and individually implanted and secured in the epimysium. Three types of muscle can be neurotized: native facial muscles, local pedicled muscles, and free transplanted muscles. Neurotization can either restore the function of the muscle being targeted or augment its function. Muscles that are commonly targeted include the orbicularis oculi, orbicularis oris, levator anguli oris, and depressor anguli oris. Neurotization may be performed several times before the desired outcome is achieved.

The success of direct muscle neurotization is related to the clinical presentation, age of the patient, and EMG findings.[65] Any facial movement from the targeted muscle, partial findings of innervation on EMG, and short denervation time (< 2 years) are favorable conditions for muscle neurotization. In adults, the use of an ipsilateral motor donor nerve does not produce a coordinated function of the reinnervated muscle when compared with the contralateral side. In children undergoing muscle rehabilitation, coordinated animation is possible because of increased cerebral plasticity.[66,67]

When performing muscle reinnervation, almost all patients experience a certain degree of synkinesis. Synkinesis is defined as the contraction of two or more muscles that usually do not contract at the same time and is the result of aberrant axonal sprouting during regeneration. In general, the better the recovery, the more severe the synkinesis. Synkinesis may also be seen in patients undergoing other types of dynamic reconstructive procedures. An example of this abnormal regeneration would be eye closure with smiling secondary to aberrant axonal growth regeneration that is due to the extensive anastomotic network between the different branches of the facial nerve. Treatment of synkinesis includes botulinum toxin injections and myectomy.

16.10 Conclusion

Facial paralysis can cause significant functional, aesthetic, and psychological disturbance for the patient. The management of these patients is challenging, and a thorough evaluation and assessment of the patient will help direct the reconstructive surgeon to the appropriate treatment modality.

References

1. **Von Doersten PG, Jackler RK.** Anterior facial nerve rerouting in cranial base surgery: a comparison of three techniques. *Otolaryngol Head Neck Surg* 1996;115:82–88.
2. **Fisch U, Esslen E.** Total intratemporal exposure of the facial nerve: pathologic findings in Bell's palsy. *Arch Otolaryngol* 1972;95:335–341.
3. **May M.** Anatomy of the facial nerve for the clinician. In: May M, ed. *The Facial Nerve.* New York, NY: Thieme Stratton; 1986:35.
4. **Davis RA, Anson BJ, Budinger JM, Kurth LR.** Surgical anatomy of the facial nerve and parotid gland based upon a study of 350 cervicofacial halves. *Surg Gynecol Obstet* 1956;102:385–412.
5. **Tzafetta K, Terzis JK.** Essays on the facial nerve: part I. Microanatomy. *Plast Reconstr Surg* 2010;125:879–889.
6. **Pitanguy I, Ramos AS.** The frontal branch of the facial nerve: the importance of its variations in face lifting. *Plast Reconstr Surg* 1966;38:352–356.
7. **Dingman RO, Grabb WC.** Surgical anatomy of the mandibular ramus of the facial nerve based on the dissection of 100 facial halves. *Plast Reconstr Surg Transp. Bull* 1962;29:266–272.
8. **Bleicher JN, Hamiel S, Gengler JS, Antimarino J.** A survey of facial paralysis: etiology and incidence. *Ear Nose Throat J* 1996;75:355–358.
9. **De Diego-Sastre JI, Prim-Espada MP, Fernández-Garcia F.** The epidemiology of Bell's palsy [in Spanish]. *Rev Neurol* 2005;41:287–290.
10. **Katusic SK, Beard CM, Wiederholt WC, Bergstralh EJ, Kurland LT.** Incidence, clinical features, and prognosis in Bell's palsy, Rochester, Minnesota, 1968–1982. *Ann Neurol* 1986;20:622–677.
11. **May M, Klein SR.** Differential diagnosis of facial nerve palsy. *Otolaryngol Clin North Am* 1991;24:613–645.
12. **Hilsinger RL Jr, Adour KK, Doty HE.** Idiopathic facial paralysis, pregnancy, and the menstrual cycle. *Ann Otol Rhinol Laryngol* 1975;84:433–442.
13. **May M, Hardin WB.** Facial palsy: interpretation of neurologic findings. *Laryngoscope* 1978;88:1352–1362.
14. **Yanagihara N, Mori H, Kozawa T, Nakamura K, Kita M.** Bell's palsy: nonrecurrent vs. recurrent and unilateral vs. bilateral. *Arch Otolaryngol* 1984;110:374–377.
15. **Falco NA, Eriksson E.** Facial nerve palsy in the newborn: incidence and outcome. *Plast Reconstr Surg* 1990;85:1–4.
16. **Smith CK, Portelli FR, Hermann LK, Walike JW.** Facial palsy caused by facial nerve tumor. *Laryngoscope* 1971;81:1542–1545.
17. **Kobayashi T.** Congenital unilateral lower lip palsy. *Acta Otolaryngol* 1979;88:303–309.

18. **Sapin SO, Miller AA, Bass HN.** Neonatal asymmetric crying facies: a new look at an old problem. *Clin Pediatr* 2005;44:109–119.
19. **Gayler GG.** An "epidemic" of congenital facial paresis and heart disease. *Pediatrics* 1967;40:666–668.
20. **Verzijl HT, van der Zwaag B, Cruysberg JR, Padberg GW.** Möbius syndrome redefined: a syndrome of rhombencephalic maldevelopment. *Neurology* 2003;61:327–333.
21. **Terzis JK, Karypidis D.** Direct tongue neurotization: the effect on speech intelligibility in patients with Möbius syndrome. *Plast Reconstr Surg* 2010;125:150–160.
22. **Keane JR.** Bilateral seventh nerve palsy: analysis of 43 cases and review of the literature. *Neurology* 1994;44:1198–1202.
23. **Kamaratos A, Kokkoris S, Protopsaltis J, *et al.*** Simultaneous bilateral facial palsy in a diabetic patient. *Diabetes Care* 2004;27:623–624.
24. **House JW, Brackmann DE.** Facial nerve grading system. *Otolaryngol Head Neck Surg* 1985;93:146–147.
25. **Hughes GB.** Prognostic tests in acute facial palsy. *Am J Otol* 1989;10:304–311.
26. **Sillman JS, Niparko JK, Lee SS, Kileny PR.** Prognostic value of evoked and standard electromyography in acute facial paralysis. *Otolaryngol Head Neck Surg* 1992;107:377–381.
27. **Hardy DG, Macfarlane R, Baguley DM, Moffat DA.** Facial nerve recovery following acoustic neuroma surgery. *Br J Neurosurg* 1989;3:675–680.
28. **Fisch U.** Maximal nerve excitability testing vs. electroneuronography. *Arch Otolaryngol* 1980;106:352–357.
29. **Hatsuyama Y.** Histological studies on the reinnervation of denervated muscle with special reference to the collateral branching. *Electromyography* 1966;6:71–72.
30. **Sullivan FM, Swan IR, Donnan PT, *et al.*** Early treatment with prednisolone or acyclovir in Bell's palsy. *N Engl J Med* 2007;357:1598–1607.
31. **Lagalla G, Logullo F, Di Bella P, Provinciali L, Ceravolo MG.** Influence of early high-dose steroid treatment on Bell's palsy evolution. *Neurol Sci* 2002;23:107–112.
32. **Gantz BJ, Rubinstein JT, Gidley P, Woodworth GG.** Surgical management of Bell's palsy. *Laryngoscope* 1999;109:1177–1188.
33. **Cabaud HE, Rodkey WG, McCarroll HR Jr, Mutz SB, Niebauer JJ.** Epineurial and perineurial fascicular nerve repairs: a critical comparison. *J Hand Surg Am* 1976;1:131–137.
34. **Dellon AL, Mackinnon SE.** Basic scientific and clinical applications of peripheral nerve regeneration. *Surg Annu* 1988;20:59–100.
35. **Chiu DT, Janecka I, Krizek TJ, Wolff M, Lovelace RE.** Autogenous vein graft as a conduit for nerve regeneration. *Surgery* 1982;91:226–233.

36. **Sunderland S, Cossar DF.** The structure of the facial nerve. *Anat Rec* 1953;116:147–165.
37. **Brown PD, Eshleman JS, Foote RL, Strome SE.** An analysis of facial nerve function in irradiated and unirradiated facial nerve grafts. *Int J Radiat Oncol Biol Phys* 2000;48:737–743.
38. **Gagnon NB, Molina-Negro P.** Facial reinnervation after facial paralysis: is it ever too late? *Arch Otorhinolaryngol* 1989;246:303–307.
39. **Carlson BM, Faulkner JA.** Reinnervation of long-term denervated rat muscle freely grafted into an innervated limb. *Exp Neurol* 1988;102:50–56.
40. **Gulati AK.** Long-term retention of regenerative capability after denervation of skeletal muscle, and dependency of late differentation on innervation. *Anat Rec* 1988;220:429–434.
41. **Rubin LR.** The anatomy of a smile: its importance in the treatment of facial paralysis. *Plast Reconstr Surg* 1974;53:384–387.
42. **Harrison DH.** Current trends in the treatment of established unilateral facial palsy. *Ann R Coll Surg Engl* 1990;72:94–98.
43. **Razfar A, Afifi AM, Manders EK, *et al.*** Ocular outcomes after gold weight placement and facial nerve resection. *Otolaryngol Head Neck Surg* 2009;140:82–85.
44. **Rofagha S, Seiff SR.** Long-term results for the use of gold eyelid load weights in the management of facial paralysis. *Plast Reconstr Surg* 2010;125:142–149.
45. **Dinces EA, Mauriello JA Jr, Kwartler JA, Franklin M.** Complications of gold weight eyelid implants for treatment of fifth and seventh nerve paralysis. *Laryngoscope* 1997;107:1617–1622.
46. **Berghaus A, Neumann K, Schrom T.** The platinum chain: a new upper-lid implant for facial palsy. *Arch Facial Plast Surg* 2003;5:166–170.
47. **Conley J, Baker DC.** Hypoglossal-facial nerve anastomosis for reinnervation of the paralyzed face. *Plast Reconstr Surg* 1979;63:63–72.
48. **Schaitkin BM.** Nerve substitution techniques: XII-VII hook-up, XII-VII jump graft, and cross-facial graft. In: May M, ed. The Facial Nerve. New York, NY: Thieme Medical Publishers; 2000:611–633.
49. **May M.** Muscle transposition for facial reanimation: indications and results. *Arch Otolaryngol* 1984;110:184–189.
50. **Tan ST.** Anterior belly of digastric muscle transfer: a useful technique in head and neck surgery. *Head Neck* 2002;24:947–954.
51. **Zuker RM, Manktelow RT.** A smile for the Möbius syndrome patient. *Ann Plast Surg* 1989;22:188–194.
52. **Zuker RM, Goldberg CS, Manktelow RT.** Facial animation in children with Möbius syndrome after segmental gracilis muscle transplant. *Plast Reconstr Surg* 2000;106:1–8.

53. **Manktelow RT, Tomat LR, Zuker RM, Chang M.** Smile reconstruction in adults with free muscle transfer innervated by the masseter motor nerve: effectiveness and cerebral adaptation. *Plast Reconstr Surg* 2006;118:885–899.
54. **Fattah A, Borschel GH, Manktelow RT, Bezuhly M, Zuker RM.** Facial palsy and reconstruction. *Plast Reconstr Surg* 2012;129:340e–352e.
55. **Harii K, Asato H, Yoshimura K, Sugawara Y, Nakatsuka T, Ueda K.** One-stage transfer of the latissimus dorsi muscle for reanimation of a paralyzed face: a new alternative. *Plast Reconstr Surg* 1998;102:941–951.
56. **Terzis JK, Olivares FS.** Long-term outcomes of free-muscle transfer for smile restoration in adults. *Plast Reconstr Surg* 2009;123:877–888.
57. **Harii K, Ohmori K, Torii S.** Free gracilis muscle transplantation, with microneurovascular anastomoses for the treatment of facial paralysis: a preliminary report. *Plast Reconstr Surg* 1976;57:133–143.
58. **Lifchez SD, Gasparri MG, Sanger JR, *et al.*** Serratus anterior in vivo contractile force study. *Plast Reconstr Surg* 2005;116:839–845.
59. **Terzis JK, Bruno W.** Outcomes with eye reanimation microsurgery. *Facial Plast Surg* 2002;18:101–112.
60. **Asaoka K, Sawamura Y.** Hypoglossal-facial nerve side-to-end anastomosis. *J Neurosurg* 1999;91:163–164.
61. **Kim DH, Connolly SE, Voorhies RM, Beuerman RW, Kline DG.** Initial evaluation of variable graft lengths and lesion lengths in the repair of nerve gaps. *J Reconstr Microsurg* 1990;6:311–316.
62. **Bae YC, Zuker RM, Manktelow RT, Wade S.** A comparison of commissure excursion following gracilis muscle transplantation for facial paralysis using a cross-face nerve graft versus the motor nerve to the masseter nerve. *Plast Reconstr Surg* 2006;117:2407–2413.
63. **Lifchez SD, Matloub HS, Gossain AK.** Cortical adaptation to restoration of smiling after free muscle transfer innervated by the nerve to the masseter. *Plast Reconstr Surg* 2005;115:1472–1479.
64. **Takushima A, Harii K, Asato H, Momosawa A.** Revisional operations improve results of neurovascular free muscle transfer for treatment of facial paralysis. *Plast Reconstr Surg* 2005;116:371–380.
65. **Terzis JK, Karypidis D.** Outcomes of direct muscle neurotization in pediatric patients with facial paralysis. *Plast Reconstr Surg* 2009;124:1486–1498.
66. **Bach-y-Rita P.** Brain plasticity as a basis for recovery of function in humans. *Neuropsychologia* 1990;28:547–554.
67. **Kiziltan ME, Uzun N, Kiziltan G, Savrun FK.** The influence of age in peripheral facial palsy on brainstem reflex excitability. *Neurol India* 2005;53:318–322.

CRANIOFACIAL APPLICATIONS IN FACIAL AESTHETIC SURGERY

17

James E. Zins, MD and Chad R. Gordon, DO

17.1 Introduction

Creating facial harmony in patients seeking cosmetic surgery can be challenging, especially in those patients with facial disproportions. Aesthetic disharmonies are often related to both soft tissue and bony structures of the face. The skeletal pillars that support the facial soft tissues in the horizontal, sagittal, and vertical directions include the zygomatic eminence, the lateral and infraorbital rims, the zygomatic arches, and the mandibular rami.[1] In the youthful face, this skeletal support system forms a ground-level foundation, fixing facial soft tissues through its retaining ligaments. In contrast, facial aging is in large part related to laxity in ligamentous attachments and associated descent of soft tissue adjacent to these points of fixation.[2,3] Although attempts at restoring facial volume and contour are most often beneficial in creating a more youthful appearance, quite often the opportunity for significant improvement in overall facial attractiveness and harmony achieved with bony alteration or contouring is overlooked. The application of craniofacial principles to aesthetic surgery is a powerful tool that works synergistically with traditional rejuvenation techniques to produce more dramatic improvements through skeletal modification (Figure 17.1).

17.2 Craniofacial Principles and Practice

Generally speaking, alteration of the bony foundation of the face allows for more consistent results than do attempts at soft-tissue contouring alone.[4]

This is especially so for results obtained with osteotomy compared with alloplastics, for augmentation in the vertical direction.[5–7] Bony reduction of the mandible or frontal bone may also be effective in the

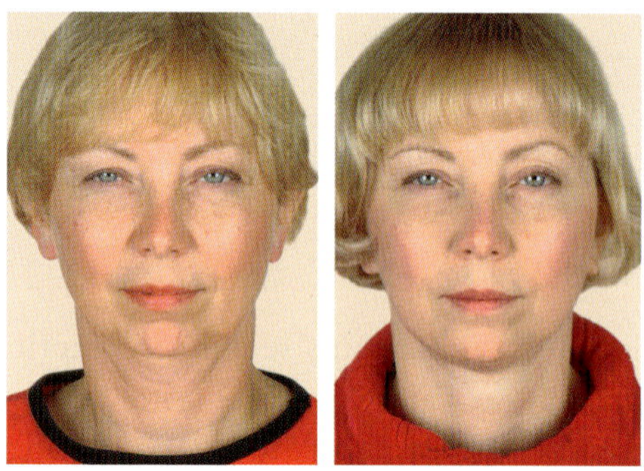

(A)

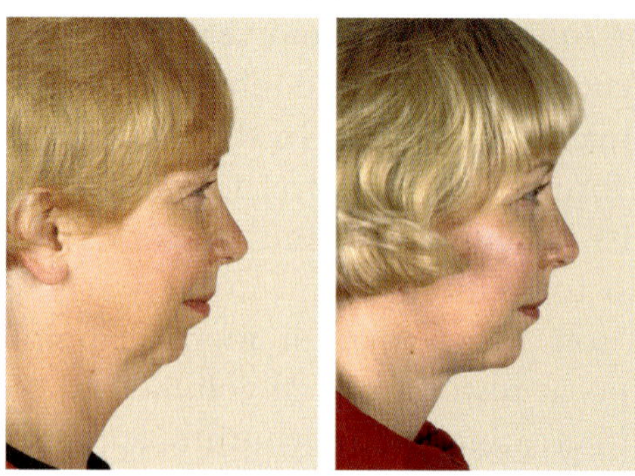

(B)

Figure 17.1. Pre- and postoperative anteroposterior (A) and profile (B) photographs showing the dramatic difference seen by applying craniofacial principles to aesthetic surgery.

appropriately selected patient, especially those presenting with conditions such as frontal sinus hyperpneumatization, benign masseteric hypertrophy, and vertical macrogenia.

When feasible, bony augmentation of the facial skeleton should be favored over reduction since reduction of skeletal support may lead to relative skin excess or ptosis. Augmentation, on the other hand, even when done beyond cephalometric norms, tends to enhance the youthful appearance.[1,6]

Orthognathic surgery can also improve both form and function in patients with congenital and developmental jaw deformities and therefore offers ideal correction. If by chance this type of surgery has been offered (i.e., vascularized osteotomies) during aesthetic consultation and the patient has confirmed that this procedure is unacceptable, then alternatives for appearance improvement, including osteotomies and implant augmentation, can be discussed. Of note, dental relation takes precedence, and therefore each patient's occlusion should be assessed briefly before discussion of genioplasty. The major factors are overjet, overbite, and incisor show at rest and repos.

Options include bone contouring, skeletal augmentation with autogenous bone grafts, alloplastic implants, and bone substitutes to the midface/lower face. The surgeon equipped with a wide armamentarium to perform these procedures will be best suited to tailor the operation to the specific needs of the patient, thereby delivering the optimal aesthetic result.[2]

17.3 Aesthetic Facial Analysis

Aesthetic surgery can be quite challenging, since perfection is often the goal. Cosmetic surgery that includes craniofacial applications offers the opportunity for dramatic improvement with a variety of minimally invasive, skin-sparing, craniofacial approaches.

Attention to detail is of paramount importance. This begins with the very first in-office consultation. A thorough history and physical examination should be accompanied by life-size photographs or computer imaging, or both. These modalities are used as a guide for the surgeon and the patient, so that both parties are in full understanding when discussing realistic postoperative expectations and potential complications.

During consultation, the face should be analyzed in the frontal, oblique, and profile views. A number of techniques can be used for soft-tissue cephalometric analysis. A commonly used analysis divides the face into three equal anatomic aesthetic zones: the first involving the area from the hairline down to the glabella, the second extending from the glabella to the columella-labial junction, and the third from the columella-labial junction to the menton (Figure 17.2). This method of analysis can be used for rapid evaluation during consultation as well as during careful photographic preoperative planning. Whitaker and Bartlett described the ideal transverse dimensions in the adult face from a craniofacial perspective, finding that the bitemporal distance is about equal to the bigonial distance, which together are both less than the bizygomatic distance (this corresponds to the oval or diamond-shaped face).[1,8]

Whitaker[1,8] and Bartlett[8] also noted that the forehead/frontal region, the zygomatic eminences, and the gonial angles should

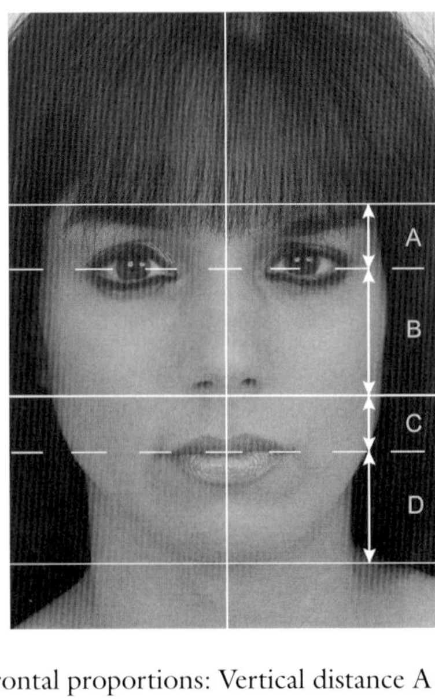

Figure 17.2. Ideal frontal proportions: Vertical distance A = C (upper lip). Vertical distance B = D. D = vertical chin length.

all be seen as high-light areas, while the temporal and buccal sulcus regions should remain as low-light areas. Also, a prominent gonial angle is often considered attractive whereas a steep mandibular plane is not. In a face with harmonious lower facial proportions on profile view, when a tangent is drawn from upper lip to lower lip, the chin falls on this tangential line (also known as Riedel's plane[9]) (Figure 17.3).

17.4 Body Dysmorphic Disorder

Surgeons performing aesthetic surgery should remain vigilant for patients desiring repetitive, unnecessary surgery. These patients, although rare, can be extremely difficult to manage, and are referred to in the literature as having either "dysmorphic personality disorder" or "body dysmorphic disorder." The mean age of onset for this psychiatric disorder is reported to be 16 (±7) years; most patients seeking

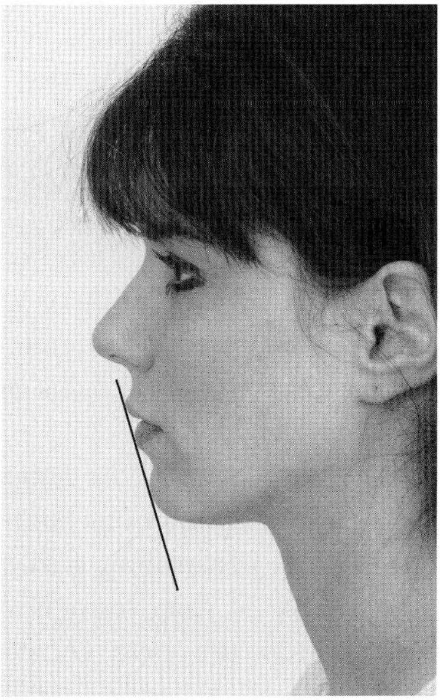

Figure 17.3. A tangent is drawn from upper to lower lip. Ideally, the soft-tissue pogonion should fall on this line.

treatment are in the 20- to 30-year-old age range.[10] The typical course is often progressive rather than episodic, and remission is unfortunately rare. Men and women are affected with equal frequency, but men have been found more likely to remain single and unmarried.[11,12] The incidence of body dysmorphic disorder in cosmetic surgery patients varies considerably in the literature, depending on a variety of factors that include patient age and type of procedures considered. This incidence has been documented to be as high as 15% of cosmetic patients in some studies.

Rhinoplasty is one of the most commonly pursued operations in this patient population.[13,14] Revealing characteristics include patients presenting with numerous photographs, having an unrealistic perception about the severity of their own cosmetic deformity, or presenting to the office with a predetermined surgical plan. Operating on these patients should be avoided, as expectations may be unattainable and postoperative satisfaction is routinely difficult to achieve.[15–17]

A variant of the dysmorphic personality is the "plastic surgery junkie." This patient is often satisfied with surgical results, but later focuses attention on other parts of the body. Perhaps this represents a happier group on a continuum of the disorder.

17.5 Contouring the Craniofacial Skeleton

Augmentation of the frontal bandeau, forehead, and bitemporal regions can all be done either endoscopically or with a bicoronal incision. If the temporal fossa needs to be augmented, the dissection should be taken along the deep temporal fascia in order to stay deep to the frontal branch of the facial nerve.[18,19]

The dissection is then taken deep to the temporalis muscle in the subperiosteal plane along the temporal bone to the level of the lateral orbital rim, as one does when performing a fronto-orbital advancement.[20,21] Because of the risk of long-term bone graft resorption, prosthetic materials are often the best choice in this situation. Augmentation can be carried out with either a solid or porous implant secured at the periphery, preventing unwanted migration, or by using methyl methacrylate or calcium phosphate-based cements. Regardless of implant material, the temporalis muscle and fascia must be redraped over the implant and properly secured back to the temporal fusion line anatomically to prevent displacement or foreshortening.[22,23]

17.5.1 *Frontal/forehead contouring*

Ousterhout characterizes the male forehead according to the degree of frontal sinus bossing.[24] The typical male forehead has varying degrees of frontal bossing that transition superiorly before becoming convex at the hairline. In contrast, an attractive female forehead is without bossing and has a continuous, mild curvature from eyebrow to hairline. A low hairline is a sign of attractiveness and youth in both males and females. Hairline lowering is often combined with forehead contouring in the transsexual population.[24,25] Anterior hairline correction may also be indicated in neurosurgical patients postcraniotomy. In these cases, the hair-bearing scalp may be widely undermined posteriorly in the subgaleal plane. It is then advanced anteriorly using cortical tunnels to hold the scalp in this position. This is the best means of lowering the anterior hairline.

The surgical feminization procedures described by Ousterhout and colleagues classify the forehead into three groups.[24] Each reconstructive method is chosen based on the thickness of the anterior wall of the frontal sinus, which mandates preoperative imaging such as a frontal radiograph and lateral cephalogram (Figure 17.4). All frontal sinus irregularities can be approached by a bicoronal incision, extending one's dissection subperiosteally laterally to the temporal fusion lines and caudally to the supraorbital neurovascular bundles. Type I patients have mild frontal sinus bossing and a thick anterior wall of the sinus that can be easily corrected with reduction by burring down the anterior wall alone.[24,25]

For individuals presenting with mild bossing and a thin anterior table (Type II), bony contouring may need to be combined with a camouflaging procedure just cephalad to the sinus prominence, using a methyl methacrylate onlay. If there is a thin anterior table as well as hyperpneumatization of the sinus (Type III) (Figures 17.5 and 17.6), then one needs to perform an osteotomy of the anterior wall of the

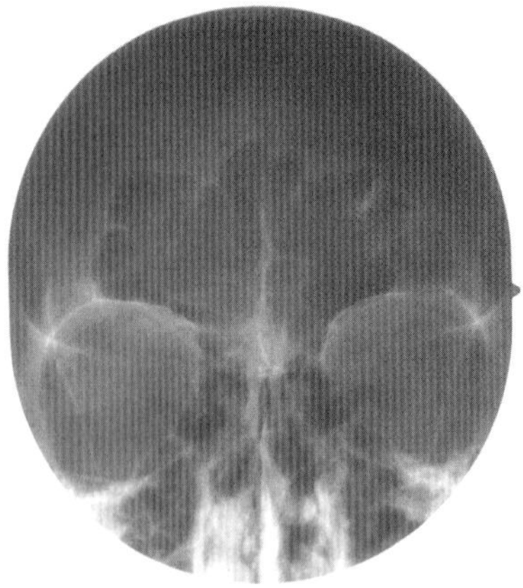

Figure 17.4. Radiograph of preoperative frontal view of patient with hyperpneumatized frontal sinus and thin anterior wall of frontal sinus (Ousterhout Type III patient). Hyperpneumatized sinus is characterized by the large translucent air spaces and scalloped edges.

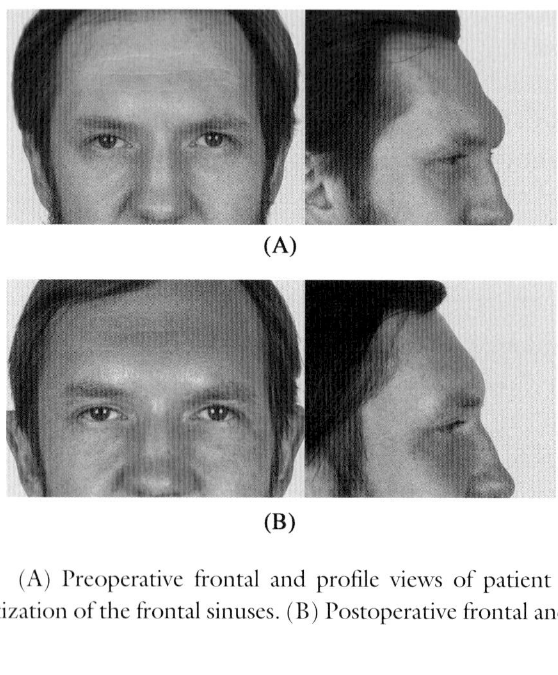

Figure 17.5. (A) Preoperative frontal and profile views of patient with Type III hyperpneumatization of the frontal sinuses. (B) Postoperative frontal and profile views.

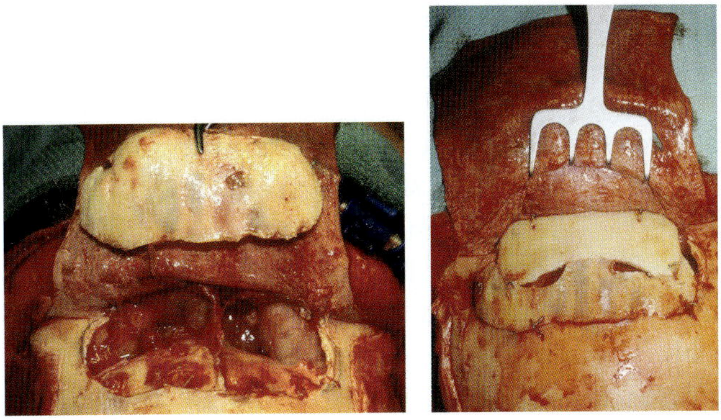

(A) (B)

Figure 17.6. (A) Intraoperative view of same patient as in Figure 17.5 with hyperpneumatized frontal sinus. Osteotomy of the anterior wall of the frontal sinus has been performed. (B) The osteotomized bone has been contoured and flattened and replaced as a bone graft. Additional cranial bone graft has been added.

sinus. The anterior wall is contoured and flattened and placed back as a bone graft, fixed with microplates, and a bone graft is added if necessary (Figure 17.6).[26]

17.5.2 *Malar (cheekbone) augmentation*

Significant improvements of the midface in terms of form and function can be achieved by orthognathic surgery. For this subset, techniques for malar augmentation commonly include autogenous bone grafts and alloplastic implants. Regardless of the technique chosen, careful analysis of the deficiency on both physical examination and radiographic evaluation affects surgical planning. One should always note the thickness of the midfacial soft-tissue envelope to help predict whether the implant or bone graft's edges will be obvious. In addition, the profile view will reveal the convex or concave parasagittal line. Parasagittal convexity is a major contributor to aesthetic harmony.[27]

Although multiple techniques have been described for preoperative midface analysis,[28–31] Terino's description of the five midface zones is the most widely used to date.[32] This classification system divides the midface zones into zone 1 (the zygomatic eminence and anterior third of the arch), zone 2 (the middle third of the arch), zone 3 (the paranasal zone), zone 4 (the posterior third of the arch, which is rarely augmented), and zone 5 (the submalar zone).

According to Terino, the most common zones requiring augmentation are zones 1, 2, and 5.[33] He believes augmenting zones 1 and 2 leads to a more angular appearance, with a well-defined midface and increased bizygomatic distance (Figure 17.7), while augmentation of zone 5 is best reserved for patients who require a fuller, more round appearance. This is a technique that we often use in facelift surgery after massive weight loss and for patients with lipodystrophy after standard triple-drug therapy for human immunodeficiency virus. Although temporal, periorbital, and facelift incisions have all been described for malar augmentation, an intraoral approach through an intraoral buccal sulcus incision is most commonly used. It allows for optimal visualization and avoids a scar. There is, on the other hand, a higher risk of implant contamination and subsequent infection using this approach. However, in most cases of implant infection, micromotion is the culprit, which confirms the need for subperiosteal dissection and screw fixation. Perioperative antibiotics covering oral flora and antibiotic irrigation are both used to minimize overall risk.[29,31,33] Also, one should always identify and protect the infraorbital nerve during dissection and augmentation to avoid nearby compression.

Some craniofacial surgeons prefer the simplicity of using alloplastic implants,[34–37] whereas others still prefer to use nonvascularized bone grafts.[38,39] Cranial bone seems to be the most preferred autogenous graft because of its long-term durability,[40–43] but long-term outcomes have demonstrated progressive and unpredictable resorption.[44,45] The amount of autogenous augmentation (reported in millimeters) is estimated preoperatively based on a lateral cephalogram or life-sized photograph (profile view), or both, and should be overcorrected by 50% intraoperatively.[2] As for alloplastic implants, they should be stabilized with rigid fixation extending from the piriform aperture to the maxillary buttress in areas of aesthetic deformity. Screw fixation decreases the overall risk for postoperative infection (i.e., micromovement) or resorption. However, given the

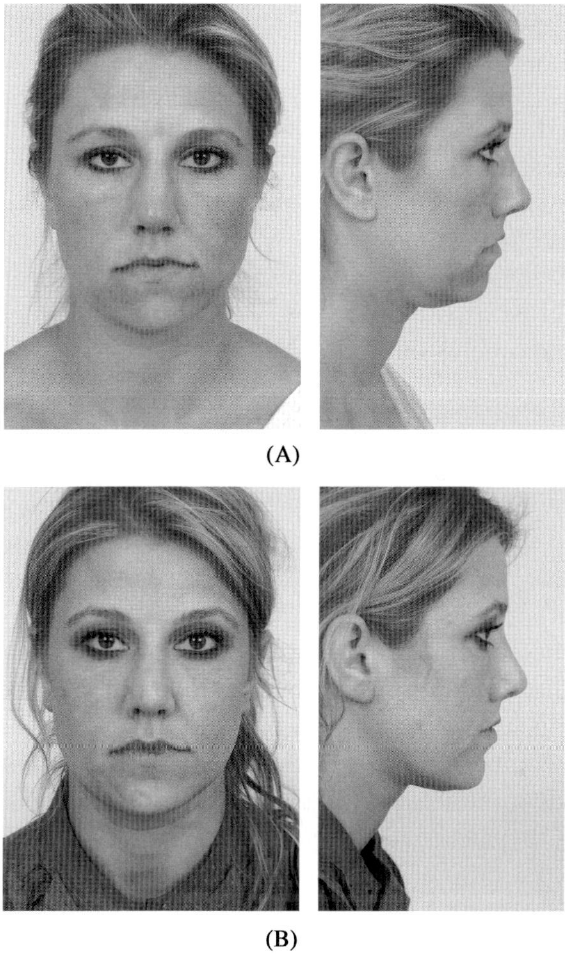

Figure 17.7. (A) Preoperative frontal view of patient with malar weakness and parasagittal concavity. (B) Postoperative view after malar augmentation of Terino zone 3.

added morbidity of in situ bone harvest and the long-term risk of resorption,[44] many find it difficult to justify the use of nonvascularized bone grafts in the cosmetic patient. Interestingly, Wolfe and Vitenas[39] and Kawamoto[40] have described the successful use of the malar osteotomies for cosmetic applications in the midface. In general, alloplastic implants have the distinct advantages of long-term stability (no resorption), ease of contouring compared with rigid bone, and lack of any additional donor site morbidity. On the other hand, alloplastic implants may cause resorption of bone at the augmented site due to micromotion — often times in situations where screw fixation was not used. Porous implants with screw fixation are, therefore, favored over solid implants since bone resorption is minimized and tissue ingrowth is optimized. Alloplastics have been successfully used in the midface region for nasal base, maxillary, and infraorbital augmentation.[26,40,46,47] Experience states that a soft tissue-to-implant ratio of 1:1 should be used by the surgeon, and standard implants can be tailored at the time of surgical correction.[48]

17.5.3 *Gonial angle augmentation*

There are multiple reasons for a patient to present with an underdeveloped bigonial angle distance (or insufficient bigonial width). These include congenital, acquired/posttraumatic, or iatrogenic (postsurgical) etiologies. Alloplastic augmentation used by some surgeons has the advantages of shorter operative times, implant long-term durability (no resorption), and the lack of donor site morbidity. Drawbacks include a higher risk of implant-related infection and subperiosteal bone resorption at the gonial angle recipient site.[48–50] Resorption is minimized with the use of porous implants such as porous polyethylene (Medpor),[35,36,51–53] which allows significant tissue ingrowth. A 1:1 ratio of soft tissue-to-implant correction is suggested when one is planning augmentation.[54] For patients with unilateral deformities (i.e., hemifacial microsomia), a customized, prefabricated implant may enhance the final result versus using an "off-the-shelf" implant. As is often the case, the additional costs associated with this approach must be justified.

Bone reduction often gives consistent results in clinical problems involving bone and soft tissue excess.[2] This is well highlighted in the case of benign masseteric hypertrophy (excessive bigonial width). This condition is actually a result of coexisting hypertrophy of both the overlying soft tissue and the mandibular gonial-angle skeleton, thereby producing a widened lower face in the transverse dimension. The most consistent and durable results can be accomplished using

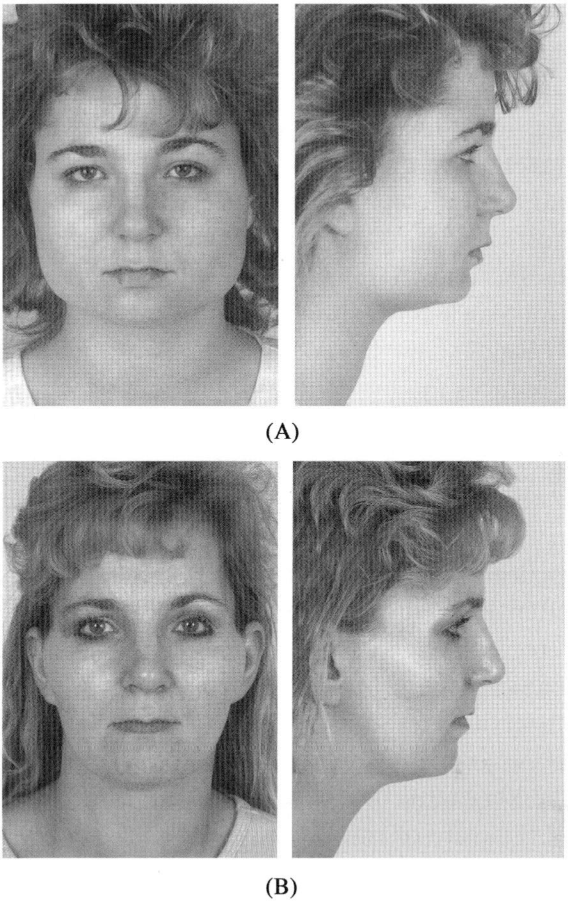

Figure 17.8. (A) Preoperative frontal and profile view of patient demonstrating benign masseteric hypertrophy and vertical microgenia. (B) Eight years postoperatively, after gonial angle reduction and vertical lengthening genioplasty (frontal and profile views).

conservative bony resection/burring of the mandibular angle via an intraoral approach, creating a more aesthetic, obtuse gonial angle[45,55–58] (Figure 17.8). If bone reduction alone is insufficient, then masseter muscle debulking may need to be done sparingly. This, however, should include only the inner portion of the masseter after a subperiosteal approach, so that one avoids injuring the facial nerve and parotid duct. Alternatively, botulinum toxin A injections have been documented to be effective in masseter muscle reduction but provide only a temporary solution, necessitating recurrent injections.[59]

The gonial angle requires the same transoral, vestibular approach used to complete a vertical ramus osteotomy.[54] The buccal incision should extend from the coronoid process to the first molar followed by a subperiosteal dissection, using an elevator to expose the mandibular ramus and body. Yaremchuk *et al.* have popularized the use of porous implants, such as Medpor, that come in a variety of thicknesses and shapes.[60] Rigid screw fixation minimizes the risk of malposition and perhaps reduces the incidence of infection, which in their hands is quite low.[61] If one is performing autogenous augmentation, one option includes using an L-shaped, split cranial bone graft harvested *in situ* from the posterior parietal skull. Even though cranial bone grafts are known to undergo some degree of resorption,[33,44,45] using the dense cortical bone of an outer table graft will surely maximize volume maintenance.[43,51,56,57] Either way, small-caliber, closed-suction drainage is recommended to prevent unwanted dead space and unnecessary fluid accumulation postoperatively.

Based on previous research analyzing the revascularization pattern of cortical bone grafts, a single piece of thick cranial bone is more durable in the long term than a combination of multiple, thin strips. An L-shaped template of the desired bone graft should be designed with slight overcorrection (in the transverse dimension by 1–2 mm) to account for expected graft resorption. Autogenous, calvarial bone grafts less than 3 cm in length or width should be harvested using an *in situ* technique, avoiding the need for a craniectomy.[49,62] This is done using a contouring burr in an area at least 2 cm lateral to the sagittal suture, allowing one to avoid the underlying sagittal sinus and arachnoid granulations. Once the boundaries of the graft are burred down to the diploë, the sagittal saw completes the harvest. It is important to always keep the edge of the blade *visible* and *parallel to the native skull* to avoid violation of the inner table.

The donor site defect may have some surrounding rough edges, which can then be contoured/burred before placing a bone substitute (implant versus bone cement) within the defect.[63] The potential deleterious biomechanical effects of in situ split cranial bone-graft harvesting have been studied, showing a loss of strength of approximately 40% directly over the donor site. Of note, there is no loss in biomechanical skull strength found in the areas away from the donor site, and there are no reported pathologic skull fractures following cranioplasty documented in the literature.[64]

When the defect is large and requires that a full-thickness cranial bone graft be harvested (>3 cm diameter) from the skull by craniectomy, the donor site should be repaired using the outer table of the split bone graft. Alternatively, methyl methacrylate or calcium phosphate cements may be used as an overlay above fixated titanium mesh, which provides a rigid fixation along the underlying defect (preventing transmission of dural pulsations to the implant material). The two main advantages to using full-thickness calvarial grafts for augmentation are their increased bone stock volume and a presumed delay of graft revascularization, which in turn minimizes graft resorption.[57] The bone graft needs to be secured with rigid fixation in order to minimize the risks of displacement/micromovement and resorption.[65]

17.5.4 *Chin augmentation/reduction*

The chin plays an important role in the perception of appropriate facial proportions in both the frontal and profile views. Chin position has a decided effect on the relative proportions of other structures of the face including the neck and nose.[66–71] Augmentation genioplasty is a predictable and powerful technique that can be achieved with either vascularized osteotomies or alloplastic implants[72] (Figure 17.9). Two-piece chin implants may provide the aesthetic surgeon with more control during implantation than the commonly used, single-piece implant. Osseous procedures include burr reduction (ostectomy), osteotomy with caudal segment repositioning, osteotomy with grafting, and osteotomy with segmental sectioning[73–78] (Figure 17.10). Overall skeletal relation *and* dental occlusion should be assessed for all genioplasty patients desiring maxillofacial rejuvenation.[79]

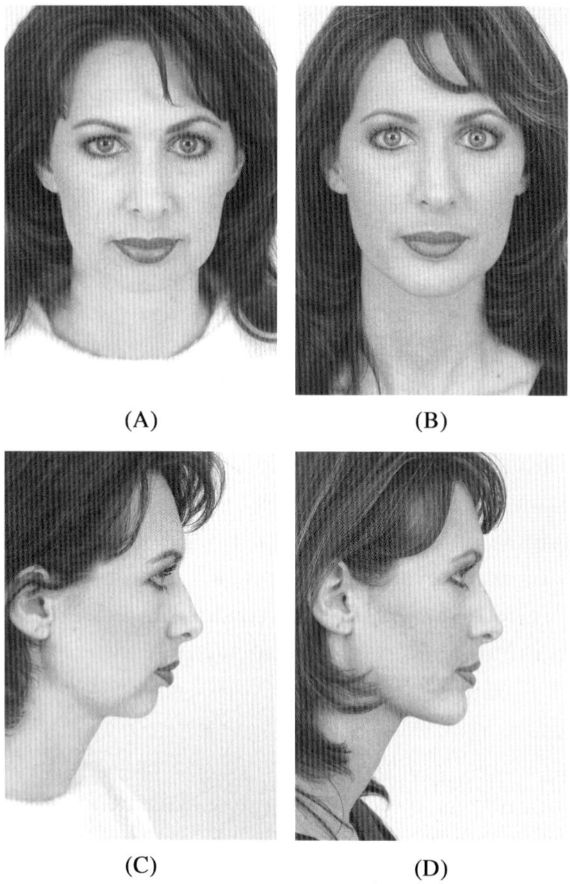

Figure 17.9. (A) Preoperative frontal view of patient with vertical and sagittal microgenia. (B) Postoperative view following horizontal advancement genioplasty. (C) Preoperative profile view. (D) Postoperative profile view.

Augmentation can also be accomplished with onlay autogenous bone grafts, but today's alloplastic implants are more commonly used. Although an alloplastic genioplasty is technically easier to execute, it is not as versatile as the osteotomy, which can address not only sagittal deficiencies but also vertical microgenia and macrogenia, as well as chin asymmetries. Horizontal genioplasties can be performed as isolated procedures or in combination with mandibular ramus osteotomies. Patients with Angle Class II malocclusions are best treated

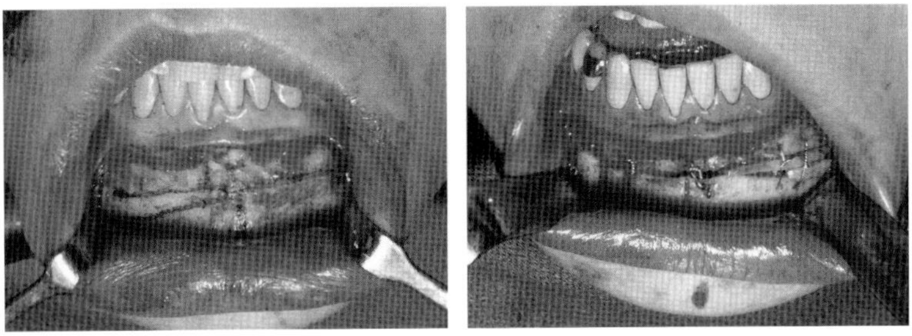

(A) (B)

Figure 17.10. (A) Bone pencil lines demonstrate planned osteotomy. (B) Osteotomy completed. Segment of bone from right side was used to lengthen left side to correct chin asymmetry.

orthognathically. But if such a treatment regimen is refused, a masking procedure with a horizontal sliding genioplasty is an acceptable alternative.[80,81]

Osseous genioplasty may be approached through a lower buccal–sulcus incision. It is important to leave the inferior soft tissues intact in order to maintain a blood supply to the caudal bone flap. The proposed midline of the osteotomy is scored with the saw before any bone cuts are made. The osteotomy should be 3 to 5 mm caudal to the mental foramen to avoid nerve injury. After the caudal segment is osteotomized, it can be moved in any dimension to improve facial proportions. It is then secured using rigid fixation (Figure 17.10). Of note, care should be taken to minimize abrupt bone-to-implant transition points, since these may increase long-term risk of abnormal soft-tissue scarring, including chin-pad displacement.[79,82]

Alloplastic genioplasty can be accomplished successfully with either a silicone or porous polyethylene implant. The submental incision is preferred over an intraoral approach because of the associated risks of implant migration, dehiscence, and infection. The implant should be placed subperiosteally over the densest portion of the mandible to minimize potential visibility, migration, and bone resorption. The chin position is slightly overcorrected since actual clinical correction is slightly less than the bony advancement carried out. There is approximately 0.8 mm of actual advancement for each millimeter of bony advancement made. Complications with alloplastic genioplasty onlay require ultimate removal of the implant or adjustment of either the implant or soft tissue. Subsequent osseous genioplasty to preserve aesthetic contour is a good option for implant malposition or soft tissue problems.[79,80,83,84]

17.5.5 *Orthognathic surgery*

The aesthetic correction of lower facial deformities using orthognathic surgery allows for simultaneous correction of both malocclusion and appearance, thereby providing stable, long-term improvements in both form and function. These techniques are discussed in Chapter 6 of this book.

17.6 Conclusion

Alteration of the bony foundation of the face using osteotomies, alloplastic implants, or bone contouring can have a dramatic effect on facial proportions and can enhance the aesthetic result.[85] A thorough familiarity with these techniques as well as facial analysis should be part of every plastic surgeon's armamentarium. When appropriate, approaches to the craniofacial skeleton allowing subperiosteal exposure should be utilized, representing the tremendous value of craniofacial practice and principles within successful aesthetic surgery.

References

1. **Whitaker LA.** Facial proportions in aesthetic surgery. In: Farkas LG, Munro IR, eds. *Anthropometric Facial Proportions in Medicine.* Springfield, IL: Charles C Thomas; 1987.
2. **Stuzin JM, Baker TJ, Gordon HL.** The relationship of the superficial and deep facial fascias: relevance to rhytidectomy and aging. *Plast Reconstr Surg* 1992;89:441–451.
3. **Stuzin JM, Baker TJ, Gordon HL, Baker TM.** Extended SMAS dissection as an approach to midface rejuvenation. *Clin Plast Surg* 1995;22:295–311.

4. **Zins JE, Castor S, Papay FA.** Contour alteration of the facial skeleton. In: Achauer B, Eriksson E, Guyuron B, *et al.*, eds. *Plastic Surgery: Indications, Operations, and Outcomes.* Vol. 5. Philadelphia, PA: Mosby; 2000:2823–2837.
5. **Flowers RS.** Alloplastic augmentation of the anterior mandible. *Clin Plast Surg* 1991;18:107–138.
6. **Rosen HM.** Surgical correction of the vertically deficient chin. *Plast Reconstr Surg* 1988;82:247–256.
7. **Rosen HM.** Definitive surgical correction of vertical maxillary deficiency. *Plast Reconstr Surg* 1990;85:215–223.
8. **Whitaker LA, Bartlett SP.** Aesthetic surgery of the facial skeleton. Perspectives in Plastic Surgery. *QMP Clinical Series* 1988;2:23–69.
9. **Riedel RA.** An analysis of dentofacial relationships. *Am J Orthod Dentofacial Orthop* 1957;43:103–119.
10. **Castelló JR, Barros J, Chinchilla A.** Body dysmorphic disorder and aesthetic surgery: case report. *Aesthetic Plast Surg* 1998;22:329–331.
11. **Cotterill JA.** Body dysmorphic disorder. *Dermatol Clin* 1996;14:457–463.
12. **Edgerton MT, Langman MW, Pruzinski T.** Plastic surgery and psychotherapy in the treatment of 100 psychologically disturbed patients. *Plast Reconstr Surg* 1991;88:594–608.
13. **Phillips KA, Diaz SF.** Gender differences in body dysmorphic disorder. *J Nerv Ment Dis* 1997;185:570–577.
14. **Phillips KA, Menard W, Fay C, Weisberg R.** Demographic characteristics, phenomenology, comorbidity, and family history in 200 individuals with body dysmorphic disorder. *Psychosomatics* 2005;46:317–325.
15. **American Psychiatric Association.** *Diagnostic and Statistical Manual of Mental Disorders.* 4th edn. Washington, DC: American Psychiatric Association; 2000.
16. **Crerand CE, Franklin ME, Sarwer DB.** Body dysmorphic disorder and cosmetic surgery. *Plast Reconstr Surg* 2006;118:167e–180e.
17. **Crerand CE, Phillips KA, Mendar W, Fay C.** Nonpsychiatric medical treatment of body dysmorphic disorder. *Psychosomatics* 2005;46:549–555.
18. **Whitaker LA, Morales L Jr., Farkas LG.** Aesthetic surgery of the supraorbital ridge and forehead structures. *Plast Reconstr Surg* 1986;78:23–32.
19. **Wolfe SA, Berkowitz S.** *Plastic Surgery of the Facial Skeleton.* Boston, MA: Little Brown; 1989.
20. **Ortiz Monasterio F.** Aesthetic surgery of the facial skeleton: the forehead. *Clin Plast Surg* 1991;18:19–27.
21. **Epker BN.** *Esthetic Maxillofacial Surgery.* Malvern, PA: Lea & Febiger; 1994.

22. **Gordon CR, Yaremchuk MJ.** Temporal augmentation with methyl methacrylate. *Aesthet Surg J* 2011;31:827–833.
23. **Yaremchuk MJ, Gordon CR.** Facial skeletal augmentation with alloplastic implants. In: Thorne CH, ed. *Grabb and Smith's Plastic Surgery.* 7th edn. New York, NY: Lippincott Williams & Wilkins; 2011.
24. **Ousterhout DK.** Feminization of the forehead: contour changing to improve female esthetics. *Plast Reconstr Surg* 1987;79:701–713.
25. **Ousterhout DK, Baker S, Zlotolow I.** Methylmethacrylate onlay implants in the treatment of forehead deformities secondary to craniosynostosis. *J Maxillofac Surg* 1980;8:228–233.
26. **Manson PN, Crawley WA, Hoopes JE.** Frontal cranioplasty: risk factors and choice of cranial vault reconstructive material. *Plast Reconstr Surg* 1986;77:888–904.
27. **Yaremchuk MJ.** Making concave faces convex [published online ahead of print June 3, 2005]. *Aesthetic Plast Surg* 2005;29:141–148. doi:10.1007/S00266-004-0139-9.
28. **Ramirez OM, Maillard GF, Musolas A.** The extended subperiosteal facelift: a definitive soft-tissue remodeling for facial rejuvenation. *Plast Reconstr Surg* 1991;88:227–238.
29. **Ramirez OM.** The subperiosteal rhytidectomy: the third-generation face-lift. *Ann Plast Surg* 1992;28:218–234.
30. **Mladick RA.** Alloplastic cheek augmentation. *Clin Plast Surg* 1991;18:29–38.
31. **Terino EO.** Implants for male aesthetic surgery. *Clin Plast Surg* 1991;18:731–749.
32. **Terino EO.** Alloplastic facial contouring by zonal principles of skeletal anatomy. *Clin Plast Surg* 1992;19:487–510.
33. **Terino EO.** Alloplastic facial contouring: surgery of the fourth plane. *Aesthetic Plast Surg* 1992;16:195–212.
34. **Flowers RS.** Aesthetic surgery in the Oriental: current trends. In: Marsh J, edn. *Current Therapy in Plastic and Reconstructive Surgery.* Philadelphia, PA: Decker; 1988.
35. **Wellisz T.** Clinical experience with Medpor porous polyethylene implant. *Aesthetic Plast Surg* 1993;17:339–344.
36. **Romano JJ, Iliff NT, Manson PN.** Use of Medpor porous polyethylene implants in 140 patients with facial fractures. *J Craniofac Surg* 1993;4:142–147.
37. **Yaremchuk MJ.** Changing concepts in the management of secondary orbital deformities. *Clin Plast Surg* 1992;19:113–124.
38. **Whitaker LA.** Aesthetic augmentation of the malar-midface structures. *Plast Reconstr Surg* 1987;80:337–346.
39. **Wolfe SA, Vitenas P Jr.** Malar augmentation using autogenous materials. *Clin Plast Surg* 1991;18:39–54.

40. **Kawamoto HK Jr.** Late posttraumatic enophthalmos: a correctable deformity? *Plast Reconstr Surg* 1982;69:423–432.
41. **Dado DV, Izquierdo R.** Absorption of onlay bone grafts in immature rabbits: membranous versus endochondral bone and bone struts versus paste. *Ann Plast Surg* 1989;23:39–48.
42. **Hardesty RA, Marsh JL.** Craniofacial onlay bone grafting: a prospective evaluation of graft morphology, orientation, and embryonic origin. *Plast Reconstr Surg* 1990;85:5–15.
43. **Smith JD, Abramson M.** Membranous vs endochondrial bone autografts. *Arch Otolaryngol* 1974;99:203–205.
44. **Zins JE, Whitaker LA.** Membranous versus endochondral bone: implications for craniofacial reconstruction. *Plast Reconstr Surg* 1983;72:778–785.
45. **Freihofer PM, Borstlap WA.** Reconstruction of the zygomatic area: a comparison between osteotomy and onlay techniques. *J Craniomaxillofac Surg* 1989;17:243–248.
46. **Bell WH.** *Modern Practice in Orthognathic and Reconstructive Surgery.* Vol. I. Philadelphia, PA: Saunders; 1992:431–439.
47. **Flowers RS.** Implants for correction of soft tissue and bony facial deformities including the posterior mandible. Paper presented at: Congress of the PanPacific Surgical Association; Honolulu, HI; 1988.
48. **Hinderer UT.** Part 3: malar implants to improve facial proportions and aging. In: Start RB, ed. *Plastic Surgery of the Head and Neck.* New York, NY: Churchill Livingstone; 1987.
49. **Kline RM Jr., Wolfe SA.** Complications associated with harvesting of cranial bone grafts. *Plast Reconstr Surg* 1995;95:5–20.
50. **Flowers RS.** Personal communication; 1992.
51. **Wellisz T, Lawrence M, Jazayeri MA, Golshani S, Zhou ZY.** The effects of alloplastic implant onlays on bone in the rabbit mandible. *Plast Reconstr Surg* 1995;96:957–963.
52. Medpor surgical implants [package insert]. College Park, GA: Porex Surgical.
53. **Wellisz T, Dougherty W, Gross J.** Craniofacial applications for the Medpor porous polyethylene flexblock implant. *J Craniofac Surg* 1992;3:101–107.
54. **Baek SM, Baek RM, Shin MS.** Refinements in aesthetic contouring of the prominent mandibular angle. *Aesthetic Plast Surg* 1994;18:283–289.
55. **Nishida M, Iizuka T.** Intraoral removal of the enlarged mandibular angle associated with masseteric hypertrophy. *J Oral Maxillofac Surg* 1995;53:1476–1479.
56. **Ousterhout DK.** Mandibular angle augmentation and reduction. *Clin Plast Surg* 1991;18:153–161.

57. **Chen NT, Glowacki J, Bucky LP, Hong HZ, Kim WK, Yaremchuk MJ.** The roles of revascularization and resorption on endurance of craniofacial onlay bone grafts in the rabbit. *Plast Reconstr Surg* 1994;93:714–724.
58. **Ozaki W, Buchman S.** Volume maintenance of onlay bone grafts in the craniofacial skeleton: micro-architecture versus embryologic origin. *Plast Reconstr Surg* 1998;102:291–299.
59. **Andrade NN, Deshpande GS.** Use of botulinum toxin (botox) in the management of masseter muscle hypertrophy: a simplified technique. *Plast Reconstr Surg* 2011;128:24e–26e.
60. **Matros E, Momoh A, Yaremchuk MJ.** The aging midfacial skeleton: implications for rejuvenation and reconstruction using implants [published online ahead of print November 18, 2009]. *Facial Plast Surg* 2009;25:252–259. doi:10.1055/s-00291-242037.
61. **Yaremchuk MJ, Doumit G, Thomas MA.** Alloplastic augmentation of the facial skeleton: an occasional adjunct or alternative to orthognathic surgery. *Plast Reconstr Surg* 2011;127:2021–2030.
62. **Zins JE, Weinzweig N, Hahn J.** A simple fail-safe method for the harvesting of cranial bone. *Plast Reconstr Surg* 1995;96:1444–1447.
63. **Afifi AM, Gordon CR, Pryor LS, Sweeney W, Papay FA, Zins JE.** Calcium phosphate cements in skull reconstruction: a meta-analysis. *Plast Reconstr Surg* 2010;126:1300–1309.
64. **Zins JE, Reger SI, Lybch T, Papay FA.** Biomechanical analysis of split cranial bone. In: Marchac D, ed. *Proceedings of the Sixth International Congress of Craniofacial Surgery*. Saint Tropez, France: Monduzzi Editore; 1995:333–335.
65. **Phillips JH, Rahn BA.** Fixation effects on membranous and endochondral onlay bone-graft resorption. *Plast Reconstr Surg* 1988;82:872–877.
66. **Peck H, Peck S.** A concept of facial esthetics. *Angle Orthod* 1970;40:284–318.
67. **Rosen HM.** Aesthetic guidelines in genioplasty: the role of facial disproportion. *Plast Reconstr Surg* 1995;95:463–472.
68. **Gonzalez-Ulloa M.** Quantitative principles in cosmetic surgery of the face (profileplasty). *Plast Reconstr Surg Transplant Bull* 1962;29:186–198.
69. **Danahey DG, Dayan SH, Benson AG, Ness JA.** Importance of chin evaluation and treatment to optimizing neck rejuvenation surgery. *Facial Plast Surg* 2001;17:91–97.
70. **Guyuron B.** *Genioplasty*. Boston, MA: Little, Brown; 1993.
71. **Zide BM, Pfeifer TM, Longaker MT.** Chin surgery: I. Augmentation — the allures and the alerts. *Plast Reconstr Surg* 1999;104:1843–1862.
72. **Spear SL, Kassan M.** Genioplasty. *Clin Plast Surg* 1989;16:695–706.

73. **Frodel JL, Sykes JM, Jones JL.** Evaluation and treatment of vertical microgenia. *Arch Facial Plast Surg* 2004;6:111–119.
74. **Hinds EC, Kent JN.** Genioplasty: the versatility of horizontal osteotomy. *J Oral Surg* 1969;27:690–700.
75. **Hohl TH, Epker BN.** Macrogenia: a study of treatment results, with surgical recommendations. *Oral Surg Oral Med Oral Pathol* 1976;41:545–567.
76. **Park HS, Ellis E III, Fonseca RJ, Reynolds ST, Mayo KH.** A retrospective study of advancement genioplasty. *Oral Surg Oral Med Oral Pathol* 1989; 67:481–489.
77. **Wessberg GA, Wolford LM, Epker BN.** Interpositional genioplasty for the short face syndrome. *J Oral Surg* 1980;38:584–590.
78. **Millard DR Jr.** Chin implants. *Plast Reconstr Surg* 1954;13:70–74.
79. **Yaremchuk M, Gordon CR.** Lip-chip deformity correction following osseous and alloplastic genioplasty. Presented at: Annual Meeting of the American Association of Plastic Surgeons; April 2011; Boca Raton, FL.
80. **Wolfe SA, Rivas-Torres MT, Marshall D.** The genioplasty and beyond: an end-game strategy for the multiply operated chin. *Plast Reconstr Surg* 2006;117:1435–1446.
81. **Guyuron B, Raszewski RL.** A critical comparison of osteoplastic and alloplastic augmentation genioplasty. *Aesthetic Plast Surg* 1990;14:199–206.
82. **Guyuron B.** Genioplasty. In: Ferrano JW, ed. *Fundamentals of Maxillofacial Surgery*. New York, NY: Springer-Verlag; 1997.
83. **Cohen SR, Mardach OL, Kawamoto HK Jr.** Chin disfigurement following removal of alloplastic chin implants. *Plast Reconstr Surg* 1991;88:62–70.
84. **Li KK, Cheney ML.** The use of sliding genioplasty for treatment of failed chin implants. *Laryngoscope* 1996;106:363–366.
85. **Yaremchuk MJ.** Aesthetic contouring of the craniofacial skeleton. In: Guyuron B, Eriksson E, Persing J, *et al.*, eds. *Plastic Surgery: Indications and Practice*. New York, NY: Elsevier; 2009:Chapter 116.

CRANIOMAXILLOFACIAL ALLOTRANSPLANTATION: FROM A BASIC SCIENCE PERSPECTIVE

18

Maria Siemionow, MD, PhD and Fatih Zor, MD

18.1 Introduction

Over the last 2 decades, the plastic surgery research laboratory at Cleveland Clinic has developed numerous craniomaxillofacial allotransplant models (in rats) evaluating various immunosuppressive protocols for tolerance induction. These include full face/scalp, hemiface, composite hemiface/calvarium, rat maxilla, composite osteomusculocutaneous hemiface/mandible/tongue, and composite midface, composite hemiface, and eyeball allotransplantation model.[1–7] Similarly, research from other laboratories has reported analogous studies in large-animal models such as nonhuman primates, pigs, dogs, and rabbits (Table 18.1). With this in mind, the craniomaxillofacial surgeon should be aware of the current state of the art in relation to basic science investigation and those animal models of importance.

Table 18.1. Animal Models of Experimental Face Transplantation.

Animal model	Animal	Year published	Center
Full face/scalp transplant model[1]	Rats	2003	Cleveland Clinic, USA
Hemiface transplant model[2]	Rats	2005	Cleveland Clinic, USA
Composite hemiface/calvarium transplant model[3]	Rats	2006	Cleveland Clinic, USA
Maxilla allotransplantation model[4]	Rats	2007	Cleveland Clinic, USA
Composite osteomusculocutaneous hemiface/mandible/tongue-flap model[5]	Rats	2006	Cleveland Clinic, USA
Composite midface model with sensory and motor neuromuscular units[6]	Rats	2010	Cleveland Clinic, USA
Composite hemiface orbita allotransplantation with optic nerve[7]	Rats	2011	Dr. Zor, Turkey
Hemifacial transplant model[8]	Dogs	2007	Dr. Shengwu, Shanghai, China
Hemifacial transplantation model[9]	Rabbits	2006	Dr. Guo, Xi'an, China
Hemifacial composite tissue allotransplantation[10]	Swine	2009	Dr. Kuo, Taiwan
Heterotopic model for facial composite tissue transplantation[11]	Primate	2008	Dr. Silverman, Baltimore, USA
Facial subunit composite tissue allografts in nonhuman primates[12]	Primate	2009	Dr. Barth, Baltimore, USA

18.2 Experimental Animal Models

18.2.1 *Small-animal models*

18.2.1.1 *Full face/scalp transplant model*

Our institution confirmed for the first time the feasibility of total facial/scalp allograft transplantation across major histocompatibility complex

(MHC) barriers in the rodent model. Transplants were performed between semi-allogeneic Lewis–Brown-Norway (LBN) ($RT1^{1+n}$) donors and Lewis (LEW) ($RT1^{1}$) recipients. In the donors, using an alloflap based on the bilateral common carotid arteries and external jugular veins, the entire facial skin and scalp flap, including both ears was harvested. In the recipient, a facial/scalp defect was created by excising facial skin, scalp, and external ears. The facial nerves and muscles, and the perioral and periorbital regions, were preserved to avoid functional deficits that could interfere with animal feeding, breathing, and eye closure. Both common carotid arteries were used to perfuse the full facial/scalp alloflap. Arterial anastomoses were performed to either the recipient's common carotid arteries (end-to-side) or external carotid arteries (end-to-end). Venous anastomoses were performed to either the external jugular vein on one side or to the anterior facial veins (end-to-end) on the contralateral side. Postoperatively, the recipient animal received cyclosporine A (CsA) monotherapy at a dose of 16 mg/kg/day, tapered to 2 mg/kg/day over 4 weeks, and was maintained at this serum level for more than 200 days.[1,13]

Recently, to improve the survival of the facial/scalp alloflaps, we have introduced a new approach by modifying the arterial anastomoses in the recipients. A single (unilateral) common carotid artery of the recipient was used to vascularize the entire transplanted facial/scalp flap. Different modifications of the arterial anastomoses were evaluated. With these modifications, postoperative mortality of the animals has been significantly reduced by avoiding the complications associated with bilateral common carotid artery anastomoses.

In this model, facial/scalp allotransplants are performed between fully allogeneic ACI ($RT1^{a}$) donors and LEW ($RT1^{1}$) recipient rats. The same CsA immunosuppressive protocol as in the previously described model resulted in more than 180 days of facial/scalp alloflap survival.[14]

18.2.1.2 *Hemiface transplant model*

To further shorten surgery time and brain ischemia time, we introduced a hemifacial allograft transplant model that is technically less challenging than the full facial/scalp model. This model has been used to test induction of operational tolerance across MHC barriers. Hemifacial allotransplants were performed between semi-allogeneic LBN ($RT1^{1+n}$) and fully allogeneic ACI ($RT1^{a}$) donors and LEW ($RT1^{1}$) recipients. Composite hemifacial/scalp alloflaps, including the external ear and scalp, based on the common carotid artery and external jugular vein, were harvested from the donors. In the recipient, the hemifacial/scalp skin was excised, including the external ear. The arterial and venous anastomoses were performed to the common carotid artery (end-to-side) and to the external jugular vein (end-to-end), respectively. The same CsA monotherapy immunosuppressive protocol was used, and 400 days of survival were achieved for semi-allogeneic transplants and 330 days for the fully MHC-mismatched hemifacial transplant recipients.[2,15,16]

18.2.1.3 *Composite hemiface/calvarium transplantation model*

A composite hemiface/calvarium transplantation model in the rat was created for the purpose of incorporating vascularized calvarial bone, based on the same vascular pedicle, as a new treatment option for extensive craniomaxillofacial deformities with large bone defects. Composite hemiface/calvarial transplants were performed across the MHC barrier between LBN and LEW rats. Hemicalvarial bone and face alloflaps were dissected on the common carotid artery and jugular vein, and were transplanted to the de-epithelialized donor faces. All rats received tapered and continuous doses of CsA monotherapy. Evaluation methods included flap angiography, daily inspection, computed tomography (CT), and bone histology. Flap angiography demonstrated an intact vascular supply to the bone. The average survival time was 154 days. No signs of rejection or flap loss were noted at 220 days posttransplant. Bone histology at days 7, 30, 63, and 100 posttransplant revealed viable bone at all time points, and CT at days 14, 30, and 100 revealed normal bones without resorption. For extensive face deformities, involving large defects of soft and bony tissue, this osteomusculocutaneous hemiface/calvarium flap model serves to evaluate new reconstructive options for covering multitissue defects in one surgical procedure.[3]

18.2.1.4 *Maxilla allotransplantation model*

A rat model was developed for investigating vascularized maxilla allotransplantation for reconstructing complex maxillary defects. Maxillary allotransplantations were performed across the MHC barrier between 10 LBN and 10 LEW recipient rats under CsA monotherapy. Grafts were dissected along Le Fort II osteotomy lines based on the common carotid artery and external jugular vein, and then transplanted to the anterior abdominal wall via microvascular anastomoses. Alloflaps were examined by CT, flow cytometry, angiography, and histology. The alloflaps survived up to 105 days without signs of rejection. A high level of donor-specific chimerism for T- and B-cell lineages was maintained. The incisors continued to grow; tooth buds, bone, cartilage, and mucosa remained intact. Moderate inflammation of the nasal and oral mucosa and keratinous metaplasia were noted histologically. This maxilla allotransplantation model allows one to study immunologic responses and demonstrates potential clinical applications based on the growth properties of the alloflap. Surviving recipients, at more than 105 days, showed no indication of flap loss, partial necrosis, or rejection. The incisors grew more than 10 mm during the follow-up period. Flow cytometry analysis of donor-specific chimerism in the peripheral blood, performed at day 105 posttransplant, revealed 12.5% of CD4FITc/RT1n-Cy7 and 5.3% of CD8PE/RT1n-Cy7 T-cell subpopulations. Analysis of the B-cell population revealed 4.7% of CD45RAPE/RT1n-Cy7 donor-derived cells in the peripheral blood of the maxilla recipients. Histologic evaluation revealed no signs of rejection and intact allograft structures, including teeth, tooth buds, tooth pulp, bone, cartilage, oral mucosa, nasal mucosa, and soft-palate musculature.[4]

18.2.1.5 *Composite osteomusculocutaneous hemiface/mandible/tongue-flap model*

An analogous model of composite osteomusculocutaneous hemiface/mandible/tongue allograft transplant evolved as an application of the face/scalp transplantation model in the rat. This alloflap incorporates a vascularized mandible, masseter, and tongue, based on the same vascular pedicle. The feasibility of composite osteomusculocutaneous hemiface/mandible/tongue transplants were tested in an isotransplant model between LEW rats and allotransplants performed across an MHC barrier using LBN donors and LEW recipients. Hemimandibular bone, masseter muscle, tongue, and hemifacial flaps were dissected on the same pedicle of the external carotid artery and jugular vein and were transplanted to the donor inguinal region. All allogeneic transplant recipients received our established protocol of CsA monotherapy. Isograft controls survived indefinitely. All hemiface/mandible/tongue allotransplants survived more than 100 days posttransplant. Flap angiography demonstrated intact vascularity to the bone. No signs of rejection and no flap loss were noted. CT and bone histology confirmed the viability of bone components of the composite allografts. The viability of the tongue was confirmed by pink color, bleeding after puncture, and histology. Hemotoxylin-eosin staining determined the presence of viable bone marrow cells within the transplanted mandible. Donor-specific chimerism at day 100 posttransplant was evaluated by the presence of donor T cells (2.7% CD4/RT1n, 1.2% CD8/RT1n) and B cells (11.5% CD45RA/RT1n). Long-term allograft acceptance was accompanied by donor-specific chimerism supported by vascularized bone marrow transplantation of the mandibular component. This model may serve as a new reconstructive option for coverage of extensive head and neck deformities involving defects of soft and bony tissues.[5,17,18]

18.2.1.6 *Composite midface transplant model with sensory and motor neuromuscular units*

A composite midface allotransplant rat model, containing sensory and motor neuromuscular units, a vascularized premaxilla, a nose with infraorbital nerve, and facial nerves for evaluation of functional recovery, was also developed. Composite midface isotransplants between LEW rats and midface allotransplants between LBN donors and LEW recipients were performed. Midfacial structures including nose, premaxillary bone segment, mystacial pad, masseter muscle, and lower lip were dissected on the same pedicle of the common carotid artery and external jugular vein. Facial and infraorbital nerves were included in the flap as motor and sensory nerves. Composite midface flaps with sensory and motor units were transplanted to the donor inguinal region and connected to femoral vessels. Standard epineural neurorraphies were performed between infraorbital donor nerves and recipient saphenous nerves and between donor facial nerves and recipient femoral nerves. All allogeneic transplant recipients received CsA monotherapy.

Return of motor function was evaluated by observation of the return of movement to the mystacial pad. Sensory recovery was observed clinically by evasive behavior and defense reactions when the transplanted whiskers were pulled. Somatosensory evoked potentials (SSEPs) and motor evoked potentials (MEPs) were used to evaluate the sensory and motor recovery, respectively.

Successful flap transplantation was accomplished in all animals, with 100% flap survival rate of more than 100 days. Clinically, all grafts were pink and pliable during the entire observation period. The incisors continued to grow; tooth buds, bone, cartilage, and mucosa remained intact. Motor recovery was observed at 21 days posttransplant and was confirmed by the movement of the mystacial pad. Clinically evasive behavior and defense reactions were observed when transplanted whiskers were pulled. CT of the composite nose flaps showed persistence of the premaxilla bone. At 100 days posttransplant, SSEP and MEP tests revealed that sensory and motor recovery reached 67% of normal latency values for infraorbital nerve and 70% for facial nerve latency values. This model allows for single-stage reconstruction of the central midface with functional recovery of the sensory and motor nerves.[6]

18.2.1.7 *Composite face and eyeball allotransplant model with optic nerve*

A composite facial allotransplant rat model has been developed, containing orbital contents that included the eyeball and optic nerve.[7] The allograft was harvested based on the common carotid artery and external jugular vein. After a midline neck incision, the submandibular gland and sternocleidomastoid muscle were resected. All branches of the external carotid artery were divided except for the superficial temporal artery and the facial artery. Dissection was performed as in the composite hemiface allotransplantation model. The upper and lower eyelids were included in the allograft. At the level of the supraorbital and infraorbital rim, the dissection plane was changed to the subperiosteal plane. With a subperiosteal dissection, all orbital contents including the periorbital fat tissue and muscles were included in the flap. The optic nerve was transected at the level of the optic foramen and was included in the allograft. The harvested allograft was transplanted to the anterior neck of the recipient rat. Standard microsurgical arterial anastomosis was performed to the common carotid artery (end-to-side), and venous anastomosis was performed to the external jugular veins of the recipient rat in an end-to-end manner. Next, nerve coaptation was performed between the great auricular nerve of the recipient rat and the optic nerve of the donor allograft using standard epineural techniques with 10/0 sutures. After allograft inset, a total tarsorrhaphy was performed with 8/0 sutures to protect the cornea of the transplanted eyeball. All transplant recipients received the CsA immunosuppression protocol monotherapy.

All transplants survived indefinitely. However, the eyeball lost its brightness in the early posttransplant period, with a minimal decrease in its volume. The volumetric analysis of the eyeball was performed at the 1st and 30th day posttransplant by magnetic resonance imaging (MRI) and indicated 35% of eyeball volume loss. The histologic evaluation of nerve sections showed severe degeneration with no evidence of regeneration. However, this model is important for further studies regarding eyeball transplantation.[7]

18.2.2 *Large-animal models*

18.2.2.1 *Dog hemifacial transplant model*

Hemifacial dog allotransplants have been evaluated and reported by Shengwu *et al.* for determining the viability of facial alloflaps based on the facial artery and external jugular vein.[8] A skin/muscle flap in the superficial myoaponeurotic system plane was harvested based on these two vessels. In the recipient animal, the arterial and venous anastomoses were performed to the recipient's lingual artery and external jugular vein, respectively. The recipient dog received CsA (4 mg/kg/day) and prednisone (1 mg/kg/day) to prevent rejection of the allograft. In this model, the hemifacial flap was acutely rejected at day 6 after transplantation.[8]

18.2.2.2 *Hemifacial transplantation model in rabbits*

Hemifacial transplants with auricle were reported by Xudong *et al.* and performed between New Zealand white rabbits and livid blue rabbits.[9] To preserve blood supply, the donor tissue was dissected beneath the mimetic muscles in order to leave the perforating branch of the mandibular artery intact. The hemifacial flaps were harvested on common carotid arteries and external jugular veins, and anastomoses were performed to the recipient's common carotid arteries and external jugular veins. Immunosuppression included CsA, prednisone, and azathioprine. Methylene blue dye injection via the arterial pedicle demonstrated that the composite alloflap had a well-established network and optimal perfusion. This experiment proved that the common carotid artery, with the branch of the external mandibular artery and auricularis magna artery, can provide a satisfactory blood supply to the hemifacial flaps in rabbits.[9]

18.2.2.3 *Swine model of hemifacial composite-tissue allotransplantation*

Kuo *et al.* reported hemifacial transplants performed between outbred miniature swine.[10] The hemifacial orthotopic transplant consisted of ear cartilage, auricular nerve, parotid gland and lymphoid tissue, muscle with a surrounding hemifacial skin paddle supplied by the carotid artery, and the external jugular vein transplanted to recipient swine. Three different experimental designs were studied: autologous hemifacial transplantation, hemifacial allotransplantation without treatment as a rejection control, and hemifacial allotransplantation with CsA treatment for 4 weeks. The transplanted faces were observed daily for signs of rejection. A biopsy of donor skin, gland lymphoid tissue, and cartilage was obtained at days 7, 14, 28, or at the time of clinically evident rejection. The results indicated that the survival of autologous hemifacial–facial transplants was 100%. Allografts without treatment were rejected between 7 and 28 days. The allografts under short-term CsA protocol revealed delayed rejection between 38 and 49 days posttransplant. The histologic examination of the allograft rejection control group revealed abundant lymphocyte infiltration, especially in lymphoid gland and alloskin at 1 week and at the time they were killed. In contrast, the CsA-treated group showed no significant rejection signs at 4 weeks posttransplant. These results demonstrated that lymphoid tissue and alloskin are both susceptible to early rejection. The experimental results described here proved this model suitable for the investigation of various preclinical strategies for facial allotransplantation.[10]

18.2.2.4 *Heterotopic primate model for facial composite-tissue transplantation*

A nonhuman primate model for heterotopic composite-tissue facial transplantation was first developed by Silverman *et al.*[11] A composite oromandibular facial segment transplant, based on the common carotid artery, was tested in cynomolgus monkeys after heterotopic transplantation to the groin of recipients. These alloflaps were anastomosed to the recipient's superficial femoral artery and vein. The immunosuppressive regimen consisted of thymoglobulin, rapamycin, and tacrolimus. Allograft survival ranged from 6 to 129 days. Histology performed in the long-term survivors at the time of necropsy revealed extensive inflammation and necrosis of the allograft skin; however, muscle and bone elements were viable, with minimal inflammation. By performing heterotopic facial transplantation, the potential morbidity of mandibular resection and orthotopic facial transplantation were avoided. In this study, the skin component of the allograft was found to be the most antigenic tissue.[11]

18.2.2.5 *Facial subunit composite-tissue allografts in nonhuman primates*

A nonhuman primate composite-tissue allotransplantation model has been developed for preclinical study by Barth *et al.*[12] Composite facial subunits of skin, muscle, and bone were transplanted between mismatched cynomolgus monkeys. The pedicles consisted of the common carotid artery and external/internal jugular veins. Facial allografts were heterotopically transplanted to the recipient's lower abdomen with end-to-side anastomoses between the common carotid artery and the common femoral artery, and between the internal/external jugular veins and the common femoral vein. Animals received tacrolimus monotherapy. Grafts were inspected daily, submitted to interval biopsies, and evaluated using MRI. Two grafts were lost within 3 to 5 days posttransplant because of venous thrombosis. Long-term success was achieved with rejection-free graft survival (60–177 days) under tacrolimus monotherapy.[12]

18.3 Immunologic Concerns

These various small- and large animal experiments, together with decades of clinical experience, have taught us that composite-tissue transplantation engenders an immune response in the host directed against the donor tissues. This inflammatory reaction, which is generated by cells and antibodies, is inevitable except in the case of grafts transplanted between identical twins. The magnitude of the response varies according to the tissue or organ transplanted and the existence of prior sensitization of the recipient against donor histocompatibility antigens. Other factors, such as the degree of mismatching for major histocompatibility antigens between donor and recipient, the age of the recipient, and as yet poorly understood genetic determinants in the recipient, may also influence long-term outcomes. However, skin, the major component of a craniomaxillofacial transplant, has been recognized for many years both experimentally and clinically as one of the most immunogenic tissues or organs that can be transplanted.[19]

18.4 Future Directions

Advances in basic science research, along with experimental applications of clinical maxillofacial transplantation, have made great strides to ensure their place in the future of reconstructive transplant surgery. There is no doubt that face transplantation has great potential in reconstructive plastic surgery. For severely disfigured patients, it is the only option that truly upholds Gillies' principle of "replacing like with like." It is the unique surgical solution for many conditions that cannot be reconstructed with autologous tissues.[20] The technical aspects of maxillofacial transplantation are no longer the factors limiting its widespread application in the clinical setting. The feasibility of the procedure has been established, and the functional outcomes have been excellent. Currently, the major remaining challenge is at the immunologic level. Although our understanding of the immune system and the development of different immunosuppressive therapies has advanced exponentially, the introduction of new, less-harmful antirejection strategies still has to be defined.

In the short term, introduction of new antirejection mechanisms could broaden the spectrum of immunosuppressive agents, reduce their toxicity, and perhaps prevent development of chronic rejection. However, the long-term goal is to induce donor-specific tolerance and to avoid the toxicity of immunosuppression. Among some of the new and potentially beneficial approaches are different types of cellular therapies such as bone marrow cells, mesenchymal stromal cells, or chimeric cells used as supportive treatments. These novel strategies could in the near future facilitate widespread application of craniomaxillofacial allotransplants, and therefore further basic science studies, such as those described here, are warranted.

References

1. **Siemionow M, Gozel-Ulusal B, Engin Ulusal A, Ozmen S, Izycki D, Zins JE.** Functional tolerance following face transplantation in the rat. *Transplantation* 2003;75:1607–1609.
2. **Siemionow MZ, Demir Y, Sari A, Klimczak A.** Facial tissue allograft transplantation. *Transplant Proc* 2005;37:201–204.

3. **Yazici I, Unal S, Siemionow M.** Composite hemiface/calvaria transplantation model in rats. *Plast Reconstr Surg* 2006;118:1321–1327.
4. **Yazici I, Carnevale K, Klimczak A, Siemionow M.** A new rat model of maxilla allotransplantation. *Ann Plast Surg* 2007;58:338–344.
5. **Kulahci Y, Klimczak A, Siemionow M.** Long term survival of composite hemiface/mandible/tongue tissue allograft permitted by donor specific chimerism. *Plast Reconstr Surg* 2006;118(Suppl):34–35.
6. **Zor F, Bozkurt M, Nair D, Siemionow M.** A new composite midface allotransplantation model with sensory and motor reinnervation. *Transpl Int* 2010;23:649–656.
7. **Polat M, Zor F, Kurt B, Ors F, Battal B, Isik S.** Evaluation of optic nerve regeneration on composite face and eyeball allotransplant model. Paper presented at: 33rd National Congress of Turkish Society of Plastic Reconstructive and Aesthetic Surgeons, September 14–18, 2011; Cesme-Izmir, Turkey.
8. **Shengwu Z, Qingfeng L, Hao J, *et al.*** Developing a canine model of composite facial/scalp allograft transplantation. *Ann Plast Surg* 2007;59:185–194.
9. **Xudong Z, Shuzhong G, Yan H, Datai W, Yunzhi N, Linxi Z.** A hemifacial transplantation model in rabbits. *Ann Plast Surg* 2006;56:665–669.
10. **Kuo YR, Shih HS, Lin CC, *et al.*** Swine hemi-facial composite tissue allotransplantation: a model to study immune rejection [published online ahead of print April 28, 2008]. *J Surg Res* 2009;153:268–273. doi: 10.1016/j.jss.2008.03.050.
11. **Silverman RP, Banks ND, Detolla LJ, *et al.*** A heterotopic primate model for facial composite tissue transplantation. *Ann Plast Surg* 2008;60:209–216.
12. **Barth RN, Bluebond-Langner R, Nam A, *et al.*** Facial subunit composite tissue allografts in nonhuman primates: I. Technical and immunosuppressive requirements for prolonged graft survival. *Plast Reconstr Surg* 2009;123:493–501.
13. **Ulusal BG, Ulusal AE, Ozmen S, Zins JE, Siemionow MZ.** A new composite facial and scalp transplantation model in rats. *Plast Reconstr Surg* 2003;112:1302–1311.
14. **Unal S, Agaoglu G, Zins J, Siemionow M.** New surgical approach in facial transplantation extends survival of allograft recipients. *Ann Plast Surg* 2005;55:297–303.
15. **Demir Y, Ozmen S, Klimczak A, Mukherjee AL, Siemionow M.** Tolerance induction in composite facial allograft transplantation in the rat model. *Plast Reconstr Surg* 2004;114:1790–1801.
16. **Siemionow M, Kulahci Y.** Facial transplantation. *Semin Plast Surg* 2007;21:259–268.
17. **Siemionow M, Kulahci Y.** Experimental models of composite tissue allograft transplants. *Semin Plast Surg* 2007;21:205–212.

18. **Bozkurt M, Kulahci Y, Nasir S, Klimczak A, Siemionow M.** Long term survival of composite hemiface/mandible/tongue tissue allograft permitted by donor specific chimerism. *Plast Reconstr Surg* 2007;120(Suppl):82.
19. **Gordon CR, Zor F, Siemionow M.** Skin area quantification in preparation for concomitant upper extremity and face transplantation: a cadaver study and literature review. *Transplantation* 2011;91:1050–1056.
20. **Gordon CR, Zor F, Cetrulo C Jr., Brandacher G, Sacks J, Lee WP.** Concomitant face and hand transplantation: perfect solution or perfect storm? *Ann Plast Surg* 2011;67:309–314.

MAXILLOFACIAL COMPOSITE TISSUE ALLOTRANSPLA-NTATION: FROM A CLINICAL PERSPECTIVE

19

Chad R. Gordon, DO; Srinivas M. Susarla, MD, DMD, MPH; James E. Zins, MD and Francis Papay, MD

19.1 Introduction

In 2008, the world's first face and maxilla transplant was performed at Cleveland Clinic.[1] In total, six osteomyocutaneous face transplants have been reported in the literature (Table 19.1).[2–5] Because of encouraging results seen thus far, there has been a dramatic rise in interest in maxillofacial allotransplantation (MFA). The craniomaxillofacial surgeon should therefore become familiar with the emerging state of the art. This chapter reviews the evolution of Le Fort-based cadaveric studies pertaining to MFA, briefly describes all clinical reports to date, and introduces a refined technique for employing orthognathic principles and practice.

19.2 Development of Cadaveric Models

For MFA, osteomyocutaneous alloflaps contain many structural components necessary for functional *and* aesthetic reconstruction when

Table 19.1. Worldwide Timeline of Maxillofacial Allotransplantation.

Date	Location	Team leader	Skeleton included
April 2007	China	Zhang	*En bloc* anterior maxillary sinus wall, zygomatic arch
December 2008	Cleveland, OH, USA	Siemionow	Vascularized Le Fort III-based (bilateral orbital floors, bilateral zygomas, anterior maxilla with central incisors, total maxillary alveolus, and anterior hard palate)
March 2009	France	Lantieri	Vascularized anterior Le Fort II-based maxilla and anterior mandible (chin)
April 2009	Boston, MA, USA	Pomahac	Vascularized Le Fort II-based maxilla
February 2010	France	Lantieri	Vascularized Le Fort II-based maxilla and mandible (angle-to-angle)
March 2010	Spain	Barret	Vascularized Le Fort III-based maxilla, bilateral zygomas, mandible

Reprinted with permission from Wolters Kluwer Health (Ref. 16). Copyright © 2012 Mutaz B. Habal, MD.

autologous technique is suboptimal or wholly inadequate. To date, numerous articles have been published on cadaveric dissections for maxillofacial composite tissue allotransplantation (CTA) (Table 19.2).[6–9] Early studies evaluated the utility of CTA versus autologous free-tissue transfer and its feasibility, focusing on autologous skin coverage boundaries, establishment of dissection parameters (sequence, timing, pertinent anatomy, and so forth), vascular pedicle length, definition, and preservation.[10–12] Additional studies have evaluated the psychosocial aspects of facial appearance/identity transfer in face transplantation and its surrounding ethical considerations.[13,14]

Table 19.2. Summary of Pertinent Le Fort-Based Maxillofacial Cadaver Studies.

Author (year)	No. cadavers studied	Le Fort type studied	Key findings	Recommendations
Baccarani (2006)	1	Le Fort III	Subperiosteal plane used for harvest of osteocutaneous flap via Le Fort III-based osteotomies	Technically feasible to include vascularized maxilla with facial alloflap
Yazici (2008)	6	Le Fort II	Key vascular structures for maxilla allograft harvest are within the masticatory space and its anterior pterygomaxillary extension	Vascular territories for maxilla allograft harvest are those in and around the infratemporal fossa, within the course of the internal maxillary artery
Pomahac (2009)	4	Le Fort III	Facial and angular blood vessels are connected to the maxillary vessels via an anastomotic framework centered about the microarchitecture (bony canals, periosteum) of the midface skeleton	The critical elements of a functional face transplant include appropriate donor selection and recipient vessel selection, meticulous graft harvest, complete graft revascularization, and restoration of motor and neurosensory function
Banks (2009)	5	Le Fort III	A single external carotid artery supplies the nasal dorsum and tip Bilateral perfusion is seen in the maxilla Ipsilateral perfusion is seen in the zygomaticomaxillary complex without notable contralateral contributions	Inclusion of the midfacial-skeletal elements (i.e., maxilla) in the design of facial allotransplants requires bilateral vascular pedicles based on the internal maxillary arteries

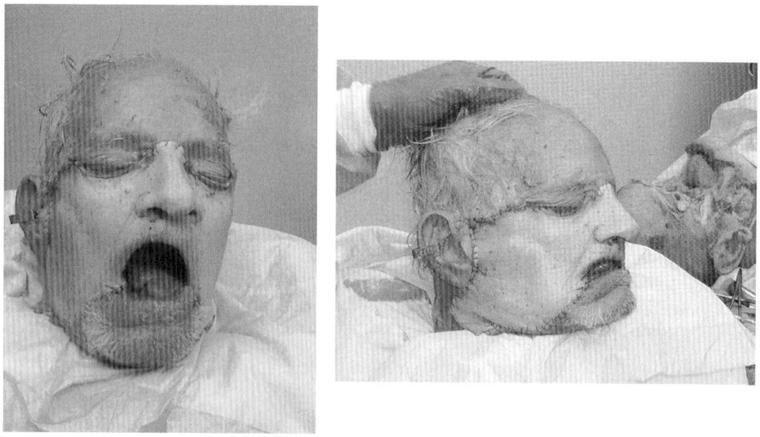

Figure 19.1. Photographs demonstrating a Le Fort III-based, maxillofacial cadaver transplant using orthognathic applications. Of note, optimal skeletal alignment, projection, and height have been maintained even though both the donor maxilla and recipient mandible were edentulous. Reprinted with permission from Wolters Kluwer Health (Ref. 21). Copyright © 2011 American Society of Plastic Surgeons.

Many plastic surgeons are now realizing that for severe, bilateral orbito-zygomaticomaxillary defects, autologous reconstructive technique may be insufficient, and patients may be better served with allotransplantation.[15] In this instance, the use of a Le Fort-based alloflap may provide a realistic alternative in the properly selected patient with respect to (1) function — i.e., structural support of facial musculature for expression, neonasal cavity for olfactory function, and so on; (2) a neopalate and maxillary dentition for mastication; and (3) a skeletal framework for improving and predicting the facial-skeletal profile and overall harmony post-transplant (Figure 19.1).[16]

In 2006, an experimental study was performed at Cleveland Clinic using 10 cadaver heads in an attempt to define critical variables such as operating time for donor flap procurement and inset, nerve coaptation, and microvascular anastamoses, as well as critical thresholds for pedicle lengths. The authors reported that the minimum time necessary for mock cadaver transplant would be approximately 5.3 hours.[11] However, the actual operative time for the maxilla-containing face transplant performed nearly 2 years later was 22 hours. The expected discrepancy related to the logistics of operating on cadaveric versus living tissue (e.g., neurovascular repair, maintaining hemostasis) and the inability to truly assess the recipient's 3-dimensional skeletal defect (due to tremendous scarring and previous autologous reconstruction), but the discrepancy served to highlight the significant obstacles associated with MFA.[17]

Soon thereafter, a complementary study followed, involving a new generation of cadaveric dissection models. The controversial concepts of "facial appearance" and "identity transfer" as they related to soft-tissue facial CTA were discussed.[13] The authors hypothesized that the recipient's facial skeleton would be the primary determinant of alloflap draping, resulting in preferred maintenance of facial contour for soft-tissue face transplantation (i.e., identity). Eight soft-tissue alloflaps were placed alternatively on two recipient molds, and the study concluded that the post-transplant appearance was a "hybrid" containing features of both donor *and* recipient. This is an important consideration, as myocutaneous facial alloflaps rely on the recipient's underlying skeleton as a final determinant with respect to final appearance, while Le Fort-based alloflaps are supported by the donor's midfacial skeleton and its retaining ligaments, thereby remaining consistent with the donor's soft-tissue appearance and skeletal relation. With proper orthognathic evaluation, the craniomaxillofacial surgeon can therefore more likely predict the post-transplant occlusion, orthognathic profile, and facial-skeletal harmony following osteomyocutaneous face transplantation.[16]

In November 2006, Baccarani *et al.* described two new cadaver techniques, one for soft tissue and one for hard tissue.[6] In the first scenario, the myocutaneous alloflap was raised via subgaleal, sub-superficial musculoaponeurotic system and subplatysmal dissection. In the second, a subperiosteal plane was used, allowing for harvest of an osteomyocutaneous alloflap utilizing Le Fort III-based osteotomies. This study was the first to show that the donor maxilla could be included with the facial alloflap, allowing for concomitant osseous/soft tissue reconstruction. A similar approach was subsequently used in the midface allotransplant performed in Cleveland, Ohio, in December 2008.[1]

Baccarani *et al.* then addressed the critical issue of donor-recipient matching, with emphasis on certain facial features.[18] Using four facial soft-tissue alloflaps and four facial skeletons, the authors demonstrated that gender, head/facial skeletal size, soft-tissue features, and skin color and texture were critical factors in preserving facial morphology post-transplant. However, a lack of available donors and institutional resources has limited the consideration of all such parameters. To address this issue, Gordon *et al.* proposed the use of a preliminary screening tool (i.e., FACES score[19]) and the establishment of registries to maximize the yield of relatively limited resources.

In 2008, Yazici *et al.* reported the first Le Fort II-based osteocutaneous face transplant model.[7] Using magnetic resonance imaging and angiographic techniques, these authors defined the vascular territories in and around the infratemporal fossa and mapped the course of the internal maxillary artery. More recent studies by others have evaluated the vascular territories pertinent to a Le Fort-based, osteocutaneous alloflap design,[8,9] both determining that bilateral vascular pedicles were in fact necessary for facial alloflaps with maxillary osseous components.

19.3 Clinical Experiences

The first published report of face transplantation containing facial skeletal components was that performed by Guo and colleagues in April 2006.[20] These surgeons reconstructed an extensive midfacial defect in a 30-year-old man who was mauled by a bear. They used a facial alloflap procured from a 25-year-old male donor. The time between injury and transplantation was 18 months. The alloflap included the right anterior maxillary sinus wall and lateral orbital rim with associated skin and soft tissue, upper lip, nose (cartilage and soft tissue), right parotid gland, and partial masseter with intraoral mucosa. Per the authors' description, the underlying bone was harvested *en bloc* rather than with Le Fort-type osteotomies. Its pedicle design included bilateral facial arteries, anterior facial veins, and bilateral facial nerves.

The preliminary operation was a technical success. The recipient subsequently required scar revisions, excision of redundant soft tissue, oral commissure reconstruction, and autologous cartilage grafting/

floor reconstruction of the right orbit. Of note, our recent experience in the cadaver lab has revealed the maintenance of orbital volume to be a critical element in Le Fort III-based allotransplantation due to its relation to (1) skeletal projection, (2) maxillary occlusive plane, and (3) inset.[21]

Poor right-sided facial nerve function was also noted by the team, with significant right eyelid lagophthalmos and poor levator labii superioris/levator anguli oris function, resulting in suboptimal smiling. There was normal skin and mucosal sensation by 5 months post-transplant. However, the patient died at 24 months post-transplant, and the cause of his death is unclear from the available literature.

In December 2008, the Cleveland Clinic eight-member team reported the world's first near-total face and maxilla transplant, reconstructing an extensive midfacial defect in a 45-year-old woman originating from ballistic trauma.[17] During the time between injury and transplant (4 years), the patient had undergone numerous attempts at reconstruction, including multiple free flaps, without acceptable results. The donor was a brain-dead 44-year-old woman. The allotransplant was a composite Le Fort III-based, midfacial skeletal allotransplant, including overlying soft tissue, entire nose, lower eyelids, upper lip, bilateral zygomas/orbital floor, bilateral parotid glands, anterior maxilla with alveolar process, central maxillary incisors, anterior hard palate, and oral mucosa. The pedicles included the bilateral external carotid arteries, external jugular/posterior facial veins, and bilateral facial nerves. The total operative time was 22 hours. To date, there have been no major complications reported with this recipient. Revisional surgeries included bilateral ectropion repair and redundant neck skin excision/redraping at 1 year. A palatal obturator was used to obliterate a 2-cm palatal defect at the interface of the donor and recipient palates.

Functionally, this patient has done relatively well. Quantitative neurosensory testing at 3 months showed reinnervation of the transplanted skin, with normal two-point discrimination at 1 year. Facial mimetics were noted to improve at 6 months, with a symmetric smile and steady improvement in upper lip/lower eyelid function. The patient experienced significant improvement in speech, nasal breathing, olfaction, and taste. Mastication and swallowing also improved,

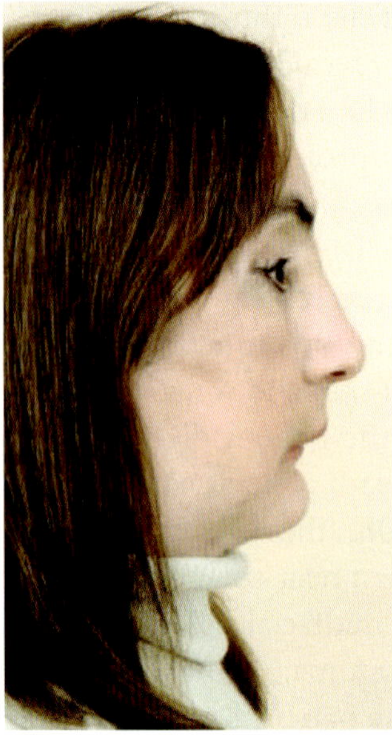

Figure 19.2. Profile view of world's first face and maxilla transplant patient with Class II skeletal relation. Reprinted with permission from Wolters Kluwer Health (Ref. 21). Copyright © 2011 American Society of Plastic Surgeons.

and soft foods and liquids were tolerated at 6 months.[22] However, she has maintained a significant Class II skeletal profile, with mandibular retrognathism and excessive overjet (Figure 19.2). This most likely occurred due to the donor's long maxilla and mismatched size in comparison with the patient's native skeleton, but certain orthognathic-based refinements as presented here may help to improve outcomes in the future, shorten operative times, reduce blood loss, and may in return reduce hospital-acquired infections.[21,23,31]

The other four osteomyocutaneous transplants reported in the literature have also yielded encouraging results. For instance, Lantieri *et al.* performed two successful maxillofacial transplantations with one involving the anterior maxilla, chin, nose and overlying soft tissue in a 27-year-old gunshot victim and the second consisting of an anterior maxilla/mandible (angle-to-angle) with soft tissue in a 33-year-old gunshot victim.[3] Both transplant recipients have reportedly done well to date.

Pomahac *et al.* reported the transplantation of a dentate maxilla/hard palate with associated skin and facial mimetic muscles, nose, and upper lip in a 59-year-old man who had suffered an electrical burn injury.[4] The patient has reportedly done well to date. Important to note here is that the recipient's native mandible was edentulous, and true functional rehabilitation will require the placement of osseointegrated mandibular implants or a removable prosthesis. Occlusal planning in this regard is highly dependent on the maxillary dentoalveolar position and maxillary occlusion. As such, the post-transplant appearance at 1 year shows an elongated upper lip with a corresponding short face syndrome and vertical maxillary deficiency (Figure 19.3).[21] This case, along with the seminal case from Cleveland, together demonstrate a role for orthognathic planning in the context of MFA as described here. With this in mind, the senior author [C.G] is currently developing a computer assisted and planning execution (CAPE) system in a translational swine transplant model.[31–35]

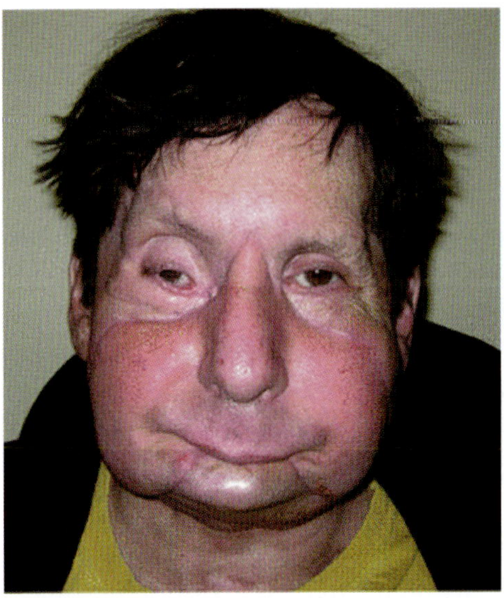

Figure 19.3. Frontal view with Boston transplant recipient with elongated upper lip suggestive of vertical maxillary deficiency. Reprinted with permission from John Wiley and Sons (Ref. 4). Copyright © 2011 The Authors Journal compilation © 2011 The American Society of Transplantation and the American Society of Transplant Surgeons.

19.4 Orthognathic Applications

The evolution of cadaveric techniques for MFA has been rapid, encouraging, and associated with notable clinical successes insofar as technical execution goes. However, there has been little to no emphasis on occlusion or facial-orthognathic harmony in pre-operative planning and/or post-operative alloflap inset.[21]

Developing a plan for the occlusion and skeleton begins with an analysis of the donor's and recipient's maxillofacial skeletons to identify pre-operative facial form and occlusion. Specifically, detailed evaluation of the maxillo-mandibular relationships should be undertaken, with linear and angular measurements focusing on sagittal, vertical, and transverse dimensions between the skeletal and dental landmarks. Recipients with missing landmarks secondary to injury require review of preinjury photographs and any available dental or orthodontic records. A firm understanding of these orthognathic tools is critical for assessing compatibility between the dental arches, and also for evaluating the need for post-transplant orthognathic corrections. Dental cast models should be generated for the *donor* maxilla and mandible as well as for the *recipient's* maxilla and mandible. In most cases, the transplant team has nearly 24 to 36 hours between donor identification and actual transplant, which may be used to obtain and evaluate occlusal models. Lateral and anterior–posterior cephalograms should be used to generate cephalometric data, allowing for a quantitative comparison between the size and position of the donor maxillofacial anatomy relative to the planned recipient. Pre-operative facial asymmetry in the recipient should also be considered, especially in the context of "facial identity." Figure 19.4 details the various components of an ideal pre-transplant orthognathic workup.

A critical difference in pre-operative planning for MFA, as compared with standard orthognathic surgery, is that *the relationship between the donor maxilla and recipient mandible is most critical.* Once the cast models are generated, the donor maxilla can be manually articulated with the recipient mandible, and size discrepancy can be evaluated. The sagittal relationship between the maxillary and mandibular arches is evaluated using cephalometric (e.g., SNA, SNB,

CLINICAL EXAMINATION
Extraoral examination:
Symmetry
Facial proportions (thirds—vertical; fifths—horizontal)
Nasal contour and projection
Malar projection
Periorbital contour
Profile (straight, convex, concave)
Vertical position of the mandible (correct if overclosed)
Chin-throat distance
Intraoral examination:
State of the dentition
Presence of crowding
Angle classification (canine and molar)
Dental midline to midsagittal plane
Overbite and overjet
Centric occlusion versus maximal intercuspation

PHOTOGRAPHS
Frontal repose
Frontal smiling
Right and left lateral (right lateral is the conventional view for planning)
Right and left 3/4 view
Superior (bird's eye) and inferior (worm's eye) views
Preinjury photographs

RADIOGRAPHS
Panoramic radiograph
Lateral and anteroposterior cephalogram
Maxillofacial computed tomogram with axial, sagittal, and coronal reformations as well as 3-dimensional reconstructions

OCCLUSAL AND SKELETAL ANALYSES
Cast dental models to assess maximal intercuspation and transverse relation
Compare donor-to-recipient on cephalometric analyses: Steiner and Harvold analysis
Overlay tracings of donor maxilla and recipient mandible

Figure 19.4. Key components of an orthognathic pretransplantation evaluation in the setting of maxillofacial transplantation. Reprinted with permission from Wolters Kluwer Health (Ref. 16). Copyright © 2012 Mutaz B. Habal, MD.

maxillary and mandibular length) and dental (e.g., overjet, Angle classification) analyses. A fundamental understanding of hierarchy of stability in orthognathic surgery will allow the transplant team leader to understand the limitations of certain post-transplant corrections. Given the potential for vascular compromise with maxillary orthognathic surgery, combined with the relative instability of maxillary transverse expansion or disimpaction, or both, detailed assessment of the potential to perform mandibular surgery for correcting post-transplant skeletal deformities is essential.

For the purpose of MFA, in particular, ideal "hybrid occlusion" may be considered to exist when (1) the condyles are in centric relation, (2) there is bilateral posterior contact, and (3) overbite/overjet

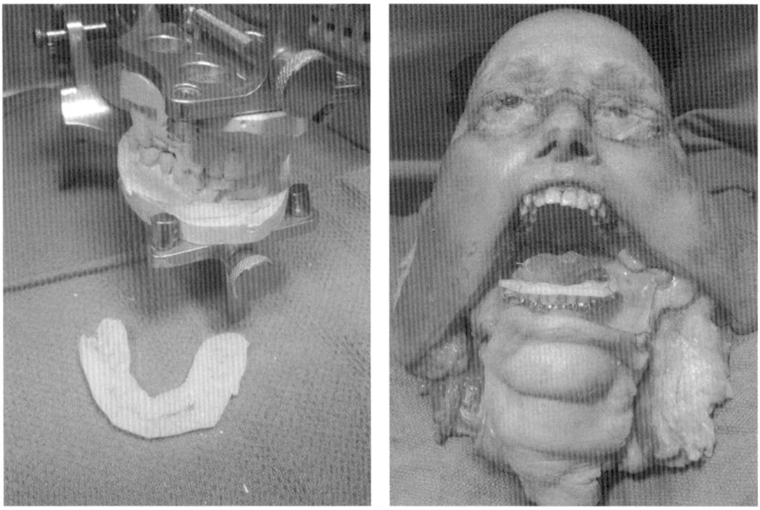

Figure 19.5. Acrylic splint used to establish intra-operative occlusion on donor/recipient models (left) and placed in situ for assistance with skeletal stabilization (right). Reprinted with permission from Wolters Kluwer Health (Ref. 21). Copyright © 2011 American Society of Plastic Surgeons.

relationships between the anterior teeth are 0 to 2 mm. Inadequate occlusion would include the presence of open bites, excessive overjet or overbite, midline asymmetry, or significant occlusal prematurities. The occlusion can be improved by selective tooth grinding to eliminate guiding and balancing interferences. We therefore recommend that an acrylic splint (i.e., "hybrid" splint) be fashioned to assist with intra-operative positioning of the skeletal segments (Figure 19.5). This may optimize and improve the efficiency of alloflap inset and decrease overall operative time.

Cephalometric analyses should also be used to facilitate the operative planning with regard to the vertical naso-orbital position relative to maxillary position. Although an ideal occlusion can be generated using articulated casts, such positioning does not account for the orbital or nasofrontal position, both of which are critical sites of rigid fixation for the Le Fort III-based alloflap. In instances where ideal positioning of the naso-orbital segments would result in an excessive vertical maxillary position (i.e., Le Fort II/III), the rotation of the

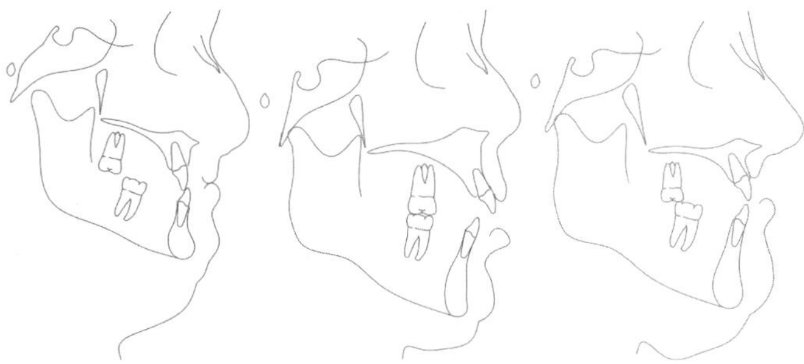

Figure 19.6. Cephalometric tracing of recipient with extensive midfacial defect, pretransplant (A), with transplanted midface alloflap and resulting skeletal Class II malocclusion (B), and with occlusal correction following mandibular advancement (C). Reprinted with permission from Wolters Kluwer Health (Ref. 21). Copyright © 2011 American Society of Plastic Surgeons.

mandible along the hinge axis should be taken into account and simulated cephalometrically, to identify any open-bite potential for when the upper facial segments are ideally positioned. In addition, if future mandibular reconstruction is anticipated, the predicted mandibular movements can be analyzed cephalometrically (Figure 19.6).

In instances where the donor and/or recipient jaws are edentulous, the same protocol can be used, with simulated occlusion achieved using Gunning-type splints for vertical dimension assessment and maxillo-mandibular fixation screws for fixation guidance. Figure 19.7 is a step-by-step algorithm for orthognathic planning in patients undergoing maxillofacial CTA.[16]

19.5 Future Directions

There have been significant advances in the evolution and practice of osteomyocutaneous face transplantation for reconstruction of defects not applicable to current technique. Preliminary results in cadaveric models and clinical examples have together highlighted many challenges.[31,32] However, published results thus far are extremely promising. A notable area for refinement in these patients is their suboptimal

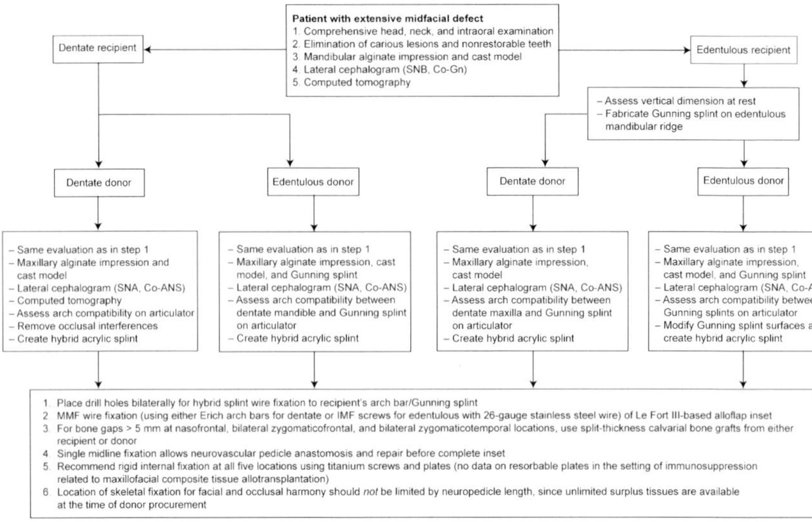

Figure 19.7. Proposed algorithm for patients undergoing maxillofacial allotransplantation. Reprinted with permission from Wolters Kluwer Health (Ref. 16). Copyright © 2012 Mutaz B. Habal, MD.

facial-skeletal harmony and profile in the context of skeletal projection and maxillomandibular relation.[21]

To our knowledge, the first two papers describing pre- and/or peri-transplant orthognathic applications related to maxillofacial transplantation were published by Gordon and colleagues in 2011 and 2012.[16,21] Concordant with this, all recipients have demonstrated significant post-transplant malocclusions, as expected given the donor-to-recipient jaw discrepancies in all three dimensions. Given that the goal of MFA is to improve function as well as form, the importance of orthognathic planning cannot be overestimated with respect to optimizing harmony, profile, and occlusion. Pre-operative planning, including generation of donor and recipient dental cast models as described herein, is essential.[16]

For instance, a transplant recipient with a midface defect and an intact native mandible should have orthognathic records and planning completed before identifying a suitable donor. Once a donor has been identified, a cast model of the donor jaw (maxilla in the case of midfacial defects) should be obtained. Compatibility of the teeth, predicted occlusion, and assessment of the transverse, vertical, and sagittal jaw relationships can all be defined in the peri-operative window using either handheld analyses or a Giletti articulator. The "best-fit" occlusion and intercuspation in each specific case, as depicted here with models, can be established using selective reduction of dental interferences, with an ultimate goal of bilateral posterior tooth contacts and overbite/overjet within 0 to 2 mm (Figure 19.8).

Subsequent to this, cephalometric planning or 3-dimensional computed tomographic reconstructions can be used to identify the degree of discordance between ideal positioning of the skeletal fixation points and the vertical position of the dentate segment. This will allow the transplant team to determine whether an ideal occlusion can be obtained with bone–bone contact at the upper facial segments, approximate the extent to which donor split-thickness calvarial grafts are required during procurement, and whether orbital or respiratory functions, or both, may be jeopardized. In addition, any significant malocclusion can therefore be anticipated and minimized, potentially allowing post-transplant correction by preferential orthodontic treatment rather than surgery. In the latter instance, orthognathic surgery in the setting of immunotherapy is not trivial, and efforts should be made to avoid gross skeletal malpositioning that necessitates such correction. Indeed, a recent published report of maxilla/mandible transplantation resulted in a less than acceptable occlusion, requiring mandibular osteotomies at 8 months post-transplant.[3]

In all, six osteomyocutaneous face transplants have been performed since 2006, all providing functional results well above expectation. Two were Le Fort III-based (Cleveland, Spain), three resembled Le Fort II design (France [two], Boston), and one was procured in *en bloc* fashion (China). All have been revolutionary in their own right, providing the disfigured recipient with varying combinations of skin, muscle, and bone. Indications now include severe facial skeletal trauma from high-velocity blast injuries, avulsion injuries, and severe thermal injury. Of note, there has been one osteomyocutaneous face transplant mortality reported to date, related to noncompliance with immunosuppression (1/6, 17%).[2]

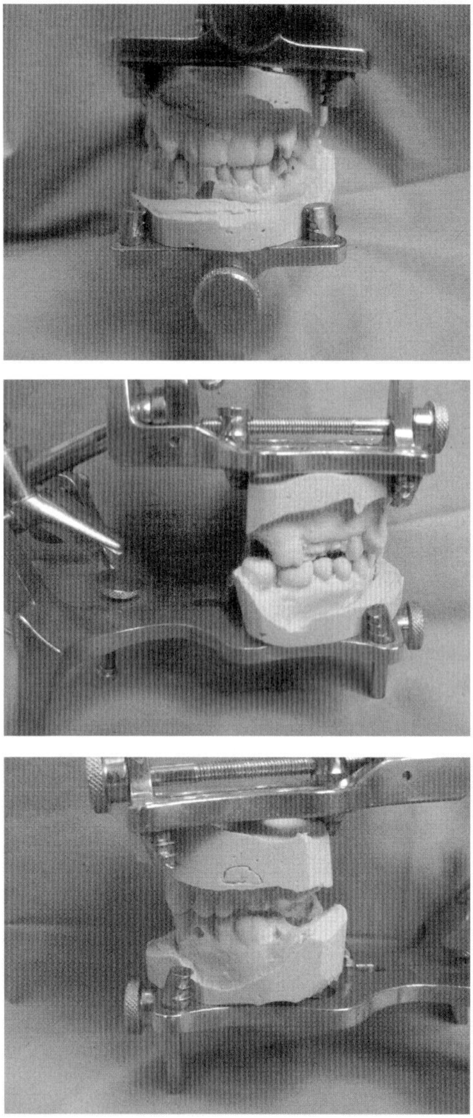

Figure 19.8. A "best-fit" occlusion with optimal intercuspation is shown for the donor maxilla and recipient mandible models. Reprinted with permission from Wolters Kluwer Health (Ref. 21). Copyright © 2011 American Society of Plastic Surgeons.

Overall function has been reported to be satisfactory in all long-term reports thus far, with functional recovery of sensation occurring by 6 months and acceptable motor function recovery by 12 months.[22] Aesthetic outcomes for both soft- and hard-tissue reconstruction have varied, most notably related to significant skeletal discrepancies in the sagittal and vertical planes (i.e., Class II skeletal profile in Cleveland, vertical maxillary deficiency in Boston).[1,4] Of note, craniofacial strategies related to obtaining optimal occlusion and skeletal relation post-transplant are under current development.[31–33,35]

The risks and benefits of MFA, which currently involves mandatory lifelong immunosuppression at levels analogous to cadaveric renal transplants, should be deliberated by a multidisciplinary team in a critical case-by-case scenario. In addition, all transplant programs should remain centered at university-based institutions led by craniomaxillofacial plastic surgeons with expertise in CTA, along with a talented team including oral maxillofacial surgeons and dentists, as depicted in our revised figure (Figure 19.9).[16,24,25]

In summary, MFA has been shown to be a viable option in the properly selected patient with bilateral orbito-zygomaticomaxillofacial

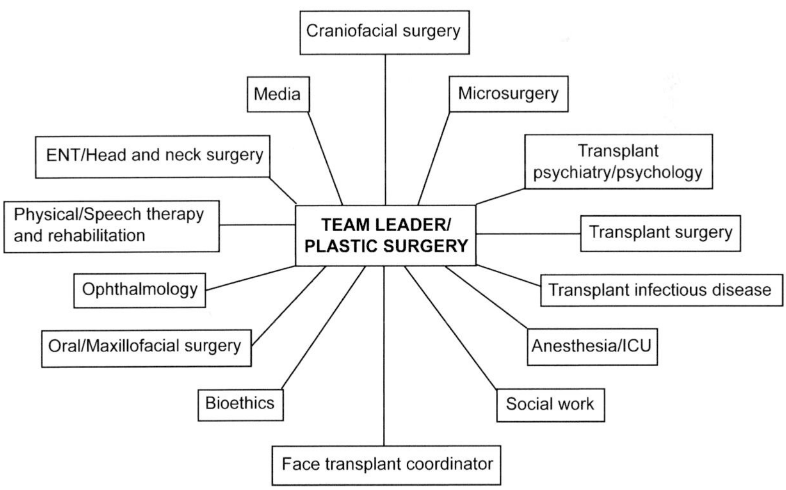

Figure 19.9. Revised team-based approach is shown for maxillofacial transplantation requiring dental expertise. Reprinted with permission from Wolters Kluwer Health (Ref. 16). Copyright © 2012 Mutaz B. Habal, MD.

deficits not amenable to standard reconstructive technique.[15] As newer immunosuppression options become available, indications for MFA will likely expand.[26] Future research evaluating the challenging ethical and psychological challenges surrounding candidate selection (i.e., blindness),[27,28] establishment of maxillofacial transplant protocols,[29] and investigation in an effort to achieve donor-specific tolerance and to eradicate the obliged lifelong immunotherapy[30] are warranted.

Acknowledgments

Dr. Gordon would like to recognize the generous funding awarded by the following organizations for the work detailed within this chapter — the American Society of Maxillofacial Surgeons (2011 Grant Research Award), the American Association of Plastic Surgeons (2012–14 Furnas' Academic Scholar Award), the Johns Hopkins' Institute for Clinical and Translational Research (2012–13 Accelerated Translational Incubator Pilot Award), and The Abell Foundation/ Johns Hopkins Alliance for Science and Technology Development/ Univ. of Maryland-Baltimore Commercial Advisory Board (2014 Abell Foundation Award).

References

1. **Alam DS, Papay F, Djohan R, *et al.*** The technical and anatomical aspects of the world's first near-total human face and maxilla transplant. *Arch Facial Plast Surg* 2009;11:369–377.
2. **Guo S, Han Y, Zhang X, *et al.*** Human facial allotransplantation: a 2-year follow-up study. *Lancet* 2008;372:631–638.
3. **Lantieri L, Hivelin M, Audard V, *et al.*** Feasibility, reproducibility, risks and benefits of face transplantation: a prospective study of outcomes. *Am J Transplant* 2011;11:367–378.
4. **Pomahac B, Pribaz J, Eriksson E, *et al.*** Restoration of facial form and function after severe disfigurement from burn injury by a composite facial allograft [published online ahead of print January 7, 2011]. *Am J Transplant* 2011;11: 386–393. doi:10.1111/j.1600-6143.2010.03368.x.

5. **Landau E.** First full face transplant successful in Spain. CNN website. Available at: http//thechart.blogs.cnn.com/2010/04/23/first-full-face-transplant-successful-in-spain. Published April 23, 2012. Accessed April 3, 2012.
6. **Baccarani A, Follmar KE, Baumeister SP, Marcus JR, Erdmann D, Levin LS.** Technical and anatomical considerations of face harvest in face transplantation. *Ann Plast Surg* 2006;57:483–488.
7. **Yazici I, Cavusoglu T, Comert A, *et al*.** Maxilla allograft for transplantation: an anatomical study. *Ann Plast Surg* 2008;61:105–113.
8. **Pomahac B, Lengele B, Ridgway EB, *et al*.** Vascular considerations in composite midfacial allotransplantation. *Plast Reconstr Surg* 2010;125:517–522.
9. **Banks ND, Hui-Chou HG, Tripathi S, *et al*.** An anatomical study of external carotid artery vascular territories in face and midface flaps for transplantation. *Plast Reconstr Surg* 2009;123:1677–1687.
10. **Siemionow M, Unal S, Agaoglu G, Sari A.** A cadaver study in preparation for facial allograft transplantation in humans: Part I. What are alternative sources for total facial defect coverage? *Plast Reconstr Surg* 2006;117:864–872.
11. **Siemionow M, Agaoglu G, Unal S.** A cadaver study in preparation for facial allograft transplantation in humans: Part II. Mock facial transplantation. *Plast Reconstr Surg* 2006;117:876–885.
12. **Follmar KE, Baccarani A, Das RR, *et al*.** Osteocutaneous face transplantation [published online ahead of print March 7, 2008]. *J Plast Reconstr Aesthet Surg* 2008;61:518–524. doi:10.1016/j.bjps.2007.12.014
13. **Siemionow M, Agaoglu G**. The issue of "facial appearance and identity transfer" after mock transplantation: a cadaver study in preparation for facial allograft transplantation in humans. *J Reconstr Microsurg* 2006;22:329–334.
14. **Pomahac B, Aflaki P, Nelson C, Balas B.** Evaluation of appearance transfer and persistence in central face transplantation: a computer simulation analysis [published online ahead of print April 23, 2009]. *J Plast Reconstr Aesthet Surg* 2010;63:733–738. doi:10.1016/j.bjps.2009.01.078.
15. **Gordon CR.** A four-type classification system for microvascular reconstruction of oncologic midface defects: but what about maxillofacial allotransplantation? *Plast Reconstr Surg* 2011;128:323–325.
16. **Gordon CR, Susarla SM, Peacock ZS, Kaban LB, Yaremchuk MJ.** Le Fort-based maxillofacial transplantation: current state of the art and a refined technique using orthognathic applications. *J Craniofac Surg* 2012;23:81–87.
17. **Siemionow M, Papay F, Alam D, *et al*.** Near-total human face transplantation for a severely disfigured patient in the USA [published online ahead of print July 14, 2009]. *Lancet* 2009;374:203–209. doi:10.1016/S0140-6736(09)61155-7.

18. **Baccarani A, Follmar KE, Das RR, *et al.*** A pilot study in sub-SMAS face transplantation: defining donor compatibility and assessing outcomes in a cadaver model. *Plast Reconstr Surg* 2007;119:121–129.
19. **Gordon CR, Siemionow M, Coffman K, *et al.*** The Cleveland Clinic FACES score: a preliminary assessment tool for identifying the optimal face transplant candidate. *J Craniofac Surg* 2009;20:1969–1974.
20. **Yi C, Guo S.** Facial transplantation: lessons so far [published online ahead of print July 14, 2009]. *Lancet* 2009;374:177–178. doi:10.1016/S0140-6736(09) 61292-7.
21. **Gordon CR, Susarla SM, Peacock ZS, *et al.*** Osteocutaneous maxillofacial allotransplantation: lessons learned from a novel cadaver study applying orthognathic principles and practice. *Plast Reconstr Surg* 2011;128:465e–479e.
22. **Gordon CR, Siemionow M, Papay F, *et al.*** The world's experience with facial transplantation: what have we learned thus far? *Ann Plast Surg* 2009;63:572–578.
23. **Gordon CR, Avery R, Abouhassan W, Siemionow M.** Cytomegalovirus and other infectious issues related to face transplantation: specific considerations, lessons learned, and future recommendations. *Plast Reconstr Surg* 2011;127: 1515–1523.
24. **Siemionow MZ, Papay F, Djohan R, *et al.*** First U.S. near-total human face transplantation: a paradigm shift for massive complex injuries. *Plast Reconstr Surg* 2010;125:111–122.
25. **Siemionow M, Gordon CR.** Institutional review board-based recommendations for medical institutions pursuing protocol approval for face transplantation. *Plast Reconstr Surg* 2010;126:1232–1239.
26. **Siemionow MZ, Zor F, Gordon CR.** Face, upper extremity, and concomitant transplantation: potential concerns and challenges ahead. *Plast Reconstr Surg* 2010;126:308–315.
27. **Paradis C, Siemionow M, Papay F, *et al.*** Ethical considerations in the first American face transplant. *Plast Reconstr Surg* 2010;126:896–901.
28. **Coffman KL, Gordon C, Siemionow M.** Psychological outcomes with face transplantation: overview and case report. *Curr Opin Organ Transplant* 2010; 15:236–240.
29. **Siemionow M, Gordon CR.** Overview of guidelines for establishing a face transplant program: a work in progress [published online ahead of print March 26, 2010]. *Am J Transplant* 2010;10:1290–1296. doi:10.1111/j.1600-6143.2010.03096.x.
30. **Horner BM, Randolph MA, Duran-Struuck R, *et al.*** Induction of tolerance to an allogeneic skin flap transplant in a preclinical large animal model. *Transplant Proc* 2009;41:539–541.

31. **Gordon CR, Murphy R, Coon D, Basafa E, Otake Y, Al Rakan M, Rada E, Susarla S, Swanson E, Fishman E, Santiago G, Brandacher G, Liacouras P, Grant G, Armand M.** Preliminary development of a workstation for craniomaxillofacial surgical procedures — introducing a computer-assisted planning and execution (CAPE) system. *J Craniofac Surg* 2014;25(1):273–283.
32. **Santiago GF, Susarla SM, Al Rakan MA, Coon D, Rada EM, Sarhane K, Shores JT, Bonawitz SC, Cooney D, Sacks J, Murphy RJ, Fishman EK, Brandacher G, Lee WPA, Liacouras P, Grant G, Armand M, Gordon CR.** Establishing cephalometric landmarks for the translational study of Le Fort-based facial transplantation in swine: Enhanced applications using computer-assisted surgery and custom cutting guides. *Plast Reconstr Surg* 2014. Jan 17. [Epub ahead of print]
33. **Al Rakan M, Shores JT, Bonawitz S, Santiago G, Christensen J, Grant G, Murphy RJ, Basafa E, Armand M, Otovic P, Eller S, Brandacher G, Gordon CR.** Ancillary procedures necessary for translational research in experimental craniomaxillofacial surgery. *J Craniofac Surg* 2014. [In Press]
34. **Grant GT, Liacouras P, Santiago G, Garcia JR, Al Rakan M, Murphy R, Armand M, Gordon CR.** Restoration of the donor face after facial allotransplantation: Digital manufacturing techniques. *Ann Plast Surg* 2014. [In Press]
35. **Gordon CR, Swanson EW, Susarla SM, Coon D, Rada E, Al Rakan M, Santiago GF, Shores JT, Bonawitz SC, Fishman E, Murphy R, Armand M, Liacouras P, Grant GT, Brandacher G, Lee WPA.** Overcoming cross-gender differences and challenges in Le Fort-based, craniomaxillofacial transplantation with enhanced computer-assisted technology. *Ann Plast Surg* 2013;71(4): 421–428.

CONGENITAL FACIAL APLASIAS: HEMIFACIAL MICROSOMIA, ROBIN SEQUENCE AND TREACHER COLLINS SYNDROME

20

Marcin Czerwinski, MD and Jeffrey A. Fearon, MD

20.1 Hemifacial Microsomia

Hemifacial microsomia is a condition that falls along the oculo-auriculo-vertebral spectrum. It comprises varying degrees of unilateral facial hypoplasia (although it may also present bilaterally), ranging from subtle asymmetries to severe facial aplasias.

20.1.1 *Epidemiology*

Hemifacial microsomia has been reported to occur in 1/3,500 to 1/5,600 live births. The male:female and right:left ratios occur[1] with an incidence of approximately 3:2. It has been suggested that roughly two-thirds of cases are unilateral and up to one-third are asymmetrically bilateral, although a 10% bilateral incidence is more likely.[2,3] Most cases are sporadic; rarely, however, the condition is familial, with both autosomal dominant and recessive transmission being reported.

Human studies have found the candidate gene at the 14q32 position. Other candidate genes have been identified in animal studies: *Hfm*, *Far*, *Goosecoid*.[4]

20.1.2 *Etiology and pathogenesis*

Numerous etiologic factors have been suggested for hemifacial microsomia, including maternal vasoactive medication use, multiple gestation, primidone embryopathy, retinoic acid embryopathy, thalidomide embryopathy, maternal diabetes (preexisting or gestational), and even military service.[4] Currently, however, vascular perturbation and neural crestopathy are thought to be the most likely mechanisms. Vascular perturbation, occurring in the distribution of the stapedial artery, has been associated with hemifacial microsomia-like features in the murine model. The stapedial artery arises as the second branch of the embryonic aorta and is transiently the main artery supplying the embryonic face.[5] Neural crestopathy seems to involve both early loss and decreased migration of neural crest cells, which are known to be progenitors of the facial skeleton.[6] The proposed final pathway for both these theories is a perturbation in chondrogenesis leading to either hypoplasia or aplasia of structures within the first and second branchial arches and the nasal placode.[5,6]

20.1.3 *Diagnosis and evaluation*

The diagnosis of hemifacial microsomia can be made solely on the basis of physical examination, although radiologic evaluations can help to further assess the degree of skeletal hypoplasia. It has been suggested that (1) concomitant ear and mandibular asymmetry (from a unilateral hypoplasia) or (2) isolated ear or mandibular asymmetry and the presence of two or more indirectly associated anomalies or a positive family history, are diagnostic.[7,8] The oculo-auriculo-vertebral spectrum includes changes in all these structures, but the term "oculo-auriculo-vertebral spectrum" is typically reserved for more mildly affected children. Hemifacial microsomia tends to fall within the middle of the spectrum. Goldenhar's syndrome, characterized by the presence of an epibulbar dermoid, falls further along the spectrum and should probably not be considered a variant.[4] Most severe form of the oculo-auriculo-vertebral spectrum is craniofacial microsomia, which includes concomitant involvement of the orbit and skull. Examination of a child with hemifacial microsomia is best performed systematically, as follows:

20.1.3.1 *Skull and forehead*

Diminished height of the forehead and associated frontal recession may be markers for craniofacial microsomia. It is important to note that hemifacial microsomia may also occur, very rarely, in combination with single-suture craniosynostosis.

20.1.3.2 *Orbit*

Subtle aplasia or inferior dystopia of the orbit may be associated with craniofacial microsomia. In rare instances, there may be complete aplasia of the orbit with associated anophthalmia. The presence of an epibulbar dermoid is a marker for Goldenhar's syndrome, and larger dermoids may impair vision by obstruction or infiltration of the cornea.[9] Ocular closure may be incomplete due to facial nerve weakness or eyelid soft-tissue deficiency.

20.1.3.3 *Ear*

Preauricular skin tags and sinuses represent the mildest form of auricular deformity, with incompletely formed and complete anotia representing the other end of the spectrum. The ear may be positioned symmetrically with respect to the opposite side, but more commonly it is anteroinferiorly displaced. Conductive hearing loss is present in up to 90% of affected children, most frequently in the moderate-severe range (40–80 dB). Sensorineural hearing loss is present in 10%.[10,11] Hearing deficits occur most commonly as the result of atresia

(60%) or stenosis (36%) of the external acoustic canal; hypoplasia or atresia of the middle ear (30%); fused, malformed, or absent ossicles (95%); or poorly developed or absent mastoid air cells (65%). The severity of external ear and mandibular deformities is proportional to middle and inner ear abnormalities.

20.1.3.4 *Zygoma*

Absence or hypoplasia of the zygomatic arch is usually readily apparent by palpation lateral to the maxilla.

20.1.3.5 *Maxilla*

Various degrees of maxillary hypoplasia may be present. A unilateral raised oral commissure suggests hemifacial microsomia. The degree of hypoplasia can be determined by having the patient bite on a tongue blade. It is important to remember that this hypoplasia is 3-dimensional. In addition to vertical shortening, the maxilla is narrower and retruded. This can be appreciated by observing the amount of rotation of the maxillary dental midline off the facial midline.

20.1.3.6 *Mandible*

The degree of mandibular hypoplasia mirrors the maxillary hypoplasia. Deviation of the chin point off the facial midline is usually the most obvious sign of hemifacial microsomia. However, a reduction in lateral facial fullness may also be noted because of the anomalous medial displacement of the hypoplastic ascending ramus. A mandible that can be rocked posteriorly on one side is indicative of aplasia of the temporomandibular joint (TMJ).

20.1.3.7 *Intraoral examination*

The amount of displacement of the maxillary and mandibular midlines off the facial midline should be noted. Dental crossbites are almost never seen; however, as the severity progresses, a lateral open bite may become present. Dental eruption may be delayed, and with more severe manifestations, tooth formation may fail. Examination of the palate may reveal asymmetric motion of the posterior palate, suggesting partial or incomplete unilateral palatal paresis. Velopharyngeal incompetence may result due to pharyngeal muscle hypoplasia or an overt or submucous orofacial cleft. Articulatory errors may be caused by malocclusions.

20.1.3.8 *Nervous system*

Examination of facial nerve function is necessary to document the degree, if any, of facial paralysis. The incidence of facial nerve weakness is between 22 and 45%.[12–14] Trigeminal nerve deficits may also be present.

20.1.3.9 *Extracranial abnormalities*

Associated extracranial abnormalities may be found in more than one-half of patients in the following organ systems[15–18]: skeletal (40%), vertebral (24%, fusions and duplications[15]); cardiac (5–58%), atrial and ventricular septal defects (32%), conotruncal defects (39%); targeted growth defects (14%); and defects of the central nervous system (5–15%), genitourinary system (5–10%), gastrointestinal system (10%), and respiratory system (10%).

20.1.4 *Classification*

Although several classification systems have been described, two are most commonly used today. The OMENS-Plus system is the most comprehensive and is helpful for research analysis[9–11] (Table 20.1). However, because of its completeness, it is more complex to use. Perhaps as a result, the most commonly referred-to clinical classification is the Pruzansky system, which focuses solely on the mandible[20] (Table 20.2). Panoramic, plain mandibular films and computed tomography (CT) allow qualitative and quantitative assessments of mandibulo-maxillary deformity and may assist with surgical planning.[21]

Table 20.1. OMENS-Plus Classification: Presence of Extracranial Anomalies.[19]

Orbit

O_0: Normal orbital size and position

O_1: Abnormal orbital size

O_2: Abnormal orbital position — superior or inferior

O_3: Abnormal orbital size and position

Mandible

M_0: Normal mandible

M_1: Mandible and glenoid fossa are small with a short ramus

M_2: Mandibular ramus is short and abnormally shaped

M_{2A}: Glenoid fossa is in an anatomically acceptable position with reference to opposite TMJ

M_{2B}: TMJ is inferiorly, medially, and anteriorly displaced with severely hypoplastic condyle

M_3: Complete absence of ramus, glenoid fossa, and TMJ

Ear

E_0: Normal ear

E_1: Mild hypoplasia and cupping with all structures present

E_2: Absence of external auditory canal with variable hypoplasia of the concha

E_3: Malpositioned lobule with absent auricle; lobular remnant usually inferiorly and anteriorly displaced

Facial nerve

N_0: No facial nerve involvement

N_1: Upper (temporal and zygomatic) facial nerve involvement

N_2: Lower (buccal, mandibular, and cervical) facial nerve involvement

N_3: All branches of the facial nerve affected

Soft tissue

S_0: No obvious subcutaneous tissue or muscle deficiency

S_1: Minimal deficiency

S_2: Moderate deficiency

S_3: Severe soft tissue deficiency

TMJ = Temporomandibular joint

Table 20.2. Mulliken Modification of Pruzansky Mandibular Hypoplasia Grading System.

Type I:	The mandible and glenoid fossa are small with a short ramus
Type II:	The mandibular ramus is short and abnormally shaped
Type IIA:	The glenoid fossa is in an acceptable functional position in reference to the opposite TMJ
Type IIB:	The TMJ is inferiorly, medially, and anteriorly displaced
Type III:	There is complete absence of ramus, glenoid fossa, and TMJ

TMJ = Temporomandibular joint

The most important initial test for any child presenting with hemifacial microsomia is polysomnography. Sleep-disordered breathing and obstructive sleep apnea are significantly more likely to occur when there is a significant degree of mandibular or TMJ hypoplasia, and any suggestion of obstructive sleep apnea needs to be further evaluated.[22] Feeding may be impaired due to hypoplastic or absent masticatory muscles, nonfunctional or absent TMJs, occlusal imbalances, or orofacial clefting (10%). Therefore, it is also important to assess oral intake and weight gain in affected infants. Additionally, the value of otology and speech therapy should be initially assessed.

20.1.5 *Treatment*

The treatment of hemifacial microsomia requires multiple specialists; therefore, it is best referred to craniofacial centers. The following is an overview of available treatment strategies.

20.1.5.1 *Ear reconstruction*

The initial surgical intervention in a child with hemifacial microsomia is ideally delayed until the child is around 8 years old, when external ear reconstruction may be performed. By age 6, the size of the ear is approximately 85% of the final adult size. However, delaying surgery until age 8 allows for growth of the costal cartilage to a size sufficient to permit creation of a sturdier, higher-profile framework. Of course, the optimal time for surgery must take into account associated psychosocial issues and is best decided by the patient and family.

Current treatment options include artificial ear prosthesis placement, alloplastic framework reconstruction, and costochondral ear reconstruction. Artificial ear prostheses require minimal surgery (for bony anchored prostheses), and can have excellent aesthetic results. However, these results are impaired by seasonal variations in color match that vary with sun exposure. They may require lifelong changes (resulting in higher costs) and are known to include long-term issues with bony anchoring. They are also subject to trauma.

Alloplastic ear implants are technically much easier to perform than autogenous reconstructions and offer reproducibly good aesthetic results. Their primary drawback is that placing artificial material under a thin skin covering has a high complication rate that likely increases with length of follow-up; therefore, they probably should be thought of only as "temporary ears."[23,24]

Costochondral ear reconstruction is currently the most widely accepted method of microtia reconstruction. This technique has the potential to provide both optimal appearance and durability. However, these multistaged reconstructions are technically challenging, with results highly dependent on the experience and skill of the surgeon. For this reason, microtia reconstruction is best referred to those with a special interest in this procedure and sufficient experience to produce reliable results. Reconstruction of the external auditory canal, tympanic membrane, and ossicles may be possible depending on the degree of aplasia. It is our opinion that for most patients with microtia, the results of this procedure do not provide sufficient justification. Moreover, the creation of an external auditory canal not only detracts from the aesthetic appearance of the ear but also requires routine lifelong cleaning by an otolaryngologist to maintain canal patency.

20.1.5.2 *Skeletal reconstruction*

Skeletal reconstruction is partially dependent on the degree of hypoplasia. There are currently three basic approaches to treating the facial skeleton: distraction osteogenesis, standard orthognathic corrections, and reconstructions using rib grafts. The following is a brief overview of the advantages and disadvantages of these general categories of treatment.

20.1.5.2.1 Distraction osteogenesis. These procedures are generally limited to treating children with milder variations of hemifacial microsomia, and are not recommended for those with absent TMJs (Pruzansky Type III). One advantage of distraction is that it allows gradual concomitant lengthening of the soft-tissue envelope. However, the primary reason for the current popularity of this technique may be that it is technically straightforward and does not require any significant orthognathic training. Distraction is associated with a fairly high complication rate, including external facial scars, injury to permanent dentition, facial nerve injury, device failures, and TMJ issues.[25–28] Aside from requiring multiple stages, the largest issue with distraction is that it does not treat the associated maxillary hypoplasia; therefore, isolated lengthening of one side of the mandible (which is already anomalously medialized) creates problematic crossbites.

20.1.5.2.2 Traditional orthognathic surgery. This surgical approach is also best reserved for children with intact TMJs. The advantage of this approach is the complete correction of both maxillary and mandibular hypoplasia while idealizing occlusion, in a single stage. The facial midline can be completely aligned, although the lateral hypoplasia will persist. The disadvantage of this technique is that it is technically more challenging. Experience with orthognathic surgery is necessary, as severe cases often require 3-dimensional repositioning of the maxilla, unaided by splint guidance.

20.1.5.2.3 Rib graft reconstruction. Agenesis of the TMJ requires rib bone and cartilage graft reconstruction. These procedures, similar to orthognathic two-jaw surgery, are technically demanding. Reconstruction of the absent TMJ requires reconstruction of both the ascending ramus and the condyle as well as the zygomatic arch and glenoid fossa. Intraoral exposures are associated with significant infection rates; therefore, extraoral approaches may be justified.

20.1.5.3 *Summary of reconstructive options*

The timing for surgical intervention may have come full circle. The traditional orthognathic correction, first proposed by Obwegeser,[29] was performed only in skeletally mature individuals. Taking into consideration the psychosocial issues associated with more significantly affected children, Munro popularized a complete orthognathic correction, including rib grafting, in younger children.[30] Subsequent experience with these early procedures has shown that rib grafts grow erratically and may both undergrow and overgrow. Treatment using distraction has also been adopted in younger children. However, it has become clear that earlier treatment provides only temporary improvement, and it seems that many children require repeat distraction and then orthognathic correction at skeletal maturity. This suggests that the ideal scenario for most children with hemifacial microsomia may be to delay surgery, whenever possible, until skeletal maturity. The most significant caveat to this recommendation would be for young children with significant sleep apnea, not amenable to more conservative measures (continuous positive airway pressure, Herbst appliances, and so forth). In these cases, rib graft reconstruction at an earlier age may be desirable to keep the mandible positioned forward, thus keeping the tongue from shifting backward during sleep in the supine position.

Selecting the best procedure for treating hemifacial microsomia requires balancing many factors. Most important is assessing each technique's potential to accomplish the surgical goals of normalizing appearance and function with as small, as safe, and as few operations as possible.[31] Final reconstructive procedures may include allogenic malar augmentation. This has been shown to produce long-lasting results, but it should not be placed before skeletal maturity because these implants will "sink" into the underlying bone with growth.[32,33] Alloplastic cheek implants create a long-lasting result but have a long-term infection risk, particularly when placed transorally. This method of reconstruction has advantages over autogenous bone graft onlays, which, while having low complication rates,[34,35] typically show resorption rates >50%. Soft-tissue augmentations with fat injections, dermal grafts, and free-tissue transfers have all been described. However, these techniques can reduce subsequent facial motion by virtue of their location and dead weight. Patients often appear better in still photographs after these procedures than in animation.

20.2 Robin Sequence

Robin sequence is a condition that typically involves mandibular hypoplasia in association with a cleft palate.

Pierre Robin was a French stomatologist who, in 1923, described a series of children with retromicrognathia, glossoptosis, and airway obstruction with or without a cleft palate.[36] The triad occurs as a developmental sequence; that is, one condition is thought to lead to another.[37,38]

20.2.1 *Epidemiology*

Robin sequence occurs in 1:2,000 to 1:20,000 live births.[39] This broad range is likely due to differences in definition and varying sensitivities of diagnostic criteria. The male-to-female ratio is roughly equal.[39–42] The anomaly may be isolated (one-half to two-thirds of cases) or syndromic (one-third to one-half of cases). Isolated Robin sequence is sporadic and infrequently may be associated with concomitant abnormalities (10–15%). Heritance rates for Robin sequence are syndrome-dependent. The most common syndromes include Stickler syndrome, Treacher Collins syndrome, and velocardiofacial syndrome; chromosomal abnormalities (T18, T21), and teratogenic syndromes.

20.2.2 *Etiology and pathogenesis*

Robin sequence is probably initiated by mandibular hypoplasia, which has been postulated to be the result of a deformation, a disruption, or a malformation.[38] For those cases involving a deformation, the growth of the mandible, while inherently normal, is physically restricted. Examples include oligohydramnios and multiple gestations. In cases involving disruption, the growth is inherently normal but exogenously disrupted, as with amniotic band sequence. In malformation, mandibular growth is inherently abnormal, and the resultant pathogenesis will be syndrome-dependent.

Some degree of airway compromise is almost universally seen with Robin sequence, and the etiology for this impaired ventilation is often multifactorial. Oropharyngeal obstruction may be caused by glossoptosis (in which a normal-sized tongue shifts posteriorly, seated in a hypoplastic mandible). Hypopharyngeal obstruction may be caused by laryngotracheomalacia. Central sleep apnea may occur due to excessive flexion of basicranium or cervical instability. Rarely, a small or abnormally configured chest may compromise the lower airway.

20.2.3 *Diagnosis and evaluation*

Diagnosis is based on a physical examination that confirms the presence of the three classic findings: retromicrognathia, glossoptosis, and airway obstruction. Some geneticists believe that cleft palate is a frequent (50–90%) part of Robin sequence but is not essential for the diagnosis, whereas others reserve the diagnosis of Robin sequence only for those with mandibular hypoplasia and a cleft. These palatal clefts involve only the secondary palate and characteristically are U-shaped, but they may assume a V-shape with growth.[43]

The initial evaluation of a child with suspected Robin sequence begins with a history and physical examination but may be supplanted by additional investigations, as indicated. The preliminary examination focuses on the degree of respiratory obstruction, seeking the pathogenesis for any observed respiratory compromise; a feeding evaluation to reveal any cleft-related difficulties or signs of aspiration; and a search for concomitant abnormalities. The presence and pathogenesis of respiratory compromise may be determined by the degree of mandibular hypoplasia as measured by upright maxillomandibular distance, identification of glossoptosis in the supine position, and a Müller maneuver (observation of the neck and chest wall with the mouth and nares occluded during inspiration). There should be a low threshold for proceeding with overnight polysomnography with the child in different positions. Any suspicion of laryngomalacia or any significant degree of airway obstruction indicates the need for upper endoscopy. Feeding ability may be judged by weight gain and by monitoring oxygen saturation levels during feeding. A swallow study is usually performed to also evaluate the child for silent aspiration, which frequently accompanies this condition. Given the relatively high incidence of gene anomalies associated with Robin sequence (most commonly Stickler syndrome), a consultation with a geneticist is necessary. Finally, an ear examination and hearing screenings are necessary, as with all children with palatal clefts.

20.2.4 *Treatment*

The most common methods of managing the airway include prone positioning, nasopharyngeal airways, tongue–lip adhesion, mandibular distraction, and tracheostomy.

20.2.4.1 *Prone positioning*

This conservative technique has been described as successful in most patients with Robin sequence (50–70%+), especially for those with milder mandibular hypoplasia.[44,45] This technique, while noninvasive, should be accompanied by continuous airway monitoring with pulse oximetry and an apnea monitor after discharge from the hospital.

20.2.4.2 *Nasopharyngeal airways*

The next step in managing a child with impaired ventilation is to place a nasopharyngeal airway. Some centers have reported consistent success with this technique. It is recommended that the airway be rotated between nares, and that the smallest effective diameter tube be used to avoid future nasal airway constriction.

20.2.4.3 *Tongue–lip adhesion*

This procedure has a relatively long history in treating Robin sequence-related airway obstruction, and has been successfully used even in those with more severe presentations.[44,45] It is important to first rule out the presence of laryngomalacia because that condition can be successfully handled only with a tracheostomy. The most common complication after a tongue–lip adhesion is a postoperative dehiscence, which may be avoided by accomplishing a secure intrinsic tongue-to-lip musculature connection. This simple and safe technique is reversed at the time of palatal closure (sometime between 9 and 11 months of age). Another disadvantage of these adhesion procedures is an initial interference with swallowing; however, this typically improves quickly in most children. Overall, this procedure has an extremely high success rate with an overall low morbidity.

20.2.4.4 *Distraction osteogenesis*

Bilateral mandibular distraction has enjoyed recent popularity for treating the airway compromise associated with mandibular hypoplasia. This technique can achieve fairly rapid lengthening of the mandible, completely alleviating airway compromise. Once again, it is important to first rule out the presence of laryngomalacia, as this condition too requires placement of a tracheostomy. Although very successful in improving ventilation, distraction has been associated with a fairly high complication rate in neonates, including visible scars, device failure, injury to the facial and inferior alveolar nerves, and nearly certain injury to permanent tooth buds.[24] Although many reports cite the effectiveness of this technique, there have been no well-designed comparisons with other less invasive techniques, nor have the effects of these early osteotomies on subsequent long-term mandibular growth been studied.

20.2.4.5 *Tracheostomy*

This procedure is ideally reserved for children with associated laryngomalacia. Its obvious advantage is that it results in an immediate obstruction-free airway. Tracheostomies are typically not needed for very long, as the mandible grows fairly quickly in the first year of life and the associated airway cartilages progressively stiffen. The disadvantages of tracheostomies include early impairments in oral feeding and work-intensive maintenance on the part of the parents. Despite these issues, this can be a lifesaving procedure.

20.2.4.6 *Ancillary treatments*

Almost all infants with Robin sequence require placement of bilateral myringotomy tubes. In cases where feeding is not effective with the infant in the upright position and use of a cleft-specific feeder, transient gavage tube feeding may be necessary. If silent aspiration is diagnosed and does not resolve after the short-term use of a nasogastric feeding tube, a temporary gastrostomy may be required (most of these are removed within the first year). Oral stimulation should be performed in all patients in whom oral feeding is not possible, to mitigate the development of oral aversions. Palatoplasties are typically delayed until just before 1 year of age, to permit growth of the mandible and thus improve the overall airway before narrowing the nasopharynx. By virtue of the thinness of the palatal leaves, the subsequent fistula rate may be higher than with traditional cleft palates. Moreover, in children with velocardiofacial syndrome, associated neuromuscular weaknesses result in high rates of persistent velopharyngeal incompetence.

Children with Robin sequence who have not undergone mandibular osteotomies typically demonstrate fairly normal subsequent growth of the mandible, although "catch-up growth" should not be expected. Thus, surgical planning is best delayed until skeletal maturity before determining the need, type, and extent of further treatments.[46] The two most common treatment options for any residual mandibular hypoplasia include osseous or alloplastic genioplasty and bilateral sagittal split osteotomies with advancement, depending on the final observed occlusal relationships.

20.3 Treacher Collins Syndrome

Treacher Collins syndrome is a condition resulting in a bilateral facial aplasia affecting the orbits, zygomas, maxilla, mandible, and associated facial soft tissues.

20.3.1 *Definition and etymology*

Edward Treacher Collins was an English ophthalmologist who, in 1900, first described a series of patients with eyelid notches and deficient malar bones.[47] In 1949, Franceschetti and Klein also described a series of patients with the syndrome; therefore, it is sometimes referred to as Treacher Collins–Franceschetti syndrome.[48] Others prefer the more descriptive term "mandibulofacial dysostosis."

20.3.2 *Epidemiology*

Treacher Collins syndrome has been reported to occur in 1:50,000 live births.[49,50] About 60% of cases represent sporadic mutations. Familial cases demonstrate autosomal dominant transmission with complete penetrance. The gene for Treacher Collins syndrome *(TCOF1)* is located at 5q32–q33.1 and encodes treacle protein (a nucleolar protein involved in rRNA transcription).[51–53]

20.3.3 *Etiology and pathogenesis*

Aside from heritance and spontaneous new mutations, retinoic acid has been the only other suggested etiologic factor.[54] The *TCOF1* mutation (more than 130 types have been described) results in a prematurely degraded treacle protein. A decreased quantity of treacle protein allows apoptosis of neural crest cells and subsequently decreases their migration into the first and second branchial arches.[51,55] This culminates in perturbation in chondrogenesis, leading to aplasia and hypoplasia of structures within the first and second branchial arches and the nasal placode.[55] The penetrance of this gene is variable, resulting in a range of phenotypic severity.

20.3.4 *Diagnosis and evaluation*

The diagnosis of Treacher Collins syndrome is based on the clinical identification of (1) downward slanting palpebral fissures and sometimes pseudocolobomas of the lower lids, (2) malar deficiencies, and (3) mandibular hypoplasia.[56] Testing for a *TCOF1* gene mutation can confirm the diagnosis.

The examination of a child with Treacher Collins syndrome begins with a careful assessment of the airway, for many children will have significant problems with ventilation and some may require tracheostomies very early in life. In addition, a feeding assessment is necessary. Not only will feeding be impaired secondary to airway obstruction, but many children may have cleft palates in addition. The facial examination is focused on the following areas:

20.3.4.1 *Orbits*

Inferior lateral orbital dystopia may occur, resulting in associated inferior displacement of the lateral canthi. As the degree of hypoplasia increases, true clefts may be palpated in the inferolateral orbital region. The medial lower-eyelid lashes will be absent in many individuals. There may be significant attenuation of the lower eyelids, giving the appearance of pseudocolobomas, which may result in problems with dry eyes and eventual corneal scarring. Amblyopia (33%) and strabismus (37%) are present with an increased frequency.[57,58]

20.3.4.2 *Zygomas*

Zygomatic arches will be absent in most children, which can be determined by facial palpation just lateral to the malar eminences.

20.3.4.3 *Ears*

Although mildly affected individuals may have normally formed ears, bilateral microtia is most often noted. Preauricular skin tags and sinuses may also be present. Conductive hearing loss occurs in up to 90% of cases, most frequently in the moderate to severe range (40–80 dB).[56] The severity of the external ear deformity does not always correlate with the type and severity of hearing loss.

20.3.4.4 *Nasal bones*

With growth, children develop a dorsal nasal hump, secondary to a clockwise rotation of the maxilla.

20.3.4.5 *Maxilla*

A central maxillary prominence may be noted, and palatal clefting is not uncommon. Velopharyngeal incompetence may be present from either an overt or submucous palatal cleft (23%).[56] Hyponasality may occur due to a high arched palate, resulting in a diminished nasal airway. There may be posterior vertical shortening of the maxilla as a component of a clockwise rotation of the jaws.

20.3.4.6 *Mandible*

Mandibular hypoplasia is a characteristic finding, and sometimes the pogonion will be rotated inferiorly so that it points downwards. A prominent antegonial notch is usually palpable. More severe presentations will result in complete aplasia of the TMJs. This may be readily ascertained by rocking the mandible posteriorly.

20.3.4.7 *Soft tissues*

Associated with the underlying skeletal aplasias, there may be significant soft-tissue hypoplasia. This is most readily seen in a line between the lateral canthus and oral commissure. A characteristic preauricular hairline may also be present.

Nager and Miller syndromes share many of their craniofacial features with Treacher Collins syndrome. In Nager syndrome, preaxial limb abnormalities include thumb hypoplasia or aplasia, radial hypoplasia or aplasia, and syndactyly. The TMJ and soft palate may be absent. Trismus of the TMJ is common.[59] In Miller syndrome, postaxial limb abnormalities are present and include little-finger hypoplasia or aplasia, ulnar hypoplasia or aplasia, syndactyly, and lower-limb abnormalities.

Ancillary testing includes overnight polysomnography and a hearing screen. Radiologic assessments, such as a panoramic radiograph, mandibular plain films, and CT allow qualitative and quantitative assessments of the skeletal aplasias but are best reserved until just before treatment.

20.3.5 *Treatment*

20.3.5.1 *Airway*

Initial treatment is focused on any potential neonatal airway compromise, and may include prone positioning, tracheostomy, or distraction osteogenesis. Prone positioning may be used in patients with mild and moderate micrognathia, allowing gravity to bring the tongue forward. Prone positioning should be accompanied by continuous monitoring of oxygen saturation. For severely affected individuals and those with laryngomalacia, tracheostomy may be lifesaving. Neonatal distraction osteogenesis has also been described for treating airway compromise, and is extremely effective for mandibular lengthening. However, as noted previously, this technique is associated with significant complication rates and may result in long-term mandibular growth inhibition.[27,28] Orotracheal intubation in patients with Treacher Collins syndrome may be extremely challenging at any age and should be undertaken only by highly experienced anesthesiologists.

20.3.5.2 *Eyelids*

Although upper-to-lower eyelid switch flaps have been described, they should be reserved for only the most severe cases; because of the associated scarring, the final appearance of these flaps, typically, is somewhat undesirable aesthetically. In general, corneal exposure is best corrected using exaggerated lateral canthopexies (or even lateral tarsorraphies when indicated).

20.3.5.3 *Ear reconstruction*

As described previously, auricular reconstruction is ideally performed at 8 years of age or later. Children with Treacher Collins syndrome have low-lying scalp hair in the auricular region and soft-tissue hypoplasia, both of which increase the challenges for auricular reconstruction.

As with hemifacial microsomia, microtia reconstruction in Treacher Collins syndrome is best referred to those, who have special interest in the procedure and sufficient experience to produce reliable results. Reconstruction of the external auditory canal, tympanic membrane, and ossicles is rarely possible in Treacher Collins syndrome; therefore, bony anchored hearing aids are often placed after external ear reconstruction. As a rule, they should not be placed before ear reconstruction as they can severely limit reconstructive options.

20.3.5.4 *Zygoma reconstruction*

Reconstruction of the zygomatic arches is ideally performed sometime after external ear reconstruction. The zygoma reaches approximately 90% of final adult size sometime between 8 and 9 years of age. Reconstructive options include both autogenous bone grafts and alloplastic implants. Autogenous bone-graft onlay augmentation has a low complication rate but >50% resorption rate, lacks growth potential, and requires a donor-site harvest, with associated potential morbidities (craniotomy, chest-wall contour deformity).[34,35,60] Pedicled calvarial bone flaps have been described. Theoretically, by virtue of carrying a blood supply, they might have a growth potential and decreased resorption rates, although these traits have yet to be demonstrated. The main drawbacks to this technique include suboptimal aesthetics (given constraints on shape and size), as well as limited mobility.[61] We prefer placing alloplastic implants at skeletal maturity, which offers greater malar projection and long-lasting results with a relatively simple procedure. These implants can be placed without prior zygomatic reconstruction. Although such implants can create aesthetically pleasing long-lasting results, they carry an infection risk (especially if placed by a transoral route instead of a preauricular approach) and, when indicated, should not be placed until skeletal maturity.[32,56]

20.3.5.5 *Jaw reconstruction*

Reconstruction of the jaw that has the milder hypoplasia is best deferred until skeletal maturity. As with skeletal reconstruction for patients with hemifacial microsomia, the choice of reconstructive techniques depends partially upon the degree of skeletal hypoplasia. The three basic approaches are distraction osteogenesis, standard orthognathic corrections, and reconstructions using rib grafts. One concern with distraction osteogenesis in Treacher Collins syndrome is that when the mandible is appropriately distracted, a posterior open bite results. This open bite gradually regresses, producing a subsequent significant relapse. In traditional orthognathic surgery, closure of the anterior open bite is often frustrated by recurrences. These can be reduced through the use of prolonged postoperative anterior dental elastics. In younger children with limited airways, bilateral sagittal mandibular osteotomies, secured by intermaxillary fixation in an Angle Class III relationship, may have high success rates but require an experienced craniofacial team for support. The intégrale osteotomy provides a counterclockwise rotation of the Le Fort II osteotomy.[62] Its advantages include reduction of the upper nasal prominence and sagittal leveling of the palatal plane. The procedure, however, can be technically challenging and often produces an unstable result. Isolated counterclockwise maxillary rotation worsens the anterior open-bite deformity and does not allow differential movements of maxilla and zygoma.

20.3.5.6 *Ancillary procedures*

At skeletal maturity, in addition to placing malar alloplasts, accessory chin augmentation with implants is often beneficial. Rhinoplasties are also best reserved until skeletal maturity, after completion of any orthognathic corrections. Dorsal nasal reduction and infracture, along with tip repositioning and reconstruction, are typically required.

References

1. **Gorlin RJ, Cohen MM Jr., Hennekam RCM.** *Syndromes of the Head and Neck*, 4th edn. New York, NY: Oxford University Press; 2001:790–798.
2. **Poswillo D.** Otomandibular deformity: pathogenesis as a guide to reconstruction. *J Maxillofac Surg* 1974;2:64–72.

3. **Grabb WC.** The first and second branchial arch syndrome. *Plast Reconstr Surg* 1965;36:485–508.
4. **Hartsfield JK.** Review of the etiologic heterogeneity of the oculo-auriculo-vertebral spectrum (hemifacial microsomia). *Orthod Craniofac Res* 2007;10:121–128.
5. **Rice DP.** Craniofacial anomalies: from development to molecular pathogenesis. *Curr Mol Med* 2005;5:699–722.
6. **Johnston MC, Bronsky PT.** Prenatal craniofacial development: new insights on normal and abnormal mechanisms. *Crit Rev Oral Biol Med* 1995;6:368–422.
7. **Cousley RR, Calvert ML.** Current concepts in the understanding and management of hemifacial microsomia. *Br J Plast Surg* 1997;50:536–551.
8. **Cousley RR.** Diagnosis of hemifacial microsomia. *Dent Update* 1993;20:416–419.
9. **Hertle RW, Nesbum K, Katowitz JA.** Visual consequences of ocular and adnexal findings in patients with Goldenhar's syndrome. *J Ophthalmic Nurs Technol* 1997;16:12–17.
10. **Rahbar R, Robson CD, Mulliken JB, *et al.*** Craniofacial, temporal bone, and audiologic abnormalities in the spectrum of hemifacial microsomia. *Arch Otolaryngol Head Neck Surg* 2001;127:265–271.
11. **Wan J, Meara JG, Kovanlikaya A, Nelson MD, Don D.** Clinical, radiological, and audiological relationships in hemifacial microsomia. *Ann Plast Surg* 2003;51:161–166.
12. **Bassila MK, Goldberg R.** The association of facial palsy and/or sensorineural hearing loss in patients with hemifacial microsomia. *Cleft Palate J* 1989;26:287–291.
13. **Carvalho GJ, Song CS, Vargervik K, Lalwani AK.** Auditory and facial nerve dysfunction in patients with hemifacial microsomia. *Arch Otolaryngol Head Neck Surg* 1999;125:209–212.
14. **Bergstrom L, Baker BB.** Syndromes associated with congenital facial paralysis. *Otolaryngol Head Neck Surg* 1981;89:336–342.
15. **Poon CC, Meara JG, Heggie AA.** Hemifacial microsomia: use of the OMENS-Plus classification at the Royal Children's Hospital of Melbourne. *Plast Reconstr Surg* 2003;111:1011–1018.
16. **Horgan JE, Padwa BL, LaBrie RA, Mulliken JB.** OMENS-Plus: analysis of craniofacial and extracraniofacial anomalies in hemifacial microsomia. *Cleft Palate Craniofac J* 1995;32:405–412.
17. **Gougoutas AJ, Singh DJ, Low DW, Bartlett SP.** Hemifacial microsomia: clinical features and pictographic representations of the OMENS classification system. *Plast Reconstr Surg* 2007;120:112e–120e.
18. **Digilio MC, Calzolari F, Capolino R, *et al.*** Congenital heart defects in patients with oculo-auriculo-vertebral spectrum (Goldenhar syndrome). *Am J Med Genet A* 2008;146A:1815–1819.

19. **Vento AR, LaBrie RA, Mulliken JB.** The OMENS classification of hemifacial microsomia. *Cleft Palate Craniofac J* 1991;28:68–77.
20. **Figueroa AA, Pruzansky S.** The external ear, mandible and other components of hemifacial microsomia. *J Maxillofac Surg* 1982;10:200–211.
21. **Fearon JA.** Hemifacial microsomia. In: VanderKolk CA, ed. *Plastic Surgery: Indications, Operations, and Outcomes.* Vol. II. St. Louis, MO: Mosby; 2000.
22. **Cloonan YK, Kifle Y, Davis S, Speltz ML, Werler MM, Starr JR.** Sleep outcomes in children with hemifacial microsomia and controls: a follow-up study [published online ahead of print July 27, 2009]. *Pediatrics* 2009;124:e313–e321. doi:10.1542/peds.2008-3488.
23. **Cenzi R, Farina A, Zuccarino L, Carinci F.** Clinical outcome of 285 Medpor grafts used for craniofacial reconstruction. *J Craniofac Surg* 2005;16:526–530.
24. **Sevin K, Askar I, Saray A, Yormuk E.** Exposure of high-density porous polyethylene (Medpor) used for contour restoration and treatment. *Br J Oral Maxillofac Surg* 2000;38:44–49.
25. **Davidson EH, Brown D, Shetye PR, *et al.*** The evolution of mandibular distraction: device selection. *Plast Reconstr Surg* 2010;126:2061–2070.
26. **Fan K, Andrews BT, Liao E, Allam K, Raposo Amaral CA, Bradley JP.** Protection of the temporomandibular joint during syndromic neonatal mandibular distraction using condylar unloading. *Plast Reconstr Surg* 2012;129:1151–1161.
27. **Troulis MJ, Kaban LB.** Complications of mandibular distraction osteogenesis. *Oral Maxillofac Surg Clin North Am* 2003;15:251 261.
28. **da Silva Freitas R, Tolazzi AR, Alonso N, Cruz GA, Busato L.** Evaluation of molar teeth and buds in patients submitted to mandible distraction: long-term results. *Plast Reconstr Surg* 2008;121:1335–1342.
29. **Obwegeser HL.** Correction of the skeletal anomalies of oto-mandibular dysostosis. *J Maxillofac Surg* 1974;2:73–92.
30. **Munro IR.** One-stage reconstruction of the temporomandibular joint in hemifacial microsomia. *Plast Reconstr Surg* 1980;66:699–710.
31. **Fearon JA.** Discussion. The evolution of mandibular distraction: device selection. *Plast Reconstr Surg* 2010;126:2071–2073.
32. **Eski M, Sengezer M, Turegun M, Deveci M, Isik S.** Contour restoration of the secondary deformities of zygomaticoorbital fractures with porous polyethylene implant. *J Craniofac Surg* 2007;18:520–525.
33. **Robiony M, Costa F, Demitri V, Politi M.** Simultaneous malaroplasty with porous polyethylene implants and orthognathic surgery for correction of malar deficiency. *J Oral Maxillofac Surg* 1998;56:734–742.
34. **Tong L, Buchman SR.** Facial bone grafts: contemporary science and thought. *J Craniomaxillofac Trauma* 2000;6:31–42.

35. **Ozaki W, Buchman SR.** Volume maintenance of onlay bone grafts in the craniofacial skeleton: micro-architecture versus embryologic origin. *Plast Reconstr Surg* 1998;102:291–299.
36. **Robin P.** La chute de la base de la langue consideree comme une nouvelle cause de gene dans la respiration nasopharyngienne. *Bull Acad Med (Paris)* 1923;89:37–41.
37. **Carey JC, Fineman RM, Ziter FA.** The Robin sequence as a consequence of malformation, dysplasia, and neuromuscular syndromes. *J Pediatr* 1982;101:858–864.
38. **Cohen MM Jr.** The Robin anomalad: its nonspecificity and associated syndromes. *J Oral Surg* 1976;34:587–593.
39. **Bush PG, Williams AJ.** Incidence of the Robin anomalad (Pierre Robin syndrome). *Br J Plast Surg* 1983;36:434–437.
40. **Sheffield LJ, Reiss JA, Strohm K, Gilding M.** A genetic follow-up study of 64 patients with the Pierre Robin complex. *Am J Med Genet* 1987;28:25–36.
41. **Holder-Espinasse M, Abadie V, Cormier-Daire V, *et al.*** Pierre Robin sequence: a series of 117 consecutive cases. *J Pediatr* 2001;139:588–590.
42. **Caouette-Laberge L, Bayet B, Larocque Y.** The Pierre Robin sequence: review of 125 cases and evolution of treatment modalities. *Plast Reconstr Surg* 1994;93:934–942.
43. **Hanson JW, Smith DW.** U-shaped palatal defect in the Robin anomalad: developmental and clinical relevance. *J Pediatr* 1975;87:30–33.
44. **Evans AK, Rahbar R, Rogers GF, Mulliken JB, Volk MS.** Robin sequence: a retrospective review of 115 patients [published online ahead of print January 26, 2006]. *Int J Pediatr Otorhinolaryngol* 2006;70:973–980. doi:10.116/j.ijporl.2005.10.016.
45. **Kirschner RE, Low DW, Randall P, *et al.*** Surgical airway management in Pierre Robin sequence: is there a role for tongue–lip adhesion? *Cleft Palate Craniofac J* 2003;40:13–18.
46. **Figueroa AA, Glupker TJ, Fitz MG, BeGole EA.** Mandible, tongue, and airway in Pierre Robin sequence: a longitudinal cephalometric study. *Cleft Palate Craniofac J* 1991;28:425–434.
47. **Treacher-Collins E.** Cases with symmetrical congenital notches in the outer part of each lower lid and defective development of malar bones. *Trans Ophthalmol Soc UK* 1900;20:190.
48. **Franceschetti A, Klein D.** The mandibulofacial dysostosis: a new hereditary syndrome. *Acta Ophthalmol (Copenh)* 1949;27:143–224.
49. **Fazen LE, Elmore J, Nadler HL.** Mandibulo-facial dysostosis (Treacher-Collins syndrome). *Am J Dis Child* 1967;113:405–410.
50. **Rovin S, Dachi SF, Borenstein DB, Cotter WB.** Mandibulofacial dysostosis: a familial study of five generations. *J Pediatr* 1964;65:215–221.

51. **Isaac C, Marsh KL, Paznekas WA, *et al.*** Characterization of the nucleolar gene product, treacle, in Treacher Collins syndrome. *Mol Biol Cell* 2000;11:3061–3071.
52. **Dixon MJ, Read AP, Donnai D, Colley A, Dixon J, Williamson R.** The gene for Treacher Collins syndrome maps to the long arm of chromosome 5. *Am J Hum Genet* 1991;49:17–22.
53. **Dixon J, Edwards SJ, Anderson I, Brass A, Scrambler PJ, Dixon MJ.** Identification of the complete coding sequence and genomic organization of the Treacher Collins syndrome gene. *Genome Res* 1997;7:223–234.
54. **Trainor PA, Dixon J, Dixon MJ.** Treacher Collins syndrome: etiology, pathogenesis and prevention [published online ahead of print December 24, 2008]. *Eur J Hum Genet* 2009;17:275–283. doi:10.1038/ejhg.2008.221.
55. **Dixon J, Trainor P, Dixon MJ.** Treacher Collins syndrome. *Orthod Craniofac Res* 2007;10:88–95.
56. **Thompson JT, Anderson PJ, David DJ.** Treacher Collins syndrome: protocol management from birth to maturity. *J Craniofac Surg* 2009;20:2028–2035.
57. **Hertle RW, Ziylan S, Katowitz JA.** Ophthalmic features and visual prognosis in the Treacher-Collins syndrome. *Br J Ophthalmol* 1993;77:642–645.
58. **Prenner JL, Binenbaum G, Carpentieri DF, *et al.*** Treacher Collins syndrome with novel ophthalmic findings and visceral anomalies. *Br J Ophthalmol* 2002;86: 472–473.
59. **Halonen K, Hukki J, Arte S, Hurmerinta K.** Craniofacial structures and dental development in three patients with Nager syndrome. *J Craniofac Surg* 2006;17:1180–1187.
60. **Posnick JC, Goldstein JA, Waitzman AA.** Surgical correction of the Treacher Collins malar deficiency: quantitative CT scan analysis of long-term results. *Plast Reconstr Surg* 1993;92:12–22.
61. **Roddi R, Vaandrager JM, van der Meulen JC.** Treacher Collins syndrome: early surgical treatment of orbitomalar malformations. *J Craniofac Surg* 1995;6:211–217.
62. **Tulasne JF, Tessier PL.** Results of the Tessier integral procedure for correction of Treacher Collins syndrome. *Cleft Palate J* 1986;23(Suppl 1):40–49.

INDEX